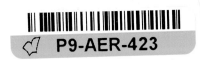

MEDICAL
BOTANY

PLANTS
AFFECTING
MAN'S
HEALTH

MEDICAL BOTANY

PLANTS AFFECTING MAN'S HEALTH

WALTER H. LEWIS
Professor of Biology, Washington University
Senior Botanist, Missouri Botanical Garden

MEMORY P. F. ELVIN-LEWIS
Associate Professor
and Chairman of Dental Microbiology
Washington University
St. Louis, Missouri

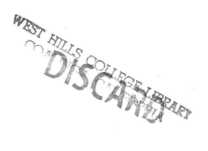
A WILEY-INTERSCIENCE PUBLICATION
JOHN WILEY & SONS
New York • Chichester • Brisbane • Toronto • Singapore

Library of Congress Cataloging in Publication Data:

Lewis, Walter Hepworth.
  Medical botany.

  "A Wiley-Interscience publication."
  Bibliography: p.
  Includes index.
  1. Botany, Medical. 2. Materia medica, Vegetable.
I. Elvin-Lewis, Memory P. F., 1933–   joint author.
II. Title. [DNLM: 1. Plants, Medicinal. QV766 L677m]

RS164.L475   615'.32   76-44376
ISBN 0-471-53320-3
ISBN 0-471-86134-0 (Paperback)

Printed in the United States of America

10 9 8 7

To our Parents

Florence† and John Wilfred

May Winnifred and Richard James†

Preface

Medical Botany is designed to bring into perspective the massive knowledge acquired by man to retain his health by using the plants around him. Man's survival has been dependent on his innate curiosity, his desire to examine by trial and error all aspects of his environment, and to conclude, for example, which materials are remedial, which ones are harmful, and which give him the greatest nourishment. This legacy exists today, but it is only partially utilized in our endless quest for well-being.

During the past century, the extraordinary results of research have unquestionably led to the success at an exponential rate that the practitioner of cosmopolitan (modern) medicine now enjoys. However, the nearly exclusive use of this research-oriented approach, with little regard for data acquired through the empirical method, has served to delay the application of many potential benefits. For example, it is unfortunate that man's first cosmopolitan tranquilizer derived from *Rauvolfia* did not come into general use until 1952, despite the long history of its use in Ayurvedic medicine in India, or that cromolyn, the miraculous prophylactic drug for asthma, has only recently been introduced, though its use in the form of *Ammi* seeds was part of Bedouin folk medicine for centuries. The rarity of these discoveries is understandable, however, for it is not always easy to retrieve such information from the many meaningless folk remedies. Whereas a few centuries ago the physician was also trained in botany, few medical scientists nowadays have this appreciation. Thus their search for medically useful elements seldom combines the ability to distinguish chemical compounds for medical value with the ability to recognize the relationship of plants used medically by different cultures. Clearly, empirical selection has led to studies resulting in the isolation and use of important active principles and these, together with synthetic derivatives of natural products, are an important source of our therapeutic armament. Nature is still mankind's greatest chemist, and many compounds that remain undiscovered in plants are beyond the imagination of even our best scientists. We hope that by bringing together information gleaned from both cosmopolitan and herbal medicine, we will encourage future discoveries along these lines.

Botanical sources for new drugs may seem endless, but are they? Should man not be concerned with the rapid destruction of our vegetation, particularly in tropical regions containing the greatest diversity of plants, often in limited quantities? Many species may be irretrievably lost now or in another generation. The answer is obvious, but those interested in natural history, conservation, and medicine must do their utmost to prevent the extinction of even a single species that might contain a compound invaluable to man's well-being.

We recognize that our attraction to self-medication has made us vulnerable to exploitation by those who foster the use of natural substances without reasonable knowledge of their scientific value. Therefore it is necessary to take away some of the mystique, dealing objectively with the many facets involved and teaching the reader who lacks medical training the language describing more fully the implications of such activities.

This book may also be used by undergraduate students, particularly those planning medical or paramedical careers and those having an appreciation for natural history and a sensitivity for environmental phenomena. It is based on a course, taught at Washington University by the authors, which lends itself to a team approach with the course master trained in botany. Students having multidisciplinary interests beyond biology and medicine have found the course valuable while studying psychology and anthropology, as have those taking liberal arts and general studies programs. The content of Medical Botany provides an interface between the more preprofessional course and that designed for a liberal educational experience.

Plants relating to man's health fall into three categories: those which injure, those which heal and nourish, and those which alter the conscious mind. Our book is divided on this basis into three sections, for normally a plant may be placed in one of these groups with little difficulty. In a minority of cases, however, typical characterization of a plant's activity as injurious, remedial, or psychoactive is questionable; for example, it may depend entirely on the concentration or amount of the plant extract being used. Thus some plants appear in two or even three categories; in these cases, the index should be helpful in locating the organism.

Some compounds that are not wholly natural (semisynthetic) or even synthetic are included, to ensure presentation of a more complete discussion. Very often the synthetic compounds have been patterned after those found in nature, and it seems logical to discuss barbiturates in relation to naturally occurring depressants or amphetamines in any discussion of stimulants.

Generally each chapter introduces the subject through a brief historical account and/or statistical review; there follows a short, reasonably nontechnical description of the system on which the plant derivatives react, including where appropriate their microbial infections, and also an account of the plants' uses in cosmopolitan (orthodox) medicine both now and in the past. Finally, most chapters contain a section on herbology that describes the plants employed in domestic or indigenous medicine. Usually this is a random sample from the vast array of plants being used domestically around the world, in addition to our emphasis on those utilized by North American Indians. However, this selection in no way implies any particular efficacy. Pertinent research literature concludes each chapter; additional references to broadly useful herbals and medically oriented botanical texts are found in Appendix II.

A difficulty for most individuals reading about many organisms under a single topic is an understanding of what is being included and how the material is organized and categorized. Our broad definition of plants includes not only those which are usually green and are classified into major groups from the seaweeds to the flowering plants, but also those which are not characteristically green. These include the bacteria and fungi. All major taxa referred to in the text are listed in Appendix I beginning with the most primitive forms and ending with the most advanced plants, all of them flowering. Since the majority of plants with known medical properties are found among this advanced group, we have arranged them in a phylogenetic system, to permit the reader to obtain some idea of their relationship. This may be of considerable practical importance for those interested in compounds common to the plants brought together by this system.

The plants and animals are usually referred to by their vernacular (common) and scientific names, often including both specific (binomial) and familial designations. Authorities for taxa are not given, but the authors for most species included may be found in either *Bergey's Manual of Determinative Bacteriology*, 8th edition, 1974, or JCT Uphof's *Dictionary of Economic Plants*, 2nd edition, 1968.

This book, which is directed to all those concerned with man's health, should be useful to the physician and the biologist and interesting to the layman. We hope that our approach will stimulate worldwide interdisciplinary studies of plants in relation to the health of man.

WALTER H. LEWIS
MEMORY P. F. ELVIN-LEWIS

St. Louis, Missouri
July 1976

Acknowledgments

We wish to express our sincere thanks to Dr. Norman R. Farnsworth, Department of Pharmacognosy and Pharmacology, University of Illinois Medical Center, Chicago, for his thorough and significant review of Chapters 1 through 9. The effort he expended represents an important contribution to *Medical Botany* and we appreciate it exceedingly. Others kindly reviewed individual chapters, and the assistance of the following persons is also very much appreciated: Dr. G. Edward Montgomery, Department of Anthropology, Washington University (Chapter 1, Plants in Medicine); Dr. John M. Kingsbury, Division of Biological Sciences, Cornell University (Chapter 2, Internal Poisons); Dr. Raymond G. Slavin, Department of Internal Medicine, St. Louis University School of Medicine (Chapter 3, Allergy); Dr. Jonathan L. Hartwell, National Cancer Institute, Bethesda, Maryland, and Dr. Robert E. Perdue, U.S. Department of Agriculture, Beltsville, Maryland (Chapter 5, Cancer); Dr. W. Maxwell Cowan, Department of Anatomy, Washington University School of Medicine (Chapter 6, Nervous System); Dr. Thomas A. Scott, Department of Biochemistry, Leeds University (Chapter 8, Metabolism); Dr. Hugh G. Berry, Department of Endodontics, Washington University School of Dental Medicine (Chapter 10, Oral Hygiene); Dr. William R. Fair, Division of Urology, Washington University School of Medicine (Chapter 13, Urogenital System); and Dr. Richard E. Schultes, Botanical Museum, Harvard University (Chapter 18, Hallucinogens). To all we extend our wholehearted thanks for their expert reviews.

Though many individuals contributed to our task, usually by helping with reference and illustrative materials, we also wish to acknowledge a few in particular: Dr. Raymond E. Altevogt; Dr. William C. Burger (Field Museum of Natural History, Chicago); Richenda E. Crawford; June Croce; Dr. William G. D'Arcy (Missouri Botanical Garden); Faith A. Darnbrough; Dr. W. Hardy Eshbaugh (Miami University, Oxford); Dr. Robert B. Faden (Field Museum of Natural History, Chicago); Ross Field Jr.; Olive Gordon; Mary C. Johnson; Dr. Yojiro Kawamura (Osaka University Dental School); Dr. Marilyn Krukowski (Washington University); Lance Lewis; Memoria F. R. M. Lewis; Dr. Alexander R. Lind (St. Louis University School of Medicine); Anita MacBryde; Dr. James Maniotis (Washington University); Dr. Frank L. Mercer (St. Louis College of Pharmacy); Dr. Stephen Molnar (Washington University); Dr. H. Wayne Nichols (Washington University); Clem Okalie; and David W. Pate. Special appreciation is extended to the librarians who helped in so many ways and without whose guidance this book never would have been completed. We cite especially Margaret S. Cummings (Washington University School of Medicine), Betty W. Galyon (Washington University Biology Department), Harriet Steuernagel (Washington University School of Dental Medicine), Helen Silverman (St. Louis College of Pharmacy), Carla Lange (Missouri Botanical Garden), and Barbara Gibson (Woodward Memorial Biomedical Library, University of British Columbia). Also, without the assistance of those in the Biomedical Communications Service Department, University of British Columbia, the photographic aspects of the book would be meager indeed. This help was both significant and generous.

Finally, we wish to recognize two whose care and patience helped bring *Medical Botany* to fruition. To Lucy Steelman (Department of Biology, Washington University), who typed the manuscript so skillfully, and to Erna R. Eisendrath (Associate Professor Emeritus of Biology, Washington University), who aided us with galley corrections and in other ways, goes our particular gratitude.

In conclusion, we recognize the two universities at which this book was completed: to our alma mater, the University of British Columbia, we thank Dr. William C. Gibson, Department of the History of Science and Medicine, Faculty of Medicine, for generous facilities and many courtesies; and to Washington University, Departments of Biology and Dental Microbiology, we acknowledge wholehearted support over many years of affiliation.

W. H. L.
M. P. F. E.-L.

Contents

Caution

This book is not intended for prescribing medication or for curing afflictions. Its purpose is not to replace the services of a physician but rather to serve as a reference for matters relating to health. We emphasize that the use of any of this information for purposes of self-treatment without consulting a physician can be dangerous.

MEDICAL BOTANY

PLANTS AFFECTING MAN'S HEALTH

Chapter 1

Plants in Medicine

The student and the teacher must always remember that what is new is not necessarily true and what is true is not necessarily new. Perhaps Pope's advice in *Essays in Criticism* (1711) is still applicable:

Be not the first by whom the new is tried
Nor yet the last to lay the old aside.

INTRODUCTION

We can choose no more appropriate people to introduce *Medical Botany* than the North American Indians (Fig. 1-1). The Indian has long been in harmony and partnership with the elements of our natural world, having used them to survive and to embellish his well-being. We chose the Indians of our continent for still another reason, however: today we are seeing an exciting revitalization of interest *in situ* in their ancient traditions of religion, in their language, and in other aspects of their culture. The young are now aflame with newly developed pride in their heritage, while the elderly are encouraged that after a century of indifference to Indian life-style, art, and science, we may be reversing some of the unfortunate attitudes found in the white population as well as among the Indians themselves.

For centuries the Indians have perpetuated an empirical science of herb-

1

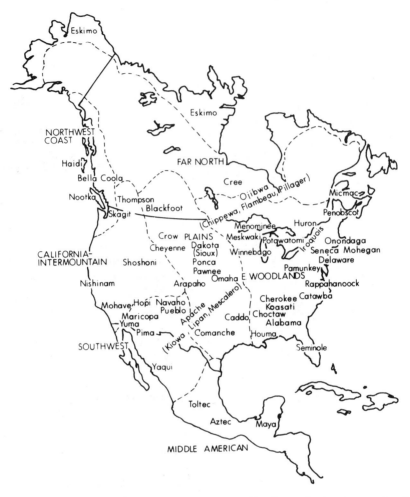

Figure 1-1   North American Indians: approximate original localities of tribes discussed in the text.

ology in relation to health which has been essentially ignored during these days of great advances in biomedicine. We must and can learn what is efficacious in their use of plants.[1] Their healing science program, encompassing traditional spiritual and mythical roles, is both elaborate and lengthy. Apprentices of Navajo medicine men, for example, learn to use medicinally nearly 200 plants, often applying them to both physical and mental afflictions. Substantiated, well-documented cases exist of herbal cures for blood poisoning, rattlesnake bites, and a variety of physical ills we cannot fully understand. Dealing with psychic phenomena, the medicine man may also obtain remarkable results as yet unexplainable. For example, a peyote user who was diagnosed a schizophrenic was apparently cured after a prolonged treatment involving the hallucinogenic plant *Datura inoxia* while working "with that part of the mind that is outside the person, and that the person doesn't really know about."[2]

Many Navajo consider that white doctors take care of certain physical needs such as infections and surgery, while their medicine men minister to the major problems of the mind and spirit. They believe such difficulties to be far more important, for during one's life both harmony and order impart strength and inner peace, which in turn assure physical safety and emotional security.

These medicine men of North America, and their counterparts in Africa (herbalists, witch doctors) and Asia (shamans), are all therapists. They treat patients and obtain results not unlike the formally trained therapists dealing with psychiatry in cosmopolitan or modern Western-derived medicine—the psychoanalysts, psychologists, psychiatric social workers, and trained counselors.[3] We often think that the village herbalist is an untrained charlatan working in the realm of magic that in no way relates to science. In the same vein, we also confuse the educational attainments of the practitioner with the therapy—M.D.'s and Ph.D.'s do scientific things, while the "uneducated" do magical things. Yet in Western cultures, mental illness was thought to be primarily caused by witches only a century ago. In other words, it is not difficult to mix a bit of illogic, fantasy, and placebo with the healing science, and at times it may be beneficial. Many people are unaware that much time and effort are expended before an individual is recognized as a herbalist or witch doctor (comparable in indigenous medicines to our pharmacist and psychiatrist), for he must train many years often under several instructors, in one region and then in another, to learn the use of herbs in several localities, the methods of preparation, and how the materials are related to various spiritual rites.

As organized as these local indigenous practices may be (e.g., the Ga Medical Association, Ghana[4]), traditional medicine is nowhere as extensive or as widely accepted as in the People's Republic of China. There, traditional medicinal techniques uniquely involving herbology and acupuncture have been fused with cosmopolitan medicine to form the New Chinese Medicine.[5] The Chinese take pride in their indigenous therapies and procedures, and "the advancement of new anti-inflammatory drugs, the bold theory of using purgative in appendicitis in conjunction with herbs and acupuncture, delicate limb and digital connection surgery, the employment of ancient Chinese herbs for the substitution of skin in treating burns, and new experimental techniques and concepts that treat man as a whole entity, all are aspects of the New Chinese Medicine."[6]

Not in harmony but in mutual conflict are the medical practices in the second most populous nation, India, and indeed in much of the Asian subcontinent. Here ancient practices known as Ayurvedic or Hindu and Unani or Muslim medicines, to which the majority of the population turn for assistance, are not treated as in China. By and large, the cosmopolitan trained physicians ignore the practices and teachings of their traditional medicines, which are nevertheless preferred by the population as a whole. This is unfortunate, for much could be shared to mutual advantage. For example, new evidence[7] of lipid permeability of skin supplies a logical scientific basis for the efficacy of the traditional Ayurvedic techniques of oil and milk herbal messages and partial baths for headaches, rheumatism, and eye ailments.

The widespread and long-standing practice of using plants in medicine in Eurasia, especially around the Mediterranean, the subcontinent, and China,[8] has been transcribed to us through the pictographs of the Egyptians, the clay tablet ideographs of the Babylonians, and the Vedic Sanskrit, as well as by the verbal communications of the secretive, fraternalistic Greek pharmicist.[9] Following the contributions to medicine of Hippocrates (460–377 BC), Dioscorides (first century AD), and Galen (AD 131–200), together with the early Arabian physicians, there was essentially a period of 1000 years during which little if any progress was achieved either in the medicinal sciences or in botany. Original data in botany accumulated during the Middle Ages, however, as plants were grown, new recipes were used, and empirical data were increased—it was the period of the great medicinal herbals.[10] In medicine, the practices of surgeons and barbers became separated during this time. These combined European developments sparked the beginning of Western cosmopolitan medicine. Writings on medicine then were used and read for their content irrespective of the period in which they had been written, for most physicians believed that the experience of the preceding generations had to be assimilated if progress was to be achieved.

This attitude toward the past of medicine changed radically in the second half of the nineteenth century when a new medical science developed and progress was achieved such as never before. The past seemed dead. To the average physician the history of medicine appeared as the history of errors. Nothing could be learned from it; to study it, to read the ancient writers, was a waste of time. Science was worshiped and the best minds turned to the laboratory with great enthusiasm.[11]

But the biomedical scientist of today who does consider early practices and procedures often finds data important to modern medical therapy and practice, as might be exemplified by the neglected field of ethnomedicine.[12] A combination of data from the empirical method and the most elaborate experimental laboratory and clinical procedures has given us a number of man's most startling and important contributions to the well-being and health of the species.

PLANTS IN MEDICINE

What examples do we have of the correlation between empirical applications and proved efficacy? What examples are there of plant products or their derivatives that directly affect man's well-being? There are a number of important reviews of these questions,[13] and following the outline of this book, we note a few significant highlights.

There is no doubt that of products harmful to man, those of plant origin are important to everyday life, whether he lives in an urban or rural area in more developed countries, or in the underdeveloped nations. In these various environments are found hundreds of plants that are injurious if ingested and are capable of causing any number of symptoms, including death. People in rural settings, of course, are exposed to nature's lethal organisms every day, but even those in more urban areas must be wary of garden plants introduced from all parts of the world. House plants often are poisonous, and children are attracted to the colorful parts of these otherwise harmless organisms in our midst. Few realize, for example, that apple seeds contain cyanide, which may be lethal in large doses; that the alkaloid taxine from the common bedding plant English yew is rapidly absorbed and causes sudden death; that the leaves and twigs of boxwood, so common as a hedging plant, produce another alkaloid, buxine, which contributes to respiratory failure in humans and domestic animals; that children using peashooters made of elderberry stems may be poisoned from exposure to this plant's alkaloids and cyanide; and that the eating of green and sprouting parts of potatoes may cause severe poisoning. Likewise, common house plants such as oleanders, caladiums, and philodendrons must be avoided, for a person ingesting the leaves of oleander, or its sweet nectar, may develop severe vomiting, irregular heartbeat, and respiratory paralysis, followed by death.

Hay fever and dermatitis result from an abnormality of our immune system known as allergy. The abundant grasses, trees, weeds, and fungi in our environment produce pollen, spores, and other materials to which we become sensitized so that on reexposure they cause discomforting symptoms that may become life-threatening. No one who has suffered from ragweed hay fever, asthma attacks, or poison ivy dermatitis can doubt the role of allergenic plants in health and productivity.

Certain plants have the disturbing quality of modifying our cells in other ways. Some give rise to mutations that may occur in our reproductive cells, permanently altering succeeding generations if these cells are utilized in reproduction. Others may affect our somatic or body cells in a way that causes congenital abnormalities, resulting in irreparable damage to the fetus. Even more insidious, some plants have the ability to induce cellular aberrations, especially in the peripheral blood, perhaps affecting the immune and clotting systems, and in some instances causing death. Plant proteins, typified by those found in the juice of the poke weed, enter the body through simple cuts and abrasions to do their damage. As a precaution, one should never handle mature poke without gloves.

Of the plants found to have remedial properties, none are more welcomed than those that help in our fight against cancer. How many thousands of lives have been saved or extended by the antineoplastic agents of microorganisms, or by the alkaloids vincristine and vinblastine of the Madagascaran annual periwinkle. The dramatic results of using these compounds in combination chemotherapy for treating Hodgkin's disease

(80% remission), acute lymphocytic leukemia (99% remission), Wilms' tumor (80% cured), Burkitt's lymphoma (50% cured), and gestational choriocarcinoma (70% cured) are testimonials to the gigantic strides achieved in the past few years when plant products have been introduced against the most terrifying of all disease complexes.

Many plant products affect the nervous system and we, like our forefathers, constantly take advantage of this property in either dulling or exciting the system. Throughout North Temperate America and Eurasia, our ancestors used willows and poplars, which contain an aspirinlike compound, to relieve fever and pain. Eventually we learned that opium alkaloids also relieve pain, and morphine became the all-important analgesic in cosmopolitan medicine. Almost as valuable to the surgeon as his knife are the curare plants (arrow poisons of South American Indians), which reversibly paralyze skeletal muscles and thus make the surgical process more effective.

Our greatest killer is heart disease, but where would we be if the useful properties of foxglove had not been known empirically and then "discovered" by a very astute botanist-physician several centuries ago? The answer should be obvious, since 3 million or more Americans daily take an extract from this plant to stay alive. Without foxglove, or other plants producing cardiotonic compounds, congestive heart failure and death would occur inevitably, and perhaps quickly for most of these people. High blood pressure at one time was also a quick killer. Before 1950 the inflexible fate of those with this disease was a stroke, heart failure, or kidney failure, but today, thanks to the use of *Rauvolfia* extracts, a large percentage of cases of hypertension can be controlled. The ability to lead a reasonably normal and healthy life despite high blood pressure entails one of the great advances in biomedical research in the twentieth century, yet it stems from an Old World plant long used in Ayurvedic medicine for its tranquilizing effect.

The mystique of what we eat and how our food affects us has been one of man's basic preoccupations. To promote more specific understanding in this area, and to elaborate on the afflictions that may arise from abuse, we have included a chapter on metabolism. In addition to the plants we eat, many plants are useful for alleviating metabolic diseases, such as gout and diabetes, examples of a clear intersection between the empirical method and biomedical research.

The treatment of glaucoma with alkaloids from the calabar bean of Nigeria, or leaves of Brazilian species of *Pilocarpus,* can prevent blindness. These compounds relieve the pressure within the eye by acting on neural receptor sites in that organ.

The oral cavity is of constant concern. When oral disease relates to tooth decay and gum disorders, we might well wonder if preventive dentistry has been adequate, especially when we observe that the teeth of the indigenous peoples of western Africa and southern Asia are free of caries. Recent research suggests that their cleaning implement—nature's toothbrush, the chewing stick—may in fact contain anticariogenic principles. Furthermore, the oil from an Indian chewing stick, when incorporated into toothpaste, has been found to promote the healing of inflamed gums. Such studies, still in their infancy, may reveal new substances that could be used by all to promote dental health.

A bewildering array of efficacious plant extracts appears to be available for the alleviation of most symptoms involving the gastrointestinal tract. Countless plants known to indigenous medicine are used for indigestion and stimulation of digestion, as antispasmodics, emetics, antieme-

tics, purgatives, antidiarrheals, anthelmintics, amebicides, carminatives, and to treat liver complaints and hemorrhoids. In most instances, commercial over-the-counter preparations are also available from the same plants. A recent research development has been the use of two derivatives of *Glycyrrhiza glabra* root, the common licorice from which candy is made, to treat peptic ulcers: ulcers are reduced in size and healing occurs even though the patient is not confined to bed. Licorice has a long history in European domestic medicine for the treating of indigestion and for alleviating (or relieving) inflamed stomachs.

Respiratory diseases include bronchial asthma and emphysema, in which bronchodilators such as plant-derived ephedrine and theophylline are indicated. To clear the lungs of sputum, patients often use expectorants, such as ipecac syrup from *Cephaelis,* creosote from American beech, or mucolytic agents from leaves of the Malabar nut tree. The latter, in very recent clinical trials, has proved efficacious. The vegetable kingdom abounds in antitussive agents, as well as substances utilized in soothing sore throats and treating colds.

Plants have had no greater impact in recent years than in the area of producing substances from which sex hormones are manufactured. They provide the basic steroidal compound for the efficient development of human sex hormones, which are now available cheaply for oral contraception and for treating menopause, improper menstruation, premenstrual tension, and testicular deficiency. Few realize the great contribution made by yams, for example, in stabilizing or decreasing world population, but perhaps no postwar development has been so relevant in changing the lifestyle of those at reproductive age.

Plants are implicated in most folk medicinal aspects of the urogenital system, but none are more extensive than those involved in sexual drive and performance. Perhaps hundreds of aphrodisiac substances are allegedly used by men of certain indigenous populations. Some are available commercially, such as the alkaloid yohimbine, from the bark of the African *Corynanthe*.

The skin is man's largest tissue, and a great many herbs have cosmetic uses in perfumes, creams, salves, soaps, oils, and shampoos. Important to his survival are plants having properties to stop bleeding and to heal wounds and burns.

Fortunately man has displayed the ingenuity to seek out deterrents, such as the antibiotics, as well as pest inhibitors, to improve his health and often save his life. Great strides in agriculture are intimately associated with pest control, whether it be insecticide, fungicide, or herbicide. Pesticides from natural plant sources, such as the pyrethroids, are preferred because they have low mammalian toxicity and are biodegradable. As we become more sophisticated in our attitude about the environment, we shall undoubtedly increase our use of plant-derived compounds.

As man appears to have long had his aphrodisiacs, whether real or imaginary, he has also had his panaceas. Some of these are imaginary, too, but the star of them all, ginseng, has been shown in recent years to aid the user under stress. Very possibly the millions dedicated to its use have an elixir after all.

Plants having psychoactive properties have always been popular. Stimulants like cocaine, chat, the beverages including coffee, tea, chocolate, and noncaffeine teas, and nicotine, all give a sense of well-being and exhilaration, of self-confidence and even power. They also alleviate fatigue and insomnia. In addition, man found plants capable of inducing hallucinations, ranging from cacti, spices, and morning glories, to mushrooms: he ingested, smoked, and sniffed them, rubbed them on the skin, and even deified them. But man also has his depressants, which include the widely enjoyed derivative of fungi, alcohol. All such drugs are enormously useful in medicine, but all are subject to abuse.

Many current and ancient texts have been scrutinized in the preparation of the cited examples of plants useful, harmful, and enjoyable to man. From these works we have gleaned what our forefathers learned the hard way and passed on to us. They performed experiments over thousands of years by trial and error, and we with broader insight and scientific expertise have a much greater opportunity to utilize these data than any who preceded us. Valuable data, however, are not always recorded. It behooves us to study the practices of indigenous populations before they are lost, either through human indifference or our relentless ability to change the vegetation around us. We hope that this book will stimulate those interested in botany and man's welfare to look closely and seriously at the field data awaiting our scrutiny.

As a guide to the literature of herbal medicine, we have compiled a list of pertinent herbals, pharmacopoeias, materia medicas, and other types of references relative to medical plants (Appendix II). Remember,

Someone once said that there are but two types of fools: one professes "This is old and therefore is good," and the other says, "This is new and therefore better."

But when judging the medical value of information regarding plants, neither view has a scientific basis.

LITERATURE CITED

1. Vogel VJ. 1970. *American Indian Medicine.* University of Oklahoma Press, Norman. 583 p.
2. McDowell E. 1973. Tending the spirit. *Wall Street J* **53**: 1, March 26.

3. Torrey EF. 1972. *The Mind Game: Witchdoctors and Psychiatrists.* Emerson Hall, New York.

4. Maclean U. 1971. *Magical Medicine.* Penguin Books, Middlesex, England. 167 p.

5. *Atlas of Common Chinese Drugs.* 1970. Revolutionary Committee of Pharmaceutical Institute, Chinese College of Medical Sciences, Peking (Farnsworth NR. Rating and Interpretation of Chinese Herbs, mimeograph, Chicago).

6. Kao FF. 1973. China, Chinese medicine, and the Chinese medical system. *Am J Chin Med* **1:** 1–59.

7. Leslie C. 1969. Modern India's ancient medicine. *Trans-action* **6:** 46–55; Marriott M. 1955. Western medicine in a village of northern India, 239–268. In BD Paul (ed), *Health, Culture and Community.* Russell Sage Foundation, New York; Montgomery E. 1976. Systems and the medical practitioners of a Tamil town. In C. Leslie (ed), *Asian Medical Systems.* University of California Press, Berkeley.

8. Alland A Jr. 1970. *Adaptation in Cultural Evolution: An Approach to Medical Anthropology.* Columbia University Press, New York and London. 203 p.

9. Stern WL. 1974. The bond between botany and medicine. *Bull Pac Trop Bot Gard* **4:** 41–60.

10. Lange C. 1969. The violet: Peter Schoffer's *Latin Herbarius. Mo Bot Gard Bull* **57**(2): 4–5; Lange C. 1970. The great herbal of John Parkinson. *Mo Bot Gard Bull* **58**(1): 4–10; Lange C. 1971. William Turner's *A New Herbal. Mo Bot Gard Bull* **59**(1): 4–7; Lange C. 1972. Hieronymus Bock's *Kreutterbuch. Mo Bot Gard Bull* **60**(1): 4–7.

11. Sigerist HE. 1951. *A History of Medicine.* Vol 1. *Primitive and Archaic Medicine.* Oxford University Press, New York.

12. Fabrega H Jr. 1975. The need for an ethnomedical science. *Science* 189: 969–975.

13. Kupchan SM. 1971. Drugs from natural products—plant sources. *Adv Chem* **108:** 1–13; Marini-Bettolo GB. 1971. New natural substances of pharmacological interest, 201–238. In H Wagner, L Hörhammer (eds), *Pharmacognosy and Phytochemistry.* Springer-Verlag. Berlin and New York.

Section One
"INJURIOUS" PLANTS

Plants harmful to man cause injury in a wide range of ways. There are many that cause serious illness and death when ingested, and almost as many result in allergies, such as hay fever, asthma, and dermatitis, when contacted over a period of time. Millions are afflicted by these debilitating abnormalities of the immune system. A much less familiar group of plants injure man by causing serious changes in his cells, which can lead to heritable mutations, abnormal fetuses, and aberrations of the blood.

These injurious plant-man relationships are discussed in Chapters 2 to 4. To fully appreciate the complexity of plants, particularly the diversity represented by the flowering plants (Angiosperms), the reader should consult the phylogenetic tree (Fig. 2-2) and Appendix I.

Chapter 2

Internal Poisons

Probably no field of scientific endeavor exists in which it is more difficult to separate fact from fiction than in the field of poisonous plants. Examination of the pertinent literature will reveal considerable confusion tending to mask an even greater amount of ignorance. Indeed, almost any plant may be judged as toxic, questionable, or edible, depending upon the reference consulted.*

Primeval man in search of food undoubtedly experienced much poisoning. He learned by trial and error that eating certain mushrooms, berries, and roots could produce various degrees of gastrointestinal discomfort or death, whereas others could be ingested safely. Certain lessons were learned quickly, and primitive, food-gathering man soon became a toxicologist of no mean ability. Eventually this knowledge was made to work for him: he prepared arrow poisons from plant extracts to bring down his game or foe, he threw crushed leaves of particular plants into water and with little effort quickly obtained a bountiful supply of stupefied fish, and he learned also to wash poison (e.g., cyanide) from a number of common, staple foods to make them edible. It probably took *Homo sapiens* but a short time to learn how to gather food with relative ease and to participate in the good life.

Man also learned that it could also be profitable to poison one another. The

* From Claus EP, Tyler VE, Brady LR. 1970. *Pharmacognosy*, ed 6, p 453. Lea & Febiger, Philadelphia. Reprinted by permission.

peoples of the Near East, Greece, and Rome developed the criminal arts to a high degree of lethal efficacy. In classical Rome, for example, mushrooms were the poison of choice and were expertly used by Agrippina, wife of Emperor Claudius and mother of Nero. Agrippina had Lollia Paulina put to death because Claudius, in a careless moment, remarked on the beauty of Lollia. Next came Marcus Silanus, whom she poisoned because Claudius was about to name him heir rather than Nero. Thus Agrippina embarked on a reign of terror in which she eliminated anyone in Rome who stood in her way. Finally, after five years, Claudius realized what she was doing and resolved to put an end to her power and her imperial desires for Nero. He decided to name Britannicus his heir, but Agrippina was more determined. She fed Claudius poisonous mushrooms, and he was dead in 12 hours without uttering a word. When the Senate deified Claudius, Nero, who was by then enthroned, remarked that mushrooms must be the food of the gods, for after eating them Claudius had become a divine dead god, and he, Nero, an emperor god.[2]

Higher plants were among those studied by Cleopatra in her search for a suicidal poison. Using her prisoners and slaves as guinea pigs, she was quite systematic. It was reported that she was not satisfied with the effects of either henbane (*Hyoscyamus niger*) or belladonna (*Atropa belladonna*), for they produced too much pain in spite of their rapid action. She was further disappointed with *Strychnos nux-vomica* from which strychnine was eventually extracted; although its action was instantaneous, it produced convulsions that left distorted facial features at death. Finally, she selected the bite of the asp (Egyptian cobra), which produced a serene and prompt death!

The art of poisoning and the need for food tasters as part of the household retinue has declined markedly, although our "Arsenic Lillys" still manage to kill husbands and even get away with it.[3] But if the practice is fading, the incidence of poisoning is increasing. Many of the victims are children exposed to pet products, art and craft materials, cosmetics, industrial cleaners, and plants. Plants, in fact, comprise the third largest category of poisonings recently reported from the Duke Poison Control Center, Durham, North Carolina.[4] This is probably because house plants have become more popular recently and many of these are unfortunately poisonous. Moreover, families are outdoors more with the renewed interest in the environment: there is more camping, picnicking, hiking, and gardening than a generation ago, and the frequency of poisoning will undoubtedly increase. With this new interest in the outdoors should go a rekindling of the desire to learn the plants, to find out which are harmful and which can be handled and eaten without danger.

CLASSIFICATION OF POISONOUS PLANTS

CHEMISTRY OF THE POISONOUS PRINCIPLE

A logical way to group poisonous plants is by their poisonous principles, which cause toxic reactions when ingested by animals. Often these principles are similar or identical chemically within a single botanical family or genus, especially if the taxa are closely allied. By this we mean that the taxonomic grouping has been arrived at and substantiated by numerous characters considered to be phylogenetically significant. These are primarily morphological (e.g., in Angiosperms, floral characters are of primary value), supplemented whenever possible with data from anatomy, cytology, chemistry, and other disciplines. Plants having many characters of similar form and origin are grouped together and a natural classification can be constructed around the data reflecting close relationships. Alternately, if similar morphological and other features between organisms are wanting, they should not be grouped together, and a natural system of classification will recognize these dissimilarities by accommodating the plants in separated taxa.

Similar morphological characters, for example, brought together various species into the Apocynaceae, long before the family was found to possess cardioactive glycosides. In fact, almost as many different genera in this family are known with compounds having digitalis-like action on the heart and circulation (Chapter 7), as all other genera in the plant kingdom. This additional characteristic would, therefore, enhance and verify a taxonomic grouping already reached on very different features. Since cardioactive glycosides are not restricted to the Apocynaceae, however, this cannot be used as an exclusive taxonomic trait of the family: all cardioactive glycosides are not apocynaceous. Indeed, the most widely used cardiac glycosides in medicine today are found in the disparate genus *Digitalis* of the Scrophulariaceae. This common characteristic between the families might, of course, suggest that they have inherited the ability to produce glycosidic compounds from a common ancestor, as could be expected from organisms judged to be related; alternately, such compounds might have evolved independently.

In this case, either explanation is logical, for the Apocynaceae and Scrophulariaceae are not unrelated (Appendix I); but a common ancestral inheritance of glycoside formation would be difficult to prove, for example, between the mono-

cotyledonous family Liliaceae (where glycosides are also found) and the dicotyledonous families under discussion. It is more logical to conclude that the cardioactive glycosides of the Liliaceae arose independently of those found in the Apocynaceae and Scrophulariaceae, an example of parallel evolution in no way reflecting true relationship. Obviously this kind of chemical classification (i.e., relying on cardiac glycosides without an understanding of the plants *per se*) could bring together wholly distinct organisms and would result in an artificial system of classification (other examples are given below).

Other difficulties exist in constructing a chemical system. As might be expected, compounds of many toxic plants remain unknown, hence could not be placed in such a system; and many plants have multiple compounds, each exerting toxic influences, which complicates the placement of many plants. Finally, since environmental factors markedly affect the presence or absence of poisonous principles, the difficulties of developing a useful scheme are increased still further.

On the other hand, it is important to recognize these principles as they occur in plants, not to construct a broad botanical classification, but rather to recognize relationships when they coincide with a natural classification based on all known data, and to initiate new or improved ideas within the framework of an existing classification. This is important to the practitioner, who can expect similar symptoms from a poisonous plant known to be closely allied to another and can respond accordingly. This technique is extremely useful in dealing with botanical families, and it may also be of value at the ordinal level and even within phylogenetic groups.

The major poisonous principles found among plants are organic compounds, such as alkaloids, diterpenes, cardiac and cyanogenic glycosides, nitro-containing compounds, oxalates, resins, and certain proteins and/or amino acids. Some plants also accumulate inorganic elements, largely from the soil, and these too may have serious effects on animals and/or man.[5]

Alkaloids

Alkaloids are a heterogeneous group of compounds difficult to define precisely. The term is a useful one, however, and it is commonly applied to basic organic nitrogenous compounds of plant origin which are physiologically active.

Thousands of different alkaloids have been characterized and many more remain for analysis. Alkaloids of similar structure are commonly found in closely related plants, but often they occur in quite distinct and unrelated plants (Table 2-1). Distribution of most alkaloids is not random among the higher plants: the Apocynaceae, Berberidaceae, Fabaceae, Papaveraceae, Ranunculaceae, Rubiaceae, and Solanaceae are outstanding families for yielding alkaloids, whereas the Lamiaceae, Rosaceae, and Gymnosperms are almost free of them.

Alkaloids appear to be active metabolites, rather than inert end products of metabolism as once supposed, but their usefulness to plants remains obscure.[6]

Glycosides

On hydrolysis, the glycosides yield one or more sugars (glycone) and one or more other compounds (aglycones). Glucose is a commonly occurring sugar. Toxicity or other major activity (many glycosides are nontoxic) is commonly associated with the aglycone moiety of these compounds. Glycosides are widespread in the plant kingdom, but only several of the more important groups are discussed.

CYANOGENIC GLYCOSIDES

The glycosides yielding hydrocyanic acid (HCN) as one product of hydrolysis are called cyanogenic. Probably the most widely distributed of these is amygdalin, which is commonly found in the Rosaceae (rose family). Amygdalin is found in large quantities in seeds of apples and pears and in the stony seeds, bark, and leaves of apricots, bitter almonds, wild and domestic cherries, peaches, and plums. In the hydrolysis of amygdalin, a two-step process (Fig. 2-1), two molecules of glucose are released, the first caused

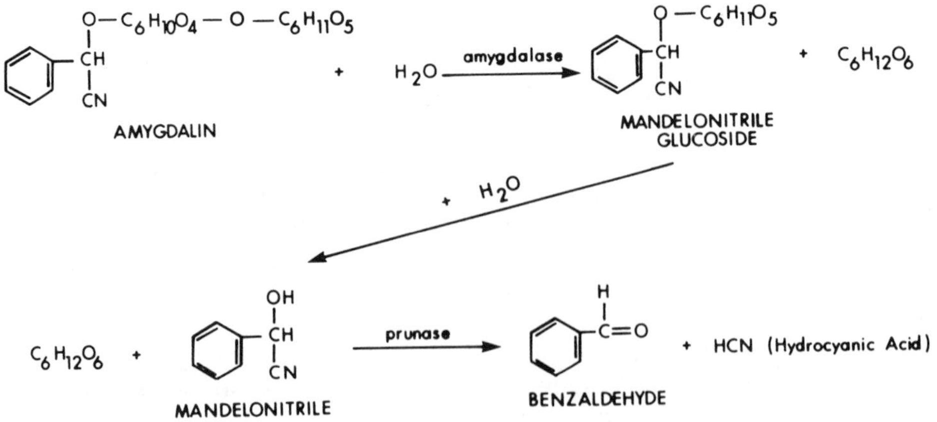

Figure 2-1 Hydrolysis of amygdalin.

Table 2-1 Major Types of Alkaloids Classified by Basic Ring Structure with Examples of Poisonous (and Other) Plants Containing Each

Alkaloid Type	Major Alkaloid	Plant		
		Family	Genus and Species	Vernacular Name
Alkaloids with heterocyclic nitrogen atoms				
Pyridine-piperidine	Coniine	APIACEAE	*Conium maculatum*	Poison hemlock
	Arecoline	ARECACEAE	*Areca catechu*	Betel nut palm
	Lobeline	CAMPANULACEAE	*Lobelia inflata*	Indian tobacco
	Piperine	PIPERACEAE	*Piper nigrum*	Pepper
	Isopelletierine	PUNICACEAE	*Punica granatum*	Pomegranate
	Nicotine	SOLANACEAE	*Nicotiana* spp., *Duboisia hopwoodii*	Tobacco
Tropane	Ecgonine (cocaine)	ERYTHROXYLACEAE	*Erythroxylum coca*	Cocaine
	Atropine, hyoscyamine, scopolamine	SOLANACEAE	*Atropa belladonna*	Belladonna
			Datura stramonium	Jimson weed
			Duboisia spp.	
			Hyoscyamus niger	Henbane
			Mandragora officinarum	Mandrake
			Withania somnifera	
Isoquinoline	Tropine			
	Berberine	BERBERIDACEAE	*Mahonia aquifolium*	Oregon grape
	Tubocurarine	MENISPERMACEAE	*Chondodendron tomentosum*	Curare component
	Morphine,[a] codeine,[a] noscapine (narcotine),[a] papaverine, thebaine[a]	PAPAVERACEAE	*Papaver somniferum*	Opium poppy
	Berberine, sanguinarine		*Argemone mexicana*	Prickly poppy
	Berberine, sanguinarine, chelidonine		*Chelidonium majus*	Celandine
	Aporphine			
	Sanguinarine		*Corydalis caseana*, *Dicentra* spp.	Fitweed Dutchman's breeches
			Sanguinaria canadensis	Bloodroot
	Hydrastine	RANUNCULACEAE	*Hydrastis canadensis*	Goldenseal
	Emetine	RUBIACEAE	*Cephaelis ipecacuanha*	Ipecac

15

Table 2-1 (Continued)

Alkaloid Type	Major Alkaloid	Plant		
		Family	Genus and Species	Vernacular Name
Quinoline	Viridicatin	FUNGUS	Penicillium viridicatum	
	Acronycine	RUTACEAE	Acronychia baueri	
	Quinine, quinidine	RUBIACEAE	Cinchona and Remijia spp.	
Indole	Ergonovine, ergotamine	FUNGUS	Claviceps purpurea	Ergot
	Psilocybin	FUNGUS	Psilocybe spp.	
	Vinblastine, vincristine	APOCYNACEAE	Catharanthus roseus	Periwinkle
	Reserpine		Rauvolfia serpentina	
	Physostigmine	FABACEAE	Physostigma venenosum	Calabar bean
	Gelsemine, sempervirine	LOGANIACEAE	Gelsemium sempervirens	Yellow jessamine
	Strychnine, brucine		Strychnos nux-vomica	Strychnine
Imidazole	Pilocarpine	RUTACEAE	Pilocarpus jaborandi	
Pyrrolizidine	Retrorsine	ASTERACEAE	Senecio spp.	Groundsel
		BORAGINACEAE	Echium plantagineum	Viper's bugloss
	Heliotrine, lasiocarpine		Heliotropium europaeum	Heliotrope
	Monocrotaline, retrorsine	FABACEAE	Crotalaria spectabilis	Rattlebox

Class	Compound	Family	Species	Common name
Quinolizidine	Sparteine	FABACEAE	Cytisus scoparius	Scotch broom
	Cytisine		Laburnum anagyroides	Golden-chain
	Lupinine		Lupinus spp.	Lupine
Steroid alkaloids	Cevadine	LILIACEAE	Schoenocaulon officinalis	
	Ester alkaloids germidine & germitrine, glycoalkaloid veratrosine		Veratrum viride	American hellebore
	Zygacine	RANUNCULACEAE	Zigadenus spp.	Death camas
	Aconitine		Aconitum spp.	Aconite
	Solanidine	SOLANACEAE	Lycopersicon esculentum	Tomato
	Solanidine		Solanum spp.	
Purine bases	Caffeine	AQUIFOLIACEAE	Ilex paraguariensis	Maté
	Caffeine	RUBIACEAE	Coffea arabica	Coffee
	Caffeine	SAPINDACEAE	Paullinia cupana	Guarana
	Caffeine	STERCULIACEAE	Cola nitida	Kola
	Caffeine	THEACEAE	Camellia sinensis	Tea
	Theobromine	STERCULIACEAE	Theobroma cacao	Chocolate

Alkaloids without heterocyclic nitrogen atoms

Class	Compound	Family	Species	Common name
Alkaloid amines	Ephedrine	EPHEDRACEAE	Ephedra sinica	
	Mescaline	CACTACEAE	Lophophora williamsii	Peyote
	Cathine	CELASTRACEAE	Catha edulis	Chat

EPHEDRINE

a Phenanthrene alkaloids derived biosynthetically from benzylisoquinoline intermediates.

by the enzyme amygdalase, the second by prunase. Free hydrocyanic acid is the violently toxic end product of hydrolysis.

The severity of poisoning from cyanide in plants depends on how much free HCN and/or cyanogenic glycoside exists in the plant. Hydrocyanic acid inhibits the action of the enzyme cytochrome oxidase, the terminal respiratory catalyst linking atmospheric oxygen with metabolic respiration. Therefore, HCN poisoning is asphyxiation at the cellular level. As little as 0.06 g has caused death in man, and the largest dose from which a person has been known to recover is 0.15 g.

A wide range of plants possess cyanogenic glycosides capable of releasing HCN. Selected examples of such plants are presented in Table 2-2, which shows a predominance of genera classified in the Rosaceae. This presentation also illustrates the great number found in the allied Fabaceae (pea family), as well as in the totally unrelated Poaceae (grass family). The cyanogenic-rich families are also indicated in boldface type in the phylogenetic tree for Angiosperms (Fig. 2-2), which further illustrates and emphasizes the wide and presumed repeatedly independent origin of cyanogenic glycosides.

ANTHRAQUINONE GLYCOSIDES

On hydrolysis, the anthraquinone glycosides yield aglycones that are anthraquinones, and either the aglycone or glycoside would be expected to have purgative activity. They include such plants as cascara (*Rhamnus purshiana*, Rhamnaceae), frangula or buckthorn (*Rhamnus frangula*), aloe (*Aloe barbadensis* and other species, Liliaceae), rhubarb (*Rheum* spp., Polygonaceae), and senna (*Cassia senna*, Fabaceae).

CARDIOACTIVE GLYCOSIDES

The cardioactive glycosides are characterized by their specific action on the cardiac muscle (Chapter 7). The aglycones are steroidal. As many as 400 cardiac glycosides have been characterized, most from the Apocynaceae (*Acokanthera, Apocynum, Nerium, Strophanthus, Tanghinia, Thevetia*), Asclepiadaceae (*Asclepias, Calotropis*), Liliaceae (*Bowiea, Convallaria, Urginea*), Moraceae (*Antiaris*), Ranunculaceae (*Adonis, Helleborus*), and Scrophulariaceae (*Digitalis, Scrophularia*). There is no close taxonomic or chemical relationship among these families, except for the Apocynaceae and Asclepiadaceae, which are often grouped together, and possibly between them and the Scrophulariaceae, suggesting a number of parallel, independent developments of these glycosides in the flowering plants.

Table 2-2   Some Important Toxic Plants Having Cyanogenic Glycosides Arranged Phylogenetically

Angiosperms: Dicotyledons
CHENOPODIACEAE. *Suckleya*
PASSIFLORACEAE. *Adenia, Passiflora*
EUPHORBIACEAE. *Manihot, Stillingia*
ROSACEAE. *Cercocarpus, Cotoneaster, Eriobotrya, Malus, Prunus, Pyrus, Rhodotypos*
FABACEAE. *Acacia, Cassia, Dolichos, Lotus, Phaseolus, Trifolium, Vicia*
SAXIFRAGACEAE. *Hydrangea*
MYRTACEAE. *Eucalyptus*
LINACEAE. *Linum*
OLACACEAE. *Ximenia*
CAPRIFOLIACEAE. *Sambucus*
BIGNONIACEAE. *Crescentia*
ASTERACEAE. *Ageratum, Bahia, Florestina*

Angiosperms: Monocotyledons
JUNCAGINACEAE. *Triglochin*
POACEAE. *Cynodon, Glyceria, Holcus, Panicum, Sorghum, Zea*

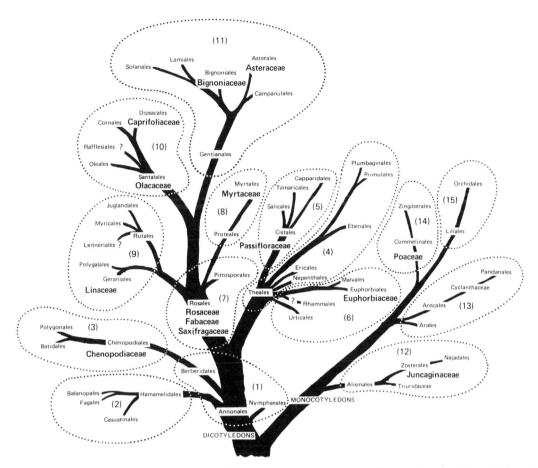

Figure 2-2   A schematic phylogenetic tree of the Angiosperms showing significant orders (endings -ales) and a few families (endings -aceae); the families in large boldface type contain plants producing hydrocyanic acid (see Appendix I for details of tree).

SAPONIN GLYCOSIDES

The saponin glycosides are widely distributed among the higher plants. Following hydrolysis they yield an aglycone (sapogenin) that is either a type of steroid or triterpene. Saponins form colloidal dispersions with water; they foam when shaken with water, and they usually have a bitter, acrid taste. They usually irritate mucous membranes, frequently destroy red blood cells by hemolysis, and are considered to be for the most part toxic, especially to cold-blooded animals (many are fish poisons).

The recent importance of plant ster-

oidal compounds, especially the steroid saponins, is their suitability as cortisone and hormone precursors. Many of the steroids developed in this way are of considerable value in the fights against arthritis (Chapter 6) and overpopulation (Chapter 13). Some of the plants having useful steroidal sapogenins include *Dioscorea* spp. (yams, Dioscoreaceae), *Agave* spp., and *Smilax* spp. (Liliaceae).

Other plants containing biologically interesting triterpene saponins and/or sapogenins are *Glycyrrhiza glabra* (licorice, Fabaceae), *Panax ginseng* (ginseng, Araliaceae), *Fagus sylvatica* (beech, Fagaceae), *Hedera helix* (English ivy,

Araliaceae), *Phytolacca americana* (poke, Phytolaccaceae), and *Medicago sativa* (alfalfa, Fabaceae).

COUMARIN GLYCOSIDES

Although coumarin is widely distributed in plants, coumarin glycosides are not common. Such glycosides are important, however, and several that are known to be poisonous are found in *Artemisia* spp. (wormwood, Asteraceae) as anthelmintics, *Viburnum prunifolium* (black haw, Caprifoliaceae) as antispasmodics, *Melilotus* spp. (sweetclovers, Fabaceae), *Aesculus* spp. (buckeyes, Hippocastanaceae), and *Daphne mezereum* (daphne, Thymelaeaceae).

There are many other kinds of glycosides, and a number of these are considered to be poisonous principles, such as those which prevent thyroid from accumulating inorganic iodine as found in broccoli, brussel sprouts, cabbage, kale, and all species of *Brassica*,[7] and irritant oils such as those obtained from mustard (seeds of Brassicaceae) and buttercup (ranunculin of Ranunculaceae).

Oxalates

Oxalic acid, the only organic acid of plants toxic to animals under natural conditions, occurs in plants as soluble (sodium and potassium) and insoluble (calcium) oxalates or acid oxalates. Although widespread in plants, the oxalates rarely reach dangerous levels. Exceptions— plants known to contain high levels of soluble oxalates—are certain *Oxalis* spp. (wood sorrel, Oxalidaceae), *Rheum rhaponticum* (rhubarb, Polygonaceae), *Rumex* spp. (dock, Polygonaceae), and *Portulaca oleracea* (purslane, Portulacaceae). Certain species of the Araceae are known to contain high levels of calcium oxalate.

Resins

Resins are amorphous products of a complex chemical nature. They are insoluble in water and do not contain nitrogen. Resins are also hard, transparent, or translucent; they soften on heating, and finally melt. Often they occur in mixtures with volatile oils (oleoresins), gums (gumresins), and sugars (glycoresins). Balsams are also resinous mixtures, containing aromatic plant acids.

Some species containing toxic resins are among the most violent poisons: members of the Apiaceae (*Cicuta*, water hemlock), Asclepiadaceae (*Asclepias*, milkweeds), Ericaceae (*Kalmia*, laurel; *Rhododendron*, rhododendron or azalea), and Meliaceae (*Melia azedarach*, chinaberry tree).

Phytotoxins

Found in a small number of plants, phytotoxins are protein molecules of high toxicity. They are similar to some bacterial toxins in structure, physiological reaction, and their action as antigens. The important ones known to the pea and spurge families are abrin (*Abrus precatorius*, Fabaceae), curcin (*Jatropha curcas*, Euphorbiaceae), ricin (*Ricinus communis*, Euphorbiaceae), robin (*Robinia pseudoacacia*, Fabaceae), and an uncharacterized phytotoxin in *Aleurites fordii* (Euphorbiaceae). In addition, a highly toxic albumin known as modeccin has been isolated from the roots of *Adenia digitata* (Passifloraceae).

Element and Nitrate Absorption

Plants may absorb and accumulate nitrate compounds, selenium, molybdenum, and other elements at levels harmful to animals. Selenium poisoning is well known where natural deposits are high and where there are plants with selenium accumulating ability, as in the western United States. Plants of the Asteraceae, Brassicaceae, and Fabaceae are important accumulators. Nitrates often reach dangerous levels in plants, particularly among crop plants such as oats, corn, and sorghum, and among the more weedy families (Asteraceae, Brassicaceae, Chenopodiaceae), and are often the direct result of excessive use of fertilizers. After digestion, the nitrates are reduced to nitrites, which are many more times toxic than nitrates, particularly in ruminants.[5]

PHYSIOLOGICAL ACTION OF POISONOUS PRINCIPLES

Of considerable merit is a classification of poisonous principles based on the physiological action of plants in animals.[8] Such a system is important to the clinician in diagnosis and therapy, although difficult to use because of complex actions involving the presence of more than one toxic principle. Nevertheless, such a scheme has potential value and should be examined at greater length, summarizing for example, the toxic elements of Chapters 5 through 14, utilizing chapter headings as major components.

PHYLOGENY OF PLANTS CONTAINING POISONOUS PRINCIPLES

As described in Appendix I, the lower and higher plants are divided on the basis of primary characters of morphology and anatomy in relation to their alternation of generations. The lower plants include the Bacteria, Algae, Fungi, and Bryophytes, and these are treated first, in that order, in most phylogenetic systems of classification. Following them are the higher plants, from the primitive Ferns through plants of increasing complexity and more

recent evolution (the Gymnosperms) and finally the dominant terrestrial plants, the Angiosperms or flowering plants.

Because of the complexity and importance of so many different kinds of Angiosperms in medical botany, the most current system of phylogeny is outlined in Appendix I with a supraorganization of families into phylogenetic groups. These are also illustrated in Fig. 2-2, which can be used by referring to the lists of Appendix I for any angiospermous family that needs phylogenetic placement. This system is used in presenting the plants that are poisonous when taken internally. Those who wish to pursue readings in classification of lower and higher plants should refer to the references of Appendix I.

INTERNAL POISONING BY PLANTS

Plants from the primitive Bacteria to the advanced Angiosperms having poisons and toxins are discussed in that sequence. The Angiosperms, which include the vast majority of harmful plants, are divided additionally into phylogenetic groups. Morphological descriptions of important common species in North America are accompanied by some discussion of their toxic principles. Among less significant species and among those not normally found in North America (usually indicated in small type), only a brief notation on poisoning in man is given; known instances of poisoning in domestic animals are sometimes included.*

* Those plants considered highly toxic to man, often resulting in death, are by and large given in large type; if commonly found in North America such plants are then described briefly. Those plants not known to cause poisoning in man, although considered a serious danger to animals, are presented in small type.

The data have been synthesized primarily from seven superb volumes on poisonous plants: N. Escobar, *Flora Tóxica de Panamá* (1972)[9]; J. W. Hardin and J. M. Arena, *Human Poisoning from Native and Cultivated Plants*, ed. 2 (1974)[10]; J. M. Kingsbury, *Poisonous Plants of the United States and Canada* (1964)[5]; W. C. Muenscher, *Poisonous Plants of the United States*, rev ed. (1951)[8]; P. M. North, *Poisonous Plants and Fungi* (1967)[11]; B. Verdcourt and E. C. Trump, *Common Poisonous Plants of East Africa* (1969)[1]; and J. M. Watt and M. G. Breyer-Brandwijk, *Medicinal and Poisonous Plants of Southern and Eastern Africa*, ed. 2 (1962).[12]

BACTERIA

The most common form of food poisoning in the United States is due to ingestion of food contaminated with *Staphylococcus aureus* enterotoxin. This heat stable, low molecular weight protein is associated with coagulase positive strains of specific phage types III and IV and is readily produced in poorly refrigerated cooked foods, such as cream-filled bakery goods and potato salad. However it imparts no changes in appearance, odor, or taste. This enterotoxin may not have any direct effect on the digestive tract; rather it is believed to exert its effect once it reaches the central nervous system through the bloodstream. Depending on the amount ingested, symptoms of acute gastrointestinal distress occur from 1 to 6 hours afterward, that usually subside within 8 hours, and recovery is complete within a few days. Shock and death are rare, and supportive rehydration therapy is necessary only when dehydration is severe in the young and debilitated.

As staphylococcal intoxication is considered the scourge of the summer picnic table, so can botulism be the ultimate disaster of the home or commercial canner. Spores of toxigenic strains of *Clostridium botulinum* (types A, B, E, and F) not killed by cooking can germinate under anaerobic conditions and produce toxin. This potent, high molecular weight protein is activated by proteolytic enzymes of the digestive tract and cleaved into toxic fragments that are absorbed into the bloodstream, where they act to stimulate denervation of the peripheral nervous system. They suppress or block the release of acetylcholine and halt cholinergic synaptic and junctional transmission at the neuromuscular junctions.

The earlier the symptoms occur, the greater the intoxication and the poorer the prognosis. Usually after an interval of 12 to 36 hours one observes symptoms of weakness, dizziness, headache, constipation, diplopia (double vision), difficulty in swallowing and speech, and accompanying oculomotor or other symmetrical motor cranial nerve paralyses. Only rarely do vomiting and diarrhea initiate illness. Death results from respiratory or cardiac failure in approximately two-thirds of cases, three to seven days after symptoms appear; mortality is higher in type A than type B or type E intoxications.

Therapy involves a regimen of induced vomiting, gastric lavage, and purgation to rid the system of unabsorbed toxin. Although rarely necessary, treatment with penicillin may be used to kill any ingested organisms that produce toxin; more important is the infusion with specific or trivalent antitoxin to inactivate toxin circulating in the bloodstream. Of limited therapeutic value is the use of atropine and guanidine, which influence the release or metabolism of acetylcholine.

ALGAE

Freshwater *Anabaena flos-aquae, Aphanizomenon flos-aquae,* and *Microcystis aeruginosa* (blue-green algae), all common in algal blooms, are undoubtedly responsible for extensive loss of life in livestock, pets, wild animals, birds, and even man. Toxicity of such blooms may result from toxic fast-death factors produced in certain blue-green algae, from products of decomposition, and from toxins produced by bacteria that are often associated with these blooms. Poisoning does not occur unless a dense bloom of toxic organisms is formed and toxic material is thus concentrated. Extensive growths of algae may be a nuisance, but most do not include large numbers of harmful organisms or enough toxic products to be dangerous.

Shellfish poisoning, which has caused hundreds of cases of severe intoxication and death, is due to the presence of specific toxic algal substances in healthy shellfish. Mussels, clams, scallops and other molluscs, and invertebrates such as crabs have been found to contain dangerous levels of toxic agents. Epidemics have occurred on both the Atlantic and Pacific coasts of North America.

Toxicity in shellfish is due to blooms of *Gonyaulax catenella* on the Pacific coast and of *G. tamarensis* on the Atlantic coast; these are Dinoflagellates that are ingested in extraordinarily large numbers by shellfish. The toxic principle produced by these Dinoflagellates is a complex nitrogenous compound known as tetrodotoxin, which accumulates in the tissues of shellfish without harming them. Cooking probably eliminates about one-third of the toxicity on the average, perhaps only leaching out the toxin, which by no means reduces poisoning below a dangerous level in many cases. These hazardous Dinoflagellate blooms, which normally appear as areas of reddish or brownish water, can also confer toxicity to shellfish at bloom levels not visible to the naked eye.

Another Dinoflagellate bloom (red tide) is conspicuously red and is associated with massive poisoning of fish and other marine animals (turtles, oysters, shrimp, crabs, dolphins). Such toxicity is linked to *Gymnodinium brevis* in Florida and *G. veneficum* in Great Britain, although the active principle is unknown. These Dinoflagellates are rapidly toxic to marine animals, however, and in many cases fish have been observed to die almost immediately after swimming in an area where the algae are numerous.

FUNGI

The fungi are found everywhere and are perhaps the most ubiquitous of all organisms. Their poisonous principles are readily divisible into those that produce toxic substances, the mycotoxins, and those such as mushrooms that possess toxins.

Mycotoxins

Eating mycotoxin-contaminated foods may result in a serious hazard to the health of man and beast.[13] The toxins often remain in food long after the fungus that produced them has died; that is, toxins can be present in food that is not visibly moldy. In addition, many mycotoxins remain toxic after food has ben cooked or processed in some way. Hazards of poisoning do not end here, however, for an even more treacherous problem exists if animal feed is contaminated by mycotoxins. Not only will many animals be lost by toxicity, but the toxins, or their metabolic products, can remain as residues in meat or can be passed into eggs or milk, that is eventually consumed in part by man.

ASPERGILLUS FLAVUS AND A. PARASITICUS

A few strains of these widely distributed species of *Aspergillus* produce a specific group of mycotoxins called aflatoxins.[14] Aflatoxin B_1, the toxin perhaps most frequently found in food, is also the most potent of the group. These fungi can produce their toxic compounds on essentially any food that will support growth. Thus any food is susceptible to aflatoxin contamination once it becomes moldy. Symptoms of poisoning become apparent at 10 to 100 ppm contamination of livestock feed. Aflatoxins are able to interact with DNA and markedly affect transcription of genetic information in animals, cells, and microorganisms. Indeed, aflatoxin B_1 is among the most potent carcinogens known (Chapter 5). The aflatoxins affect chiefly the liver, and it appears that children are the most susceptible to this kind of poisoning.

The presence of these toxigenic fungi on foods, both human and livestock, presents a significant potential risk to all. Techniques for minimizing food contamination, especially in warm humid regions of the world where fungi grow well, is of utmost importance if the hazards of aflatoxins are to be reduced. The old axiom, prevention is the best cure, certainly applies here.

CLAVICEPS PURPUREA (ERGOT)

The use of ergot in childbirth and in controlling uterine hemorrhage gained wide acceptance long before it came into general use by physicians and midwives (Chapter 13). Poisoning by ergot has an equally long history, involving incidents, particularly during the Middle and Dark

Ages, when human suffering and death have been incalculable (Chapter 18).

Ergotism, or St. Anthony's fire, is caused by the fungus *Claviceps purpurea,* which parasitizes cereal grains and is ingested by man through flour milled from contaminated rye and other cereals. The baking of bread, for example, does not alter the alkaloids produced by ergot, and ingestion of small amounts daily over a period of several weeks or longer results in chronic poisoning. The alkaloids ergonovine and ergotamine act by contracting arterioles and the smooth muscles of the digestive tract, giving rise to gangrene of the extremities, vomiting, muscle twitchings, and a staggering gait. Ingestion of large amounts of ergot results in convulsive ergotism and death unless the source of contamination is decreased or removed. In the case of livestock, source elimination can be difficult because ergot grows on common range and weedy grasses—for example, *Agropyron* spp. (wheat and quack grasses), *Agrostis alba* (redtop), *Elymus* spp. (wild rye), *Poa* spp. (blue or June grasses)—and may be a constant and continuing threat.

Ergot alkaloids also contain lysergic acid in combination with various amine-bearing structures. Thus hallucinations are an additional symptom of ergotism in man (Chapter 18).

Mushrooms (Basidiomycetes)[15] (Fig. 2-3a)

Direct internal poisoning by mushrooms is a serious danger particularly for those in the North Temperate zone where toxic species are numerous and often abundant. If man were not inquisitive, this frequency would present no problem. But there has always existed, and probably always will exist a group of adventuresome and dedicated if not invariably well-educated amateur mycologists. In playing

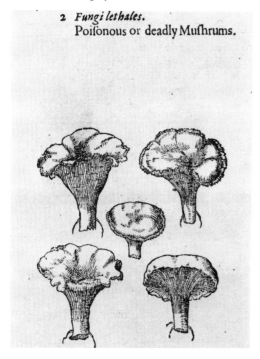

2 Fungi lethales.
Poifonous or deadly Mufhrums.

Figure 2-3a *Fungi lethales,* (from J Gerard, *The Her-ball,* 1597).

this deadly game the amateur collector must be well-versed because:

There are old mushroom hunters
And there are bold mushroom hunters
But there are no old, bold mushroom hunters.

Amanita phalloides and its close relatives account for about 90% of all fatalities. Fungi causing poisoning in man may induce enteritis (*Entoloma sinuatum, Russula* spp., *Lactarius* spp., *Boletus satanus*) or cell destruction (*Amanita phalloides* and other species, *Gyromitra esculenta, Lepiota helveola*), affect the nervous system (*Amanita muscaria, A. pantherina, Clitocybe* spp., *Inocybe* spp.), or produce hallucinations. These symptoms are discussed further in Chapter 18. Poisoning in domestic and wild animals is rare, occurring mostly from species of *Amanita*. Cattle, dogs,

and cats are only infrequently reported as being poisoned by fungi.

Amanita phalloides (death cup). This species is found in deciduous woods and is fairly common in North America and Europe. One or two mushrooms ingested cooked or raw produce no symptoms for about 10 hours; then suddenly the patient is seized by extreme abdominal pain, vomiting, diarrhea, and excessive thirst. Pain is excruciating, loss of strength is rapid, and is usually accompanied by convulsions and coma. Death that follows in 50 to 90% of the cases can occur as early as 48 hours, although it is more usual after 4 to 6 days in children and 6 to 8 days in adults. Liver damage is found in the majority of patients who recover.

Poisoning. The toxins of this and

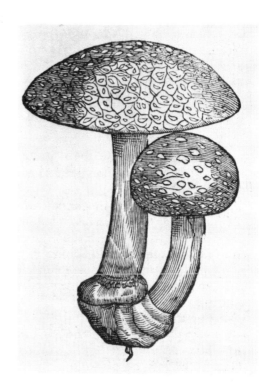

Figure 2-3b *Amanita muscaria* (from J Gerard, *The Herball,* ed 2, 1636).

closely related species are polypeptides, including phalloidin, which produces degenerative changes in the kidney, liver, and cardiac muscles, and several amanitins, which produce hypoglycemia and are responsible for the major symptoms.

Gyromitra esculenta (false morel or lorchel), looks like the highly prized edible morel. It is poisonous to some individuals, but not to others; some may eat the mushroom for years, then suddenly become susceptible to poisoning. The effects of this plant and of Lepiota helveola (poisonous lepiota) resemble mild poisoning by Amanita phalloides.

Entoloma sinuatum (livid agaric) is known to cause severe or fatal poisoning in Europe. Symptoms are chiefly violent sickness and diarrhea, generally within one-half hour of eating, gradually causing great weakness. Damage to the liver is frequent. Similarly, Russula emetica (sickener), Lactarius torminosus (woolly milk cap), and Boletus satanus (devil's boletus) result in gastroenteritis, which may be either severe to the point of fatality, or mild.

Amanita muscaria (fly agaric) (Fig. 2-3b) see Chapter 18, Hallucinogens. The fly agaric occurs through the North Temperate zone, commonly in wooded areas. It is found singly or in groups, sometimes in circles (the fairy rings) and frequently around birch trees. Fatalities are rare; the main symptoms are malaise, vomiting and diarrhea, slow pulse, rapid breathing, and hallucination.

Poisoning. Muscarine is present in only small amounts, and although originally isolated from fly agaric, the neurological effects of poisoning by this species more nearly resemble the central nervous system stimulation of atropine. So-called mycoatropine of fly agaric is a mixture of two isoxazole derivates, ibotenic acid and muscimol, both psychoactive compounds, with muscimol about five times as active. A third active principle is muscazone, an oxazole derivative.

Amanita pantherina (panther cap) is similar to A. muscaria, but it produces more severe symptoms. Other fungi having major effects on the nervous system include Clitocybe and Inocybe spp., which contain as much as 3% (dry weight) of muscarine. Symptoms of muscarine poisoning may occur quite rapidly (increased salivation, perspiration, abdominal pain, diarrhea, slow pulse, constricted pupil, asthmatic breathing, and cardiac or respiratory failure in severe cases), but fatalities are infrequent. Hallucinations do not occur.

Lichens

Parmelia molliuscula, a ground lichen, is toxic to cattle and sheep; the toxic principle is usnic acid.

FERNS (AND FERN ALLIES)

EQUISETACEAE

Equisetum arvense and E. palustre (horsetails) (Fig. 2-4a) are toxic to cattle and horses, but less frequently injurious to other livestock. Thiaminase is the major toxic component.

POLYPODIACEAE

Notholaena sinuata (jimmy fern). Ingestion by sheep usually results in a mortality rate of about 25%.

Onoclea sensibilis (sensitive fern). Poisoning of horses has been reported.

Pteridium aquilinum (bracken) contains thiaminase, which destroys thiamine and results in a vitamin B_1 deficiency and causes serious poisoning, particularly in

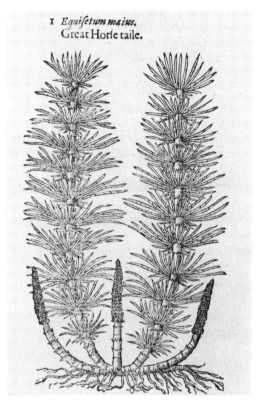

I Equiſetum maius.
Great Horſe taile.

Figure 2-4a *Equisetum telmateia* (from J Gerard, *The Herball, 1597*).

horses and cattle. Extracts have carcinogenic and mutagenic properties; in sufficient concentrations they are acutely toxic to a wide range of domestic animals. Toxicity is passed through the milk of cows and is a potential health hazard where cattle eat bracken.[16] The carcinogenic principle is shikimic acid.

GYMNOSPERMS

CUPRESSACEAE

Cupressus macrocarpa (Monterey cypress). Leaves induce unusual pregnancy difficulties and abortion in cattle.

Juniperus virginiana (red cedar or juniper) and other species are considered toxic to livestock.

CYCADACEAE

Cycas circinalis (fern palm), *Dioon edule* (chamal), *Macrozamia miquelii*, *Microcycas* spp., and *Zamia integrifolia* (coontie) possess fleshy seeds that are poisonous, but if the harmful azoxy glycosides are washed out, the seeds can be eaten. These plant parts are especially poisonous to cattle and *Zamia* is particularly toxic.

PINACEAE

Pinus ponderosa (western yellow pine) and *P. taeda* (loblolly pine). Needle consumption has caused abortion (*P. ponderosa*) and death (*P. taeda*) in cattle.

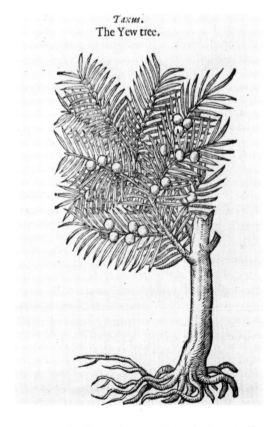

Taxus.
The Yew tree.

Figure 2-4b *Taxus baccata* (from J Gerard, *The Herball,* ed 2, 1636).

TAXACEAE

Taxus spp. (yew). Evergreen shrubs or trees, the bark thin and flaking, the branches horizontal; leaves linear, dark green above, yellow-green below, to about 1 inch long, two-ranked on branches; "flowers" yellowish, inconspicuous; seeds solitary, ovoid, and nearly surrounded by a bright scarlet fleshy cup (aril).

Taxus baccata (English yew, Fig. 2-4*b*) and *T. cuspidata* (Japanese yew) are widely cultivated, and a number of other species are native to North America.

Poisoning. The alkaloid taxine in the bark, leaves, and seeds of all species is rapidly absorbed from the intestine. Death is sudden, and survival after poisoning is uncommon. Children should be warned to avoid the alluring bright colored aril-seed. Mortality of livestock is well known.

ANGIOSPERMS

The Angiosperms contain by far the most numerous and diverse toxic materials. Almost all members of some families appear toxic at some stage of development of one or more parts of the plant. Such families as the Apocynaceae, Asclepiadaceae, Euphorbiaceae, and Sapotaceae (all having caustic white latex), are generally dangerous ingestants, as are the Fabaceae (which contain many tannins, and toxic glycosides and alkaloids), the Solanaceae (commonly having toxic tropane and other alkaloids), and the Papaveraceae (which have many poisonous isoquinoline alkaloids). Some of these most dangerous families, however, are among the most important ones medicinally, for in small, controlled doses any one of these potentially lethal compounds may be of great medicinal value. Not all large, diverse families, however, possess poisonous principles. Why, for example, do the many alkaloids in the large family Rubiaceae appear to have so few harmful properties?

The dicotyledonous families are given first (phylogenetic groups 1–11) followed by the monocotyledons (phylogenetic groups 12–15), which have few toxic compounds except in the Liliaceae. The list emphasizes the toxic plants found in North America and Europe. While not ignoring the important ones from tropical regions, the compilation is far from complete and does not pretend to be encyclopedic. As a student guide to toxicity in flowering plants, however, the list is sufficiently inclusive to illustrate the importance of natural poisons to man's well-being.

Dicotyledons

PHYLOGENETIC GROUP 1

ANNONACEAE (Custard Apple)

Annona cherimola (custard apple) seeds and stem cortex extracts are used as fish poisons and insecticides.

MYRISTICACEAE (Nutmeg)

Myristica fragrans: see Chapter 18, Hallucinogens.

ARISTOLOCHIACEAE (Birthwort)

Aristolochia petersiana from eastern Africa and perhaps all species of Dutchman's pipe are poisonous to both man and livestock. A few leaves are said to be sufficient to kill a goat. *Aristolochia grandiflora* in Panama is known to kill deer and has been used by criminals for poisoning.

CALYCANTHACEAE (Calycanthus)

Calycanthus floridus (Carolina allspice) contains calycanthine (similar to strychnine) and is reported to have poisoned cattle in Tennessee.

LAURACEAE (Laurel)

Persea americana (avocado) leaves, fruit, bark, and seeds have poisoned cattle, horses, goats, rabbits, canaries, and fish.

PIPERACEAE (Pepper)

Piper darienensis leaves poison fish in Panama.

MENISPERMACEAE (Moonseed)

Chondodendron tomentosum (pareira). A chief ingredient of South American Indian arrow poisons or curare, contains the neurologically active bis-isoquinoline alkaloid tubocurarine. Extracts of the inner bark and wood of pareira, one or more species of *Strychnos,* and sometimes other species, are boiled by the Indians to a gummy mass containing the crude poisons. This mass readily sticks to arrows, which are often constructed to detach and remain in the shallow wound; thus the arrow tip is not pulled out as the wounded animal crashes through the forest. With the arrow neatly in place, the prey never goes far.

Menispermum canadense (moonseed). Perennial twining vine with smooth stems; leaves alternate, palmately lobed with three to five rounded lobes (looking somewhat like a grape leaf), the petioles usually twisted; flowers small in axillary clusters, greenish-white; fruit small, purple, globular drupes occurring in grapelike clusters, but with only one crescent-shaped grooved seed. Moonseeds are found throughout eastern North America.
   Poisoning. The toxic principles are isoquinoline alkaloids, including dauricine with a curarelike action, which have caused fatalities to children eating the fruit. Birds, however, are known to eat the fruit and seeds without harm.

RANUNCULACEAE (Buttercup)

Aconitum spp. (aconite, monkshood). Herbaceous perennial with ascending or nearly trailing stems; leaves bright green, alternate palmately three to nine lobed commonly five lobed; flowers in terminal racemes or panicles, white to deep bluish-purple, the upper part helmet shaped; fruit of three to five many-seeded follicles.

Aconitum reclinatum (white flowers) and *A. uncinatum* (blue flowers) are native to eastern North America; *A. columbianum* occurs in western Canada south to California and New Mexico; *A. napellus* (blue flowers) is European and commonly cultivated; *A. vulparia* (Fig. 2-5a) is of Eu-

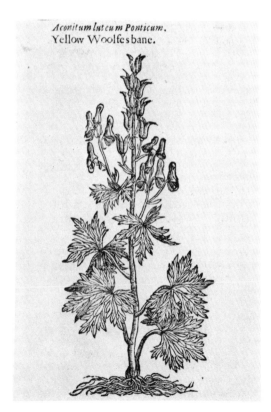

Figure 2-5a   *Aconitum vulparia* (from J Gerard, *The Herball,* ed 2, 1636).

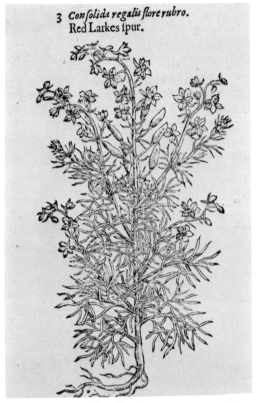

Figure 2-5b *Delphinium* sp. (from J Gerard, *The Herball,* 1597).

rasian origin and is used as a narcotic in Chinese medicine.

Poisoning. All parts of the plant contain the alkaloid aconitine, as well as other alkaloids. The root is the most dangerous part but the leaves are greatest in toxicity just before flowering. The main symptom of poisoning is numbness, followed by paralysis of the lower then upper extremities, leaving the mind clear. Weak pulse, respiratory paralysis, and convulsions are typical, with death occurring in about 2 hours.

In ancient times a decoction was given to criminals as fatal punishment and, on the Greek island of Ceos, infirm old men were compelled to take a draught of aconite.

Actaea spp. (baneberry). Herbaceous perennial to 3 feet tall with a stout rhizome; large coarsely divided pinnately compound leaves, the leaflets having toothed margins; small white flowers in long-stalked terminal racemes; berries white, red, or black. *Actaea pachypoda* (white berries) and *A. rubra* (red berries) are eastern North American, *A. arguta* is largely western North American, and *A. spicata* (black berries) is European.

Poisoning. All parts of the plant are toxic, probably because of an essential oil. Chief symptoms are quickening of the heart, gastroenteritis, and dizziness; symptoms usually disappear after 3 hours. As few as six berries can result in severe symptoms, but fatalities are rare.

Adonis spp. (pheasants-eye) is lethal to horses and sheep, although symptoms in livestock usually are those of severe gastroenteritis. Some species contain a cardioactive glycoside, adonidin.

Anemone spp. (windflower) contain protoanemonin, an irritant toxic principle, and are potentially hazardous to livestock.

Aquilegia vulgaris and other species of columbine are probably all poisonous giving an effect similar to that of aconite. Seeds have been reported to be fatal to children.

Caltha palustris (marsh marigold) is similar to the buttercups in effect of poisoning and contains the same irritant oil.

Clematis spp. (virgin's-bower) has substances resembling protoanemonin, and it may be fatal (the juice taken internally acts as a violent purgative).

Delphinium spp. (larkspur, Fig. 2-5b). Annual or perennial herbs up to 4 feet tall; leaves finely and usually deeply palmately divided often on long petioles; flowers in a terminal raceme, white, rose, or bluish-purple, each flower with a backward projecting spur; fruit a many-seeded follicle.

Species of *Delphinium* occur throughout North America and Eurasia; a number are frequently cultivated, such as *D. ajacis* from Europe.

Poisoning. Alkaloids delphinine, ajacine, and others occur mostly in the seeds and in young plants. Ingestion may cause stomach upset and nervous symptoms; death may occur if the plant is eaten in large quantities, especially by children. Larkspur poisoning of cattle is widespread and is a major hazard in the western United States.

Eranthis hyemalis (water aconite), containing poisonous alkaloids, is toxic to livestock.

Helleborus foetidus, H. niger (Christmas rose), and *H. viridis* all contain cardiac glycosides that cause violent purging, delirium, convulsions, and death from respiratory failure. The main cardiac stimulant is hellebrin. Poisoning in livestock is largely from hay contaminated with *Helleborus* species, because the glycosides are not destroyed by drying and storage.

Pulsatilla vulgaris (pasque flower), which contains protoanemonin, is potentially dangerous to livestock.

Ranunculus spp. (buttercup) poisoning due to the irritant yellow oil protoanemonin is very rare in man, and because buttercups are distasteful to grazing animals also, poisoning of them is infrequent. Hay containing *Ranunculus* is not dangerous because protoanemonin is unstable on drying.

BERBERIDACEAE (Barberry)

Caulophyllum thalictroides (blue cohosh). Perennial glabrous herb with knotty rootstock; stem erect, terminated by a small raceme or panicle of yellowish-green flowers, and just below a large three-parted compound sessile leaf;

seed dark blue. The species is common in rich woods in eastern North America.

Poisoning. Leaves and seeds contain the alkaloid methylcytisine as well as uncharacterized glycosides; children have been poisoned by eating the blue seeds.

Podophyllum peltatum (May apple). Perennial herb having a creeping rhizome and thick fibrous root; stems single, one or two leaved, the latter with one flower in the fork; leaves large, rounded, five to nine lobed; single flowers nodding, six to rarely nine white petals, stamens numerous; fruit a large fleshy berry turning yellow when ripe. May apples are common spring flowers in eastern North American woods.

Poisoning. Podophyllotoxin and related lignans, the active poisonous principles, are found throughout the plant but mainly in the roots (except in the ripe fruit, which can be eaten without harm), and will cause gastroenteritis. Children have been poisoned by eating too many unripe fruit.

PAPAVERACEAE (Poppy)

Argemone mexicana (prickly poppy). Coarse annual to 3 feet tall with erect, usually branched, stems, the herb whitish green and with yellow juice; leaves prickly and thistlelike, alternate, the leaf base clasping the stem; flowers single, terminal, and showy, with four to six delicate, pale yellow to orange petals; fruit a prickly capsule opening near the top and having many small seeds. Prickly poppies are widely distributed in weedy habitats in temperate and tropic regions. *Argemone intermedia* and *A. glauca* have the same properties as the common species.

Poisoning. Toxic alkaloids sanguinarine, berberine, protopine, and others are found in the whole plant or the seeds. Since the plant is distasteful to animals, cases of poisoning are rare, although stock losses have been reported in Australia. A greater problem is contamination of feed and home-ground grains by seeds: in India, for example, wheat so contaminated resulted in an epidemic of dropsy.

Chelidonium majus (celandine poppy) has extremely acrid, orange-yellow juice and is only rarely ingested by animals or man (reportedly leaves have been eaten by those who mistook them for parsley). The plant contains many of the poppy alkaloids (chelidonine, sanguinarine, berberine, protopine, etc.), and loss of life has been recorded in Europe, but not in eastern North America, where it has become naturalized.

Corydalis caseana (fitweed), rich in apomorphine, protoberberine, protopine, and other isoquinoline alkaloids, has caused great losses among livestock. It is toxic to sheep and cattle but not distasteful to them. A number of other weedy species in North America are suspected of being toxic (*C. aurea*, *C. flavula*), but tubers of some species are eaten in Eurasia.

Dicentra spp. (Dutchman's breeches), having the same isoquinoline alkaloids as *Corydalis*, and being similarly toxic to livestock, have not been known to cause loss of life in man. The genus is widely cultivated (*D. spectabilis*) and common in rich woods in North America (*D. cucullaria, D. canadensis, D. formosa*).

Papaver spp. (poppy) are distasteful to livestock and rarely cause poisoning, although they contain numerous potentially toxic alkaloids (besides those noted under *Chelidonium*, occasionally morphine, codeine, papaverine). A number of species are widely cultivated: *P. nudicaule* (Iceland poppy), *P. orientale* (Oriental poppy), *P. rhoeas* (corn poppy), and also *P. somniferum* (opium poppy), which is duscussed in Chapter 19.

Sanguinaria canadensis (bloodroot), containing the physiologically active compound sanguinarine, does not appear to have poisoned humans or livestock in North America (see comments under *Argemone mexicana*).

PHYLOGENETIC GROUP 2

FAGACEAE (Beech)

Fagus spp. (beech) nuts occasionally cause poisoning in man and in domestic animals. Reports from Europe (*F. sylvaticus*) and North America (*F. grandifolia*) indicate gastrointestinal distress, probably due to the presence of a saponin glycoside.

Quercus spp. (oak) poisoning of livestock eating excessive amounts of raw acorns, young leaves, and other tree parts has been reported, possibly due to high concentrations of tannins and probably other toxic principles.

PHYLOGENETIC GROUP 3

PHYTOLACCACEAE (Poke)

Petiveria alliacea is reputedly toxic to cattle and has been used as fish poison.

Phytolacca americana (poke). Tall shrublike herbaceous perennial from a very large, fleshy taproot, the stems to 9 feet tall, glabrous, purple or green; leaves alternate, simple, ovate, petiolate, to 1 foot long; flowers many, small, greenish-white in drooping or erect racemes; fruit a shiny, round, purplish-black, juicy berry. A common weed throughout eastern North America.

Poisoning. The roots and seeds are especially toxic. The toxic principles are triterpene saponins, one of which has been identified as phytolaccigenin. Additional toxic principles are unidentified mitogens (see Chapter 4). Ingestion of the berries produces severe gastrointestinal disturbances accompanied by weakened pulse and respiration; death occurs if the dose is sufficient. Young leaves and stems are frequently eaten as cooked greens that are prepared by first soaking in salt water, followed by cooking well in two changes of water.

However, because of the mitogenic properties of poke, the use of this species as a potherb should be avoided. Gloves should always be worn to protect the hands from absorbing any harmful principles when removing especially the mature weed from gardens and other places.

NYCTAGINACEAE (Four-o'clock)

Mirabilis jalapa (four-o'clock), commonly cultivated as an ornamental, causes gastroenteritis in children when roots or seeds are eaten.

CACTACEAE (Cactus)

Lophophora williamsii (peyote) and other cacti: see Chapter 18, Hallucinogens.

PORTULACACEAE (Purslane)

Portulaca oleracea (purslane) produces acute oxalate poisoning of sheep in Australia.

CHENOPODIACEAE (Goosefoot)

Suckleya suckleyana (poison suckleya), having hydrocyanic acid potential, is lethal to cattle and possibly sheep in Colorado and New Mexico.

AMARANTHACEAE (Amaranth)

Amaranthus palmeri and *A. retroflexus* (pigweeds) accumulate high concentrations of nitrates, especially when growing on heavily fertilized soil, and have been implicated in cattle and horse poisoning.

CARYOPHYLLACEAE (Pink)

Agrostemma githago (corn cockle), Fig. 2-6a). Erect weedy annual to 3 feet tall, the stems with silky hairs and branched; leaves opposite, narrow and up to 4 inches long, covered with white hairs; flowers large (about 1 inch across), solitary, the five corolla lobes pink or purplish-red and the calyx of five hairy, long pointed tips; fruit a capsule with numerous black seeds. The species is native

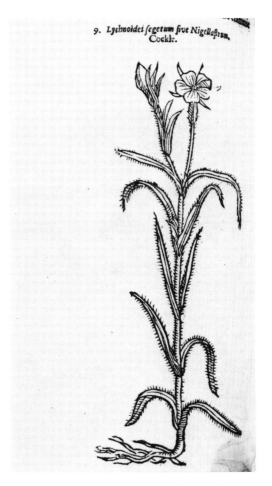

Figure 2-6a *Agrostemma githago* (from J Parkinson, *Theatrum Botanicum*, 1640).

to Europe and has become widely established in North America as a weed of waste and cultivated areas.

Poisoning. All parts, but especially the seeds, contain the sapogenin githagenin, which may be the toxic principle causing severe gastrointestinal irritation. The species may contaminate home-ground corn, oats, or wheat, and poisoning may result from eating flour made from such mixtures.

Drymaria arenarioides (alfombrilla) and *D. pachyphylla* (inkweed) from the southwestern United States and Mexico may poison cattle, sheep, and goats.

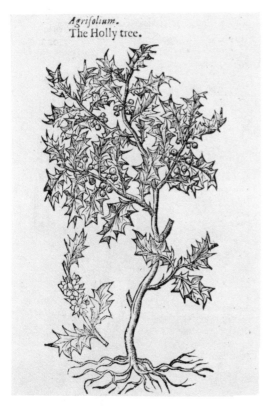

Agrifolium.
The Holly tree.

Figure 2-6b *Ilex aquifolium* (from J Gerard, *The Herball,* ed 2, 1636).

Saponaria officinalis (soapwort) and *S. vaccaria* (cow cockle), containing githagenin in seeds, are potentially hazardous to livestock.

POLYGONACEAE (Buckwheat)

Polygonum punctatum (water smart-weed), containing about 7% calcium oxalate in leaves, is poisonous to man and may be fatal to livestock.

Rheum rhaponticum (rhubarb). Perennial to 4 feet tall; roundish leaves, large, five-veined, glabrous, downy beneath and with long fleshy petioles; flowers in dense panicles. Of Siberian origin, rhubarb is widely cultivated in gardens in the temperate zones of the Old and New Worlds.
Poisoning. Leaf blades, sometimes consumed as a vegetable, have resulted

in fatal poisonings. Blood clotting is impaired, and vomiting and diarrhea are caused by the soluble oxalates. Pigs and goats are also poisoned by the leaf blades. The petiole, however, is pleasantly acidic and edible.

Rumex spp. (dock, sorrel), containing soluble oxalates, are toxic if eaten in large quantities by livestock, particularly sheep, and ingestion may result in death.

PHYLOGENETIC GROUP 4

AQUIFOLIACEAE (Holly)

Ilex spp. (holly). Shrub or small tree; leaves alternate, simple, spine-tipped, evergreen; flowers small and white; fruit a red or black berry-like drupe. *Ilex aquifolium* (Fig. 2-6b) of Europe and *I. opaca* native to eastern North America are widely cultivated and extensively used for Christmas decorations.
Poisoning. The berries of these species are poisonous, though not fatally, being violently emetic and purgative; thus they should be considered dangerous to children. The active principle is unknown. It is noteworthy that leaves of *I. vomitoria,* containing an appreciable amount of caffeine, were used by Indians and early settlers in the southeastern United States to brew yaupon tea.

CLUSIACEAE (St. John's-wort)

Hypericum perforatum (St. John's wort) is poisonous to animals as reported from New Jersey, North Africa, and Australia (also causes photosensitivity in animals).

Mammea americana (mamey) seeds are highly toxic to insects, fish, and hungry animals, particularly pigs.

Clusia rosea (balsam apple), having yellow milky latex, is violently and dangerously purgative; the fruit is considered poisonous.

ERICACEAE (Heath)

Agauria salicifolia leaves poison sheep and goats in eastern Africa with symptoms similar to those produced by andromedotoxin, a diterpene widespread in the family and known to be the toxic principle of other Ericaceae.

Kalmia latifolia (mountain laurel). Large, dense evergreen shrubs; leaves mostly alternate, elliptic, to 5 inches long, coriaceous, margin not toothed, dark green above and bright green below; flowers in terminal corymbs, showy, white to rose with purple markings; fruit a capsule. Mountain laurel occurs in moist woods of eastern Canada, south in the Appalachian Mountains and the Piedmont region. Other species include *K. angustifolia* (lambkill) and *K. polifolia* (pale laurel).

Poisoning. All parts, including pollen, contain andromedotoxin, a toxic diterpene causing slow pulse, lowering of blood pressure, lack of coordination, convulsions, progressive paralysis, and death. Arbutin, a glycoside of hydroquinone, is also present and indicated in the poisoning. Poisonous honey is made by bees attracted to this plant, and children have been poisoned by sucking flowers and making a decoction from leaves. The Delaware Indians used mountain laurel to commit sucide. Relatively severe losses of livestock have been reported. Many other members of the heath family are toxic and react much as *Kalmia latifolia* in poisoned animals. These include *Ledum columbianum* (Pacific Labrador tea), *L. glandulosum* (western Labrador tea), *Leucothoe davisiae* (Sierra laurel), *Menziesia ferruginea* (mock azalea), *Pieris japonica* (Japanese pieris), and *Rhododendron* spp. (rhododendron, azalea).

Pernettya spp. berries poison man, producing symptoms of drunkenness and paralysis, as well as sensations of cold. Cattle are poisoned by the leaves.

THEOPHRASTACEAE

All parts of *Jacquinia macrocarpa* are employed as a fish poison in tropical America.

PRIMULACEAE (Primrose)

Anagallis arvensis (scarlet pimpernel) has been implicated in poisoning of sheep in Australia and calves in Pennsylvania.

PHYLOGENETIC GROUP 5

FLACOURTIACEAE

Ryania spp., all parts and probably all species, are extremely toxic, acting as a violent gastric poison on warm- and cold-blooded animals. An alkaloid, ryanodine, has been isolated from the roots and stems of *R. speciosa* and is the toxic principle.

VIOLACEAE (Violet)

Viola odorata rhizomes and seeds cause severe gastroenteritis, nervousness, and respiratory and circulatory depression that may reach serious proportions if the dose is large.

PASSIFLORACEAE (Passion Flower)

Adenia volkensii is considered a serious human poison in eastern Africa and may contain both a cyanogenic glycoside and a phytotoxin like the southern Africa *A. digitata*.

Passiflora quadrangularis roots, leaves, fruits, and immature seeds, containing hydrocyanic acid and an uncharacterized principle called passiflorine, may be both psychoactive and poisonous.

CUCURBITACEAE (Gourd)

Bryonia cretica subsp. *dioica* (bryony) contains a glycoside bryonidin and a brown resin bryoresin in roots and berries, which are primarily responsible for poisoning. The poisonous principles are probably cucurbitacins, known to occur widely in the Cucurbitaceae. It has been estimated that 15 berries could be fatal to a child.

Cayaponia racemosa root is poisonous to cattle and has a strong purgative action in man. Most cucurbitacins are known to be purgative and would be expected to be present in this species.

Cucurbita lagenaria (gourd) fruit pulp ingested to get rid of roundworms killed two children in Cuba; seeds are considered very toxic.

Melothria scabra fruit and roots are very poisonous to domestic animals.

Momordica charantia (wild balsam apple). Creeping or climbing vine to 15 feet long; leaves alternate, palmately lobed up to 5 inches across; flowers yellow, tubular, nearly 1 inch in diameter; fruit to 5 inches long, tapering, very warty, orange or yellow at maturity, the seeds and pulp red. Of tropical origin, the species has become naturalized in the southern United States; often cultivated in the southern Midwest, the unripe fruit is eaten and used in home remedies for treating colds.

Poisoning. The seeds and wall of the fruit contain a resin, a saponic glycoside yielding elaterin (a cucurbitacin), and alkaloids that cause vomiting and diarrhea.

DATISCACEAE (Datisca)

Datisca glomerata (Durango root) is highly toxic to cattle and sheep. Toxic cucurbitacins are known to be present in many *Datisca* species.

CAPPARIDACEAE (Caper)

Capparis fascicularis and *C. tomentosa* leaves, bark, roots, and fruit have caused human as well as livestock deaths in eastern Africa.

Courbonia glauca root extracts have caused several human deaths in eastern Africa.

BRASSICACEAE (Mustard)

Armoracia rusticana (horseradish) can be fatal to livestock feeding on tops or roots; it is known to cause bloody vomiting and diarrhea in man after eating large quantities. Mustard oil containing isothiocyanates is considered the poisonous principle.

Barbarea vulgaris (yellow rocket) can cause poisoning in horses.

Brassica spp. (broccoli, cabbage, charlock, kale, rape, turnip, black mustard) may cause serious loss of livestock, especially rape poisoning.

Descurainia pinnata (tansy mustard). Poisoning of cattle from this plant is known in the southwestern United States.

Erysimum cheiranthoides (wormseed mustard) was reportedly responsible for loss of hogs in Canada.

Raphanus raphanistrum (wild radish) can be dangerous to livestock, and there are reports of losses of lambs from France, cattle from Australia, and elsewhere.

PHYLOGENETIC GROUP 6

STERCULIACEAE

Theobroma cacao (cacao tree). Cocoa fruit waste products may cause theobromine poisoning with death resulting from sudden heart failure.

MALVACEAE (Mallow)

Gossypium spp. (cotton). Cottonseed meal, the residue left after the cottonseed oils have been pressed out, can be poisonous to cattle, sheep, and pigs because of the presence of a sesquiterpene phenol, gossypol.

MORACEAE (Mulberry)

Antiaris toxicaria (upas tree). Latex, containing two cardioactive glycosides antiarin x and z, is extremely toxic and is used in tropical Asia as a principal poison for arrows and darts. As an instrument of execution it is unmatched. For example, it was used in Java in 1776 to punish 13 concubines of the king who were convicted of infidelity. The girls were lashed to posts, their breasts bared, and an awllike instrument poisoned with the latex of upas lanced the unhappy women about the middle of their breasts. All died within 5 minutes in great agony.

Maclura pomifera (Osage orange) is suspected of causing livestock loss in Arkansas and Texas.

Morus rubra (red mulberry): in excess fruit mildly intoxicating.

CANNABACEAE (Hemp)

Cannabis sativa (marihuana): see Chapter 18, Hallucinogens.

EUPHORBIACEAE (Spurge)

Aleurites fordii (tung oil tree). Small deciduous tree up to 25 feet tall, the branches stout and often in whorls; leaves alternate, simple, palmately veined and cordate, to 10 inches long, the margins smooth, long-petiolate; flowers pink to white, petals five to seven; fruit pendant, 2 to 3 inches in diameter, brown at maturity, the seeds three to seven with rough seed coats. Native to China and widely cultivated in the Old and New Worlds, the species is found in commercial plantings along the Gulf Coast and as ornamentals. Other species are less toxic.
  Poisoning. Uncharacterized saponins and a phytotoxin principle of the seeds and other plant parts produce severe gastroenteritis in humans. A single seed can result in serious illness. Poisoning in cattle is not uncommon.

Croton spp. (marans), many of which contain croton oil predominantly in seeds but also in leaves and stems, are powerful purgatives. Death occurs in man and domestic animals on ingestion of small amounts.

Euphorbia spp. (spurges, snow-on-the-mountain, crown-of-thorns, poinsettia, candelabra tree, pencil tree). Upright or prostrate herbs or shrubs with milky, acrid juice, often cactuslike; leaves simple, alternate or opposite, some leathery; flower cluster in cup-shaped structures, greenish, often with glands; fruit a three-lobed capsule extending from the cup and commonly the long stalk pendant. There are numerous species native to North America. The milky sap of these and many cultivated species, such as *E. milii* (crown-of-thorns), *E. pulcherrima* (poinsettia), and *E. tirucallii* (pencil tree), contains toxic principles that will cause severe poisoning if ingested in quantity. The toxic principles of most irritant *Euphorbia* species are known to be complex esters related to the diterpene phoabol. Many of these compounds are also cocarcinogens. Reported deaths are rare. Livestock can be seriously affected.

Excoecaria venenifera: milky latex is very poisonous and particularly injurious to the eyes. Ingestion of the plant has killed camels in Kenya.

Hippomane mancinella (manchineel tree). Usually a small tree to 20 feet tall, occasionally to 50 feet with milky juice; leaves alternate, ovate, dark green, to 6 inches long, the margins finely serrate; flowers in spikes, small, greenish; fruit a green or yellowish-green drupe about 1½ inches in diameter. Native to Central America, the West Indies, and the Gulf Coast, the tree has been almost eliminated in the United States because of its widely known toxicity; the species is now restricted to remote areas of this country like the Everglades.

Poisoning. Ingestion of a few seeds may cause poisoning accompanied by severe gastroenteritic symptoms. The oil in the seed is purgative; the toxic principle is not known. The milky sap is extremely caustic to the skin.

Hura crepitans (sandbox tree) of tropical America is occasionally planted as an ornamental. The milky juice and seeds cause severe vomiting and diarrhea when eaten. The toxic principle is the irritant and carcinogenic diterpene huratoxin. Seeds of *H. polyandra* in Mexico are used to poison coyotes and as a violent purgative; the milky juice is used for poisoning fish.

Jatropha curcas (purging nut). Coarse shrub or short-lived tree to 15 feet tall with smooth stems mostly green; leaves alternate, long-petioled, palmately veined, cordate, about 6 inches in diameter, usually three to five lobed; flowers small, yellow; fruit an ovoid capsule, brownish-black at maturity and with two to three black seeds. Native to the American tropics, widely distributed elsewhere; in Florida it is cultivated. Other poisonous species include *J. gossypifolia* (bellyache bush), *J. integerrima* (peregrina), and *J. multifida* (physic nut or coral plant).

Poisoning. The toxic fruits or seeds, containing a purgative oil and the phytotoxin curcin, are often eaten by children, causing nausea, vomiting, diarrhea, and coma a few hours after eating. It is considered a serious cause of poisoning in southern Florida. A number of cytotoxic diterpenes, such as jatropham, have been isolated from *Jatropha* species.

Manihot esculenta (cassava, manioc, tapioca). Raw roots and leaves can have high concentrations of hydrocyanic acid sufficient to cause death from cyanide poisoning. Acute poisoning can be avoided if the roots are peeled and several changes of cooking water are employed during preparation for eating.

Mercurialis annua (annual mercury), introduced from Europe and found occasionally throughout North America, and the European *M. perennis,* possess a volatile oil that causes severe gastroenteritis in man and livestock. Leaves eaten as a vegetable cause poisoning.

Pedilanthus tithymaloides (redbird-cactus), a cultivated, succulent shrub with milky juice from tropical America, causes severe poisoning if any part of the plant is eaten.

Phyllanthus abnormis is toxic to cattle, sheep, and goats; *P. engleri* roots mixed with *Albizia petersiana* and smoked have caused unconsciousness and even death in Tanzania, and the bark is reputedly used as a suicidal agent.

Poinsettia, see *Euphorbia pulcherrima,* leaves of which have been responsible for the loss of human life.

Reverchonia arenaria (reverchonia) of the southwestern United States is poisonous to sheep.

Ricinis communis (castor bean, castor-oil plant). Shrublike annual to 12 feet tall with branches green to reddish-purple; leaves alternate, simple, palmately lobed with 5 to 12 lobes, to 30 inches wide, long petiole, margins toothed; flowers green, the male clusters on the upper, the female clusters on the lower part of the plant; fruit a spiny capsule, oval, green or red, with three brownish mottled seeds ½ to ¾ inch in diameter. Probably of African origin, *R. communis* occurs throughout the tropics and extends into the warmer temperate regions. It is widely cultivated as an ornamental.

Poisoning. Seeds contain the highly poisonous phytotoxin ricin, which if chewed will cause nausea, muscle spasms, purgation, convulsions, and death; kidney dysfunction (uremia) is common. Two to four seeds seriously poison man, eight usually being fatal. Because of the hard seed coat, poisoning is unlikely unless the seed is chewed. The plant is toxic to all livestock.

Sapium spp. Latex is poisonous to man; also used as an arrow poison in Central America.

Stillingia treculeana (queen's delight). Leaves and stems, containing hydrocyanic acid, are poisonous to sheep.

Synadenium grantii. During the Mau Mau uprising in Kenya in the 1950s, this species was suspected of being put to malicious use when 33 steers were poisoned and 8 died. The animals developed swellings along the chest, belly, and upper limbs. Lesions were attributed to stabbing with a sharp instrument, introducing the acute irritant into the animals.[1]

DICHAPETALACEAE

Dichapetalum spp. are extremely poisonous to livestock because they contain fluoroacetic acid, which is converted into a toxic substance by enzymes.

THYMELAEACEAE (Mezereum)

Daphne mezereum (daphne). Deciduous shrub to 4 feet tall; leaves alternate, simple, lanceolate, and hairless; flowers in lateral clusters of two to five on branches of the preceding year appearing before the leaves, purplish-rose or rarely white; fruit a red or rarely yellow drupe ¼ inch in diameter. Widely culti-

vated and sparingly naturalized from Europe.

Poisoning. Only a few of the attractive fruits will kill a child. They contain a coumarin glycoside and a diterpene mezerein that cause burning of the throat and stomach, internal bleeding, weakness, coma, and death. The diterpene mezerein is also carcinogenic in animals. The danger from this species and others (*D. laureola*) is great. Very likely the bark and fruit of *Dirca palustris* (leatherwood) native to North America is also poisonous.

Gnidia kraussiana young leaves and flowering tops (greatest toxicity when in flower) are very poisonous, and ingestion of only small amounts is sufficient to kill. Extracts are used in western Africa as arrow poisons, fish poisons, and also in criminal activities. The toxic mezerein found in *Daphne* species is also present in species of *Gnidia*.

BUXACEAE (Boxwood)

Buxus sempervirens (boxwood). Evergreen shrub up to 15 feet tall; leaves opposite, simple, oval, up to ¾ inch long, dark glossy green above, light green below; flowers small and white; fruit a capsule with shiny black seeds. Native to Eurasia, boxwood is cultivated as a hedging plant or shrub, particularly in eastern North America.

Poisoning. The alkaloid buxine (as well as several related alkaloids) and a volatile oil in the leaves and twigs, cause vomiting and diarrhea; death from respiratory failure follows ingestion of large amounts. Boxwood may cause death among all classes of livestock (sheep, horses, pigs, cattle, camels).

RHAMNACEAE (Buckthorn)

Karwinskia humboldtiana (coyotillo). Woody shrub or small tree to 20 feet tall;

leaves usually opposite, elliptic-ovate, 1 to 3 inches long with distinct straight veins; flowers small, greenish, in axillary clusters; fruit an ovoid drupe turning brownish-black at maturity, about ½ inch in diameter. The species is found in southwestern Texas, southern California, and Mexico on dry gravelly hills and in canyons.

Poisoning. The toxic principle of the fruit is an incompletely characterized quinone. However it causes paralysis in man, and nausea, progressive weakness, and death in cattle and sheep.

Rhamnus cathartica (common or purging buckthorn) and *R. frangula* (alder buckthorn) berries contain purgative anthraquinone glycosides, which cause violent purgation and collapse. Poisoning is rare, but the fruit is dangerous to children. The species are native to Europe but are cultivated in North America.

PHYLOGENETIC GROUP 7

ROSACEAE (Rose)

Cercocarpus montanus (mountain mahogany) is implicated in the loss of livestock (western United States and Mexico), probably because of higher than average concentrations of cyanogenic glycosides.

Cotoneaster spp. Shrubs without spines; leaves entire; flowers small, in cymes or corymbs, or solitary, the 5 petals white or pink, the stamens about 20; fruit red or black drupe with mealy flesh and stony wall surrounding 2 to 5 seeds. The closely allied genus *Pyracantha* is an evergreen shrub usually bearing spines and fruits bright red, orange, or yellow, having 5 stony-walled seeds. Both genera are native to Europe though widely cultivated in temperate areas. In North America one can find *Cotoneaster acuminatus, C. horizontalis, C. simonsii,* and *Pyracantha coc-*

cinea. In England these species are reported as common causes of poisoning in children, probably due to the presence of cyanogenic glycosides.

Malus spp. (apple). Seeds of *Malus domestica* (the major source of commercial apples) and other species, contain the cyanogenic glycoside amygdalin, which yields hydrocyanic acid (prussic acid) on hydrolysis. A man who enjoyed apple seeds saved a cupful of them, which he proceeded to eat all at once; he died of cyanide poisoning. Therefore, do not eat large quantities of apple seeds, but enjoy the rest of the apple!

Prunus spp. (apricot, bitter almond, cherry, cherry laurel, peach, plum). *Prunus serotina* (wild black cherry) is a tree, often small but becoming large (to 90 feet) with age, the bark rough and dark with a bitter taste; leaves alternate, simple, with in-curving teeth at the margins, the petiole with two glands just below the shiny leaf blade; flowers small, white, with five petals and numerous stamens occurring in racemes; fruit a black drupe about ½ inch in diameter. This species occurs throughout eastern North America, often as a weed along fences and waste areas.

Poisoning. *Prunus serotina* is the most dangerous of the eastern wild cherries. All parts, but especially the bark, leaves, and seeds, contain the cyanogenic glycoside amygdalin (and the closely allied prulaurasin and prunasin), which gives hydrocyanic acid on hydrolysis. The resulting cyanide poisoning leads to difficulty in breathing, spasms, coma, and even sudden, unexpected death. Children have been poisoned chewing and sucking twigs, eating seeds, and making a tea of leaves. All classes of livestock have been killed by ingesting leaves. All species of wild cherries are poisonous, although the fleshy portion of the fruit is edible. In addition, native and cultivated forms of apricots (*P. armeniaca*), bitter almonds (*P. dulcis,* Fig. 2-7a but not the sweet almond variety), cherry laurel (*P. laurocerasus,* Fig. 2-7b), peach (*P. persica*), and plum (*P. domestica*) contain amygdalin in their stony seeds, bark, and leaves, and ingestion should be avoided. For example, 50 to 70 bitter almond nuts are fatal for adults, 7 to 10 are fatal for children, and 3 will cause severe poisoning.

Pyrus communis (pear) seeds as well as those found in other species contain amygdalin; seeds from pears, like apple seeds, should not be eaten.

Rhodotypos tetrapetala (jetbead) seeds, within shiny black drupes in clusters of

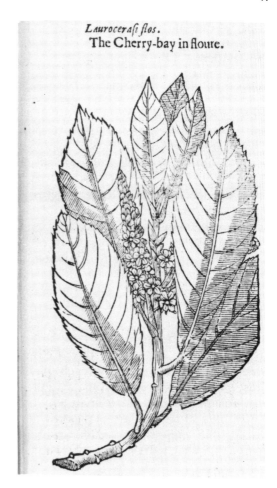

Figure 2-7b *Prunus laurocerasus* (from J Gerard, *The Herball,* ed 2, 1636).

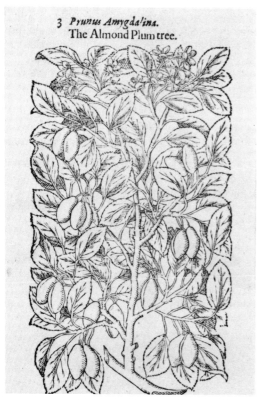

Figure 2-7a *Prunus dulcis* (from J Gerard, *The Herball,* 1597).

four persisting through the winter, contain amygdalin and should not be eaten.

Sorbus spp. (mountain ash). Fruit and perhaps other parts of *S. aucuparia* have been implicated in poisoning of children. A compound shown to cause cancer in animals has been isolated from mountain ash.

CONNARACEAE (Connard)

Rourea glabra (tropical America) and *R. volubilis* (Philippines). Fruits and seeds are very poisonous to carniverous animals; murderers have crushed *R. glabra* seeds, made a paste, and mixed it with corn mash to kill their victims.

FABACEAE (Pea)

Abrus precatorius (rosary pea). Perennial vine with twining stems to 20 feet tall; leaves alternate with 8 to 15 leaflets; flowers numerous, small, white or red to purple; fruit a legume to 1½ inches long; the ovoid seeds, about ⅜ long, are glossy scarlet over three-quarters and jet black over the remainder of the area. A common pantropical vine, it is found as a weed in Florida. The attractive toxic seeds are used as beads and sold in Latin America and the West Indies to tourists. The seeds are of potential danger because children are attracted to them.

Poisoning. The seeds contain abrin, an exceedingly poisonous phytotoxin, which will cause severe stomach pain, nausea, severe diarrhea, coma, circulatory collapse, and death depending on the amount of seed, thoroughly chewed, that has been ingested. Livestock and humans are equally vulnerable.

Acacia berlandieri (guajillo) from southwestern Texas and Mexico, *A. georginae* from Australia, and other species are known to cause poisoning in livestock when large amounts of leaves and fruit are consumed. Others are known to possess cyanogenic glycosides.

Albizia anthelmintica bark decoctions are used as anthelmintics and purgatives, and overdoses have resulted in death in Africa.

Andira inermis bark and seeds are toxic and may cause death. They have been used as a fish poison. The alkaloid andirine has been isolated from this species and may be the toxic principle.

Arachis hypogaea (peanut) meal may be toxic as a result of contamination with aflatoxin from the fungus *Aspergillus flavus.*

Astragalus spp. (milk vetches, poison vetches, locoweeds) are common in North America and can be dangerous to livestock. Some species accumulate selenium, others possess "locaine" (an uncharacterized toxic component), and still others produce toxic substances as yet undefined; all have significant poisoning effects on a wide range of livestock.

Baptisia leucantha (false indigo) and other species are responsible for livestock losses, particularly of horses.

Caesalpinia pulcherrima leaves are used as a fish poison in Guatemala and Panama, and the seeds have been used to poison criminals.

Canavalia ensiformis (jack bean), native to the West Indies, may be lethal to cattle in large quantities. The seeds contain the mitogen concanavalin A.

Cassia spp. are toxic though not fatal to sheep and other animals in the United States; elsewhere fatalities to hogs, sheep, and cattle have been reported, as well as human deaths from overdoses of herbal remedies involving *Cassia.* Some species are known to contain hydrocyanic acid. Most species contain anthraquinones, which are also toxic in overdose.

Centrosema plumieri bark is employed as a fish poison in Colombia and Central America.

Crotalaria spp. (rattlebox) poisoning occurs in horses from *C. sagittalis,* and in a wide range of livestock from *C. incana, C. retusa, C. spectabilis,* and *C. verrucosa;* they contain the toxic alkaloid monocrotaline.

Cytisus scoparius (Scotch broom), introduced to North America from Europe, possesses among others the alkaloids sparteine and isosparteine. Ingestion may result in mild animal poisoning, but large quantities must be consumed for serious effects to occur. Sparteine is well known for its abortive properties.

Dalbergia nitidula and *D. stuhlmannii* root decoctions, being used as herbal medicines, have resulted in the death of many patients in eastern Africa.

Dolichos lablab (hyacinth bean) and other

species of this Old World genus contain a glycoside in their fruit; boiling removes the possibility of cyanide poisoning. Saponins are also present. Livestock are suspected of being poisoned in Africa by various *Dolichos* species.

Entada polystachia is poisonous to cattle.

Enterolobium cyclocarpum is a tree whose sawdust kills fish and cattle when it contaminates streams.

Erythrina spp. (coral bean) possess alkaloids having curarelike action and perhaps causing death if the bark or seeds are taken internally. Crushed stems are sometimes employed as fish poisons. Some species of coral bean are native to the warmer parts of the United States, and other species are cultivated as ornamentals; because of their attractive seeds, all should be considered of potential danger, especially to children.

Erythrophleum suaveolens bark is very poisonous and was formerly widely used throughout Africa by witch doctors in trials of ordeal. Death results from respiratory and cardiac arrests; a number of alkaloids displaying digitalislike action have been isolated (cassaidine, cassaine, etc.).

Gliricidia sepium roots, leaves, and seeds have been used to poison rodents; the plant is toxic to dogs, and leaves are dangerous to horses.

Gymnocladus dioica (Kentucky coffee tree). Large, rough-barked tree to 80 feet tall; leaves alternate, to 3 feet long, pinnately compound, the leaflets ovate with smooth margins; flowers whitish, in terminal racemes; fruit an oblong, flattened, hard legume to 6 inches long and 1¾ inches wide with four to seven hard and flat seeds. Native to eastern North America, the tree is common in rich woods and is also cultivated.
  Poisoning. The seeds and pulp contain the alkaloid cytisine, which

results in gastrointestinal disorders, irregular pulse, and coma. Fatalities in livestock are recorded.

Indigofera endecaphylla (creeping indigo) poisoning of livestock in the tropics is reported.

Laburnum anagyroides (golden rain), Fig. 2-8a. Shrub or small tree to 30 feet tall; leaves alternate, trifoliate, light green, long-petioled; flowers golden yellow, the long racemes hanging from the branches; fruit a long flat legume with up to eight dark brown seeds. Native to central Europe and the Balkans, *L. anagyroides* is cultivated in the northern United States and Canada.
  Poisoning. The bark, leaves, flowers,

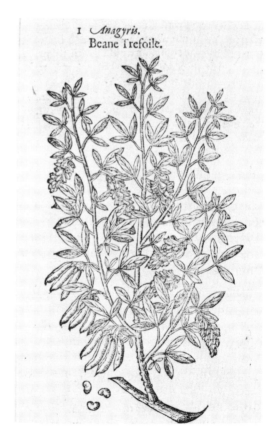

Figure 2-8a *Laburnum anagyroides* (from J Gerard, *The Herball*, 1597).

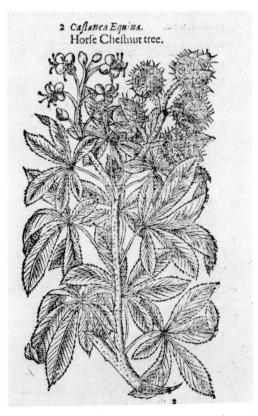

2 *Castanea Equina.*
Horse Chestnut tree.

Figure 2-8b *Aesculus hippocastanum* (from J Gerard, *The Herball,* 1597).

and seeds contain the alkaloid cytisine, whose effects are similar to those described for *Gymnocladus dioica.* In Britain this species results in many cases of poisoning and death in man; children, for example, eat the seeds, mistaking them for peas.

Lathyrus spp. (vetchlings) at one time caused much poisoning in Europe, but epidemics of lathyrism are virtually unknown today. Livestock show much variation in susceptibility, although the horse is most commonly poisoned. The seeds of *Lathyrus hirsutus* (caley pea), *L. incanus* (wild pea), *L. odoratus* (sweet pea), *L. pusillus* (singletary pea), and *L. sylvestris* (everlasting pea) may also result in poisoning.

Lespedeza stipulacea (lespedeza) may result in the death of cattle, following uncontrollable hemorrhage.

Leucaena glauca (koa haole or tan-tan) poisoning of livestock is due to mimosine in the seeds and young leaves.

Lonchocarpus floribundus and *L. sericeus* are used as fish poisons, and the first species is cultivated for that purpose.

Lotus corniculatus (birdsfoot trefoil) occasionally produces toxic amounts of a cyanogenic principle.

Lupinus spp. (lupine) possess many alkaloids, those of the quinolizidine group being most common. Sheep are frequently poisoned in the Rocky Mountain area, but losses of cattle and horses are much less frequent.

Melilotus officinalis (yellow sweetclover) poisoning, largely in cattle after eating moldy sweetclover hay, is linked to the presence of a fungus and bishydroxycoumarin (dicoumaral). Hemorrhages occur internally and externally, and death is sudden.

Mundulea sericea bark and seeds make one of the best known native fish poisons in eastern Africa. Rotenone is the toxic principle.

Ormosia coccinea seeds, if chewed, are dangerously poisonous.

Pachyrrhizus erosus seeds, which contain saponins, rotenone, and pachyrrhizid, are toxic to man; they are used as a source of fish poison and as an insecticide.

Phaseolus lunatus (lima bean) contains a cyanogenic glycoside phaseolunatin in very small amounts in the large, white lima beans grown commercially in the United States. However a number of tropical varieties, smaller in size, possess phaseolunatin and the enzyme capable of releasing hydrocyanic acid at levels considered dangerous. Cooking does not altogether destroy these compounds.

Physostigma venenosum (calabar or ordeal bean) is exceedingly poisonous due to the alkaloid physostigmine (eserine) (Chapter 9); *P. mesoponticum* of eastern Africa is also lethal to man.

Piscidia guaricensis and *P. piscipula* roots, bark, and leaves are used as fish poisons; fruits from *P. piscipula* have been used in tropical America as an arrow poison.

Poinciana gilliesii. Green seed pods cause gastrointestinal tract irritation.

Pongamia pinnata (pongam) cultivated in southern United States (Florida and California) may be poisonous; it is used in parts of India to poison fish.

Prosopis juliflora (mesquite). Ingestion over long periods will result in death of cattle.

Psoralea argophylla (scurf pea). Seeds are suspected of causing severe poisoning of a child. The toxic principles are probably coumarins, which are well-known constituents of this genus.

Robinia pseudo-acacia (black locust). Large shrub or tree to 75 feet tall, the stems long and straight, coarse-barked, the branches with spines paired below the leaf base; leaves alternate, pinnately compound, the leaflets elliptic to ovate, 3 to 10 paired; flowers white, showy, fragrant, in drooping racemes; fruit a many-seeded flat legume. Black locust is native to eastern North America and has become naturalized in the Pacific coast area; it is also cultivated.
Poisoning. A highly poisonous phytotoxin, robin, and a glycoside, robitin, found in the inner bark, young leaves, and seeds, are responsible for human poisoning, especially of children (sucking twigs, and eating inner bark and seeds). A wide range of livestock have been poisoned, but fatalities are rare.

Sesbania spp. (coffeebean, rattlebox, sesbane). Herb to shrub up to 12 feet tall, unarmed, rarely branched; leaves al-ternate, to 1 foot long, pinnately compound; flowers in axillary racemes usually shorter than the foliage, yellowish orange to red; fruit a linear legume. Several species are found in the southern United States: *S. vesicaria* from the West Indies has yellowish flowers often tinged pink or red; *S. drummondii* also has yellow flowers many with red lines; and *S. punicea,* bearing red or orange-red flowers, is naturalized from South America.
Poisoning. Seeds contain saponins that result in diarrhea, rapid pulse, respiratory failure, and even death. Flowers are also poisonous. Sheep, goats, cattle, and birds are poisoned.

Sophora secundiflora (mescal bean). Seeds contain cytisine belonging to the group of lupine alkaloids that cause nausea, convulsions, and death through respiratory failure. Toxic to livestock as well as fatal to children, the beans also possess hallucinogenic properties (see Chapter 18).

Tephrosia cinerea, yielding rotenone and the toxic principle tephrosin, is used in Venezuela and Africa as a fish poison.

Trifolium spp. (clovers) occasionally cause toxicity in livestock, but fatalities are rare; *T. repens* (white clover), having a cyanogenic glycoside, is the major offender.

Vicia faba (broad bean). A coarse, erect annual vine without tendrils; leaves alternate, the large obtuse leaflets in one to three pairs; flowers large, white with blackish blotches, one to several in the leaf axils; fruit up to 14 inches long, a thick many-seeded legume, the large seeds compressed or globular, and variously colored from green to purple or black. *Vicia faba* is widely cultivated in Canada and often grown as an ornamental vine in the United States. It is of European origin and often cultivated there.

Poisoning. Seeds may cause severe hemolytic anemia several days following ingestion and a similar condition following inhalation of pollen. This condition, known as favism, is produced by an inherited enzymatic deficiency frequent among peoples of the Mediterranean area (Italian, Greek, Semitic). Although the genetic trait is found in only 1% of whites as a whole, it occurs in about 15% of all blacks. Individuals who are not deficient in glucose-6-phosphate dehydrogenase may eat broad beans or inhale pollen without fear of collapse. Other species of *Vicia* may cause loss of livestock in part through the existence of cyanogenic potential.

Wisteria floribunda (Japanese wisteria) and *W. sinensis* (Chinese wisteria). Climbing deciduous shrubs; leaves alternate, pinnately, compound, the leaflets three to nine paired; flowers in terminal, pendant racemes, purple or less commonly white, showy; fruit a long, compressed legume with one to eight large seeds. The Chinese wisteria in particular is commonly cultivated and locally naturalized in the southern United States and in Europe. A number of children have been poisoned by eating seeds of legumes, the symptoms consisting of gastroenteritis, repeated vomiting, abdominal pains, diarrhea, and also clinical dehydration in the more severe cases. Two seeds will cause serious illness in a child.

SAXIFRAGACEAE (Saxifrage)

Hydrangea spp. (hydrangea) leaves and buds contain a cyanogenic glycoside, hydrangin, which may cause gastroenteritis after eating. Horses are similarly affected.

CORIARIACEAE

Coriaria sarmentosa seeds and shoots are poisonous to livestock in New Zealand;

C. thymifolia fruits are very toxic, and children have been poisoned by them.

PHYLOGENETIC GROUP 8

COMBRETACEAE (Combretum)

Terminalia sericea root decoction has caused the death of several individuals in eastern Africa.

MYRTACEAE (Myrtle)

Eucalyptus cladocalyx (eucalyptus), having a high hydrocyanic acid content, has caused serious loss of sheep in Australia.

Rhodomyrtus macrocarpa (finger cherry). Fruit, containing high quantities of saponin, causes temporary or permanent blindness if eaten. The species is native to Australia and is considered a serious menance there.

PHYLOGENETIC GROUP 9

LINACEAE (Flax)

Linum usitatissimum (flax) leaves and seed chaff contain the cyanogenic glycoside linamarin, from which the enzyme linamarase is capable of releasing cyanide. Cattle and sheep have been poisoned in North Dakota; *Linum rigidum* from Kansas, *L. lewisii* from Colorado, and *L. neomexicanum,* containing a saponin, have also been implicated in livestock poisoning. In Europe *L. catharticum* (purging flax) is abundant and is therefore a potential hazard to livestock. Cucurbitacins are known to be present in *Linum* species, perhaps accounting for some of the toxic effects.

ERYTHROXYLACEAE (Coca)

Erythroxylum coca (cocaine): See Chapter 17, Stimulants.

ZYGOPHYLLACEAE (Caltrop)

Guaiacum officinale (lignum vitae). Resin in wood and fruit is poisonous if eaten in quantity.

Tribulus cistoides is reported as toxic to livestock in Australia and Colombia.

OXALIDACEAE (Wood Sorrel)

Oxalis spp. (wood sorrel) possess soluble oxalates that in animals may result in colic, depression, coma, and even death, provided enough is consumed to ensure that the substances reach a toxic level. *Oxalis pes-caprae* has been implicated in sheep loss in Australia, and *O. acetosella* and *O. corniculata* are known to be lethal elsewhere.

MALPIGHIACEAE (Malpighia)

Byrsonima crassifolia is used as a fish poison in Venezuela.

Galphimia glauca leaf and branch extracts are poisonous and are used as insecticides.

POLYGALACEAE (Milkwort)

Securidaca longepedunculata roots, containing saponins (5%), are fatal in overdose.

RUTACEAE (Rue)

Citrus aurantium (sour orange). Bitter orange peel when eaten in quantity will cause violent colic, convulsions, and even death in children who ingest large amounts of rind.

Pilocarpus alvaradoi leaves, containing the imidazole alkaloid pilocarpine, are poisonous to cattle and donkeys.

SIMAROUBACEAE (Quassia)

Balanites aegyptiaca bark, containing a saponin, is used as a fish poison. It is valuable because it is nontoxic to man and other warm-blooded animals.

MELIACEAE (Mahogany)

Melia azedarach (chinaberry tree). Poisoning usually results from eating the fruit; the leaves less commonly have this effect. Toxicity to man, livestock, and fish is associated with a resinous fraction. The Chinaberry is native to Asia but is widely planted as an ornamental and has freely escaped.

Turraea robusta is poisonous to cattle in eastern Africa.

ANACARDIACEAE (Cashew)

Anacardium rhinocarpus stem bark is used as a fish poison in Panama.

Mangifera indica (mango). Old leaves ingested over a prolonged period will cause death in cattle.

SAPINDACEAE (Soapberry)

Blighia sapida (akee), native of western Africa and cultivated in the West Indies and also Florida, causes "vomiting sickness," especially in children, following ingestion of the fruit wall, seeds, white aril of the unripe fruit, or rancid aril. The sickness is characterized by marked hypoglycemia and a mortality rate ranging from 40 to 80% (toxic principles hypoglycin A and B).

Paullinia spp. Stems, leaves, and roots are used as a piscicide in Central and South America; the fish so obtained can be eaten without danger. In addition, *P. cururu* is used to prepare a type of curare, and *P. pinnata* roots and stems have been employed to produce a slow-acting poison that some Amazonian inhabitants use on their enemies.

Sapindus saponaria. Crushed seeds are valued as a fish poison by Venezuelan Indians.

Serjania paucidentata. Stems are used to poison fish.

Zanha africana. Root medicines in overdose may cause death.

MELIANTHACEAE (Melianthus)

Bersama abyssinica leaves cause death among cows in Uganda, and extracts of the roots have been used for suicidal purposes in Zambia.

ACERACEAE (Maple)

Acer rubrum (red maple) leaves have caused death of cattle and horses in West Virginia.

HIPPOCASTANACEAE (Buckeye)

Aesculus spp. (buckeye, horsechestnut). Trees and shrubs; leaves opposite, deciduous, palmately compound with five to nine leaflets, long petiolate, the leaflets serrate; flowers red, white, or usually yellow, four to five lobed, in many-flowered terminal panicles; fruit a three-parted leathery capsule, often spiny, enclosing one to six large brown seeds with a pale scar. The majority of species are found in the North Temperate zone, and *Aesculus hippocastanum* (horsechestnut, Fig. 2-8*b*) is the best known species (native to Eurasia and widely cultivated). About 25 species, however, are native to North America.

Poisoning. Leaves, bark, flowers, young twigs, and seeds contain the lactone glycoside, esculin, a hydroxy derivate of coumarin. Children as well as livestock have been poisoned after ingesting these plant parts.

PHYLOGENETIC GROUP 10

CELASTRACEAE (Staff-tree)

Catha edulis (chat): see Chapter 17, Stimulants.

Celastrus scandens (climbing bittersweet) and other species are undoubtedly poisonous. The fruit is particularly attractive to young children because of the contrasting colors of seeds and flesh, and since the plants are commonly brought into the home for dry arrangements, they must be kept out of reach.

Elaeodendron buchananii leaves have resulted in many deaths of livestock in eastern Africa; sheep also appear particularly vulnerable.

Euonymus spp. Shrub or woody climbers with many-branched stems; leaves opposite and simple; flowers small and greenish with four sepals and petals; fruit a bright red capsule splitting into four lobes, each with a seed covered by a yellow to red aril. Two species are commonly cultivated, *E. atropurpureus* (burning bush) and *E. europaeus* (spindle tree); these along with a number of native species are probably all toxic.

Poisoning. The poisonous constituent, still to be identified, is found in the bark, leaves, and fruit. Peptide and sesquiterpene alkaloids recently found in many *Euonymus* species may be the toxic principles, but this has not been proved. Ingestion of fruit results in vomiting and diarrhea followed in 12 hours by unconsciousness. Children are attracted to the colorful fruit; livestock to the leaves.

OLACACEAE (Olax)

Ximenia americana contains hydrocyanic acid which, depending on the age of the plant and the environmental conditions, may be sufficiently concentrated to cause cyanide poisoning in cattle.

LORANTHACEAE (Mistletoe)

Phoradendron serotinum (mistletoe). Evergreen, perennial, semiparasitic shrub with green branches growing largely on deciduous trees; leaves opposite, simple, oblong, and leathery; fruit a small white berry. This species is common in eastern North America; *P. villosum* is parasitic on oaks largely in the Pacific coast region, and other mistletoes, including the European *Viscum album,* are widespread.

Poisoning. The berries contain toxic amines and proteins that may cause gastroenteritis if eaten in large quantities. At Christmas, when the plant may be brought into the home, the berries should be kept out of reach of children.

OLEACEAE (Olive)

Ligustrum vulgare (common privet). Deciduous shrub or small tree with smooth bark; leaves opposite, simple, entire, lanceolate, shortly petiolate; flowers small, white, in panicles; fruit a cluster of purplish-black berries. Native to the Old World, privet has been commonly planted for hedges in North America and also has escaped.
Poisoning. Berries and possibly leaves contain a glycoside causing gastroenteritis in children who eat the fruit. Cases of poisoning are rare. Horses and sheep have been fatally poisoned.

VITACEAE (Grape)

Parthenocissus quinquefolia (Virginia creeper), a common vine of eastern North America having small blue berries, is suspected of causing poisoning and death in children who eat the berries. Similarly the Asian *P. tricuspidata* (Boston ivy), which is widely cultivated and adorns many buildings in North America, ought to be suspect.

ARALIACEAE (Ginseng)

Aralia spinosa (Hercules' club) is suspected of poisoning livestock in Maryland.

Hedera helix (English ivy). A native of Europe, ivy is a frequently planted ornamental vine used commonly as a ground cover. The leaves and berries contain the triterpene sapogenin hederagenin, which causes vomiting, diarrhea, and nervous depression, though the symptoms are considered serious only in small children. Poisoning of cattle has been reported from leaf clippings.

APIACEAE (Carrot)

Aethusa cynapium (fool's parsley). Contains poisonous alkaloids producing symptoms similar to those of *Conium maculatum,* but death is unlikely in healthy individuals. Introduced from Eurasia, the plant is naturalized in eastern North America.

Berula erecta (water parsnip) is extremely poisonous and in Africa has caused the death of cattle within an hour. This species, which is also found in North America, should be examined carefully for toxic principles.

Cicuta maculata (water hemlock). Biennial herb with fleshy tuberiform fingerlike roots, the stem to 7 feet tall often mottled purplish below, stout, and hollow except at the nodes; leaves alternate, the blade two to three pinnately divided, about 2 feet long, the petiole clasping the stem, the leaflets narrow, 1 to 4 inches long; flowers small, white, in terminal umbels; fruit small, ovoid and ribbed. Poisonous plants of North Temperate regions: *Cicuta maculata* is found in moist areas of eastern North America, and *C. virosa* (cowbane) in similar localities in Europe.
Poisoning. The root is particularly dangerous, a mouthful being sufficient to kill an adult. The poisonous principle, cicutoxin, is also found in the aboveground parts and should be considered dangerous. Roots are mistaken for parsnips and the small tuberous rootlets for potatoes. Children making peashooters from the hollow stems have been poisoned, and livestock fatalities have been reported (fresh root the size of a walnut is reputed to kill healthy cattle).

Conium maculatum (poison hemlock). Similar to water hemlock but separated by its more finely divided leaves (smallest divisions up to ¾ inch broad) compared with the more broadly divided leaves of

Cicuta maculata (smallest divisions usually ¾ to 3 inches broad). Native to Eurasia and northern Africa, the species has been introduced to North America, where it inhabits waste places, marshes, and so on.

Poisoning. All parts, especially young leaves, unripe fruit, and roots, contain the poisonous alkaloid coniine, as well as other alkaloids. Symptoms of poisoning include vomiting and diarrhea, inflammation of the gastrointestinal tract, mental confusion, convulsions, and death. When the plant is mistaken for parsley (young green leaves contain the highest quantity of active principle) or for anise seeds, and eaten, as it frequently is, death often results; and it is dangerous for children to make peashooters from the hollow stems. The species is dangerous to livestock, although the alkaloids are destroyed by drying, thus are of little danger as hay.

Eryngium foetidum is considered poisonous to cattle in Colombia.

Oenanthe spp. (water dropworts), common in Europe, contain a resin that is poisonous to man and livestock.

Sium suave (water parsnip) is suspected of poisoning a wide range of livestock throughout much of North America, where it is native.

CAPRIFOLIACEAE (Honeysuckle)

Sambucus spp. (elderberry). Coarse shrub to 12 feet tall, the wood soft and piths large; leaves opposite between long internodes, pinnately compound, the leaflets 5 to 11 per leaf, serrate; flowers in compound terminal cymes, small, 5 lobed, white; fruit small, juicy and berrylike, red or black. Shrubs largely of temperate zones of which *Sambucus australis* (southern South America), *S. canadensis* (eastern North America), *S.*

ebulus (Eurasia and northern Africa), *S. nigra* (Europe), *S. pubens* (northern North America and mountains), *S. simpsonii* (Gulf Coast), and *S. valerandi* (temperate Asia, North and South America, southwest Australia) illustrate the wide range of the genus. *Sambucus javanica* of tropical Asia further shows diversity of habitat.

Poisoning. Most parts of the plant, possibly of all species, contain uncharacterized poisonous alkaloids and cyanogenic glycosides. Children have been poisoned by using peashooters made from stems and by eating unripe or uncooked berries. Flowers and ripe fruit are edible.

PHYLOGENETIC GROUP 11

LOGANIACEAE (Logania)

Gelsemium sempervirens (Carolina or yellow jessamine). Woody perennial vine, the main stem gray, wiry, trailing or very high-climbing; leaves opposite, short-petioled, entire, lanceolate, to 2 inches long; flowers clear yellow, fragrant, tubular with five lobes, about 1 inch long, flowering in the early spring; fruit a short-beaked capsule nearly 1 inch long. The species is native to the southern United States coastal plain from Florida and Virginia to Texas. It was formerly used as a central nervous system depressant. Leaves of the subtropical Asian *G. rigens* are used in committing suicide, especially by women.

Poisoning. The indole alkaloids gelsemine and sempervirine concentrate in the roots and the flower nectar, ingestion of which produce profuse sweating, weakness, convulsions, respiratory failure, and death. Children have been severely poisoned by sucking nectar from the flowers or chewing the leaves. It is poisonous to all classes of livestock.

Spigelia anthelmia has been used as a

human poisoning with toxic effects similar to strychnine.

Strychnos nux-vomica (strychnine tree) and *S. ignatii* (poison nut) of tropical Asia. The dried ripe seeds yield the indole alkaloids strychnine and brucine, which are the main toxic constituents. All parts of the plants including the flowers contain strychnine, which is extremely toxic and fatal to man at doses of from 60 to 90 mg. South American Indians use other species of *Strynchos* (*S. toxifera, S. castelanei, S. crevauxii*) to make their deadly "flying arrows" or curare (see Menispermaceae: *Chondodendron*).

APOCYNACEAE (Dogbane)

Acokanthera spp. (but commonly *A. longiflora* and *A. schimperi*) provide the main ingredient of arrow poisons in Africa; all parts are poisonous (except the ripe fruit) but are more toxic during the dry season, and contain cardioactive glycosides ouabain, G-strophanthin, and acokantherin. Livestock die quickly after ingestion.

Adenium obesum (desert rose) contains several cardiac glycosides and is used as a fish and arrow poison in eastern Africa. It is very toxic to livestock.

Allamanda cathartica (yellow allamanda) of Brazil, and commonly cultivated as an ornamental in the southern United States, is poisonous, especially the fruit and sap of stems and leaves.

Apocynum cannabinum (dogbane) and *A. androsaemifolium* (spreading dogbane), contain the cardioactive glycoside cymarin, which is responsible for toxic symptoms in livestock ingesting either of these species.

Catharanthus roseus (periwinkle) is toxic to cattle, but it has value as a chemotherapeutic agent (Chapter 5).

Ervatamia coronaria (grape jasmine) from India, grown as an ornamental, has alkaloids known to cause loss of life.

Nerium indicum and *N. oleander* (oleanders). Evergreen shrub or small tree having thick clear gummy sap; leaves opposite or in whorls of three, leathery, entire, oblong-lanceolate with a sharp point and prominent midrib, to 10 inches long; flowers in large clusters at the tip of branches, white or pink to deep red, about 1 to 3 inches in diameter. These oleanders are native to the Mediterranean region and to tropical Asia, respectively; *N. oleander* is commonly cultivated.

Poisoning. All parts of *Nerium* spp. contain cardioactive glycosides, and oleandrin from *N. oleander* leaves, the prominent glycoside, has been used to treat cardiac insufficiency. Ingestion can be dangerous and may result in severe vomiting and bloody diarrhea, irregular heartbeat, drowsiness, unconsciousness, respiratory paralysis, and death. Children have been poisoned by chewing leaves and by sucking the nectar from flowers; poisoning is not restricted to the young, for adults have been poisoned after eating hotdogs and other meats roasted on oleander stems used as skewers.

Ochrosia elliptica (ochrosia plum). Fruit is considered poisonous.

Rauvolfia tetraphylla (bitterash). Roots contain the major alkaloids reserpine, tetraphylline, and tetraphyllicine. Fowl fed leaves and bark are poisoned. Root extracts of *R. rosea* from Tanzania are used as an ingredient in arrow poisons.

Schizozygia caffaeoides fruit contains the alkaloid schizozygine, which is said to be very poisonous.

Strophanthus spp. seed extracts, containing the cardiotonic agent strophanthin, are used in modern medicine when immediate relief from heart failure is needed (Chapter 7). Native populations in Africa have used the seeds of these species widely as arrow poisons, and a majority are known to cause serious poisoning when ingested by man and domestic animals alike.

Tanghinia venenifera (Tanghin) of Madagascar. Seeds are notoriously poisonous. They contain tanghin, a cardiac glycoside characterized by digitalislike activity. The seeds have a long history as an ordeal poison for judgments of all kinds of crimes from murder, conspiracy, and witch doctory, to stealing or for settling a debt. Forced to drink a draft or be killed by a soldier's spear, the accused was judged innocent by the ruling regime if he swallowed in a gulp and promptly vomited; but if afraid, he would sip slowly and die almost immediately. Guilt, of course, was predetermined, and since death was related to the strength of the extract, the judge could decide well in advance which way he wanted the trial to go! Such ordeals became infamous, and the French, who colonized the island, destroyed all the tanghin trees they could find.

Thevetia peruviana (yellow oleander) contains the cardiac glycosides cerebrin, neriifolin, and thevetin, which produce symptoms similar to those of fatal *Digitalis* poisoning. All parts of the plant are dangerous, and most fatalities are the result of misuse of decoctions in folk medicine. On Oahu, Hawaii, *T. peruviana* is considered the most frequent cause of fatal or dangerous poisoning in man attributed to plants.

Urechites spp. (yellow nightshade). Seed pods eaten in quantity will cause heart failure.

ASCLEPIADACEAE (Milkweed)

Asclepias spp. (milkweeds) are dangerous to sheep, cattle, goats, horses, and domestic fowl. The cardiac glycosides known to be present in almost all species of this genus result in severe poisoning, not only to livestock but to man as well.

Calotropis procera (giant milkweed). Latex, containing the cardiac glycoside calotropin, is extremely potent and is used on arrows in Africa. Minute amounts are said to produce death. It has also been used for murders and suicides in tropical America.

Cryptostegia grandiflora (rubber vine) has caused human fatalities in India.

Gomphocarpus physocarpus leaves and flowering umbels have been shown to be poisonous to sheep.

Sarcostemma viminale latex is a fish poison.

GENTIANACEAE (Gentian)

Centaurium beyrichii (rock centaury) and *C. calycosum* (Buckley centaury) are implicated in sheep losses in Texas and Mexico.

BIGNONIACEAE (Bignonia)

Crescentia cujete (calabash tree). Pulp of fruit, having hydrocyanic acid, is a purgative; it is toxic to birds and small mammals.

Tanaecium exitiosum of Colombia is very poisonous to cattle.

SCROPHULARIACEAE (Snapdragon)

Digitalis purpurea (foxglove). Erect biennial herb to 6 feet tall with downy stems; leaves alternate, simple, serrate, with few leaves on the flowering stem; flowers in showy long raceme, pendulous, corolla tubular to 3 inches long, purple to white and spotted inside the lower part of the tube; fruit a dry capsule with numerous small seeds. Foxgloves are native to Europe but are cultivated as an ornamental or for commerce, or infrequently naturalized.

Poisoning. A source of cardiac glycosides used in controlled doses for treatment of heart diseases (Chapter 7), poisoning can result from overdose of medication or when children eat the seeds or leaves, or suck the flowers. Symptoms include vomiting and purging, severe headache, irregular heartbeat and pulse, convulsion, and death, which occurs suddenly.

Scrophularia aquatica (water figwort) contains a cardiac glycoside that may cause violent purging in animals. Poisoning is rare, for as with *Digitalis,* the unpleasant taste and odor deter ingestion.

SOLANACEAE (Potato): see Chapter 18, Hallucinogens.

Atropa belladonna (belladonna, deadly

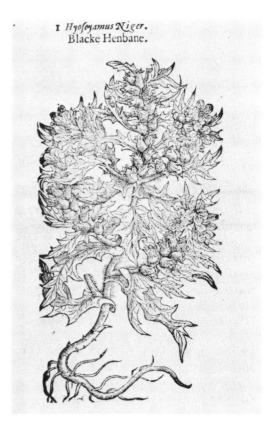

Figure 2-9b *Hyoscyamus niger* (from J Gerard, The *Herball,* ed 2, 1636).

nightshade, Fig. 2-9a). Coarse herb to 5 feet tall with a thick perennating root and branched stout stems; leaves alternate or in unequal pairs, simple, ovate, dark green; flowers solitary, nodding, five parted, brownish-purple, tubular and about 1 inch long; fruit a green or red (immature), purple to black (mature) glossy berry about the size of cherries with a persistent five-lobed calyx. Belladonna is native to Europe and Asia Minor; it is cultivated on occasion in North America.

Poisoning. All parts are dangerous to man, but the black berries are most commonly eaten, particularly by children. Roots and leaves contain L-hyoscyamine, ($\pm$)-hyoscyamine (atropine) and scopolamine (roots also include apoatropine, belladonnine, and cuscohygrine), and

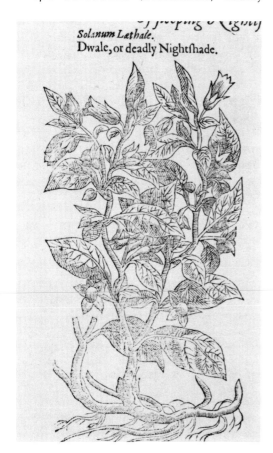

Figure 2-9a *Atropa belladonna* (from J Gerard, The *Herball,* 1597).

these alkaloids in overdose can be fatal to man. The main symptoms are flushed skin, dilated pupils, dry mouth, delirium, and death from respiratory failure. Poisoning among livestock and other animals is rare. However, atropine and the other solanaceous alkaloids are useful drugs when used in correct doses.

Cestrum spp. (jessamines) presumably contain alkaloids similar to those of Atropa belladonna and also cause poisoning accompanied by similar symptoms. Most species are native to tropical America; Cestrum nocturnum (night-blooming jessamine) extends into southern Florida and Texas, and a number are cultivated in the southern United States. Poisoning of children and pets is recorded.

Datura stramonium (jimson weed, thorn apple). Large annual up to 5 feet tall, branching at the apex, the stems green to purplish; leaves alternate, simple, to 8 inches long, irregular-toothed, and varying in size and shape; flowers white to violet, solitary, funnel-shaped, and usually from the center of a forked branch; fruit an ovoid capsule bearing many sharp spines and numerous wrinkled black seeds. This subcosmopolitan weed is common to waste areas, pastures, and roadsides throughout North America. Other poisonous species, some known as Brugmansia, include Datura candida from Colombia; D. metaloides from the southwestern United States and Mexico; D. metel (Hindu datura, downy thorn apple) native to India but introduced and cultivated widely; and D. suaveolens (angel's trumpet), cultivated in warmer regions.

Poisoning. The chief constituents of the leaves, unripe capsules, and especially the seeds are scopolamine and largely L-hyoscyamine. Many fatalities have occurred, especially among children, who are attracted to the capsules and ingest them. Even small amounts of leaves or seeds can be fatal, with symptoms similar to those recorded for belladonna. Livestock poisoning is rare, probably because the ill-smelling daturas are distasteful.

Hyoscyamus niger (black henbane, Fig. 2-9b). Coarse annual or biennial herb to 5 feet tall, the stems erect, branching, and hairy; leaves alternate, simple, oblong and coarsely lobed, hairy, up to 8 inches long, sessile; flowers in the leaf axils, the corolla greenish-yellow generally with purple veins, five-lobed and tubular; fruit a globular capsule enclosed by a persistent five-lobed calyx. Native to Eurasia and northern Africa, this species is also cultivated widely and is naturalized in parts of North America. Other species are Hyoscyamus muticus, known from Egypt to India, and grown commercially in California (for hyoscyamine), and H. reticulatus from India.

Poisoning. Hyoscyamine, and to a lesser degree scopolamine, are the chief alkaloids present in all the plant parts. Poisoning with this plant produces effects similar to those described for belladonna; but because the plant is not very common and has such an unpleasant taste, reports are infrequent.

Lycium halimifolium (matrimony vine) poisons calves and sheep.

Lycopersicon esculentum (tomato) leaves and stems have proved toxic to livestock, and also to children after taking a decoction prepared from the leaves.

Nicandra physalodes (apple-of-Peru) is closely allied to Physalis and is suspected of having similar poisonous properties.

Nicotiana tabacum (tobacco), native to tropical America and cultivated widely, contains the toxic alkaloid nicotine, which causes vomiting and diarrhea, slow pulse, collapse, and respiratory failure.

Deaths from eating the leaves as boiled greens are known, and livestock have also died following ingestion of the plant. Probably all species of *Nicotiana* contain nicotine (e.g., *N. alata* of South America, *N. attenuata* and *N. quadrivalvis* of the western United States, *N. rustica* of Mexico, and *N. trigonophylla* of the southwestern United States and Mexico, and all "wild" tobaccos that have been smoked by native populations). See also Chapter 17.

Physalis spp. (ground cherry) leaves and unripe fruit have been suspected of poisoning sheep.

Solandra spp. (trumpet flower), possessing toxic alkaloids of the solanine type, may produce poisoning if ingested by man.

Solanum spp. (nightshade, potato, Jerusalem cherry). Annual or perennial herbs and shrubs; leaves alternate, usually simple, the margins entire or slightly serrated, sometimes lobed; flowers with a five-lobed calyx and corolla spreading, the conspicuous yellow anthers erect and grouped conically around the stigma; fruit a berry. *Solanum* is a large genus particularly common in warmer regions. Some of the more significant poisonous species are *S. americanum* (black nightshade) of eastern North America, *S. alternato-pinnatum* of South America, *S. carolinense* (horse nettle) of eastern North America, *S. nigrum* (black nightshade) of Europe and widely naturalized, *S. pseudo-capsicum* (Jerusalem cherry) of Mexico (widely cultivated and prized for its ornamental bright red berries), *S. rostratum* (Buffalo bur) of central North America and naturalized, *S. sodomeum* (apple of Sodom) of the Mediterranean region, *S. triflorum* (three-flowered nightshade) of central North America and naturalized, and *S. tuberosum* (potato) of Andean South America and widely cultivated. In fact, it is generally accepted that the fruit of most species of *Solanum* is potentially dangerous.

Posioning. Several distinct glycoalkaloids (e.g., solanine) are responsible for poisoning in *Solanum,* and on hydrolysis these compounds yield either di- or trisaccharides and one of several alkamine aglycones that are steroidal. The intact glycoalkaloid is irritant, and the steroid alkamine is responsible for the major nervous symptoms. Thus the exact symptoms found in a given instance depend on the balance between the irritant (glycoalkaloid) and nervous (alkamine) effect. Effects of irritation include nausea and vomiting, abdominal pain, and constipation or diarrhea; the nervous effects are apathy, drowsiness, salivation, weakness or paralysis, circulatory and respiratory depression, unconsciousness, and death. The most poisonous part of the plant is the unripe fruit, but stems, leaves, and roots are also dangerous. The ripe fruit of a number of species is completely harmless and is used as food (e.g., *S. burbankii*), but that of other species may be very toxic. Poisoning of children and livestock is widespread, and fatalities are not uncommon. Eating green and sprouting potatoes may cause severe poisoning; one should never eat potatoes if they look green below the skin (or if spoiled), and discard all sprouts.

CONVOLVULACEAE (Morning Glory)

Argyreia, Ipomoea, Rivea: see Chapter 18, Hallucinogens.

Operculina tuberosa roots are poisonous to deer, horses, and cattle, but not to goats.

BORAGINACEAE (Borage)

Amsinckia intermedia (tarweed), containing a pyrrolizidine alkaloid liver toxin (amsinckine), has poisoned horses, pigs, and cattle in western North America.

Cynoglossum officinale (hound's tongue), native to Europe but naturalized throughout North America, contains a poisonous alkaloid that is thought to be responsible for an increase in livestock poisoning in England.

Echium vulgare (viper's bugloss) and *Heliotropium europaeum* (heliotrope), like tarweed, contain a pyrrolizidine alkaloid that affects livestock through liver toxicity and atrophy, often resulting in death.

VERBENACEAE (Vervain)

Aloysia lycioides (whitebrush) is suspected of toxicity to horses in Texas.

Duranta repens (golden dewdrop) berries contain a saponin that has caused fatalities among children who eat them.

Lantana camara (lantana). Perennial herb having square stems and a few spines to about 5 feet tall; leaves opposite or in whorls of three, petioled, ovate, up to 5 inches long, dentate, aromatic on crushing; flowers in dense, flat-topped clusters, small, tubular with four lobes, white, yellow, or pink, often darkening in color with age; fruit a greenish-blue or black, fleshy, small, one-seeded drupe. Native to tropical America and the Gulf Coast, *Lantana camara* is cultivated commonly as an ornamental.
   Poisoning. The toxic principle found in the fruit is a triterpene derivative, lantadene A. Children have been fatally poisoned, the acute symptoms resembling those of atropine poisoning.

LAMIACEAE (Mint)

Glechoma hederacea (ground ivy), if ingested in quantity, is toxic to horses.

Hoslundia opposita bark has proved fatal when used to prepare a stomach medicine. Sheep are also killed by this aromatic shrub.

Salvia reflexa (annual sage) may cause death in cattle.

CAMPANULACEAE (Bluebell)

Isotoma longiflora, containing isotomin (producing paralysis of heart), is poisonous to livestock.

Lobelia spp. Annual or perennial herbs, erect, mostly unbranched; leaves alternate, simple, mostly lanceolate; flowers in terminal racemes, strongly zygomorphic, the corolla tubular and two lipped, white, blue, or red; fruit a capsule. Several species of *Lobelia* are native to eastern North America: *L. cardinalis* (cardinal flower) with showy, deep red flowers; *L. inflata* (Indian tobacco) with inconspicuous blue flowers; and *L. siphilitica* (great lobelia) with showy blue flowers.
   Poisoning. As many as 14 pyridine alkaloids have been isolated from *L. inflata;* lobeline is the major one. Overdoses of the plant or its extracts will cause vomiting, paralysis, depressed temperature, coma, and death in man.

ASTERACEAE (Aster)
Almost all members of the aster family contain sesquiterpene lactones, many of which are cytotoxic.

Ageratum conzyoides, containing hydrocyanic acid, coumarin, and an alkaloid, is poisonous to rabbits and cows.

Arnica montana, A. fulgens (arnica), and other species, long used in medicine as an irritant, may be ingested by children, who suffer severe gastroenteritis, decrease in pulse rate, and collapse.

Artemisia filifolia, A. spinescens (sagebrush), and other species yielding volatile oils, may be toxic to livestock if heavily grazed.

Aster spp. (aster) as secondary selenium absorbers may prove dangerous to livestock in hay.

Baccharis pteronioides (yerba-de-pasmo) is toxic to sheep and cattle.

Bahia oppositifolia (plains bahia), having a cyanogenic glycoside, produces symptoms similar to cyanide poisoning in sheep and steers.

Baileya multiradiata (desert baileya) may result in severe toxicity and death among sheep.

Centaurea solstitialis (yellow star thistle). Ingestion is responsible for a nervous "chewing disease" in horses, which eventually results in death through starvation or thirst.

Chrysothamnus nauseosus (rubber rabbitbush) is toxic to livestock.

Clibadium surinamense leaves and seeds are used as fish poisons in Guyana. The Guyanese employ easy methods to secure all varieties of fish in almost unlimited quantity. The smaller fish are easily caught by throwing pellets of crushed leaves of *C. surinamense* (connami) into the water. The fish greedily devour the pellets, become narcotized, and float helplessly on the surface. They are rapidly picked up by the Indians before the effect passes off and are used either as bait for larger fish or directly for food.

Conyza coulteri (conyza) leaves are fatal to sheep.

Dichrocephala chrysanthemifolia is poisonous to sheep in Kenya, producing symptoms similar to those of ergot poisoning.

Eupatorium rugosum (white snakeroot). Showy perennial herb to 4 feet tall, the stems erect and stiff from a shallow mat of fibrous roots; leaves opposite, ovate, long-petioled, to 6 inches long, coarsely serrated; flowers white, small, arranged in composite heads in terminal corymbs; fruit a small achene. A variable weed of eastern North America.

Poisoning. The toxic principle of white snakeroot is apparently an unstable alcohol, designated tremetol, in combination with an incompletely characterized resin acid. A disease known as "milk sickness" was traced to the ingestion of dairy products derived from livestock poisoned by this species. Tremetol is readily excreted in milk. "Milk sickness" was common in early colonial times, and it became one of the most dreaded diseases from North Carolina and Virginia to the Midwest until the early nineteenth century. Drinking such milk or eating other contaminated dairy products results in weakness, nausea and vomiting, constipation, tremors, prostration, delirium, and even death for many. Mortality ranges between 10 and 25%, but the massive loss of life of former times cannot occur with current processing methods.

Florestina tripteris leaves, containing hydrocyanic acid, are reportedly fatal to sheep.

Flourensia cernua (tarbush) fruit has caused death in sheep and goats.

Franseria discolor (white ragweed) may cause loss of stock by nitrate poisoning.

Gutierrezia spp. (broomweed) leaves, containing a saponin, are severely toxic to most livestock.

Haplopappus heterophyllus (rayless goldenrod) contains tremetol, which is responsible for "milk sickness." Loss of livestock has been severe in parts of the southwestern United States because of this species, and ingestion of milk from animals that eat *Haplopappus* has resulted in human poisoning (see *Eupatorium*).

Helenium spp. (sneezeweed) contains dugaldin, a glycoside, responsible for heavy losses of stock, particularly sheep. In some years, thousands of sheep die in Colorado and Utah from sneezewood poisoning.

Hymenoxys odorata (bitterweed) and *H. richardsonii* (pingue). Ingestion has resulted in significant loss of sheep and less commonly, cattle and goats.

Lactuca scariola (wild lettuce) is toxic to cattle when the plants are young and eaten in large quantities. Mature plants appear to be nontoxic.

Neurolaena lobata leaves and stems are used as fish poisons and insecticides in the islands of the West Indies.

Oonopsis spp. (goldenweed) accumulate selenium, and livestock may show symptoms of selenium poisoning following ingestion of these plants.

Oxytenia acerosa (copperweed) increases in toxicity with age; significant cattle poisoning occurs in the fall.

Psilostrophe spp. (paperflowers) are toxic to sheep.

Rudbeckia laciniata (cone flower) and *R. hirta* (black-eyed susan) have been associated with poisoning of pigs, sheep, and cattle.

Salmea scandens is widely employed as a fish poison among the Indians of Panama.

Sartwellia flaveriae (sartwellia) causes serious liver damage in cattle, goats, and sheep.

Senecio spp. (groundsel) contain hepatotoxic pyrrolizidine alkaloids, which result in acute illness and death of livestock in many parts of the world. Many species of this large genus are toxic. Human poisoning has been reported in Africa and in the West Indies.

Silybum marianum (variegated thistle) accumulates nitrates, which can cause poisoning of cattle and sheep.

Solidago spp. (goldenrods) appear to be toxic to sheep. The toxic principles have been identified as diterpenes.

Tanacetum vulgare (tansy) oil is toxic to man in overdose. A tea made from the leaves and flowering tops is probably sufficiently dilute to permit ingestion.

Tetradymia spp. (horsebushes) produce liver damage in sheep.

Viguiera annua (annual goldeneye) poisons cattle; the principle is either cyanide or nitrate.

Xanthium spp. (cocklebur), many of which contain the poisonous principle hydroquinone in their seeds and seedlings, reportedly poison all classes of domestic livestock.

Xylorrhiza spp. (woody asters) accumulate selenium and ingestion of these results in extensive loss of sheep.

Monocotyledons

PHYLOGENETIC GROUP 12

JUNCAGINACEAE (Arrow Grass)

Triglochin maritima and *T. palustris* (arrow grasses) contain a cyanogenic glycoside giving symptoms and lesions in livestock typical of cyanide poisoning.

PHYLOGENETIC GROUP 13

ARACEAE (Arum)

Arum maculatum (lords-and-ladies). Roots and berries have poisoned children in Europe, probably because of high oxalate content or formic acid.

Arisaema spp. (jack-in-the-pulpit), *Calla palustris* (wild calla), and *Symplocarpus foetidus* (skunk cabbage) accumulate needlelike crystals of calcium oxalate, principally in the rhizomes. If the crystals are taken into the mouth, they become embedded in the mucous membranes, evoke irritation, and cause a burning sensation. Mortality is not known, although death has been produced experimentally in animals by administration of extracts of these species.

Alocasia indica, *Anthurium* spp., *Caladium* spp., *Colocasia antiquorum* (elephant's-ear), *Dieffenbachia picta* and *D. seguine* (dumbcanes), *Monstera deliciosa*, *Philodendron* spp., and *Xanthosoma* spp. are all cultivated aroids, and many are house plants. Their tissues contain irritant juice and/or crystals of calcium oxalate, giving rise to severe discomfort if ingested; often there is severe swelling of throat and mouth, which could lead to asphyxiation. Burning sensation in the mouth and throat is caused by an enzyme or asparagine in species of *Dieffenbachia*. Loss of life is infrequent, but ingestion of leaves and stems of these common house plants should be avoided.

TYPHACEAE (Cattail)

Typha latifolia (cattail) is suspected in fatal poisoning of horses in Indiana.

PHYLOGENETIC GROUP 14

JUNCACEAE (Rush)

Juncus inflexus (hard rush) poisoning has resulted in death of cattle in Europe.

CYPERACEAE (Sedge)

Scirpus americanus (bulrush) is suspected of producing pulmonary emphysema in Wyoming cattle and of poisoning cattle in Australia.

POACEAE (Grass)
The toxicity of some grass species may be that of a fungus associated with the grass and not the grass itself, as for example the fungi found on *Festuca arundinacea* (tall fescue) and *Hordeum vulgare* (barley).

Avena sativa (oats), having high nitrate content and fungal contaminants, may cause serious loss of cattle and horses after ingesting this type of hay.

Cynodon dactylon (Bermuda grass). Poisoning of cattle in the southeastern United States and Oklahoma is probably due to high concentrations of hydrocyanic acid, which may be produced under certain environmental conditions.

Glyceria striata (fowl mannagrass), producing a cyanogenic glycoside, is incriminated in the death of calves in Maryland.

Hilaria rigida (galleta grass) is implicated in cattle losses in California.

Holcus lanatus (velvet grass) is potentially dangerous to livestock because of the presence of cyanogenic glycosides.

Hordeum jubatum (squirreltail grass) may result in mechanical injury and death, particularly to sheep, as a result of bristles penetrating the delicate tissues of the oral cavity. This is sufficient to prevent feeding or to cause blindness and thus animals are unable to find feed.

Lolium temulentum (darnel). Toxicity may be related to a parasitic fungus or to the alkaloids temuline and loliine.

Panicum maximum (Guinea grass) contains hydrocyanic acid under poor soil and growing conditions and may be poisonous to cattle in the dry season. As the rainy season progresses, it is reported from Colombia, danger of poisoning disappears.

Setaria lutescens (foxtail grass) can cause major mechanical injury, especially among horses.

Sorghum spp. (Johnson grass, Sudan grass, sorghum) contain cyanogenic glycosides (e.g., dhurrin). Thus the potential of cyanide poisoning exists for livestock; the forage sorghums and Sudan grass also accumulate toxic levels of nitrates that likewise may result in poisoning.

Stipa robusta (sleepygrass). Toxicity to horses has been reported in New Mexico.

Zea mays (corn) tends to accumulate nitrates, which may result in poisoning of cattle. Under particular environmental conditions, a cyanogenic glycoside may also be produced.

PHYLOGENETIC GROUP 15

LILIACEAE (Lily)

Agave lecheguilla (lechuguilla). Leaves have been known to poison range animals, with morbidity reaching 30% in severe outbreaks. This usually occurs under drought conditions.

Allium spp. (onion) may cause poisoning in cattle and horses following ingestion.

Amianthium muscaetoxicum (staggergrass), containing an uncharacterized alkaloid similar to that known for *Zigadenus,* has resulted in many deaths of cattle.

Boophone distichia has been used as an arrow poison by the Bushmen of Africa.

Bowiea volubilis of eastern and southern Africa has long been known to be poisonous. The bulb contains a cardiotonic principle, as well as the alkaloid bowieine, which may be identical with colchicine. The plant has been reported to be lethal to man and domestic animals.

Colchicum autumnale (autumn crocus, meadow saffron). Bulbous plants with a large glossy brown corm; leaves long and narrow, appearing in the spring and then withering; flowers commonly light purple, large, in clusters appearing in the fall. Native to Europe and northern Africa, this species is cultivated widely in temperate areas.

Poisoning. Colchicine and other alkaloids are found throughout the plant with the highest concentrations in the seeds and corms. The main symptoms of poisoning are burning of the throat and stomach, vomiting, purging, weak-quick pulse, kidney failure, and respiratory failure commonly resulting in death. Fatalities are reported following administration of this plant for gout and rheumatism, as well as after erroneously eating the corms in place of onions, and by children who have eaten the flowers.

Convallaria majalis (lily-of-the-valley), native to Europe and widely cultivated as an ornamental, contains more than 20 cardiac glycosides, convallatoxin being the most significant. There are no current examples of poisoning, but because of the plant's constituents and wide availability, it is potentially dangerous.

Crinum longiflorum (spider lily). Bulbs are toxic and should be kept from children.

Endymion non-scriptus (bluebell). When eaten, bulbs result in abdominal pain, diarrhea, and weak, slow pulse. Recovery is slow. Poisoning is rare.

Erythronium spp. (dogtooth violet) bulbs are known to poison poultry.

Fritillaria meleagris (fritillaria) contains a heart-depressant alkaloid and has caused poisoning in Europe.

Galanthus nivalis (snowdrop) bulbs are reportedly poisonous to livestock.

Gloriosa superba (glory lily) rhizomes are very poisonous, containing colchicine and/or colchicinelike alkaloids, such as the highly toxic bitter superbine. The glory lily has been used for suicidal purposes in India and Burma. In eastern Africa the powdered rhizome of *G. simplex* is used by native poisoners. Probably all parts of these plants are poisonous to livestock.

Hippeastrum equestre (Barbados lily). Bulbs have been known to poison humans and animals, causing death in 2 to 3 hours.

Hyacinthus orientalis (garden hyacinth). Bulbs are reported to cause severe purgation in cattle.

Hymenocallis literalis (spider lily). Bulbs contain the alkaloid lycorine, which is toxic.

Lachnanthes tinctoria (redroot) is said to be poisonous to hogs.

Melanthium virginicum (bunchflower) may poison sheep, cattle, and horses.

Narcissus spp. (narcissus, daffodil, jonquil). Bulbs may cause poisoning if eaten in quantity.

Nolina texana (sacahuista). Flowers cause serious poisoning in cattle and sheep.

Ornithogalum umbellatum (star of Bethlehem, Fig. 2-10a). Onionlike herbaceous perennial from a bulb; leaves linear with a light green midrib, erect, basally inserted at the bulb; flowers on a long leafless stalk, showy, white and starlike, perianth six-parted. Native to the Mediterranean region; cultivated and naturalized in eastern North America.

Poisoning. All parts contain cardiac glycosides, which can cause nausea and gastroenteritis. Children have been poisoned by eating flowers and bulbs from this plant. The bulbs are toxic to livestock; more than 1000 sheep which ate them were lost in a single year in Maryland. *Ornithogalum longibracteatum* of eastern Africa is also considered extremely poisonous.

Paris quadrifolia (herb Paris), which is lit-

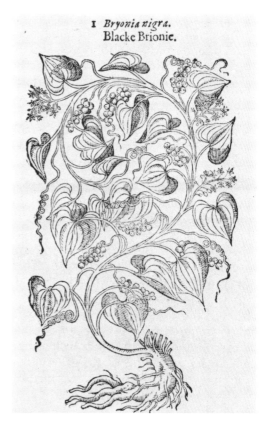

Figure 2-10b *Tamus communis* (from J Gerard, *The Herball*, 1597).

tle known, contains a saponinlike substance, particularly in its berries and seeds, and is potentially dangerous to children.

Polygonatum spp. (Solomon's seal), having an anthraquinone in the berries, are known to cause vomiting and diarrhea.

Tulipa spp. (tulip). Bulbs cause severe purgation in cattle.

Urginea maritima (squill). Bulbs contain cardiotonic glycosides having digitalislike effects, but poisoning in man and stock is rare. However *U. altissima*, native to tropical and southern Africa, is considered dangerous to livestock, and *U. brachystachys* is used to make an arrow poison. Verdcourt and Trump[1] outline the procedure used by the Nvika tribe in

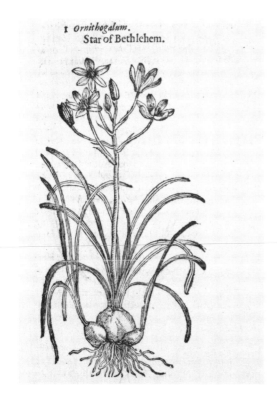

Figure 2-10a *Ornithogalum umbellatum* (from J Gerard, *The Herball*, ed 2, 1636).

Tanzania. First bulbs are pounded and the fibers dried in the sun. The fibers are again pounded with a little water, and the paste is allowed to dry on the arrows. Humans are reported to die about 3 hours after being hit by an arrow if the poison remains in the body. Recovery is often effected, however, if an arrow that has only slightly penetrated the body is removed and the wound washed with soda or wood ash and hot water.

Veratrum spp. (false hellebore), containing many alkaloids, have major effects on the heart and vessels. Blood pressure is lowered, arterioles are dilated, and a general cardiac depressant effect (Chapter 7) is caused by these alkaloids. Most cases of poisoning have been through the misuse of medical preparations; scattered reports exist of poisoning in cattle, sheep, and fowl, as well as man (e.g., mass poisoning of Korean soldiers from soup made of *Veratrum japonicum*).

Zephyranthes atamasco (rain lily). Bulbs are chiefly responsible for poisoning in cattle and horses ("staggers").

Zigadenus spp. (death camas). Perennial glabrous herbs from thick underground bulbs or rhizomes, the stem to 3 feet tall terminating in the inflorescence, unbranched, sparingly leafy; leaves several to many, narrow and grasslike; flowers in terminal racemes or panicles, white, cream, or pink, the six-parted perianth spreading with one to two yellowish glands at the base; fruit a three-parted capsule. Found throughout North America, all 15 species of *Zigadenus* are considered poisonous.

Poisoning. A number of alkaloids similar to those found in *Veratrum* (e.g., zygacine), and mainly located in the bulb, are responsible for the poisonous symptoms: vomiting, diarrhea, gastroenteritis, decreased heartbeat, and subnormal temperature. Children have been poisoned by eating bulbs and flowers; livestock fatalities are also known.

DIOSCOREACEAE (Yam)

Dioscorea spp. (yams) are important foods when properly prepared. Washing and/or boiling removes the poisonous saponins, which if not eliminated could cause fatal poisoning. Yams are a major source of diosgenin, a steroid precursor used in making birth control pills (Chapter 13).

Tamus communis (black bryony, Fig. 2-10*b*). Roots and berries on ingestion produce symptoms of an irritant purgative. Death may come rapidly. Children are attracted to the berries from this European species, sometimes with fatal results.

IRIDACEAE (Iris)

Iris foetidissima, I. pseudoacorus, and *I. versicolor* (irises) contain a glycoside that is poisonous to livestock when ingested in sufficient quantity. Fortunately toxic reports are rare.

LITERATURE CITED

1. Verdcourt B, Trump EC. 1969. *Common Poisonous Plants of East Africa.* Collins, St. James' Place, London. 254 p.

2. Jensen LB. 1970. *Poisoning Misadventures.* Charles C Thomas, Springfield, Ill. 202 p.

3. Where is Arsenic Lilly? *Time* **28** August 1972: 32.

4. Poisoning incidence increases. 1973. *Mod Med* **41**(13): 120.

5. Kingsbury JM. 1964. *Poisonous Plants of the United States and Canada.* Prentice-Hall, Englewood Cliffs, NJ. 626 p.

6. Robinson T. 1959. Alkaloids. *Sci Am* **201**(1): 113–121; Robinson T. 1974. Metabolism and function of alkaloids in plants. *Science* **184:** 430–435.

7. Greer MA, Astwood EB. 1948. The antithyroid effect of certain foods in man as determined

with radioactive iodine. *Endocrinology* **43**: 105–119.

8. Muenscher WC. 1951. *Poisonous Plants of the United States,* rev ed. Macmillan, New York. 227 p.

9. Escobar N. 1972. *Flora Tóxica de Panamá.* Editorial Universitaria, Panama. 279 p.

10. Hardin JM, Arena JM. 1974. *Human Poisoning from Native and Cultivated Plants,* ed 2. Duke University Press, Durham, NC. 194 p.

11. North PM. 1967. *Poisonous Plants and Fungi.* Blandford Press, London. 161 p.

12. Watt JM, Breyer-Brandwijk MG. 1962. *Medicinal and Poisonous Plants of Southern and Eastern Africa,* ed 2. E & S Livingstone, Edinburgh and London. 1457 p.

13. Wogan GN (ed). 1965. *Mycotoxins in Foodstuffs.* MIT Press, Cambridge, Mass. 291 p.

14. Goldblatt LA (ed). 1969. *Aflatoxin.* Academic Press, New York and London. 472 p.

15. Smith AH. 1949. *Mushrooms in Their Natural Habitats,* 2 vols. Sawyer's, Portland, Ore; Smith AH. 1963. *The Mushroom Hunter's Field Guide Revised and Enlarged.* University of Michigan Press, Ann Arbor.

16. Evans IA, Jones RS, Mainwaring-Burton R. 1972. Passage of bracken fern toxicity into milk. *Nature* **237**: 107–108.

A number of general references on poisonous plants, particularly in relation to specific regions, should be noted. Most American states and Canadian provinces also have such manuals.

Allen PH. 1943. Poisonous and injurious plants of Panama. *Am J Trop Med* **23**: 1–76.

Arena JM. 1974. *Poisoning.* ed 3. Charles C Thomas, Springfield, Ill. 804 p.

Blohm H. 1962. *Poisonous Plants of Venezuela.* Wissenschaftliche Verlagsgesellschaft, Stuttgart. 136 p.

Bodin F, Cheinisse CF. 1970. *Poisons.* McGraw-Hill, New York and Toronto. 255 p.

Chopra RN, Badhwar RL, Ghosh S. 1965. *Poisonous Plants of India.* Manager of Publications, New Delhi.

Connor HE, Adams NM. 1951. *The Poisonous Plants in New Zealand.* Government Printer, Wellington.

Dalziel JM. 1937. *The Useful Plants of West Tropical Africa.* Crown Agents for the Colonies, London.

Duncan WH. 1958. *Poisonous Plants in the Southeastern United States.* The author, Athens, Ga.

Gardner CA, Bennetts HW. 1956. *The Toxic Plants of Western Australia.* West Australian Newspapers, Perth.

Fanshawe DB, Hough CD. 1967. *Poisonous Plants of Zambia.* Forest Res Bull No 1 (rev), Government Printer, 24 p.

Heiser, CB Jr. 1969. *Nightshades: The Paradoxical Plants.* WH Freeman, San Francisco. 200 p.

Howard RA, De Wolf GP Jr, Pride GH. 1974. Poisonous plants. *Arnoldia* **34**(2): 41–96.

Howes FN. 1930. Fish-poison plants. *Kew Bull* **1930**(4): 129–153.

Hurst E. 1942. *The Poison Plants of New South Wales.* Snelling Printing Works, Sydney.

Kingsbury JM. 1965. *Deadly Harvest, A Guide to Common Poisonous Plants.* Holt, Rinehart & Winston, New York. 128 p.

Kosma JJ. 1969. *Killer Plants, A Poisonous Plant Guide.* Milestone Publ Co, Jacksonville, Ill. 50 p.

Martínez M. 1959. *Las Plantas Medicinales de México,* ed 4. Ediciones Botas, Mexico, DF.

Meléndez EN. 1964. *Plantas Medicinales de Puerto Rico.* Universidad de Puerto Rico, Estado Experimental Agrícola Bol 176. 245 p.

Morton J. 1971. *Plants Poisonous to People in Florida.* Hurricane House, Miami. 116 p.

Oakes AJ, Butcher JO. 1962. *Poisonous and Injurious Plants of the U.S. Virgin Islands.* US Department of Agriculture Misc Publ No 882, Government Printing Office, Washington, DC.

Pertchik B, Pertchik H. 1951. *Flowering Trees of the Caribbean.* Holt, Rinehart & Winston, New York.

Quisumbing E. 1951. *Medicinal Plants of the Philippines.* Bureau of Printing, Manila.

Robb GL. 1957. The ordeal poisons of Madagascar and Africa. *Bot Mus Leafl Harvard Univ* **17**: 265–316.

Rusby HH. 1918. The recognition at sight of poisonous and medicinal properties in unknown plants. *J Am Pharm Ass* **7**: 770–784.

Shone DK, Drummond RB. 1965. Poisonous plants of Rhodesia. *Rhod Agr J* **62**(4).

Webb LJ. 1948. *Guide to the Medicinal and Poisonous Plants of Queensland.* Scientific and Industrial Research Bulletin 232. Commonwealth of Australia Printing Office, Melbourne. 202 p.

Youngken HW Jr. 1964. *Common Poisonous Plants of New England.* US Public Health Service Publ No 1220, Government Printing Office, Washington, DC.

Chapter 3
Allergy

In the last century, when allergies were first recognized, the public believed that they were caused by invisible emanations produced by new hay. A second generally accepted premise was that most cases of hay fever originated in the middle or upper classes of society. As Beard wrote in 1876, "Hay-fever is . . . a disease of the fashionable and thoughtful—the price of wealth and culture, a part of the penalty of a fine organization and an in-door life."[1]

Much more is known of the etiology of allergy today, as its 31 million sufferers in the United States from all walks of life can attest.[2] Hay fever, largely caused by pollen and spores, afflicts no fewer than 13 million victims who endure physical and psychological misery at some time during the year, but mainly from spring until autumn. Among adults, 33 million disability days annually can be attributed to hay fever and asthma alone, while children lose no less than 36 million school days because of allergies. In North America, the greatest culprits are the ragweeds (*Ambrosia*) in the aster family (Asteraceae); in Europe and in more equatorial zones, however, grasses (Poaceae) are responsible for many cases of allergy. Since fungi are found everywhere, their spores are a constant cause of seasonal and perennial allergic rhinitis and asthma worldwide.

Perhaps the immune system, with its ability to distinguish abnormal from cellular proteins (antigens), was an adaptation to eliminate genetic mistakes occurring during ontogenic processes as well as to protect the body from disease. As the system developed many mechanisms evolved that increased the efficiency of recognition and elimination of foreign protein.

Usually an immune response can be elicited after contact and recognition of an antigen by several cell types belonging to the reticuloendothelial system in a manner like that proposed in Fig. 3-1. This results in the production of immunoreactive cells and modified serum globulins

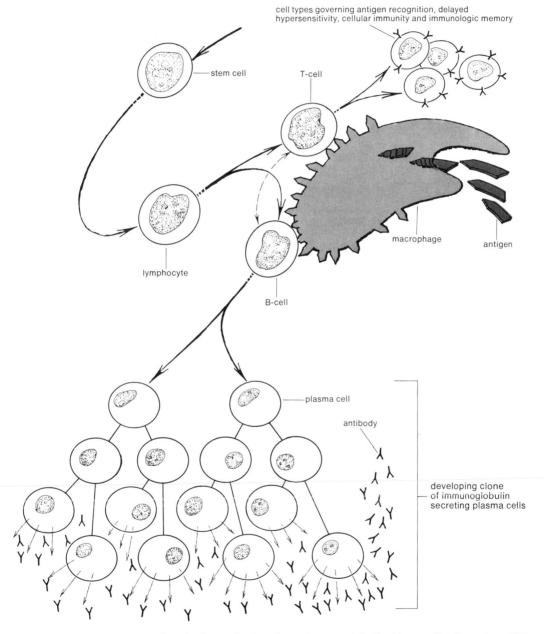

Figure 3-1 Present concept of antibody production (from *Immunoglobulin Abnormality Detection*, 1974, p 13, Fig 8, Courtesy of Millipore Corporation).

(antibodies, immunoglobulins: Fig. 3-2) that can act alone, or with other phagocytic cells, to eliminate from the body specific antigens in the form of foreign proteins, toxins, tumor cells, and infectious agents. Some of these cells then persist for a long time and are the basis for the accelerated immune responses characteristic of subsequent antigen contact.

Probably one of the most common abnormalities of the immune system is the development of the allergic state. This atopic condition is often genetically predisposed, and its evolution is related to factors such as allergen recognition through possession of specific receptor sites, changes in the proportion and types of immunoglobulins produced, and differences in inherent tissue sensitivity to

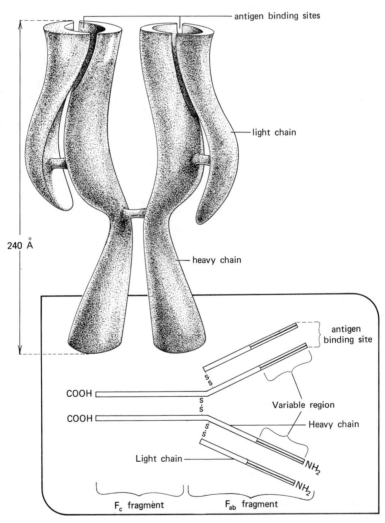

Figure 3-2 Basic antibody structure (IgG). An antibody molecule consists of four polypeptide chains, two "heavy" chains and two "light" chains joined by disulfide bonds. The N-terminals (variable regions) of a light chain and a heavy chain form the antigen binding site (Fab). Antibody molecules are divalent, that is, they have two antigen binding sites per antibody molecule. The Fc region interacts with complement and cell membranes. (From *Immunoglobulin Abnormality Detection*, 1974, p 8, Fig 5, Courtesy of Millipore Corporation.)

allergenically mediated substances. Depending on the overall mechanism involved and the speed and type of reactions observed, five types (I-V) have been distinguished (see Glossary under hypersensitivity). Of these, examples of Types I to IV are discussed in the text, with Type II incorporated into the section on Drug Sensitivity Reactions (p. 87).

ANTIBODY—MEDIATED (IMMEDIATE TYPE) HYPERSENSITIVITY (TYPE I)

Immediate hypersensitivity is related to the development of reaginic antibodies, usually Immunoglobulin E (IgE), and less often IgG, in sufficient quantities to evoke the symptoms of hay fever, asthma, hives, and anaphylactic shock. These antibodies are produced following allergen contact, locally within plasma cells embedded in the mucosa of target areas of the nasopharynx and the respiratory and gastrointestinal tracts, as well as elsewhere in the lymphatic system. After diffusing into the tissue fluid and serum the antibodies attach to mast cells, basophils, and platelets. Allergen then binds to this cell-bound reagin, triggering the release of histamine and other vasoactive substances (kinins, serotonin, slow reacting substances) that cause the allergic symptoms of bronchospasm, vasodilation, smooth muscle contraction, and increased bronchial and nasal secretion. However, clinical manifestations are often not apparent until repeated exposures to the allergen have increased the number of cells involved.

An inciting allergen can be identified from among a host of possible candidates by several provocative *in vivo* tests. The most frequently employed are skin tests that involve the introduction of dilute concentrations of allergen into the skin by intradermal injection or through pricking. If a specific reaginic antibody is present in the skin, the characteristic wheal and erythema of a cutaneous anaphylaxis reaction appear within a few minutes. More rarely, tests using the conjunctiva or nasal mucosa as target organs have also been found effectual. Since the induction of systemic anaphylactic shock is always a possibility during such testing, however, it is recommended that the procedures always be carried out under careful medical supervision and that an antianaphylactic drug (i.e., epinephrine) be available.

Sensitive *in vitro* tests are also now employed. The radioallergosorbent test (RAST) is based on binding antibody to antigen in a system containing radiolabeled anti-antibody (anti-IgG, anti-IgE, anti-IgA). When necessary, the use of different radioactive iodine isotopes as labels allows for the simultaneous detection of reaginic IgE and blocking IgG in a patient's serum. Other tests have been devised that detect reaginic antibody through its ability to release histamine from mast cells or nonallergic donor leukocytes in the presence of allergen. Results of the passive leukocyte sensitizing test (PLS) have been used to link fluctuation in serum reagin content to the seasonal prevalence of allergen such as ragweed.

Allergic symptoms may be reduced by immunotherapy consisting of careful injection of small amounts of the allergen (often into site that is not the target area, e.g., upper arm instead of respiratory tract) to elicit specific blocking antibodies (IgA or IgG), or a white cell response. In some way this response binds the allergens and prevents reagin-allergen complexes from forming (hyposensitization), reduces the amount of IgE from being formed (tolerance) or, by neutralization of reagin with excess antigen (desensitization), reduces the amount of IgE antibody available in target areas.

In seasonal spore and pollen allergies,

hyposensitization may be attempted pre-seasonally, ensuring that blocking antibodies are at their highest titer during the provocative period, since treatment during the symptomatic period (coseasonal) is less satisfactory. For allergies that occur throughout the year, such as those elicited with fungal spores, it may be necessary to maintain treatment year-round.

Anaphylactic Shock

Systemic anaphylaxis, a rare event in man, is the most severe of all allergic reactions. Typically, it can occur after an inciting dose has been given intravenously to a hypersensitive individual, but it has also been noted after oral, subcutaneous, or intramuscular administration. It is characterized by sudden vasomotor collapse leading to shock, paroxysmal bronchoconstriction, and, if treatment is not undertaken immediately, death. Most cases have been associated with serum therapy (serum sickness), penicillin therapy, and insect stings (especially the wasp, bee, and hornet). However, the following case history underlines the danger of chamomile tea ingestion by an individual known to have ragweed and *Chrysanthemum* atopic disease and other allergies.[4]

Within minutes of drinking a few sips of chamomile tea, the 35-year-old woman developed abdominal cramps, thickness of the tongue, and a tight sensation in the throat. This was followed by angioedema of the lips and eyes, diffuse pruritus, and a full sensation in the ears. There was no vomiting, diarrhea, sneezing, or wheezing. Fortunately, diphenhydramine was administered immediately and a steroid shortly thereafter. The symptoms cleared gradually over the next few hours and disappeared overnight. A subsequent scratch test with chamomile tea produced a large wheal and flare reaction with pseudopod formation. Similar reactions were also elicited among other ragweed patients, although none gave a history of chamomile tea ingestion. This suggests that allergens are shared among members of the family of which ragweed and *Chrysanthemum* are a part.

Prevention is empirical, but atopic individuals should be aware of the increased risk and should avoid agents having known anaphylactic potential, such as penicillin or chamomile tea.

Allergic Rhinitis (Hay Fever)[5]

Characteristic symptoms of hay fever, induced following exposure of the nasal mucosa to the allergen through inhalation, include profuse watery nasal discharge with sneezing, frequently accompanied by redness, irritated and watery eyes, and headache.

The inciting allergens are often found in windborne plant structures called aeroallergens. The spores from fungi and even certain algae may persist through the year, especially under warm humid conditions; but particularly in temperate regions, wind-pollinated plants elicit symptoms during certain flowering periods (Table 3-1). In North America there are three peaks in the pattern of seasonal rhinitis: the first occurs in the spring when trees shed their pollen; the second, during the summer months, involves pollen from many grasses as well as late flowering trees and weeds; and the last peak, in the autumn, is typified by weed and secondarily by grass pollen grains. Ragweed pollen (*Ambrosia*) predominates during this time and is the most allergenic pollen found in North America.

In tropical areas both perennial and seasonal patterns can also be observed with this disorder. Fungal spores and grass pollen are common aeroallergens,

Table 3-1 Aeroallergens (Largely North American) Causing Allergic Rhinitis, Bronchial Asthma, and/or Hypersensitivity Pneumonitis

ALGAE
  Chlorella, Chlorococcum
FUNGI
Phycomycetes: Mucorales
  Absidia, Cunninghamella, Mucor, Rhizopus, Syncephalastrum
Phycomycetes: Peronsporales
  Plasmopara (downy mildew)
Ascomycetes
  Yeast. *Saccharomyces*
  Powdery Mildew. *Erysiphe*
  Perithecial fungi. *Chaetomium*
  Ascostromatic fungi. *Pleospora*
Basidiomycetes: Tremellales (jelly fungi)
  Bullera, Sporobolomyces
Basidiomycetes: Uredinales (rusts)
  Puccinia, Uromyces
Basidiomycetes: Ustilaginales (smuts)
  Tilletia, Ustilago
Deuteromycetes (FUNGI IMPERFECTI)
CRYPTOCOCCACEAE (false yeast). *Candida, Cryptococcus, Rhodotorula, Torulopsis*
DEMATIACEAE. *Alternaria, Cladosporium (Hormodendrum), Curvularia, Helminthosporium, Nigrospora, Pullularia, Spondylocladium, Stemphylium*
MONILIACEAE. *Aspergillus, Botrytis, Geotrichum, Gliocladium, Monilia, Mycogone, Paecilomyces, Penicillium, Sporotrichum, Trichoderma, Trichothecium, Verticillium*
SPHAERIOIDACEAE. *Phoma*
TUBERCULARIACEAE. *Epicoccum, Fusarium*

GYMNOSPERMS
  Ginkgo biloba (ginkgo or maidenhair tree),[a] *Juniperus mexicana* (mountain cedar), *J. virginiana* (red cedar),[a] *Pinus contorta* (lodgepole pine),[b] *Thuja plicata* (western red cedar);[b] for others implicated in the San Francisco area, see Yoo[6]

ANGIOSPERMS: DICOTYLEDONS
ACERACEAE (Maple). *Acer* (box elder, maple)
AMARANTHACEAE (Amaranth). *Acnida* (water hemp), *Amaranthus* (amaranth, pigweed)
APIACEAE (Carrot). *Anthriscus* (hedge parsley),[a,c] *Heracleum* (hogweed)[a,c]
ASTERACEAE (Aster or Composite)
  AMBROSIEAE (Ragweed tribe). *Ambrosia* (ragweed), *Dicoria, Hymenoclea* (greasebush), *Iva* (marsh elder, poverty weed), *Xanthium* (cocklebur)
  ANTHEMIDEAE (Mayweed tribe). *Artemisia* (mugwort, sagebrush, wormwood), *Chrysanthemum* (ox-eye daisy)[c]
  ASTEREAE (Aster tribe). *Aster,*[c] *Callistephus* (China aster),[c] *Solidago* (goldenrod)[c]
  CICHORIEAE (Chicory tribe). *Taraxacum* (dandelion)[c]
BETULACEAE (Birch). *Alnus* (alder), *Betula* (birch), *Carpinus* (American hornbeam or blue beech), *Corylus* (hazelnut, filbert), *Ostrya* (hop hornbeam or ironwood)
BRASSICACEAE (Mustard). *Sinapsis* (charlock)[c]
CANNABACEAE (Hemp). *Cannabis* (marihuana), *Humulus* (hop)
CARICACEAE. *Carica papaya* (papaya)[b,c]
CASUARINACEAE (Casuarina). *Casuarina*
CHENOPODIACEAE (Goosefoot). *Allenrolfia* (burrow weed),[a] *Atriplex* (orach, saltbush, wing scale), *Bassia* (smotherweed), *Beta* (sugar beet),[a] *Chenopodium* (goosefoot, lamb's quarters), *Dondia* (sea blite), *Eurotia* (white or winter sage), *Kochia* (burning bush or tumbleweed), *Salsola* (Russian thistle or saltwort), *Sarcobatus* (greasewood)
EUPHORBIACEAE (Spurge). *Mercurialis* (Mercury)
FABACEAE (Pea). *Acacia* (acacia), *Prosopis* (mesquite)
FAGACEAE (Beech). *Fagus* (beech), *Quercus* (oak)
HAMAMELIDACEAE. *Liquidambar* (sweet gum)[a]
JUGLANDACEAE (Walnut). *Carya* (hickory, pecan), *Juglans* (butternut, walnut)
LAMIACEAE (Mint). *Leonotis nepetaefolia* (hollowstalk)[c]
MORACEAE (Mulberry). *Broussonetia* (paper mulberry), *Maclura* (Osage orange), *Morus* (Mulberry)
MYRICACEAE (Sweet Gale). *Comptonia* (sweet fern), *Myrica* (wax myrtle)
MYRTACEAE (Myrtle). *Eucalyptus* (gum tree)[a]
OLEACEAE (Olive). *Fraxinus* (ash), *Ligustrum* (privet), *Olea* (olive), *Syringa* (lilac)[a]

Table 3-1   (Continued)

PLANTAGINACEAE (Plantain). *Plantago*
PLATANACEAE (Plane Tree). *Platanus* (syca-
more or plane tree)
POLYGONACEAE (Knotweed). *Fagopyrum*
(buckwheat),[b,d] *Rheum* (rhubarb), *Rumex*
(dock, sorrel)
RANUNCULACEAE (Buttercup). *Ranuncu-
lus*[a,c]
ROSACEAE (Rose). *Rosa*,[c] *Spiraea*[a,c]
SALICACEAE (Willow). *Populus* (aspen or
poplar), *Salix* (willow)
SCROPHULARIACEAE (Figwort). *Leucophyl-
lum* (canizo),[c] *Verbascum* (Mullein)[c]
SIMAROUBACEAE (Quassia). *Ailanthus*
(tree-of-heaven)
TILIACEAE (Linden). *Tilia* (basswood, linden)
ULMACEAE (Elm). *Celtis* (hackberry), *Ulmus*
(elm)

URTICACEAE (Nettle). *Parietaria* (pellitory-
of-the-wall), *Urtica* (Nettle)
ANGIOSPERMS: MONOCOTYLEDONS
ARECACEAE (Palm). *Phoenix dactylifera*
(date palm)
CYPERACEAE (Sedge). *Carex* (sedge),[a] *Erio-
phorum* (cottongrass)[a]
JUNCACEAE (Rush). *Juncus* (rush),[a] *Luzula*
(wood rush)[a]
POACEAE (Grass). *Agropyron* (western
wheat), *Agrostis* (redtop), *Anthoxanthum*
(sweet vernal), *Avena* (oats), *Bouteloua* (blue
grana or mesquite grass), *Cynodon* (Bermuda), *Dactylis* (orchard), *Digitaria* (crab),
Distichlis (salt), *Festuca* (fescue), *Holcus* (velvet), *Koeleria* (crested hair), *Lolium* (ray or
rye), *Phleum* (timothy), *Poa* (blue, June), *Secale* (rye), *Sorghum* (Johnson), *Zea* (corn)
TYPHACEAE (Cattail). *Typha*

[a] Suspected of causing an allergic reaction.
[b] Especially causing bronchial asthma.
[c] May cause an allergic reaction following accidental contact with the flowers, or if the
sensitized individual is adjacent to plants that are typically entomophylous.
[d] Buckwheat flour as inhalant or ingestant allergen.

whereas those from weeds and wind-
pollinated trees are of secondary importance. However the determination of
aeroallergens in the more equatorial
zones requires further study.

Although the majority of plants that induce allergic rhinitis are wind pollinated,
a number of plants that are typically
pollinated by animals (insects, birds, bats)
have also been implicated. For example,
old-fashioned roses, which are infrequently found in gardens today, are
often heavily scented and their anthers
are exposed by the loose and open form
of the floral bud. Thus their attractiveness
frequently used to lead to sensitization
through inhalation of the pollen, and the
term rose-fever or rose-cold was used to
describe plant-associated rhinitis. Cultivated roses today rarely have much
perfume, and the majority have a tight
cone-shaped floral bud; thus few people
sniff roses, and even fewer are exposed

to the pollen from the hidden anthers.
For other typically entomophilous plants
implicated in allergic rhinitis and asthma,
see Table 3-1, footnote c.

POLLEN AND THEIR ALLERGENS

The morphological diversity of windborne pollen varies from smooth-walled
grains having a single pore, as found
among the grasses, to the very spiny
grains of ragweed, and the multiporate
apertures typical of pigweed. Size and
shape also vary. These features, as well as
their wall structure, are related to dis-
persal mechanisms and their significance
as aeroallergens.[7]

The majority of allergens are found in
the walls of pollen and spores, but their
purpose is not to elicit allergy; rather,
they act as recognition proteins to stimulate the growth of the sperm-containing
pollen tubes on specific "female" parts of

the flower. These proteins are concentrated below the apertures in the *intine* or inner wall as well as in the hard, rigid, outer wall or *exine* in minute micropores or even chambers. They are water soluble, and when in contact with the "female" part of the flower, or the mucosa of man, the protein may be released within a few seconds.[8]

Some of these proteins have been isolated only recently. For example, the fraction designated antigen E is the major allergenic protein of ragweed (*Ambrosia*). Others include antigens K, Ra, Ra3, and Ra5. Among the grasses, a number of allergens have also been identified, such as allergens A and B for timothy (*Phleum pratense*) and alpha, beta, and gamma allergens in rye (*Lolium perenne*). Also, a number of active fractions have been isolated from alder (*Alnus glutinosa*). However, the majority of specific allergens remain uncharacterized.[9]

SPORE AND POLLEN INCITANTS IN MAN

Many kinds of fungi and flowering plants are responsible for allergic rhinitis (Table 3-1). The most important fungal allergens are found in the Deuteromycetes, particularly the families Dematiaceae and Moniliaceae, which include such ubiquitous genera as *Alternaria* (Fig. 3-3), *Cladosporium, Aspergillus,* and *Penicillium.* Of these, *Alternaria* possesses the most allergenic substances and affects the greatest number of individuals, especially in the Midwestern United States.[10] Even though they produce abundant amounts of windborne pollen, the Gymnosperms rarely elicit allergic rhinitis, whereas most windborne pollen grains from Angiosperms are common incitors (Fig. 3-4). Overall, the most troublesome trees in North America are the oaks (*Quercus*), hickories (*Carya*), and elms (*Ulmus*), but weedy urban box elder (*Acer*) pollen has recently been shown to have the highest level of allergenicity among tree pollen.[11]

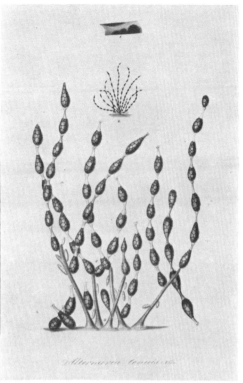

Figure 3-3 *Alternaria tenuis* (from *Flore Illustrée de mucédinées d'Europe,* plate 7, 1840).

The grass family (Poaceae) is one of the most important causes of allergy throughout the world. Many grass pollen grains are highly allergenic, e.g. redtop (*Agrostis*), sweet vernal (*Anthoxanthum*), orchard (*Dactylis*), crab (*Digitaria:* Fig. 3-5a), and timothy (*Phleum:* Fig 3-5b).[12] Of the weedy families, the Asteraceae, containing the ragweeds (*Ambrosia:* Fig. 3-6a), Marsh elders (*Iva*), cockleburs (*Xanthium*), and sagebrushes (*Artemisia*), and the Chenopodiaceae, including lamb's quarters (*Chenopodium*), burning bushes (*Kochia*), and Russian thistles (*Salsola:* Fig 3-6b), are notable examples. Of these, ragweed pollen not only affects more of the population in North America than any other plant, it also has the most potent allergens.[13]

Table 3-2 summarizes the significant aeroallergens, considered by geographic

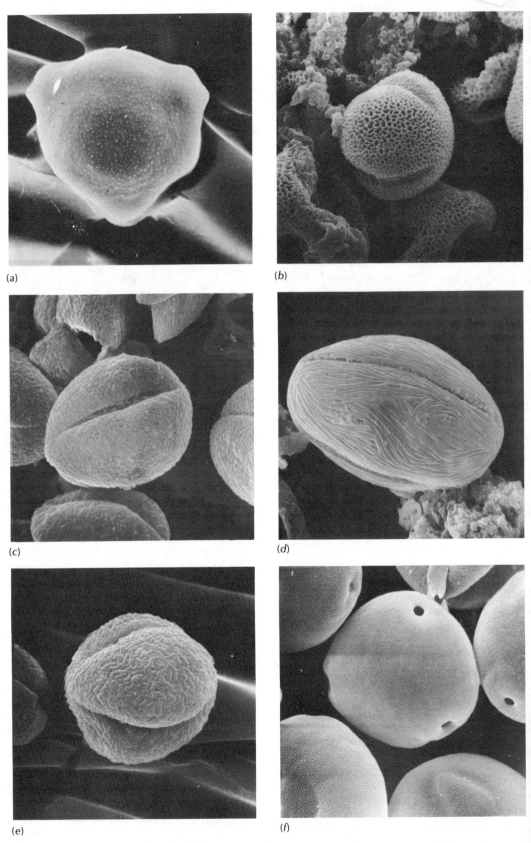

(a)

(b)

(c)

(d)

(e)

(f)

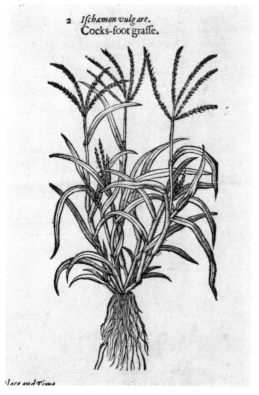

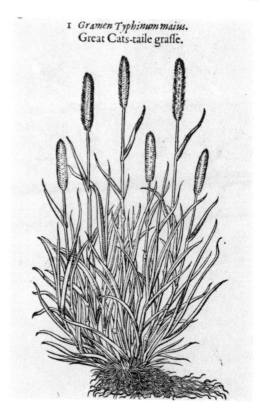

Figure 3-5a *Digitaria ischaemum* (from J Gerard, *The Herball*, ed 2, 1636).

Figure 3-5b *Phleum pratense* (from J Gerard, *The Herball*, 1597).

area and major pollen types for the continental United States.

THERAPY

The control and treatment of allergic rhinitis falls into three major categories. The first is related to controlling contact with allergic material. Often referred to as environmental control, this function might include the elimination of the affecting plants, the filtering of aeroallergens by appropriate air conditioning, and probably more important, moving away from the location of the offending allergens. It is surely relevant to consider the allergic person when plantings in urban developments are being designed.

Why, for example, should shade trees known to incite allergy be planted when others are available?

Another prophylactic measure is hyposensitization of the patient with the affecting allergen. This regimen, administered by an allergist, involves injection of increasing amounts of the allergen to develop a high titer of blocking antibodies prior to normal exposure. Today this is the most satisfactory form of prophylactic treatment, but its effect is directly related to the potency of the allergen in the antigens administered.

Finally, as an adjunct to hyposensitization, acute symptoms are also treated by the administration of antihistamines and vasoconstrictors such as ephedrine

Figure 3-4 Scanning electron micrographs of pollen grains, about ×1900. (a) *Betula nigra* (river or red birch); (b) *Platanus occidentalis* (sycamore); (c,e) *Acer negundo* (box elder); (d) *Acer rubrum* (red maple); (f) *Carya glabra* (pignut hickory).

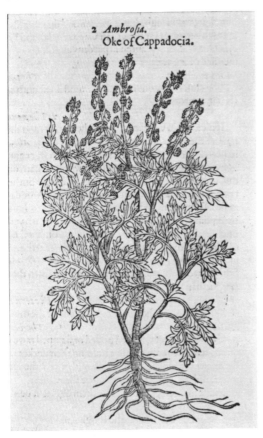

Figure 3-6a *Ambrosia artemisifolia* (from J Gerard, *The Herball,* 1597).

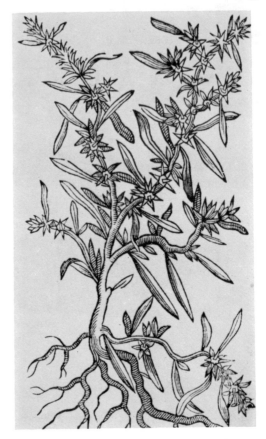

Figure 3-6b *Salsola kali* (from J Parkinson, *Theatrum Botanicum,* 1640).

(*Ephedra sinica*). Corticosteroid therapy, which may be employed to terminate a single severe attack, is often effective, though not curative. Prolonged use of steroids may be dangerous, and possible benefits must always be weighted against deleterious effects.[15]

Asthma[16]

Attacks of bronchial asthma are usually precipitated by inhalation of the specific allergen, and this form of allergy often has a more chronic course than that seen in allergic rhinitis even though the eliciting agents may be the same. Histamine and perhaps serotonin, are involved in symptoms that are characterized by bronchospasm and accompanied with ex-cessive viscid bronchial secretion, which produces the asthmatic "wheezing." Extrinsic asthma occurs typically in children and young adults and is often aggravated by emotional factors. It is considered to be an IgE mediated disease caused by the inhalation of aeroallergens such as pollen, spores, feathers and animal danders (Fig. 3-7). Although not a common aeroallergen, pollen from the lodgepole pine of Colorado (*Pinus contorta*) has also been known to cause bronchial asthma.

The mechanism for induction of intrinsic asthma is somewhat more obscure and is generally found in an older age group. The likely agents are allergic reactions to infectious materials, such as bacteria or viruses, or the inflammatory

Table 3-2 Higher Plants of Allergic Significance in Continental United States[a]

Geographic Area	Trees	Grasses	Weeds	Major Pollen
Northeastern. New England, New York, New Jersey, Pennsylvania	Birch, elm, maple, oak, poplar	Annual blue, June, orchard, sweet vernal, timothy	Short and giant ragweed, plantain	Ragweeds, grasses
Middle Atlantic. Delaware, Maryland, Washington D.C.	Birch, hickory, maple, oak, paper mulberry, sycamore	Orchard, timothy	Short and giant ragweed, plantain	Ragweeds, orchard grass
Virginias and Carolinas	Elm, maple, oak, pecan, red cedar	Annual blue, Bermuda, June, orchard	Short ragweed, sorrel, dock	Short ragweed, Bermuda grass, pecan
Southern. Florida and Georgia to eastern Texas, including Texas, Arkansas, and southern Missouri	Birch, cottonwood, elm, oak, paper mulberry, pecan, poplar, privet, red cedar	Bermuda, orchard, timothy	Giant and short ragweed, pigweed, Russian thistle, water hemp	Bermuda grass, pecan, ragweeds
North Central. Ohio and Kentucky to northern Missouri, Iowa, Wisconsin, and Michigan	Ash, cottonwood, elm, maple, oak	June, orchard, timothy	Short ragweed	Short ragweed
Plains and prairies. Minnesota, Dakotas, eastern Montana, Nebraska, Kansas	Elm, oak	Bermuda, bluegrass, orchard, redtop, timothy	Giant, short and western ragweeds, Russian thistle	Ragweeds, Russian thistle
Rocky Mountains. Idaho, western Montana, Wyoming, Colorado, Utah	Birch, box elder, cottonwood, Rocky Mountain cedar	Fescue, June, orchard, redtop, timothy	Ragweed, sagebrush, Russian thistle	Russian thistle, sagebrush
Pacific Northwest. Washington, Oregon, Nevada, northern California	Acacia, alder, box elder, birch, cottonwood, oak, walnut	Bluegrass, fescue, oats, orchard, redtop, timothy, velvet, western rye	Dock, pigweed, Russian thistle, saltbrush, sagebrush, sorrel	
Southwest. western Texas, Nevada, New Mexico, Arizona	Cottonwood, mountain cedar, mulberry, olive	Bermuda, Johnson	Amaranth, canyon ragweed, Russian thistle, saltbush	Amaranth, Bermuda grass, goosefoot, mountain cedar
Southern California	Elm, oak, olive, walnut	Bermuda, salt grass	Dock, lamb's quarters, pigweed, Russian thistle, sage, saltbush, sea blite	Bermuda grass, saltgrass

[a] Adopted from MB Rhyne.[14]

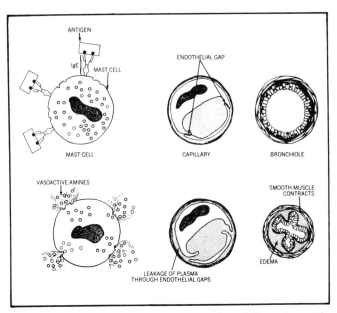

Figure 3-7   The IgE mediated release and action of vasoactive amines. IgE attaches to the surface of mast cell membranes by its Fc fragment. After combining with antigen, vasoactive amines are released from mast cell granules. This increases permeability through endothelial gaps and causes general contraction of smooth muscle, specifically around bronchioles. (From *Scope® Monograph on Immunology*, p. 46, fig 47, 1972, by permission of the Upjohn Company, Kalamazoo, Michigan.)

processes they elicit. Unlike extrinsic asthma antigens cannot be demonstrated and thus skin testing is of no value. The separation of purely extrinsic from intrinsic asthma can be diagnostically difficult whenever allergic phenomena are combined with infectious factors.

Possibly another IgE-mediated, Type I disease is the coffeebean and castorbean workers disease that is characterized by rhinitis, asthma, and dermatitis following inhalation of the hapten, chlorogenic acid. As it is widespread in plants and is concentrated in coffeebeans and castorbeans, chlorogenic acid may act more as a universal allergen than was first suspected.

HYPERSENSITIVITY PNEUMONITIS (TYPE III)

Another type of allergic respiratory condition, known as hypersensitivity pneumonitis or extrinsic allergic alveolitis, is often associated with specific professions. In these instances, animal, vegetable or bacterial enzyme material may induce the disease. For example, inhalation of *Thermoactinomyces vulgaris* or fungal spores of *Microsporum faeni,* which can contaminate hay, moldy sugar cane, or mushroom compost, have been causally related to farmer's (thresher's) lung, bagassosis, and mushroomworker's lung. In a similar way, *Cryptostroma corticale* has been associated with maple bark disease of woodworkers, *Penicillium caseii* to cheeseworker's disease, *Aspergillus clavatus* and *A. fumigatus* to brewer's lung disease, and *Graphium* and *Aureobasidium pullulans* to sequoiosis. By inhalation of the enzyme of *Bacillus subtilis,* those who work with detergents may also develop an allergic pneumonitis. Diseases produced by inhalation of airborne algae such as *Gloeocapsa* and *Chlorella,* are of more general incidence, however. Wood and paper mill workers may also develop bronchial asthma through sawdust inhalation of the Gymnosperms, redwood (*Sequoia sempervirens*), western red cedar (*Thuja plicata*), cedar of Lebanon (*Cedrus libani*), and the Angiosperms, iroko or African oak (*Chlorophora excelsa*), Nicaragua rosewood (*Dalbergia retusa*), and other exotic woods. The immunopathology suggests that a mixture of many types of immune or allergic reactions may be involved in extrinsic allergic alveolitis and thus is classified as Type III.[17]

It is also possible that symptoms similar to those of allergic respiratory illness may be elicited by inhalation of airborne leaf hairs. Such a series of cases was recently reported among gardeners who had tended saplings of Oriental sycamores or the tree of Hippocrates (*Platanus orientalis*) at a medical school campus. It is interesting that Dioscorides centuries ago had noted watery eyes, sneezing, an irritating sensation in the nasal passages, soreness of the throat, an irritating dry cough, and other similar symptoms.[19]

THERAPY

A regimen of environmental control and hyposensitization is normally prescribed for pollinosis. Currently, three basic drugs have preempted ephedrine for use in the control of asthmatic attacks: epinephrine (adrenalin) and its congeners administered by aerosol, the methylxanthines administered intravenously for acute attacks and orally for chronic asthma, and the steroids (cortisone) for severe and intractable states, in combination with other drugs mentioned. In prophylaxis, particularly where hyposensitization fails, cromolyn sodium is used; this new compound, obtained from the seeds of *Ammi visnaga* (Apiaceae), is believed to affect the release of vasoactive substances and therefore, through a regimen of frequent inhalation, acts to prevent or modify the

asthma.[20] This plant, known as khella from its native Mediterranean region, has a long history of use as an antiasthmatic among the Arab peoples, who also believe it is useful in the treatment of angina pectoris.

Although other plants used in domestic medicine to treat asthma have rarely been studied, the recent Indian research using the leaves of *Tylophora indica* (Asclepiadaceae) furnishes an interesting exception.[21] It is claimed that complete to moderate relief of nasobronchial allergic symptoms can be maintained up to one week after ingestion of but a few leaves of the plant. Typical of members of this family, *T. indica* is, however, very toxic and also has blistering or vesicant properties.

Ingestant Allergy[22]

Symptoms from ingesting a potential allergen can vary from urticaria to vomiting, diarrhea, and intestinal wall edema. It is sometimes difficult to differentiate between true atopy and toxicity, since clinical symptoms can be initiated by interaction of substances in foods with several different mediating systems. Therefore the appearance of hives (urticaria) after consumption of strawberries and citrus fruits can be traced to direct chemical mast cell degranulation; those of coeliac disease with intolerance to gluten (gliadin in wheat); and gastrointestinal upset associated with milk are traceable to inherited disaccharidase (lactase) deficiencies. Furthermore, several foodstuffs, particularly shellfish and mushrooms, contain notorious poisons. In susceptible persons, moreover, ricin (a phytotoxin from peanuts and castor beans), gossypol, aflatoxins, histamine, or tyramine (in cheese or yeast products) may also produce symptoms. It is also possible that certain nonallergenic components in food can trigger built-in labilities of mediator systems or can activate the complement system (C1 and C3: see Glossary) to generate anaphylatoxin-like agents.

Likewise, physiological age may also have a bearing on an individual's ability to absorb or reject certain allergens. Many food allergies of childhood are altered as the digestive system matures. Among cereals, for example, skin test reactions with rice indicate that there is a lower degree of reactivity among the few children affected; the opposite is true among adults, and higher reactivity involving greater frequency is typical.[23] Any ingestant may prove to have an allergic potential; skin testing, the usual method of determining such susceptibility, may not accurately reflect the true allergic state. Rather, susceptibility is better determined by demonstrating symptoms after deliberate feeding tests. Therapy related to the ingestant is used thereafter. Other techniques include using the rectal mucosa as a shock organ or feeding the test ingestant in dilute form and observing changes in the intestinal tract by X-ray.

Among the active allergens isolated from food, there is good evidence that tomato allergens fall into the same category of active glycoproteins described for inhalant allergens, as do the ovomucoids of egg white, whereas allergens of fish are simple amines.

The major symptom of ingestant hypersensitivity is urticaria, in which wheals and erythematous areas of the skin cause intense pruritus and discomfort. Local edema (angioedema) sometimes accompanies urticaria, and this condition may be life threatening if it affects the mucosa of the pharynx or larynx, since this may result in severe respiratory obstruction.

Atopic dermatitis, a common infant and childhood affliction, is often the first indicator of allergic predisposition. This infantile or atopic eczema may be clinically present as a persistent, pruritic dermatitis that may be papular, exudative, or lichenified, involving the head, neck, and flexor aspects of the trunk and extremities. Most provoking allergens are difficult to identify, varying from animal epidermal allergens (hair) to various foods in the diet.

THERAPY

Whenever it is possible to identify the allergen, avoidance is the best therapy. Otherwise, ephedrine is administered orally, and topical steroids are applied if skin lesions are severe. Antihistamines are useful when pruritus complicates atopic dermatosis or if there is urticaria.

When angioedema is a complicating factor, epinephrine is most useful and can be used concurrently with intravenous antihistamine and steroids for severe cases that involve the larynx.

Dermatitis[24]

IRRITANT DERMATITIS

Plants can mediate inflammatory reactions of the skin, which mimic in many ways the "wheal and erythematous flare" of immediate hypersensitivity, or the more severe reactions associated with the delayed response. In some instances this effect is attributable to the nature of the plant itself, that is, spines, thorns, bristles, and hairs causing mechanical injury. Moreover, the needle-sharp calcium oxalate crystals found in the outer layers of many *Narcissus* species and hyacinth bulbs can elicit the formation of wheals (bulb fingers), a symptom suggestive of histamine release. However most forms of irriation are related to specific substances produced by plants and the mechanism for the adverse reaction is usually unclear.

Of the many plants that transfer their toxins by means of stinging hairs, the nettles (*Urtica dioica* and *Laportea cana-*

densis) contain histaminelike substances found in bladders within the leaf. A more severe reaction is elicited by another species of Urticaceae, *Urera baccifera,* which is found in tropical America. The material in its spinelike hairs causes considerable pain followed by numbness lasting for several days. Similarly, the spurge nettle, *Cnidoscolus stimulosus* (Euphorbiaceae), can elicit painful irritation and itching following transfer of a caustic irritant. Perhaps the most painful reaction of all comes from *Mucuna pruriens* (Fabaceae), whose barbed spines covering the seed pods contain a highly irritating proteolytic enzyme called mucunain. Poisoning can take place long after the pods have dried, even from herbarium collections. However, the ultimate in adaptation is exemplified by *Gurania guaransenia* (Cucurbitaceae), which in addition to its own stinging hairs, harbors a butterfly larva having similar devices.

The sap of other plants, itself caustic and corrosive, results in severe inflammatory reactions, including blistering of the skin on contact. Many of these plants are tropical, although a number are widely cultivated (Table 3-3).

A characteristic of several of these irritant plant families is their milky or yellowish latex, usually found throughout the plant. Although some latex-possessing plants are harmless, a majority cause either irritant or contact dermatitis, and as a general precaution they all should be avoided. Apart from dermatitis, a hazard to those who prune or tend horticultural varieties, is the eye damage and blindness that can result from contact between the eye and the caustic sap.

Several of these irritant factors have been characterized. Members of the Brassicaceae contain sinigrin; this glucoside is harmless if dried, but it can be converted into an irritant mustard oil in the presence of water. A decomposition product of another glucoside, anemonin,

has been isolated from the buttercup (*Ranunculus*) and produces blisters on the face and around the lips of children who may chew the leaves or stems of injured plants. Furthermore, the pineapple (*Ananas comosus,* Bromeliaceae) possesses a proteolytic enzyme, bromelain, which causes separation of the superficial layers of the skin and increases skin and capillary permeability in a manner not unlike that found in the allergic wheal and flare reaction.

PHOTODERMATITIS

Photosensitization contact dermatitis is often caused by plants containing photosensitizing compounds related to furocoumarin.[25] After exposure to the appropriate furocoumarin in the plant, followed by exposure to ultraviolet radiation of a wavelength greater than 3200 Å (usually sunlight), the characteristic sunburnlike rash develops. For example, contact with *Phebalium argentium* (Rutaceae) leaves produces an erythematous blush within 24 hours and a blister by 48 hours. After healing, a white atrophic-looking area remains surrounded by a ring of dark brown pigment, leaving a recognizable area on the skin for years. Phototoxic reactions also occur in patients on sulfonamide therapy as well as in up to 40% of individuals that have received large doses of the tetracycline, declomycin.

Not all plant products known to be photosensitizing have been categorized as either phototoxic or photoallergic, although those containing the furocoumarins are considered phototoxic. Phototoxic reactions occur in most individuals by activation of such substances as the furocoumarins by photons, resulting in free radical formation that leads, by means of photochemical reactions, to cell damage, characteristic erythema, and bulla formation. Most of these compounds are tricyclic resonating aromatic

Table 3-3   Plants Primarily Responsible for Irritant Dermatitis

ANNONACEAE
   Annona (blindness from juice of crushed seeds)
APOCYNACEAE
   Plumeria,[a] corrosive juice often milky or yellowish
ARACEAE (calcium oxalate crystals and/or irritant, acrid sap)
   Alocasia (giant elephant's ear), *Arisaema* (jack-in-the-pulpit), *Arum* (lords-and-ladies), *Caladium*, *Colocasia*, *Dieffenbachia* (dumbcane), *Monstera*, *Philodendron*, *Xanthosoma* (elephant's ear)
ARALIACEAE
   Aralia (devil's walking stick), irritant hairs
BORAGINACEAE
   Cynoglossum (hound's tongue), irritant hairs
BRASSICACEAE (irritant oils)[a]
   Brassica
BROMELIACEAE
   Ananas (pineapple), proteolytic enzyme
CAMPANULACEAE
   Isotoma, milky latex
CAPPARIDACEAE
   Crataeva, blistering sap
CARICACEAE
   Carica (papaya)[b], latex
ELAEOCARPACEAE
   Sloanea, irritant bristles
EUPHORBIACEAE (irritant hairs)
   Cnidoscolus (spurge nettle), *Dalechampia*, *Jatropha*, *Tragia*
FABACEAE
   Acacia (bull horn), thorns harboring stinging ants, *Mucuna* (cowitch), proteolytic enzyme from hairs
HYDROPHYLLACEAE
   Wigandia, irritant hairs

LAMIACEAE
   Leonotis (hollowstalk), leaf
LILIACEAE
   Allium (garlic)[a], juice blistering, *Hyacinthus* (hyacinth), calcium oxalate crystals, *Narcissus* (daffodil, jonquil, narcissus), calcium oxalate crystals
LOASACEAE
   Gronovia (pica-pica), stinging hairs, *Loasa*, stinging hairs
MORACEAE
   Cecropia, harboring stinging ants, *Maclura* (Osage orange)[a], milky latex
MORINGACEAE
   Moringa, crushed leaves
PAPAVERACEAE (sap, often yellowish)
   Chelidonium (celandine poppy),[a] *Dicentra* (bleeding heart),[a] *Sanguinaria* (bloodroot)[a]
POACEAE (irritant bristles)
   Bambusa vulgaris, *Guadua*
POLYGONACEAE (crushed leaves and stems)
   Polygonum (smartweed), *Rumex* (dock)[a]
RANUNCULACEAE (sap)
   Ranunculus (buttercup)
SAPOTACEAE (milky sap)
   Calocarpum, *Manilkara*
SOLANACEAE (irritant spines)
   Capsicum frutescens (bird or wild pepper), *Solanum* (buffalo bur, horse nettle)
STERCULIACEAE (irritant hairs in fruit)
   Sterculia (Panama tree)
THYMELAEACEAE (sap)
   Daphne, *Dirca* (leatherwood)
URTICACEAE (stinging hairs or spines with caustic irritant)
   Fleurya, *Hesperocnide* (western stinging nettle), *Laportea* (wood nettle), *Urera*, *Urtica* (stinging nettle)
VITACEAE
   Cissus, juice of fruit

[a] Reaction is probably, in part, contact dermatitis.
[b] Used in meat tenderizing.

compounds that are not particularly reactive and have a molecular weight of about 200–500.

In genetically predisposed individuals, photoreactivation of the photosensitizing molecule of photoallergen causes the formation of a new substance, a photohapten. The conjugation of the photohapten with suitable proteins in the skin produces a complete photoantigen that elicits spongiosis and intradermal vesicle formation characteristic of allergic contact dermatitis (see Delayed Hypersensitivity in the following section).

This group is characterized by a halogenated phenol, coupled with another halogenated aromatic ring that is sometimes also hydroxylated. Photoallergy differs from phototoxicity reaction in several respects. Not only are these reactions rarer, the amount required to elicit the response is smaller, as well. Often the same substance can produce ordinary contact allergic dermatitis in the absence of light, and cross-sensitization between immunologically related substances has been demonstrated. Flareups can also occur at unexposed sites distant from the area of initial contact. In all cases, an incubation period is required before photoallergy is elicited. Ragweed oleoresin is a known plant photoallergen.

Not many plant families contain species with these photosensitizing compounds. In man they include the Fabaceae, Moraceae, Clusiaceae, Chenopodiaceae, Rosaceae, Ranunculaceae, and the Liverwort genus *Frullania,* but the compounds are most widespread in the families Apiaceae and Rutaceae (Table 3-4).[26] Photosensitivity reactions in animals are caused by a host of other plants including many grasses (Bermuda grass, oats, sorghum), legumes (alfalfa, alsike clover), and others.[27]

Table 3-4   Higher Plants that Provoke Photodermatitis in Man

Family and Species	Vernacular Name
APIACEAE	
Ammi majus	Artrillal
Anethum graveolens	Dill
Angelica spp.	Angelica
Apium graveolens	Celery
Daucus carota	Carrot
Foeniculum vulgare	Fennel
Heracleum spp.	Giant hogweed, cow parsnip
Pastinaca sativa	Parsnip
Peucedanum spp.	Masterwort
CLUSIACEAE. *Hypericum* spp.	St. John's wort
BRASSICACEAE. *Brassica* spp.	Mustard
FABACEAE. *Psoralea corylifolia*	Bavachi
CHENOPODIACEAE. *Chenopodium* spp.	Goosefoot
MORACEAE. *Ficus carica*	Fig
RANUNCULACEAE. *Ranunculus* spp.	Buttercup
ROSACEAE. *Agrimonia eupatoria*	Agrimony
RUTACEAE	
Dictamnus albus	Gas plant
Citrus spp.	Bergamot, lime, sour orange
Phebalium argenteum	
Ruta graveolens	Common rue

CELLULAR—MEDIATED (DELAYED TYPE) HYPERSENSITIVITY (TYPE IV)

Delayed hypersensitivity may take days or weeks to develop; often prolonged contact with an antigen is necessary, and the reaction depends on the formation of specifically modified lymphocytes from the thymus-dependent series (T cells). Through specific receptors or other mechanisms, these cells are capable of responding specifically to antigens deposited at a local site and also of mobilizing nonsensitized phagocytic cells to localize there and participate with them in tissue destruction. Unlike immediate hypersensitivity, a reaction is not apparent for 12–24 hours, when inflammation and necrosis appear in the affected area.

To test for contact hypersensitivity, the candidate allergen is usually applied as a patch to the unbroken skin and observed for 24 hours for characteristic changes. The results of attempts to provoke tolerance by deliberate desensitization through administration of repeated injection of antigen are often short-lived and frequently precipitate severe allergic reactions.

Substances of plant origin or chemicals including heavy metals can act as haptens to mediate a delayed hypersensitivity response after prolonged or repeated contact with the skin. Sensitization is dependent on attachment of the chemical to the structural proteins of the skin, which results in a change of the skin proteins. Alone or through release of substances from epidermal cells, this type of antigenic alteration can stimulate a specific inflammatory response that produces, after 24–48 hours, symptoms of pruritis, burning or stinging, erythematous macules, papules, vesicles, exudation, and crusting.

The sensitizing substances of most plants are found in the oleoresin fraction, which includes volatile oils, resins, and balsams (Table 3-5). Occasionally, water glycosides and other aqueous fractions may be the sensitizing materials.

The most dangerous examples are members of the Anacardiaceae, which are widespread throughout North America and Asia. It has been estimated that at least 70% of the population of the United States would acquire *Toxicodendron* dermatitis on casual exposure to poison oak, poison ivy, or poison sumac. Prolonged exposure would probably render even more of the population sensitive. These plants also have been known to elicit severe reactions in the oral cavity and gastrointestinal tract if ingested, and in the respiratory tract, if inhaled. The active principle is an oleoresin (urushiol), which

Table 3-5 Plants Causing Contact Dermatitis

Chemical Classification	Primary Component	Family and Species	Comments
VOLATILE (ESSENTIAL) OILS			
Hydrocarbons			
Terpenes			
Acyclic	Myrcene	CANNABACEAE *Humulus lupulus* (hops)	Lupulin (glandular hairs)
Monocyclic	Limonene	APIACEAE *Anethum graveolens* (dill) *Apium graveolens* (celery) *Carum carvi* (caraway) RUTACEAE *Citrus* spp. (peels of bitter orange, lemon, lime; bergamot)	Also ketone carvone Neroli oil, orange flower oil; also terpene alcohols and aldehydes
	Phellandrene	BURSERACEAE *Canarium luzonicum* (elemi oil) LAMIACEAE *Mentha spicata* (spearmint) LAURACEAE *Cinnamomum zeylanicum* (cinnamon)	Also limonene, pinene, ketone, and alcohols

Table 3-5 (Continued)

Chemical Classification	Primary Component	Family and Species	Comments
		PINACEAE	
		Abies balsamea (balsam fir)	Canada balsam oil
Dicyclic	Pinene	PINACEAE	
		Pinus spp. (pine) and other Gymnosperms	Chief component of turpentine oil
Sesquiterpenes	Cadinene		
	Selinene		
	Zingiberene		
Alcohols (acyclic, terpene, and sesquiterpene alcohols)	Geraniol	GERANIACEAE	
		Pelargonium odoratissimum	
	Linalool	BURSERACEAE	
		Bursera aloexylon	Linaloe
		APIACEAE	
		Coriandrum sativum	Coriander oil
	Citronellol	MYRTACEAE	
		Eucalyptus citriodora (lemon-scented gum)	
		ROSACEAE	
		Rosa alba, R. centifolia, R. damascena, R. gallica	Rose oil
		GERANIACEAE	
		Pelargonium odoratissimum, P. radula	Geranium oil
	Borneol	ZINGIBERACEAE	
		Elettaria cardamomum	Cardamon seed
	Santalol (sesquiterpene)	SANTALACEAE	
		Santalum album (sandalwood)	
Aldehydes	Citral (geranial)	POACEAE	
		Cymbopogon nardus	Citronella oil
	Citronellal	*C. nardus*	Citronella oil
Ketones	Camphor	ASTERACEAE	
		Blumea balsamifera (Ngai camphor), *Chrysanthemum parthenium* (feverfew)	
		DIPTEROCARPACEAE	
		Dryobalanops aromatica (Borneo camphor)	Borneol
		LAURACEAE	
		Cinnamomum camphora	Camphor
	Carvone	LAMIACEAE	
		Mentha spicata, M. cardiaca (spearmints)	Spearmint oil also contains terpenes, alcohol
		APIACEAE	
		Carum carvi	Caraway oil also contains terpene limonene
	Irone	IRIDACEAE	
		Iris germanica, I. pallida	Orris oil

Table 3-5 (Continued)

Chemical Classification	Primary Component	Family and Species	Comments
	Pulegone	LAMIACEAE	
		Hedeoma pulegioides	Pennyroyal oil
	Thujone	ASTERACEAE	
		Artemisia absinthium (wormwood)	Absinthe oil
		Tanacetum vulgare (tansy)	Many essential oils isolated
Phenols	Anethole	APIACEAE	
		Foeniculum vulgare	Fennel oil, also contains ketones and terpenes
	Eugenol	MYRTACEAE	
		Eugenia caryophyllus	Clove oil
	Safrole	LAURACEAE	
		Sassafras albidum	Sassafras oil (80% safrole) suspected of contact dermatitis
	Thymol	LAMIACEAE	
		Thymus vulgaris	Thyme oil also includes terpenes and alcohols
Oxides	Ascaridol	CHENOPODIACEAE	
		Chenopodium ambrosioides var. *anthelminticum* (wormseed)	Chenopodium oil suspected of contact dermatitis
	Cineole (eucalyptol)	MYRTACEAE	
		Eucalyptus globulus	Eucalyptus oil
		Melaleuca leucadendron	Cajuput oil
		LAMIACEAE	
		Rosmarinus officinalis	Rosemary oil
Lactones (many sesquiterpenes)		LIVERWORT	
		Frullania nisquallensis	Perhaps also due to usnic acid
		ASTERACEAE (tribes Anthemideae, Helenieae, Heliantheae)	
		Ambrosia (ragweed)	
		Anthemis (chamomile)	
		Arctium (burdock)	
		Artemisia (mugwort, sagebrush, wormwood)	
		Chrysanthemum	
		Cynara (artichoke)	
		Eupatorium (boneset)	
		Gaillardia	
		Helenium (sneezeweed)	
		Tagetes (marigold)	
		Xanthium (cocklebur)	
Quinones	Primin	PRIMULACEAE	
		Primula obconica (primrose)	Glandular hairs, the head containing the irritant primin
	Thymoquinone	CUPRESSACEAE	
		Libocedrus decurrens (California incense cedar)	

Table 3-5   (Continued)

Chemical Classification	Primary Component	Family and Species	Comments
RESINS AND RESIN COMBINATIONS			
Oleoresins	Urushiol (containing 3-pentadecylcatechol)	ANACARDIACEAE *Anacardium melan-orrhoea* (rengas tree), *A. occidentale* (cashew) *Comocladia dodonaea* (Christmas bush) *Mangifera indica* (mango) *Metopium toxiferum* (coral sumac, poison wood) *Schinus molle* (Brazil pepper-tree), *S. tere-binthifolius* *Toxicodendron diversi-lobium* (western poison oak), *T. radicans* (poison ivy), *T. rydbergii* (Rydberg's poison ivy), *T. toxicarium* (eastern poison oak), *T. vernix* (poison sumac)[a]	
	Capsaicin	SOLANACEAE *Capsicum frutescens* (capsicum or Cayenne pepper)	
	Asafoetida	APIACEAE *Ferula* spp.	Gum asafetida
OLEORESINS (pollen dermatitis)		*Acer* (box elder, maple) *Ambrosia* (ragweed) *Erigeron* (mare's tail) *Fraxinus* (ash) *Iva* (Marsh elder) *Mangifera* (mango) *Populus* (poplar) *Ulmus* (elm) *Xanthium* (cocklebur)	
Balsams	Benzoin (benzoresin)	STYRACACEAE *Styrax benzoin* and other spp.	Friar's balsam; also benzoic, cinnamic, and balsamic acids
	Cinnamein	FABACEAE *Myroxylon pereirae* (Peruvian balsam)	Also resin esters, vanillin (aldehyde), etc.
	Resin esters	*M. balsamum* (Tolu balsam)	
	Storesin	HAMAMELIDACEAE *Liquidambar orientalis* (Oriental sweet gum)	Levant storax
		L. styraciflua (American sweet gum)	Cinnamic acid, cinnamein, resin esters

[a] For the monographic treatment of *Toxicodendron*, see Gillis.[28]

85

contains catechols and other phenolic resins and acts as a powerful hapten; and its persistence in the necrotic blister contributes a source for further irritation and initiation of new lesions. Its presence in all parts of the plant, and its stability in dead and dried parts, makes these plants as hazardous in the winter as in the summer. Furthermore, the oleoresin may be carried to sensitive individuals through smoke, dust, contaminated articles, and the hair of animals.

The greatest hazard are plants that are introduced beyond their native range and become aggressive weeds. Farm workers are especially vulnerable, and contact with such plants can cause severe and prolonged allergic contact dermatitis. Thus, for example, in every part of India where the New World species feverfew (*Parthenium hysterophorus*, Asteraceae) has become widely disseminated, a lichenfied eczema associated with postinflammatory hyperpigmentation and hypopigmentation has reached epidemic proportions. A similar affliction has also been noted among farmers coming in contact with the Mexican marigold (*Tagetes minuta*, Asteraceae), which is common in both southeastern Africa and subtropical America.

Besides the species listed in Table 3-5, many others have been implicated in contact dermatitis, even though for the most part the offending compounds have not been identified. Differentiation between irritant and contact dermatitis is sometimes difficult, as indicated in Table 3-3 (footnote a), and a number of the plants listed below, particularly in the families Apocynaceae and Euphorbiaceae, may in fact possess compounds that are very irritating as well as capable of eliciting an allergic reaction.

ARALIACEAE: *Hedera* (ivy), *Polyscias* (aralia).
APOCYNACEAE (milky latex): *Allamanda*, *Apocynum* (dogbane), *Nerium* (oleander), *Rauvolfia, Rhabdadenia, Thevetia* (yellow oleander).
ASCLEPIADACEAE (milky latex): *Asclepias* (milkweed), *Calotropis* (crown flower), *Cryptostegia*.
BIGNONIACEAE: *Campsis* (trumpet creeper).
BUXACEAE: *Buxus* (boxwood).
COMMELINACEAE: *Rhoeo* (oyster plant), *Setcreasla* (purple queen).
EUPHORBIACEAE (often caustic milky latex): *Codiaeum, Croton, Euphorbia* (Fig. 3-8a: pencil tree, poinsettia, spotted spurge), *Hippomane* (manchineel tree), *Hura* (sandbox tree), *Pedilanthus* (redbird-cactus).
GINKGOACEAE: *Ginkgo* (maidenhair tree).
HYDROPHYLLACEAE: *Phacelia*.
LORANTHACEAE: *Phoradendron* (mistletoe).
MAGNOLIACEAE: *Magnolia*.
MORACEAE: *Cecropia*.
ORCHIDACEAE: *Cypripedium* (ladyslipper).
POACEAE: *Cynodon* (Bermuda grass), *Digitaria* (crab grass), *Secale* (rye: Fig. 3-8b).
RANUNCULACEAE: *Anemone, Clematis, Delphinium* (larkspur).
SALICACEAE: *Populus* (poplar).
SAPINDACEAE: *Sapindus* (soap berry).
SOLANACEAE: *Datura* (jimson weed).
ULMACEAE: *Ulmus* (elm).

Lower plants are also implicated. In addition to the liverwort *Frullania* noted in Table 3-5, usnic acid from Lichens, the alga *Lyngbya majuscula*, phytotoxin from blue-green algal blooms, and topical use of the antibiotics penicillin, streptomycin, and neomycin in particular, have all been implicated in contact dermatitis. The antibiotics have a high sensitization potential and should be avoided.

Therapy depends on the severity of the dermatitis. For mild, localized dermatitis, oral antihistamines and topical corticosteroids can be used. In the acute, inflammatory stage, a soothing application of aluminum acetate (Burow's solution) is helpful. For more severe, generalized involvement, oral corticosteroids given over a 5–10 day period is the treatment of choice (see Chapter 14 for domestic and native remedies).

DRUG SENSITIVITY REACTIONS

Atopy that develops from the therapeutic administration of drugs may take many forms depending on the type of drug involved, the duration of contact, and the method of administration. Moreover, from clinical symptoms it may not always be possible to differentiate between drug toxicity or allergic phenomena.

Penicillin with its antigenic benzyl pen-

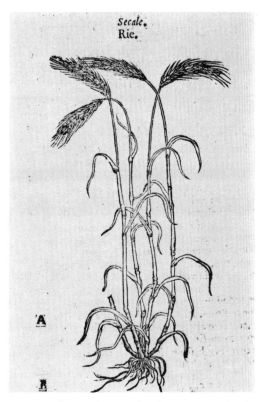

Figure 3-8b *Secale cereale* (from J Gerard, *The Herball,* ed 2, 1636).

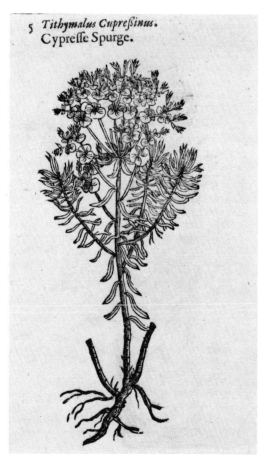

Figure 3-8a *Euphorbia cyparissias* (from J Gerard, *The Herball,* ed 2, 1636).

icilloyl antigenic determinants and other haptenic moieties is perhaps the worst offender, and some type of allergy appears in from 0.5% to 18% of patients using this drug therapeutically. The likelihood of these reactions occurring increases with age, the number of injections, the larger the doses given, and the way it is administered (with a greater risk through injection rather than orally).

Type I reactions are the most common and usually appear shortly after administration as hives (2–48 hours) or generalized anaphylaxis (20 minutes). When large intravenous doses of benzylpenicillin have been given a hemolytic anemia suggestive of a Type II reaction has also been known to develop. The somewhat later appearing (3–5 weeks), maculopapular eruptions are, however, most likely Type III reactions, whereas the delayed cutaneous responses are of Type IV. The cephalosporins with their common 7-amino-cephalosporonic acid nucleus have cross-allergenicity with penicillin and have been known to cause thrombocytopenia, a Type II reaction. Similar Type II reactions have also been reported for quinidine, amidopyrine, chlorpromazine, chloramphenicol, and the sulfonamides. Type IV reactions including maculopapular skin eruptions, fever, and hepatic dysfunction have been associated with sulfonamide therapy as well as in patients receiving para aminosalicylic acid (PAS). Because at least 5% of patients were so afflicted, ethambutol has now replaced PAS in tuberculosis therapy.

In patients with a history of antibiotic hypersensitivity it is not recommended to use the offending drug at all. Too often, allergic symptoms can only become aggravated or life threatening. Nowadays alternatives to penicillin are available that in most instances can be used as a satisfactory substitute without fear of eliciting an allergic response. For symptomatic treatment, antihistamines and corticosteroids are used, and if systemic anaphylaxis occurs, epinephrine is administered. As over two-thirds of the cases of anaphylaxis develop obstructive edema of the respiratory tract, tracheostomy should be considered to prevent death.[3, 29]

LITERATURE CITED

1. Beard GM. 1876. *Hay-Fever; or Summer Catarrh.* New York.

2. *Allergy Defined.* 1972. National Institute of Allergy and Infectious Diseases. Department of Health, Education, & Welfare Publ No (NIH)72-281, Government Printing Office, Washington, DC.

3. Eisen HN. 1973. Immunology, 349–595. In Davis BD, Dulbecco R, Eisen HN et al (eds), *Microbiology,* ed 2. Harper & Row, New York; Good RA, Fisher DW (eds). 1971. *Immunobiology.* Sinauer Associates, Stamford, Conn. 305 p; Gordon BL II, Ford DK. 1971. *Essentials of Immunology.* F. A. Davis Co., Philadelphia. 218 p; Guttmann RD, David JR, Linquist RR et al. (eds), 1970; Sell S. 1975. *Immunology, Immunopathology, and Immunity,* ed 2. Harper & Row, New York, 384 p.; *Scope Monograph on Immunology.* Upjohn Co, Kalamazoo, Mich. 60 p; Wilson D. 1972. *Body and Antibody.* Knopf, New York. 331 p.; Bellanti JH. 1971. *Immunology.* WB Saunders, Philadelphia. 584 p; Roitt I. 1974. *Essential Immunology,* ed 2. Blackwell, Oxford. 260 p.

4. Benner MH, Lee HJ. 1973. Anaphylactic reaction to chamomile tea. *J Allergy Clin Immunol* **52:** 307–308.

5. Berrens L. 1971. *The Chemistry of Atopic Allergens.* Monographs in Allergy, Vol 7. S Krager, Basel, 298 p; Samter M, Durham OC (eds). 1955. *Regional Allergy of the United States, Canada, Mexico and Cuba.* Charles C Thomas, Springfield, Ill. 395 p; Sheldon JM, Lovell RG, Mathew KP. 1967. *A Manual of Clinical Allergy,* ed 2. WB Saunders, Philadelphia. 550 p.

6. Yoo T-J, Spitz E, McGeirity JL. 1974. Allergy to Cupressaceae pollen. *J Allergy Clin Immunol* **53:** 71–72.

7. Wodehouse RP. 1935. *Pollen Grains.* McGraw-Hill, New York. 574 p.

8. Lewis WH. 1976. Pollen exine morphology and its adaptive significance. *Sida* (in press).

9. King TP, Norman PS, Lichtenstein LM. 1967. Studies on ragweed pollen allergens. V. *Ann Allergy* **25:** 541–553; Johnson P, Marsh DG. 1966. Allergens from common rye grass pollen (*Lolium perenne*)—I. *Immunochemistry* **3:** 91–100; Malley A, Reed CE, Lietze A. 1962. Isolation of allergens from timothy pollen. *J Allergy* **33:** 84–93.

10. Lewis WH, Imber WE, Maniotis J. 1975. Allergy epidemiology in the St Louis, Missouri area. I. Fungi. *Ann Allergy* **34:** 374–384.

11. Lewis WH, Imber WE. 1975. Allergy epidemiology in the St Louis, Missouri area. III. Trees. *Ann Allergy* **35:** 113–119.

12. Lewis WH, Imber WE. 1975. Allergy epidemiology in the St Louis, Missouri area. II. Grasses. *Ann Allergy* **35:** 42–50.

13. Lewis WH, Imber WE. 1975. Allergy epidemiology in the St Louis, Missouri area. IV. Weeds. *Ann Allergy* **35:** 180–187.

14. Rhyne MB. 1969. Skin testing: concepts and realities. *Pediatr Clin N Am* **16:** 227–241.

15. Lieberman P, Patterson R, Kunske R. 1972. Complications of long-term steroid therapy for asthma. *J Allergy Clin Immunol* **49:** 329–336; Miyamoto T, Yoshida T, Osawa N et al. 1972. Adrenal response and side reactions after long-term corticosteroid therapy in bronchial asthma. *Ann Allergy* **30:** 587–594.

16. Austen KR, Lichtenstein LM. 1973. *Asthma.* Academic Press, New York and London. 324 p.

17. Eaton KK. 1973. Respiratory allergy to exotic wood dust. *Clin Allergy* **3:** 307–310.

18. Layton L, Panzani R, von Helms LT. 1970. Cross-reactivity in primary respiratory allergy to Castorbean (*Ricinus communis*). *Int Arch Allergy* **37:** 67–75.

19. Ross AF, Mitchell JC. 1974. Respiratory irritation by leaf hairs of the tree *Platanus*. *Ann Allergy* **32:** 94–97.

20. Cohen EP. 1973. New asthma treatment enables sufferers to ward off attacks. *Today's Health* **51**(9): 21–23.

21. Shivpuri DN, Menon MPS, Prakash D. 1969. A crossover double-blind study on *Tylophora indica* in the treatment of asthma and allergic rhinitis. *J Allergy* **43:** 145–150; Shivpuri DN, Agarwal MK. 1973. Effect of *Tylophora indica* on bronchial tolerance to inhalation challenges with specific allergens. *Ann Allergy* **31:** 287–294.

22. Rinkel HJ, Randolph TG, Zeller M. 1951. *Food Allergy.* Charles C Thomas, Springfield, Ill. 492 p.

23. Lewis WH, Imber WE. 1975. Allergy epidemiology in the St. Louis, Missouri area. V. Cereal ingestants. *Ann Allergy* **35:** 251–254.

24. Fisher AA. 1973. *Contact Dermatitis,* ed. 2. Lea & Febiger, Philadelphia. 448 p; Lampe KF, Fagerstrom R. 1968. *Plant Toxicity and Dermatitis.* Williams & Wilkins, Baltimore. 231 p; Weber LF. 1937. External causes of dermatitis. *Arch Dermatol Syphilol* **35:** 129–179; Verhagen AR, Myaga JM. 1974. Contact dermatitis from *Tagetes minuta. Arch Dermatol* **110:** 441–444; Lonkar A, Mitchell JC, Calnan CD. 1974. Contact dermatitis from *Parthenium hysterophorus. Trans St John's Hosp Dermatol Soc* **60:** 43–53.

25. Pathak MA, Farrington D Jr, Fitzpatrick TB. 1962. The presently known distribution of furocoumarins (psoralens) in plants. *J Invest Derm* **39:** 225–239.

26. Van Dijk E, Berrens L. 1964. Plants as an etiological factor in phytophotodermatitis. *Dermatologica* **129:** 321–328.

27. Kingsbury JM. 1964. *Poisonous Plants of the United States and Canada.* Prentice-Hall, Englewood Cliffs, NJ. 626 p.

28. Gillis WT. 1971. The systematics and ecology of Poison-ivy and of Poison-oaks (*Toxicodendron,* Anacardiaceae). *Rhodora* **73:** 72–159, 161–237, 370–443, 465–540.

29. Armstrong D, Grieco MH, Louria DB and Smith L. (eds). 1975. *Infectious Diseases: Diagnosis and Treatment.* Medcom Press, New York, NY. 307 p.

Chapter 4

Cell Modifiers: Mutagens, Teratogens, and Lectins

Poke or pokeberry (*Phytolacca americana*) (Fig. 4-1) has long been a favorite spring potherb in the southern United States. The young leaves and stems are boiled, usually twice, and eaten as a green vegetable, like spinach. Occasionally a few young leaves are added to salads at this time of year to give a tang to otherwise bland, predominantly iceberg lettuce, fare. In southern Missouri, for example, poke is planted in rows as a part of perennial vegetable gardens to ensure the availability of sufficient leaves for use throughout the spring and into the summer. Others remove the plants from flower beds and waste areas from spring until fall. Difficult to eradicate because of a long perennial taproot, these weeds are a constant annoyance to the fastidious gardener.

There are about 20 species of *Phytolacca,* cosmopolitan in distribution but principally found in warmer regions, and many of us are exposed internally as well as externally to the toxic principles found throughout these plants. Fortunately cooking, properly done, destroys phytolaccatoxin, and apparently the young growth has little toxin present; but apart from potential dangers of poisoning (Chapter 2), poke present a much more

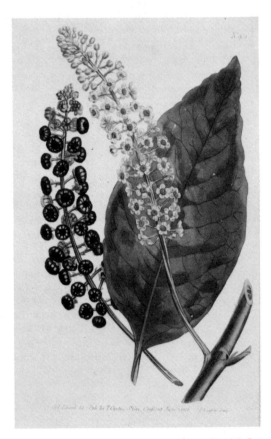

Figure 4-1 *Phytolacca americana* (from *Curtis's Botanical Magazine* **24:** 931, 1806).

insidious risk to our health. The plants possess mitogens, compounds that can be absorbed through skin abrasions, causing serious blood aberrations. *Phytolacca* species should not be handled except with caution and one should always wear gloves.

The details of plant products affecting animal cells are discussed as mutagéns, teratogens, and lectins including mitogens.

MUTAGENS

If a drug produced heritable alterations in reproductive cells (gametes), the constitution of the new individual formed from such gametes would be altered. Permanent changes in the genotype (i.e., mutations) are produced by radiation and/or by chemical agents, which are known as mutagens. There is a growing concern that in addition to a spontaneous low-level degree of mutation, presumably carried out in all species, man is unknowingly and increasingly exposed to many potential mutagens in his environment. As we continue to synthesize additional potential mutagens, of which certain amounts will contaminate the environment, this hazard will undoubtedly become greater. Irreversible mutations that accumulate from generation to generation, through exposure to environmental mutagens, are serious enough to direct attention to the causes of mutation, and the detection of mutagenic agents before they are released into our environment.

KINDS OF MUTATION

1. Basic nucleotide compounds of DNA (adenine, guanine, cytosine, thymine) can each be replaced, for example, the original guanine replaced by another guanine. This transformation would be the smallest and least dramatic of potential mutations.

2. More drastic would be the loss or addition of nucleotides from the DNA molecule so that replication of genetic material would be profoundly disturbed.

3. Alterations of the genotype may occur at all levels. Thus whole molecules of DNA and observable segments of chromosomes may be deleted, inverted, or exchanged. Many such mutations are lethal to cells.

4. Nondisjunction of chromosomes gives rise to unequal numbers of chromosomes in cells following either mitosis or meiosis; this often occurs following spindle fiber disturbance. The consequence of such aneuploidy may be drastic; the addition of a third chromosome 21 in our karyotype for instance results in mongolism.

5. Polyploidy or an increase in whole sets of chromosomes, usually following spindle fiber disturbances, is a widespread heritable mutation in plants that has been instrumental in the explosive speciation among Angiosperms.

MUTAGENS IN MAN AND OTHER ANIMALS

Mutations give rise to inherited effects only in the germ line. Therefore the hazards of mutagenesis normally concern young populations, and the period of youth on the average lasts about 30 reproductive years. The number of chromosomal replications leading to the sex cells varies markedly, however, between male (950 times) and female (70 times) over a generation.[1] In the male, the risk of agents acting on replication DNA or on the mitotic and meiotic processes spans the entire reproductive life, but in the female these effects occur primarily during fetal life when oocytes are differentiating, and only secondarily during the limited number of meiotic divisions as the ova are formed. Clearly, the potential hazard from mutated male gametes is far greater than the danger from females.

Known mutagens in domestic and experimental animals (Table 4-1) include

Table 4-1   Mutagens and Teratogens of Plant Origin

Major Plant Group/ Major Chemical Classification	Active Compound	Mutagen	Teratogen	Plant
BACTERIA				
"Antibiotic"	Actinomycin D		×	Streptomyces antibioticus, S. chrysomallus
	Azaserine	×		Streptomyces fragilis
	Chromomycin		×	Streptomyces griseus, S. olivochromogenes
	Daunomycin	×		Streptomyces peuceticus
	Mitomycin C	×	×	Streptomyces caespitosus
	Phleomycin	×	×	Streptomyces verticillatus
	Streptomycin		×	Streptomyces griseus, S. bikiniensis, S. olivaceus, S. mashuensis, etc.
	Streptonigrin	×	×	Streptomyces flocculus
	Streptozoticin	×		Streptomyces achromogenes
	Tetracycline		×	Streptomyces aureofaciens, S. viridifaciens, S. feofaciens, etc.
"Infection"			×	Treponema pallidum (syphilis)
FUNGI				
"Aflatoxin"	Aflatoxin B$_1$[a,b] (and 7 others)	×	×	Aspergillus flavus, A. parasiticus; Penicillium puberulum
"Antibiotic"	Patulin[a]	×		Aspergillus clavatus, A. claviforme; Penicillium espansum, P. leucopus, P. meliniis, P. patulum
	Penicillin		×	Penicillium notatum
Indole alkaloid	Lysergic acid diethylamide (LSD)	×?	×?	Claviceps purpurea (ergot)
GYMNOSPERM				
Glycoside	Cycasin[a,b]	×	×	Cycas circinalis, C. revoluta
ANGIOSPERMS				
Alkaloids				
Amine	Colchicine	×	×[c]	Colchicum autumnale (autumn crocus)

Table 4-1 (Continued)

Major Plant Group/ Major Chemical Classification	Active Compound	Mutagen	Teratogen	Plant
	Mescaline		×	*Lophophora williamsii* (peyote)
Imidazole	Pilocarpine		×	*Pilocarpus* spp.
Indole	Reserpine		×	*Rauvolfia serpentina*
	Vinblastine, vincristine		×	*Catharanthus roseus* (periwinkle)
Isoquinoline	D-Tubocurarine		×	*Chondodendron tomentosum*
Purine	Caffeine		×	*Coffea* (coffees), *Cola* (cola nuts), *Camellia sinensis* (tea), *Ilex paraguaensis* (maté), *Theobroma cacao* (chocolate)
Pyridine	Nicotine	×	×	*Nicotiana tabacum* (tobacco ingestion and possibly smoking)
Pyrrolizidine	Heliotrine, lasiocarpine, retrosine[a,b]	×	×	*Amsinckia* (fiddleneck or tarweed), *Crotalaria* (rattlebox), *Senecio* (groundsel or ragwort)
Quinoline	Quinine		×[d]	*Cinchona* spp.
Quinolizidine	Cytisine		×	*Sophora stenophylla*
Steroidal	Anagyrine		×	*Lupinus caudatus* (lupine)
	Cyclobuxine		×	*Buxus sempervirens* (boxwood)
	Cyclopamine, cycloposine, jervine		×	*Veratrum californicum* (false hellebore)
	Malouetine		×	*Malouetia bequaertiana*
Amino acids	Aminonitriles		×	?*Astragalus pubentissimus* (locoweed), *Lathyrus odoratus* (sweet pea), ?*Oxytropis muricata*
	Indospicine		×	*Indigofera spicata* (creeping indigo)
	Mimosine		×	*Leucaena leucocephala*
Carbohydrates	Ethyl alcohol		×	Fermentation by yeasts of sugars from grapes, grains, etc.
	Sucrose		×[e]	*Beta vulgaris* (sugar beet), *Saccharum officinarum* (sugar cane), and other sources
Corticosteroid			×[d]	Cortisone (derived from *Dioscorea*)
Glycosides	?Amygdalin (hydrolyzes to HCN)		×	*Prunus serotina* (wild black cherry)

Table 4-1   (Continued)

Major Plant Group/ Major Chemical Classification	Active Compound	Mutagen	Teratogen	Plant
	Sinigrin (yielding allylisothiocyanate)	×		*Brassica carinata* (Ethiopian mustard), *B. nigra* (black mustard), *B. oleracea* (broccoli, brussel sprouts, cabbage, cauliflower, kale, etc.); *Armoracia rusticana* (horseradish); *Sinapis alba* (white mustard), *S. arvensis* (charlock)
Phytotoxin	Ricin		×	*Ricinus communis* (castor bean)
Resin	Podophyllotoxin		×[c]	*Podophyllum peltatum* (May apple) and many other plants
Vitamins	A, B$_{12}$, and C deficiencies		×	
	D excess		×[d]	
Volatile oils Aldehyde	Citronellal	×		*Citrus limon* (lemon); *Cymbopogon citratus* and *C. flexuosus* (sources of lemongrass oil), *C. nardus* (source of citronella oil); *Eucalyptus citriodora, Melissa officinalis* (common balm)

[a] Also known to be carcinogenic (for others see Chapter 5, Cancer).
[b] Also known to be hepatotoxic.
[c] Mitotic poison that kills fetuses selectively but is not necessarily teratogenic for survivors; besides these there are apomorphine, camphor, coumarin, emetine, papaverine, penicillin, quinine, and vinblastine.
[d] Known or suspected under particular circumstances to be mutagenic or teratogenic in man.
[e] Sucrose is also known to stimulate somatic mutations (aneuploidy and polyploidy) in plants.[4]

aflatoxins and antibiotics of fungal origin, and glycosides, alkaloids, and volatile oils from flowering plants.[2] Very little is known about mutagenicity in man. However ethyl alcohol and nicotine are mutagenic in various organisms, and since humanity is exposed to these compounds in large amounts over long periods of time, the mutagenic effects they might have are worthy of speculation. Likewise, we consume large quantities of the alkaloid caffeine in coffee, tea, chocolate, and soft drinks. The substance is known to be mutagenic in bacteria, fungi, higher plants, fruit flies, mice, and human cells *in vitro*. Its effect on man is equivocal,[3] but some researchers believe that caffeine may prove to be one of the most dangerous mutagens, particularly among males.

TERATOGENS

Chemical compounds can have effects on the somatic cells of growing embryos that produce defects of organ systems. Usually the individual alone is affected; thus most congenital abnormalities are not inherited. Many factors cause defects in embryos at doses not producing serious maternal toxicity or disturbance of placental function. For example, vitamin deficiencies or mild virus diseases such as rubella during pregnancy may be sufficient to cause irreparable damage to the fetus during a critical gestation period.

Congenital malformations in human populations have been recognized since prehistoric times.[5] They were once attributed to divine or satanic intervention, to hybridization with other species, or to frightening experiences during pregnancy. There is still much irrationality toward congenital deformity, a tragedy of human life far greater than spontaneous abortions and stillbirths.

The most horrifying example of congenital abnormaltiy in humans occurred following the introduction of the synthetic compound thalidomide in the late 1950s in Europe and elsewhere. It was an effective tranquilizing agent and hypnotic, and seemingly nontoxic. Among numerous clinical trials before release of the drug was a series of attempts to induce congenital abnormalities in rabbits, but the results were negative. Shortly after the introduction of thalidomide in Hamburg, Germany, however, there were a surprising number of infants born with phocomelia, a shortening or absence of limbs. Not a single case had been seen from 1949–1959; but in 1959 there was one case, in 1960 there were 30 reports, and 154 cases appeared in 1961. In all instances pregnant women had taken thalidomide between the third and eighth week of pregnancy, often in very small doses. It has subsequently been found that when thalidomide is taken 35 to 36 days after the last menstrual period (about 21–22 days of gestation), the embryos fail to develop external ears and paralysis of cranial nerves occur. Three to five days later, the phocomelia effect is at its maximum, and this is a time during which many expectant mothers are unaware of their pregnancy.

Thalidomide was withdrawn from the market late in 1961. Fortunately, it was never approved for use in the United States, but elsewhere the number of deformed offspring related to the use of this drug is estimated at 10,000.

Besides thalidomide, what are the chemical teratogens whose activities are so accentuated during the first trimester of pregnancy? They are numerous and they are diverse enough to signal caution whenever a drug is administered to a woman of childbearing age, a woman known to be pregnant during this period should never be given such medication unless the need is pressing. Among the compounds known and suspected of teratogenesis in man and other animals (Table 4-17), the antibiotics from fungi and the alkaloids from flowering plants predominate. The activity of a number of these in man include the following effects.

Antibiotics.[6] From *Actinomyces* and *Streptomyces*—infant malformations.

Aspirin.[7] Higher percentage of defective offspring delivered by mothers taking salicylate preparations during the first trimester than by those who did not.

Corticosteroids and cortisone.[8] Base material mostly *Dioscorea* (yams) and other plants—low incidence of cleft palate; see also cyclopamine from *Veratrum californicum* (Table 4-1), which includes cyclopia in ewes.

LSD (lysergic acid diethylamide).[9] Prepared from lysergic acid obtained from *Claviceps purpurea* (ergot) but not known to occur naturally—there is probably no direct relationship between the use of LSD and teratogenesis.

Quinine.[10] Alkaloid from *Cinchona*—implicated in visual and auditory defects including congenital deafness; also directly neurotoxic to the eighth cranial nerve.

The reader is referred to the discussions and references in Goldstein et al.,[1] the catalog by Shepard,[11] and the reviews on the effects of teratogens in man[12] and animals[13] for further details.

Individual drugs may be harmful, but what are the results of combining them? Interaction between teratogenic agents in the rat is well illustrated by the effects individually of cortisone (abnormality absent) and X-rays (5.2% abnormality); when combined, the level of defects reached 18.8%.[14] This synergism was even more pronounced in mice . . . and what of man?

Thus genetic factors, such as a predisposition to teratogenesis (e.g., differing percentage of cleft palates in offspring of mouse strains treated with cortisone[15]), may account for about 20% of congenital defects; perhaps 20% occur following accidental exposure to teratogens; and about 60% of the abnormalities among the unborn are due to the combined effects of chemical teratogens and individual genetic composition.

LECTINS (INCLUDING MITOGENS)[16]

When certain vegetable proteins known as lectins contact functional cell membrane glycoproteins bearing polysaccharide side chains, they can combine to form bridges between cells, causing agglutination *in vivo*; they can induce preferential killing of tumor (transformed) cells; and when also acting as mitogens, they can stimulate B and T lymphoid cells to divide and mature. Furthermore, their mitogenic activity may

be reversed by appropriate saccharide inhibitors,[18] if applied for a critical period before the final events of mitogenesis occur. Plants containing lectins are listed in Table 4-2. Lectins have also been found in certain invertebrate species, viruses, and bacteria, and they are used experimentally to define the composition of cell surface carbohydrates.[19] Such studies involve the microanalysis of cell surface components used to understand the differences between normal and malignant cells, to evaluate ontogenic changes taking place during development, and to study immunochemical interactions at cell surfaces.[20]

Those lectins that are mitogenic are nonspecific in that they are able to stimulate transformation of immunologically competent cells in nonsensitized hosts; however they are selective in their ability to trigger T and B cell differentiation and often are used in this way to identify T or B cell types within a population. For example, T cells respond to the phytohemagglutinin (PHA) from the kidney bean, *Phaseolus vulgaris* (Fig. 4-2a), the solubilized form of concanavalin A (Con-A) from the jack bean, *Canavalia ensiformis,* as well as mitogens isolated from the lentil, *Lens culinaris* (Fig. 4-2b), and *Wisteria floribunda.* Since stimulation of B cells occurs only when Con-A and PHA proteins are insolubilized and are attached to large particles, such as Sephadex beads, mitogenesis may be triggered by cell surface events not requiring transport of the mitogen into the cell cytoplasm. B cells are also stimulated by the tuberculin skin testing purified protein derivative (PPD) of *Mycobacterium tuberculosis* cultures and by lipopolysaccharide endotoxin of Gram negative bacteria whose lipid moiety binds to lipids of the lymphocytic membrane. However, a broader range of cell-stimulating activity has been attributed to certain cyclopropenoid fatty

Table 4-2 Plants with Lectinic (Including Mitogenic) Properties

Organism	Vernacular Name	Principal Specificity[a]
FUNGI		
Agaricus bisporus, A. campestris[b]		Sialoglycoprotein
ANGIOSPERMS: DICOTYLEDONS		
Phylogenetic Group 3		
PHYTOLACCACEAE. *Phytolacca americana* (and other spp.) (PWM)[b]	Poke	
CHENOPODIACEAE		
Bassia decurrens[b]		
Rhagodia crassifolia[b]		
AMARANTHACEAE. *Amaranthus caudatus*	Inca wheat	β-D-Galp[d]
Phylogenetic Group 4		
BRASSICACEAE. *Iberis* spp.		anti-M (RBC site)
ERICACEAE. *Gaultheria procumbens*[b,c]	Wintergreen	
Phylogenetic Group 5		
CUCURBITACEAE. *Momordica charantia*	Balsam pear	Polysaccharide
Phylogenetic Group 6		
STERCULIACEAE. *Sterculia foetida* (sterculic acid)[b]		
MORACEAE. *Maclura pomifera*	Osage orange	D-Galactosyl-
EUPHORBIACEAE. *Ricinus communis*	Castor bean	D-Galactosyl-
Phylogenetic Group 7		
FABACEAE		
Subf. CAESALPINIOIDEAE		
Griffonia (Bandeiracea) simplicifolia		Mono- and oligosaccharides
Bauhinia carronii[b]	Queensland bean tree	
B. purpurea	Camel's foot tree	β-D-Galp
Subf. FABOIDEAE		
Abrus precatorius	Rosary pea	Polysaccharide
Arachis hypogaea	Peanut or groundnut	β-D-Galp, anti-T (RBC site)
Canavalia ensiformis (Con-A)[b]	Jack bean	α-D-Mannose
Crotalaria juncea	Sunn or san hemp	Polysaccharide
Cytisus sessilifolium	Broom	Mono- and oligosaccharides
Dolichos biflorus		α-D-GalpNAc, anti-A_1 (RBC site)
Glycine max (Soja hispida)	Soybean	D-Galactosyl-
Lathyrus odoratus[b]	Sweet pea	Polysaccharide
Lens culinaris[b]	Lentil	α-D-Mannose, sialoglycoprotein
Lotus tetragonolobus	Winged pea	α-L-Fucosyl-
Phaseolus lunatus	Lima bean	Glycoprotein, anti-A (RBC site)
P. vulgaris (PHA)[b]	Kidney or common bean	β-D-Galp

Table 4-2 (Continued)

Organism	Vernacular Name	Principal Specificity[a]
Pisum sativum	Garden pea	Mono- and oligosaccharides
Robinia pseudo-acacia	Black locust	Sialoglycoprotein
Sophora japonica	Japanese pagoda tree	Glycoprotein
Ulex europaeus	Gorse	α-L-Fucosyl-, anti-H (RBC site)
Vicia cracca	Gerard vetch	α-D-GalpNAc
V. graminea	Vetch	β-D-Galp, anti-N (RBC site)
Wisteria floribunda[b]	Japanese wisteria	
W. sinensis[b]	Chinese wisteria	D-Galactosyl-
Phylogenetic Group 9		
JUGLANDACEAE. Juglans nigra[b,c]	Black walnut	
Phylogenetic Group 10		
CELASTRACEAE. Euonymus europaeus	Spindle tree	D-Galactosyl-
LORANTHACEAE. Viscum album	European mistletoe	D-Galactosyl-
Phylogenetic Group 11		
SOLANACEAE		
Datura stramonium	Jimson weed	
Solanum tuberosum	Potato	Nondefined hydrophobic bond
LAMIACEAE		
Moluccella laevis		D-Galactosyl-, anti-A + N (RBC site)
Salvia sclarea		anti-Tn (RBC site)
ANGIOSPERMS: MONOCOTYLEDONS		
Phylogenetic Group 14		
POACEAE. Triticum aestivum (WGA)	Common wheat (wheat germ)	Mono- and oligosaccharides

[a] Obtained largely from Kornfeld and Kornfeld (1974),[17] Lis, Lotan, and Sharon (1974),[18] Pardoe (1974).[19]

[b] Known to act as mitogens.

[c] Personal communication from BE Barker and P Farnes, Rhode Island Hospital, Providence.

[d] Galp = galactose pyranosyl-.

acids in *Sterculia foetida* (sterculic and malvalic acids).[21] Both T and B cell mitogenesis can, however, be induced by the mitogen of poke (*Phytolacca americana*). Whenever B cells are mitogen activated, it is possible for them to produce the immunoglobulins for which they are genetically programmed.

The mechanism of mitogen stimulation remains obscure, but the need for a cross-linkage to take place between mitogenic molecules and specific receptor sites on the surface of the molecule has been proposed. Aggregation of such mitogen receptors and connecting trans-membrane-linked, membrane-associated complexes is assumed to be the cell signal for the initiation of various metabolic and transport changes associated with control of cell division, and this results in mitogenesis.

Lectins, particularly mitogenic lectins,

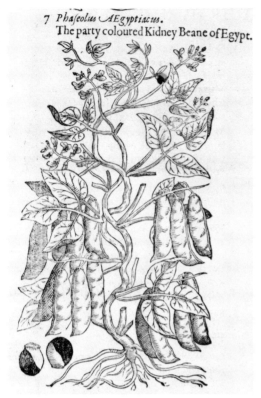

Figure 4-2a *Phaseolus vulgaris* (from J Gerard, *The Herball,* 1597).

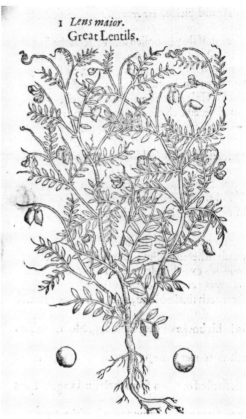

Figure 4-2b *Lens culinaris* (from J Gerard, *The Herball,* 1597).

can also modify a variety of physiological processes of lymphocytes in such a way that cytotoxicity is induced. The abilities to induce mitogenesis and cytotoxicity apparently are not related. Concanavalin A can induce mitogenesis and either stimulate or inhibit cytotoxicity, depending on concentration, whereas *Phaseolus vulgaris* PHA stimulates both mitogenesis and cell-mediated cytotoxicity. Cytotoxicity may also be the result of mitogen-induced lymphotoxins released from the cell, although this is not always the case.

ACTIVITY IN VIVO

The first clues of mitogenic induction by plants occurred during a routine patho-logical examination of tissue from a child who had died of poke berry ingestion. Death had occurred after a stormy and unresponsive course characterized by gastrointestinal and progressive neurologic dysfunction.[22] Sections of the brain revealed periovascular infiltrates of cerebral vessels in which many atypical mononuclear cells, plasma cells, and dividing cells were encountered. Subsequent studies of other cases relating to exposure to poke juice by ingestion or absorption through fresh cuts and abrasions also showed that a wide range of hematological aberrations could be induced. In these cases the immune system was triggered, and plasmacytosis and nonspecific elevation of IgG levels and eosinophilia were observed. Also, abnormal properties in blood platelets occur through platelet phagocytosis and thrombocytopenia.[23]

Furthermore, a delay in homograft rejection has been observed when *Phaseolus vulgaris* PHA was injected before homografts in experimental animals. This phenomenon is not prolonged over strong histocompatibility barriers but is enhanced by concurrent administration of antilymphocytic serum. These results suggest a possible use for PHA in inducing immune tolerance during transplantation. Moreover, *P. vulgaris* PHA has been found to enhance the antitumor effect of cultured lymphocytes and, therefore, may be useful in antitumor therapy (p. 137).

Studies with Concanavalin A have also demonstrated a pronounced effect on delayed hypersensitivity. Moreover, Con-A treatment, which is similar to PHA, not only prolongs skin allograft survival, it stimulates release of a migration inhibition factor by nonimmune lymphocytes.

FUNCTION IN THE PLANT

As Table 4-2 reveals, the majority of lectins associated with plants are found among members of the Fabaceae (pea family). Their role in these genera may be linked to an ability to agglutinate nitrogen-fixing bacteria at root hair sites. The facility of PHA to agglutinate *Rhizopus phaseoli,* and its concentration below and in root nodules, indicates such a function.[24] A selective advantage among lectin-containing plants, which are able to fix nitrogen by agglutinating bacteria to their roots, may partly explain their widespread occurrence in the Fabaceae. Other plants having nitrogen-fixing bacteria should be searched for potential lectins (e.g., *Psychotria,* Rubiaceae), as well as plants having very poisonous phytotoxins, proteins that seem to predominate among plants already examined.

LITERATURE CITED

1. Goldstein A, Aronow L, Kalman SM. 1969. *Principles of Drug Action,* reprinted. Harper & Row, New York: Chapter 10, Chemical Mutagenesis (pp 618–668); Chapter 12, Chemical Teratogenesis (pp. 711–734).

2. Fishbein L, Flamm WG, Falk HL. 1970. *Chemical Mutagens.* Academic Press, New York and London. 364 p; Hollaender A (ed). 1971. *Chemical Mutagens.* 2 vols. Plenum Press, New York and London.

3. Kihlman BA (ed). 1974. Caffeine as an environmental mutagen and the problem of synergistic effects. *Mut Res* (Special Issue) **26:** 51–155; Kuhlmann W, Fromme H-G, Heege E-M, et al. 1968. The mutagenic action of caffeine in higher organisms. *Cancer Res* **28:** 2375–2389.

4. Lewis WH, Walker SA. 1974. Chromosome abnormalities stimulated by excess sucrose. *J Hered* **65:** 193–194.

5. Barrow MV. 1970. A brief history of teratology to the early 20th century. *Teratology* **4:** 119–130.

6. Carter MP, Wilson F. 1965. Antibiotics in early pregnancy and congenital malformations. *Dev Med Child Neur* **7:** 353–359.

7. Richards DLG. 1969. Congenital malformations and environmental influences in pregnancy. *Brit J Prev Soc Med* **23:** 218–225.

8. Bongiovanni AM, McFadden AJ. 1960. Steroids during pregnancy and possible fetal consequences. *Fertil Steril* **11:** 181–186; Serment H, Ruf H. 1968. Corticotherapie et grossesse. *Bull Fed Soc Gynecol Obstet Lang Fr* **20:** 77–85.

9. Long SY. 1972. Does LSD induce chromosomal damage and malformations? A review of the literature. *Teratology* **6:** 75–90.

10. Robinson GC, Brommitt JR, Miller JR. 1963. Hearing loss in infants and preschool children. II. Etiological considerations. *Pediatrics* **32:** 115–124.

11. Shepard TH. 1973. *Catalog of Teratogenic Agents.* Johns Hopkins University Press, Baltimore and London. 211 p.

12. Wilson JG. 1973. Present status of drugs as teratogens in man. *Teratology* **7:** 3–16.

13. Keeler RF. 1972. Known and suspected teratogenic hazards in range plants. *Clin Toxicol* **5:** 529–565.

14. Wilson JG. 1964. Teratogenic interactions of chemical agents in the rat. *J Pharm Exp Ther* **144:** 429–436.

15. Fraser FC, Fainstat TD. 1951. Production of congenital defects in the offspring of pregnant

mice treated with cortisone. *Pediatrics* **8:** 527–533.

16. Nicolson GL. 1974. Interaction of lectins with animal cell surfaces. *Int Rev Cytol* **39:** 89–190.

17. Kornfeld R, Kornfeld S. 1974. Structure of membrane receptors for plant lectins. *Ann NY Acad Sci* **234:** 276–282.

18. Lis H, Lotan R, Sharon N. 1974. Synthesis and use of affinity chromatography columns for the purification of plant lectins. *Ann NY Acad Sci* **234:** 232–237.

19. Pardoe GI. 1974. Heterophile receptors of erythrocytes and leukocytes. *Ann NY Acad Sci* **234:** 239–259.

20. Bird GWG. 1974. Plant and other agglutinins in the study of some human erythrocyte membrane anomalies. *Ann NY Acad Sci* **234:** 129–138.

21. Scarpelli DG. 1974. Mitogenic activity of ster-culic acid, a cydopropenoid fatty acid. *Science* **185:** 958–959.

22. Barker BE. 1969. Phytomitogens and lymphocyte blastogenesis. *Hemic Cells in Vitro* **4:** 64–79.

23. Barker BE, Farnes P, Fanger H. 1965. Mitogenic activity in *Phytolacca americana* (Pokeweed). *Lancet* **1:** 170; Barker BE, Farnes P, LaMarche PH. 1966. Peripheral blood plasmacytosis following systemic exposure to *Phytolacca americana* (Pokeweed). *Pediatrics* **38:** 490–493; Barker BE, Farnes P, LaMarche PH. 1967. Haematological effects of Pokeweed. *Lancet* **1:** 437.

24. Hamblin J, Kent SP. 1973. Possible role of phytohaemagglutinin in *Phaseolus vulgaris* L. *Nature (New Biol)* **245:** 28–30.

Section Two
"REMEDIAL" PLANTS

This section discusses those plants that are beneficial to man: they help him when he is ill, they nourish him, and they aid his agriculture. These functions are stressed as they apply to plants used by the North American Indian, although many plants important to indigenous and cosmopolitan medicines elsewhere in the world are also included.

Throughout this book a broad definition of plants prevails and includes bacteria and fungi, as well as typically green plants. Thus infections are mentioned in a cursory way in each chapter where significant, and where essential for an understanding of the designated therapy. Each chapter contains a brief discussion of the morphology and physiology of the human system involved, presented with little jargon, so that the nonscientist and layman may more easily comprehend the description and function of that system.* The format of the section follows the arrangement found in most texts on internal medicine, with just enough detail given for a glimpse of that subject.

Reference to the Glossary, to a good dictionary or to any text on pharmacology

---

* More detailed descriptive portions of most chapters are presented in small type. These should give the interested reader a better understanding of the functioning of each system in relation to plants and plant products, but they are not essential for obtaining an overview of "remedial" plants.

and internal medicine will aid the reader. We have consulted, besides the research literature, many general texts and references, of which the following have been used most frequently:

AMA Drug Evaluations, ed 2. 1973. Prepared by the AMA Department of Drugs, Publishing Sciences Group, Acton, Mass. 1032 p.

Burgen ASV, Mitchell JF. 1972. *Gaddum's Pharmacology,* ed 7. Oxford University Press, London. 251 p.

Burger A (ed). 1960. *Medicinal Chemistry,* ed 2. Wiley-Interscience, New York. 1243 p.

Claus EP, Tyler VE, Brady LR. 1970. *Pharmacognosy,* ed 6. Lea & Febiger, Philadelphia. 518 p.

Osol A, Farrar GE et al. 1947. *The Dispensatory of the United States of America,* ed 24. Lippincott, Philadelphia. 1928 p.

Today's Drugs, Vols 1–3, 1970, 1971, 1973. British Medical Association, London.

Plants remedial to man in one way or another are discussed in Chapters 5 through 16.

Chapter 5

Cancer

Cancer is not only the most feared of human maladies, it is also the most baffling. Man's recent research into the complex of several hundred different types of cancer has produced limited success[1]: 40 years ago less than one-fifth of all known victims survived five years after diagnosis; now one-third live at least that long. Yet each year in the United States, there are more than 665,000 new cases of cancer and about 365,000 deaths from this disease. The direct medical expenses involved are estimated at $3 billion, but the agony to patients and the heartache for families and friends represent far greater and more serious costs. Americans are not alone in their suffering; the whole world shares these experiences.[2]

Overall, the incidence of cancer is decreasing in women in the United States. Between 1947 and 1971 the rate has dropped from 294 per 100,000 to 256, although breast cancer remains a constant threat. For men the peril is rising. During the same period the cancer rate in males increased from 280 per 100,000 to 304, and the death rate rose by nearly 40%. Lung cancer was the biggest factor in this increase, accounting for about 63,000 male deaths in 1975[3] (Fig. 5-1).

DESCRIPTION

But what is cancer? Cancer is the rapid and uncontrolled formation of abnormal

Cancer Incidence by Site and Sex*

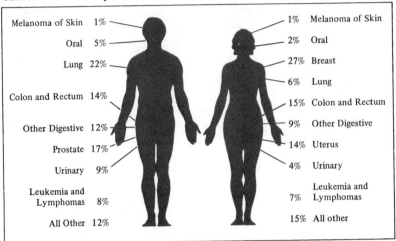

*Excluding non-melanoma skin cancer and carcinoma in situ of uterine cervix.

Cancer Deaths by Site and Sex

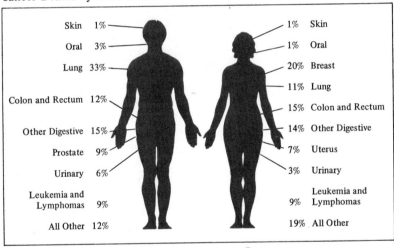

Figure 5-1 Incidence and mortality of cancer by site and sex. (From E Silverberg and Al Holleb, "Cancer incidence by site and sex," Ca **25**(1): 2–21, 1975. Copyrighted© American Cancer Society, Inc. and reprinted with their permission.)

cells in the body. Since the abnormal cells are no longer controlled by the genetic plan governing the orderly division of normal cells, they divide frequently in a disorderly fashion, often with varying chromosome numbers. The cancerous cells mass together to form a growth or proliferate individually throughout the body. Either way they serve no useful function.

Furthermore, cancerous cells may interfere with the function of the organ or tissue in which they are found. They sometimes invade neighboring tissues also, and in metastasis they enter the bloodstream, to be carried to more distant parts of the body where other similar growths (metastases) are formed. Malignant cells also spread throughout the body through lymphatic vessels, which drain lymph from organs and tissues.

Cancer is, therefore, a general term comprising all types of malignancy. Within this generalization a number of basic varieties are readily distinguished.

Carcinoma. This is a type of cancer beginning in the cells covering the skin or tissues forming the mucous membranes (e.g., the lining of the stomach and intestines). Such covering or lining cells are epithelial tissues and, depending on their locality, a number of carcinomas may exist in the body: adenoglandular carcinoma originating in the epithelial cells of glands, ducts, and mucous membranes; mucoid carcinoma, found frequently in the stomach, colon and rectum consisting of cells that form and secrete mucin; and squamous carcinoma arising from the thickened epithelium of the skin or the lining of the esophagus.

Sarcoma. This is a type of cancer arising in the connective tissues of the body, including the muscles, fibrous tissues, cartilage, bone, and lymphatic and fatty tissues. Sarcomas are often very malignant, increasing rapidly in size, invading neighboring tissues and the blood stream, and often liberally supplied with blood vessels. Sarcomas may be named from the tissue of origin. Thus a fibrosarcoma arises from the fibrous sheath of a large muscle, a chondrosarcoma from cartilage, an osteogenic sarcoma from a bone, and a lymphosarcoma from the lymph nodes.

Melanoma. This type of cancer is found in the skin, especially on the lower limbs, head, and neck. The malignant melanoma is one of the worst forms of cancer, for it often spreads rapidly through the blood stream and lymphatic vessels to form metastases in many parts of the body. The tumor is frequently a mole that is black because it contains the pigment melanin.

Teratoma. Teratomas arise from embryonic cells that may be present in the ovary, testicle, and (less frequently) other areas. Tumors from them may represent any type of immature tissue having the neoplastic power of progressive independent growth.

Leukemia. This type of cancer consists of a neoplastic change in blood-forming tissues (e.g., bone marrow, spleen, thymus), usually accompanied by a flooding into the blood and tissues of an excess of white blood cells, many of them immature and abnormal.

The cancers described next occur most frequently. The reader should refer to a textbook on pathology for further details. In depth discussions of each type of cancer, including epidemiology (Fig. 5-2), etiology, and control or cure of cancer, can be found in *Cancer Medicine* and other general references.[4]

SKIN CANCER

Although more than 300,000 new cases of skin cancer are discovered in the United States each year, the death rate is low and many patients are permanently cured. The present phenomenal cure rate of 95%, with the exception of melanomas, is no doubt related to the early detection and treatment of the cured cases when they are still in their precancerous forms (keratosis, occupational dermatoses, radiation dermatitis, xeroderma pigmentosum, leukoplakia). The appearance of these early lesions has often been associated with such inciting factors as excessive exposure to sunlight, X-rays, arsenicals, and tar products, local chronic irritants, including pipe smoking, and chronic recurrent lesions (herpesvirus I & II infections).

There are many rare forms of skin cancer; the three basic types, however, are as follows.

1. *Basal cell (rodent ulcer) carcinoma* develops from a small red or yellowish pimple that spreads slowly, particularly over the surface of the face, but it rarely metastasizes. Involvement of the eye is usually more serious.

2. *Squamous cell carcinoma* develops as a nodular mass or ulcer, which can penetrate

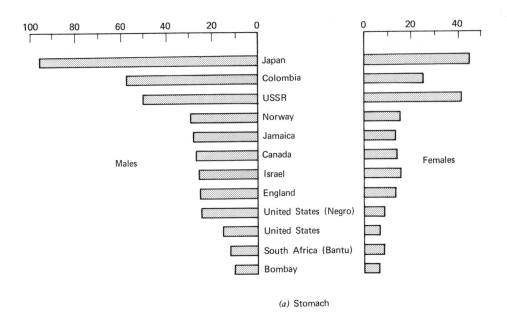

(a) Stomach

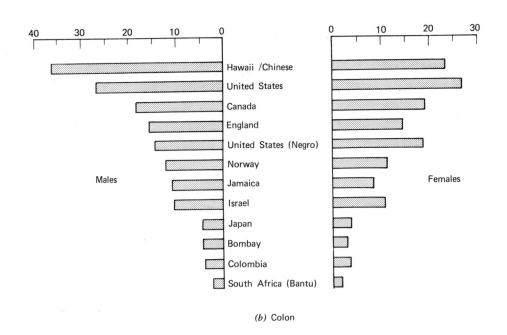

(b) Colon

Figure 5-2 Histograms showing geographic variations in incidence of cancer of (a) Stomach. (b) Colon. (c) Skin. (d) Skin (excluding melanoma). (e) Leukemia. (f) Bronchus and trachea. (g) Prostate.. (h) Breast. Incidence data expressed in rates of 100,000 per annum. (From J Higginson and CS Muir, "Epidemiology," in JF Holland and E Frei III (eds), *Cancer Medicine*, p 241–306, Lea & Febiger, Philadelphia, and reprinted with permission.)

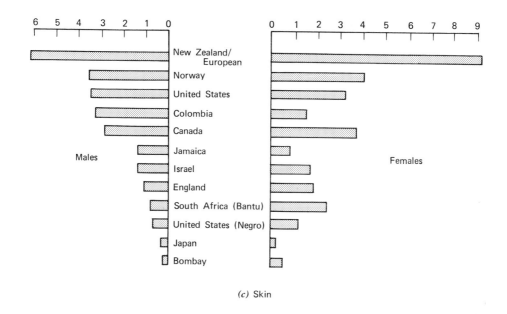

(c) Skin

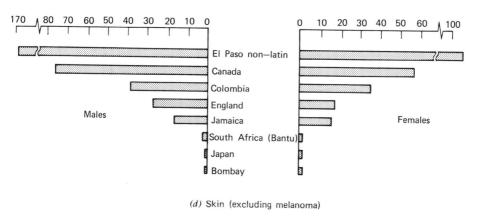

(d) Skin (excluding melanoma)

Figure 5-2 (Continued)

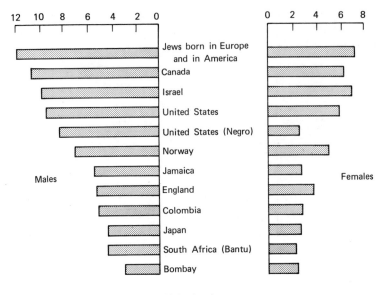

(e) Leukemia

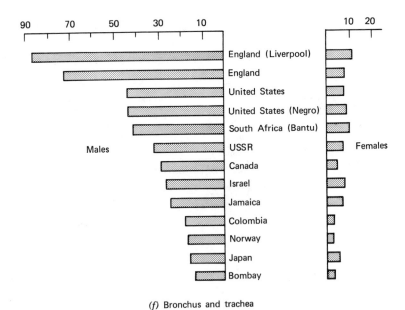

(f) Bronchus and trachea

Figure 5-2 (Continued)

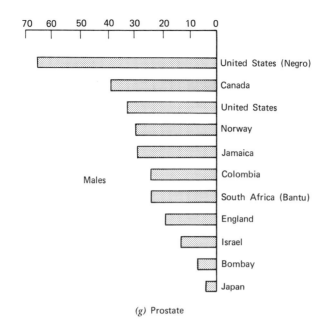

70 60 50 40 30 20 10   0

United States (Negro)

Canada

United States

Norway

Jamaica

Males

Colombia

South Africa (Bantu)

England

Israel

Bombay

Japan

(g) Prostate

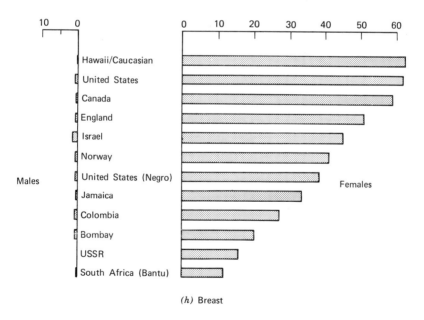

10   0   0   10   20   30   40   50   60

Hawaii/Caucasian

United States

Canada

England

Israel

Norway

Males

United States (Negro)   Females

Jamaica

Colombia

Bombay

USSR

South Africa (Bantu)

(h) Breast

Figure 5-2 (Continued)

cartilage or bones; it metastasizes to lymph nodes and through blood to many organs—most frequently the lower lip, mouth, tongue, larynx, cervix, bladder, and esophagus.

3. *Malignant melanoma or melanocarcinoma* develops *de novo* or from an existing mole and is characterized by the appearance of red, white, and especially blue patches within a brown or black lesion. It may also appear as an indented or notched border around a lesion, or as a highly irregular surface on a suspect lesion. It readily metastasizes and invades through the blood and lymphatics early. Presently the cure rate is only 50%, although the therapeutic use of Bacillus Calmette-Guerin (BCG) may improve this rate.

CANCER OF THE ORAL CAVITY

Early recognition and treatment of premalignant conditions, such as chronic dental ulcers due to physical irritants, leukoplakia, and glossitis, no doubt account for the low incidence of oral cancers. Tongue, cheek, hard and soft palate, and gum cancers are usually characterized by bleeding, painful, hard-edged, ulcerated, warty growths or by hard surfaces that metastasize to regional lymph nodes.

CANCER OF THE LUNG

Although many types of lung cancer are known, the very high mortality rate seen in men has been associated with primary carcinoma of the lung. These cancers are mainly bronchogenic in origin and may be squamous or undifferentiated (anaplastic). General respiratory symptoms make differential clinical diagnosis difficult. However if the more common bronchial sarcoma (60% incidence) is diagnosed early enough to allow its removal before lymphatic metastases occur, prognosis is good. On the other hand, the ability of anaplastic or adenocarcinomatous tumors to metastasize quickly makes for a much poorer prognosis. Metastases may result from direct invasion or extension through the lymphatics and bloodstream, resulting in dissemi-

nation to the liver, bones, adrenal glands, kidney, brain, pericardium, and heart.

Incitations have been related not only to continuous exposure to carcinogens present in tobacco or industrial pollutants, but more specifically to the industries using chromates, arsenicals, asbestos, and radioactive ores.

BREAST CANCER

Breast cancer, very common among females, is extremely rare in males. Several varieties exist, although the very malignant, hard, nodular, scirrhotic carcinoma is seen most frequently. Prognosis is poor if not eradicated, since this cancer has the ability to spread rapidly through the pectoral muscles and into the lungs, to axillary and other lymph nodes, and through the lymphatics to the liver. Dissemination through the bloodstream may also give rise to involvement of the bone marrow.

Several inciting factors are believed to be important. They include hereditary susceptibility, irritation related to inadequate drainage of milk caused by failure to nurse after pregnancy, estrogen disturbances, trauma, and fibrocystic disease. The possibility of the existence of an incitant virus, similar to that seen in mammary carcinoma in animals and capable of being transmitted through nursing, has become an area of active controversy.

COLON AND RECTAL CANCER

Carcinomas of the colon and rectum are fairly common and may begin as polypoid, sessile, or ulcerative neoplasms. Obstruction of the lumen results from an annular constrictive growth or a papillary form projecting into the bowel space. Sigmoid and rectal cancer occur most frequently (55–75%) in males, and those found in the colon (20%) occur slightly more commonly in females. Early spread to the lymphatics is often seen with the ulcerative forms. If metastatic dissemination is late, however, surgical cure is possible.

Certain environmental factors have been

implicated, although their exact etiology has yet to be determined. Ackerman[5] has suggested that increased incidence of colon cancer among American, Canadian, and British populations may be due to habitual prolonged stool retention, which would result in exposure of the colon to carcinogens produced by the interaction of fecal bacteria and certain food constituents.

OTHER DIGESTIVE TRACT NEOPLASMS

A neoplasm found frequently in parts of Africa, but less commonly elsewhere, is esophageal cancer. It occurs predominantly in males and has a morbidity rate closely approximating its mortality rate. The majority of these tumors are squamous carcinomas occurring in the lower and middle third of the viscus. Stenosis and obstruction of the lumen result from growth of the infiltrating scirrhous forms around the esophagus or from the extension of a soft, bulky ulcerating medullary type tumor. Polypoid forms are less common. Because of the inaccessibility of the area affected, prognosis is poor and metastases may occur to the liver, lung, and lymph nodes. Consumption of strong alcoholic drinks, eating food grown in molybdenum-deficient soils (which promote nitrate accumulation and are a potential source of nitrosamines in plants), "beedi" smoking (see Table 17-3), and professional exposure to brass and bronze are among the environmental factors associated with esophageal cancer.

Adenocarcinomas are the most common form of stomach and intestinal tumors. Susceptibility may be related to heredity, to having type A or O blood, and to conditions such as chronic gastritis, chronic gastric ulcer, and adenomatous polyps. The majority of carcinomas develop from mucus-secreting cells of the antrum and pylorus, especially along the lesser curvature. The most frequent form of gastric carcinoma is the ulcerative or penetrating type, although the soft, bulky polypoid or fungating tumor is relatively common; the diffuse, spreading, or infiltrating scirrhous variety is seen only rarely. The frequent appearance

of adenocarcinoma among those living on seaboards like Japan, Chile, and Iceland is striking, but the common factor, probably residing in some food, has yet to be determined. Malignant tumors of the small intestine and appendix are rare, although carcinoids that are benign argentaffin tumors can metastasize to the liver and produce carcinoid syndrome with accompanying serotonin production.

UTERINE AND CERVICAL CANCER

Although the rate of cervical cancer is high among certain segments of the population, early diagnosis through routine Pap smears has reduced the death rate considerably. Approximately 95% of the cells are squamous cell carcinomas; the remainder are adenocarcinomas. Prognosis after surgery usually depends on the degree of invasiveness; the best results are expected with carcinoma *in situ*, and the worst come when cancerous cells have massively invaded the parametrium and have extended into the wall of the pelvis. Numerous epidemiologic studies suggest that this cancer may be regarded as a venereal disease caused by a biologic agent (probably herpesvirus II) rather than a chemical substance. Not only is its incidence higher among more promiscuous patients, but it is also frequently seen among those whose consorts have penile carcinoma.

Conversely, adenocarcinomas arising from the endometrial glands of the body of the uterus are much less common and frequently occur in infertile women who have some genetic or endocrine dysfunction. The development of breast cancer among these patients appears to be greater, suggesting an etiology or predisposition completely different from that characteristic of cervical cancer. Choriocarcinomas, which arise from fetal membranes and have the ability to invade and destroy maternal tissues extensively, are very rare but extremely malignant. The incidence appears to be higher in Nigeria and Singapore, although the etiology remains obscure.

PROSTATIC CANCER

Adenocarcinomas of the prostate occur with increasing frequency after the fourth decade, but these cancers may be asymptomatic or associated with senile atrophy of the gland at any age. Early metastases of malignant forms result in the invasion of capsular perineural lymphatics followed by hematogenous metastases to the bones, lungs, and liver. The incidence is highest among the American Negro and lowest among the Japanese. Epidemiologic surveys link genetics, industrial exposure to cadmium, and air pollution to the etiology of prostate cancer, although viral infections have not been eliminated.

URINARY TRACT CANCER

Adult kidney cancers of various degrees of malignancy are almost entirely parenchymal adenocarcinomas and squamous cancers of the renal pelvis. They are commonly found among cigarette smokers and those exposed to industrial and environmental pollution. There are no painful symptoms until hematogenous spread results in metastatic tumors of the lungs or liver. The incidence of bladder cancer is much higher in males than in females. The predominance of transitional carcinomas or recurrent papillomas in Europe and North America and of squamous carcinoma in Africa suggest different etiologies. Incidence is related to exposure to tobacco, as indicated, and to coffee, bilharziasis, and carcinogenic chemicals, such as 2-napthylamine and other aromatic amines.

LEUKEMIA AND LYMPHOMA

There is a marked variance in incidence of lymphosarcomas and reticulosarcomas. Although the incidence of Burkitt's lymphoma among children is highest in holoendemic malaria areas of the world, such as Africa and New Guinea, this lymphoma of the jaws or abdomen is less rare elsewhere than originally supposed. Its relationship to Epstein-Barr virus infection, infectious mononucleosis, Hodg-kin's disease, nasopharyngeal carcinomas, and leukemias is an active area of research.

Another malignant lymphoma, Hodgkin's disease, has a much more constant attack rate between countries. It is somewhat more common in males than in females and occurs most frequently during the second decade of life. A viral etiology, presumed to be Epstein-Barr virus, has been implicated but not proved. Similar distributions of leukemia have been reported, although variations of incidence may differ from one part of the country to another. In the United States the peak of acute lymphocytic leukemia occurs among children between 3 and 4 years of age; then the rate falls until the age of 35, when the incidence of predominantly chronic lymphocytic leukemia appears to rise. Its absence or low incidence in most Asian countries suggests the involvement of genetic factors.

In addition, retrovirus (oncornavirus, leukovirus) particles similar to those found in animal leukemias have been discovered, although a causal relationship has yet to be established. The ability of radiation to induce both chronic myeloid leukemia and acute leukemia has been well documented, and the decline of these diseases in recent years may be a result of a reduction in using prenatal X-rays. Cases have been low, but acute leukemias have also been associated with exposure to such chemicals as benzene and chloramphenicol.

CARCINOGENESIS

Throughout the ages, theories relating to the causes of cancer have been as numerous as the cures proposed for them. With the sophisticated tools and techniques of modern molecular biology, some of the mystery surrounding this enigma has been stripped away, although the information that has been gleaned still incites active controversy. Acceptance of new ideas has been slow, particularly because some are completely antithetic to those generally considered correct. No simple answer is anticipated, and it is likely that a combination of many of the theories now currently in vogue will lead to new discoveries and the final solution.

ONCOVIRUSES

The contention that human cancers are induced by viruses rests on analogy with observations in other species, particularly laboratory animals. Unfortunately Koch's postulates cannot always be applied to humans, given the necessity for isolation, induction of infection, and reisolation of the etiologic agent. Not only are malignant transformations leading to cancer dependent on subtle interactions between the virus or viruses and the cell infected, they also depend on factors affecting the susceptibility and resistance inherent to the host itself. Under these circumstances, investigators have been reluctant to attribute the ability to induce cancer to an infectious agent or agents. This is especially true when only virus antigens alone, but not infectious viruses, are detected in tumor cells. Nevertheless, once the role of several viruses or virus groups has been clearly delineated, it is likely that the viruses now under serious investigation as cancer etiologic agents will be joined by others.[6]

Among the RNA viruses, many retroviruses have been known to incite certain cancers in animals, and evidence is accumulating that similar human strains may be responsible for especially mammary cancer, as well as leukemias, lipomas, fibrosarcomas, and osteosarcomas in man. Although many DNA virus groups have been shown to have oncogenic potential, in man, the herpesvirus group with herpes simplex I and II (cervical carcinoma, cancer of the lip) and Epstein-Barr virus (Burkitt's lymphoma, nasopharyngeal carcinoma, leukemia, and lymphomas) have afforded the greatest attention and are closer by far to acceptance than are others. The relationship of the papova and adenoviruses to cancers in man has yet to be established.

Two cancer theories propose the involvement of oncoviruses. One infers that exogenous viral infection occurs and that reverse transcriptase is required (with RNA viruses) to integrate the viral genome into the host genome,[7] whereas the other considers that oncogenes, some of which may represent proviruses, are inherited through the germ line and merely require derepression for expression.[8] Whether oncoviruses incite or merely utilize reverse transcriptase remains an area of active controversy, and Temin argues in his protovirus theory[9] that viruses have little to do with directly causing cancer and that cell transformation results through misevolution. Therefore, reverse transcriptase is present in normal cells to play a role in differentiation. Temin also considers that only the potential for malignant transformation is vertically transmitted from parent to child.

The role of carcinogens such as natural products, chemicals, irradiation, and aging, therefore, would be to activate proviruses or oncogenes already present in the cell or to exert some effect on the ontogenic controls existent in mature cells. It is now recognized that certain oncoviruses and carcinogens incite certain changes in the cell. Malignant transformations are characterized by the appearance of specific proteins such as enzymes or substances related to early virus infection, the presence of tumor antigens usually associated with the cell membrane, an increase in the rate of multiplication, a change in cell morphology, and the ability to incite further malignancies when introduced into a new host. Tumor antigens associated with oncovirus are readily reproducible and identifiable. On the other hand, the variation elicited by even one carcinogen may represent the random derepression of many potential oncosites.

The ability of radiation to induce malignancies, especially those associated with radioactive elements, such as ^{32}P[10] in leukemias and radium[11] with osteosarcomas or carcinomas in tissues adjacent to bone, has been well documented. This is also true of ultraviolet rays, X-rays,[12] and a variety of particulate irradiations. Radiation, or the free radicals or ions it induces, can affect functional controls in the cell or increase the rate of cell mutations so that chromosomal abnormalities, leading to cell death, aneuploidy, polyploidy, or chromosomal fragmentation, result.[13] Then, according to current cancer theories, malignant cells would develop by the derepression or induction of latent oncoviruses, oncogenic factors, or ontogenic controls. Although it is likely that malignancies appearing in the aged may be more closely related to loss of immunocompetency,[14] it is also possible that catabolic products accumulating during aging act in a similar fashion to radiation. Since age-induced chromosome abnormalities have been observed in somatic cells of certain populations of *Claytonia virginica,*[15] this plant may serve as a useful tool for the study of such phenomena without the added complication of immunologic factors associated with animals.

CHEMICAL CARCINOGENS

The carcinogenic potential was first reported by Sir John Hill, a physician and botanist who in 1761 associated the excessive use of snuff from *Nicotiana tabacum* with the appearance of fatal malignant polyps of the nose.[16] Later, in 1775, Percival Pott linked scrotal skin cancers or "soot warts" to a combination of the type of work done by English chimney sweeps and their infrequent bathing habits.[17] Subsequently, certain polycyclic aromatic hydrocarbons were found to be responsible for the carcinogenic effect of coal tar derivatives, and the synthesis of many potent carcinogens, especially 9,10-dimethyl-1,2-benzanthracene, followed.[18] In this respect skin cancers were later associated with the medicinal application of coal tar and creosote preparations,[19] and gastrointestinal cancer to the heavy laxative use of mineral oils containing these hydrocarbons.[20]

A feature of these chemicals is their ability to bind to DNA[21] and to produce cancer in the tissue with which they are placed in contact. The increase of lung cancer is no doubt related to the presence in tobacco and in polluted atmospheres of such carcinogenic hydrocarbons as 3,4-benzypyrene.[22]

Recently similar carcinogenic activity was noted for the heterocyclic compound 4-nitroquinoline-1-oxide and its relatives.[23] In plants these compounds act as growth-promoting hormones, and their ability to elicit neoplasms may account for the higher incidence of stomach and intestinal tumors found among vegetarians.[24] The lower incidence of such tumors in the small intestine may be the result of the presence of high levels of benzyprehydralase, an enzyme responsible for the natural breakdown of those compounds in man. The discovery of heterocyclic compounds in rural soils in varying concentrations (10–130 mg/g) is no doubt a reflection of the amount of plant decomposition rather than soot fallout from afar.[25]

Amines and amides of certain precarcinogenic aromatic amines may be activated in the host by N-hydroxylation.[26] Moreover, the carcinogenic disalkylaryltriazenes are activated by enzymatic dealkylation, and the carcinogenic nitrosamines are activated nonenzymatically through reactions with sulfhydryl groups. These substances are found in nature or associated with particular industries and often have a unique specificity for one type of organ. For example, bladder cancer found among aniline dye workers has been attributed to 2-naphthylamine. Other chemicals posing carcinogenic hazards are benzidine and the more complex amines auramine and fuchsin.[23,27]

It has been proposed that urinary cancer develops also in men not exposed to such amines because of the possible production of endogenous carcinogens related to abnormal tryptophan metabolism (e.g., orthohydrozyamines[28]). Similarly, metabolic alteration after ingestion or injection of the simple aliphatic compound urethran (ethyl carbamate), which yields several kinds of electrophils including free radicals that react with cystein and cytosine RNA, may result in lung tumors.[29] Also, carbon tetrachloride, which binds both protein and nucleic acid,[30] and ethinonine, which ethylates RNA,[31] have been found to be hepatocarcinogenic for the rat. A variety of tumors may result from the ingestion of 2-acetylaminofluorine, which is deacetylated in the intestine to the potent carcinogen n-hydroxy-2-acetylfluorine.[32]

Alkylating agents, also used in the treatment of cancer, are nearly always carcinogenic in laboratory animals.[33] In man, the therapeutic use of melphan and cyclophosphamide has been causally related to acute leukemia, particularly among multiple myeloma patients.[34]

Carcinogenic alkylating agents are administered in their final reactive forms. They generally take part in substitution, nucleophilic, and bimolecular reactions, where relatively positive or electrophilic atoms in the alkylating agent combine with corresponding negative or nucleophilic atoms in the molecules of the cells affected. The result with DNA would be irreversible losses or changes in the genetic information in DNA, whereas alterations in the recognition of one type of RNA for another type of RNA, or for proteins, could create critical effects in function of the cell.[33,34] It is possible that the combined or sequential reactions on different nucleic acids and proteins are responsible for the subtle loss of growth control in viable cells; such alteration in growth could also produce repression and depression of genetic information. Their tendency to react with water and protein before entering the cell reduces their carcinogenic capabilities, but frequent concentrated applications are usually necessary to affect a malignancy.[23] Certain potent carcinogens do exist, however: uracil mustard,[35] and propanesultone[36] can effectively induce murine tumors in lungs and nerves, respectively.

Corollary evidence exists to support the assumption that there is a relationship between increased levels of certain metals in water supplies and the incidence of malignancies. Like many chemical carcinogens, ionic forms of elements such as beryllium, cadmium, lead, and nickel have the ability to react with various neutrophiles.[23] Epidemiological studies among white and nonwhite males and females have indicated that oropharyngeal and bowel cancers related to industrial exposure to nickel are highest among nonwhite populations,[37] whereas a weaker correlation has been noted between exposure to beryllium and bone cancers in white populations.[38] On the other hand, no racial or sexual difference among populations with renal, stomach, intestinal, and ovarian cancers has been found to be related to increases of lead in the water supply. There appears to be some controversy regarding the carcinogenicity of cadmium, although Berg and Burbank[37] suggest a strong correlation, especially for cancers of the intestine and bowel. But with regard to arsenic concentrations, no biological interpretation can explain mortality associated with cancers of the eye and larynx or of myeloid leukemia.[37] In evaluating future data, consideration should also be given to the distribution of plants used for food that not only concentrate these elements during growth but also absorb them from water during cooking.

Also, exposure to asbestos has been related to diffuse pleural mesothelia,[39] and inhalation of asbestos may be contributory to lung cancer. Combined exposure to cigarette smoke greatly increases asbestos workers' risk of death from lung cancer.[40]

Many other chemical carcinogens are known, and still others will be found in the years ahead. The reader is referred to *Carcinogenesis Abstracts,* published monthly by the National Cancer Institute.

CARCINOGENIC (ONCOGENIC) NATURAL PRODUCTS

Fungi, Bacteria, and Algae

Certain metabolites from molds and bacteria are potential carcinogens and may present a hazard to man. In 1942 Nelson and his co-workers[41] reported the development of multiple fibromas in the ears of rats fed rye contaminated with *Claviceps purpurea.* Although regressions were achieved when ergot was removed from the animals' diet, studies of this reversible phenomenon have yet to be made.

Hepatotoxic and hepatomalignant substances were first linked to *Penicillium islandicum* contaminating a bitter, yellow rice fed to rats.[42] Later another hepatotoxic factor was isolated from metabolites of *P. rubrum.*[45] Also, the antibiotic griseofulvin formed by *P. griseofulvin* and used to treat human fungal skin infections was found to induce hepatotoxic symptoms, hepatomas, and skin tumors in mice.[44]

Similar compounds were associated with toxin-producing strains of *Aspergillus flavus* and *A. parasiticus.* Potent aflatoxins B and G from these species may be detected in trace amounts in peanut butters, in milk from cows fed peanut meal, and in maize contaminated with mold.[45] The direct ingestion of aflatoxins through moldy foods has now been related to the high incidence of liver tumors in central and southern Africa and Asia. Children appear to be most susceptible to aflatoxin and mycotoxin poisoning, and a Thai pediatric disease referred to as Reyes syndrome, and characterized by acute encephalitis and degeneration of the liver and other visceral organs, may be a result of acute aflatoxin B_1 toxicity. To prevent further dissemination of these substances, a concerted worldwide effort is underway to prevent mold contamination of food and forage products. Also under active investigation is the ability of aflatoxins to interact with DNA and markedly affect transcription of genetic information.[46]

Other fungal metabolites, some associated with the common edible mushroom *Agaricus bisporus,* have been found to be structurally similar to known synthetic carcinogens,[47] as has the synthetic carcinogen ethionine, which is a metabolite of the common gut bacterium *Escherichia coli.*[48] However the role of ethionine-producing bacteria in the induction of cecal and intestinal malignancies has yet to be defined.[27]

Seaweeds (e.g., carrageenan, a sulfated polygalactose from the Irish moss *Chondrus crispus*[72]) will also induce sarcomas at the site of injections.

Gymnosperms

From the seeds and roots of cycads, primitive cone-bearing plants common to the tropics and subtropics, are extracted cycasin and its metabolite methylazoxymethanol, a highly toxic moiety related to the nitrosamines.[49] Native populations have long known of the toxicity of these plants, and the people of Guam, for instance, prepare a nontoxic cycad flour for consumption.[50] But crude cycad meal containing cycasin, which is fed to rats, mice, and hamsters, results in hepatic, renal and, occasionally, intestinal neoplasms. If the animal's bacterial flora is able to convert the metabolite of cycasin, the rate of tumor development will reach almost 100%.[51] This depends, of course, on the amount of bacterial flora in the animal's gut.

Species known to contain seeds with carcinogenic agents are *Cycas circinalis* (cycasin, from Guam and tropical Africa), *C. revoluta* (cycasin and neocycasin, from Java), and the widely cultivated *Encephalartos barkeri* (macrozamin, from Africa), and *Macrozamia spiralis* (macrozamin, from Australia).

Angiosperms

TANNINS

An association between tannins and neoplasia in humans has been noted recently among the workers in the boot and shoe industry, where the incidence of nasal cancer was high in those exposed to the dust and cuttings of leather.[52] The leather was generally cured with tannins derived from many plants. A second association has been reported between tannins and malignancies of the sinuses found in significant levels among woodworkers.[53] Such woods as mahogany and redwood (a Gymnosperm), widely used by these workers, are rich in tannins.

Do these correlations suggest that tannins may be responsible for certain nasopharyngeal tumors? Morton believes that they do, and her additional correlary evidence is convincing.[54] A study was made among inhabitants of Curacao where *Krameria ixina,* a plant rich in tannins, was used in a concoction that was drunk daily in the treatment of liver ailments. Of the 44 inhabitants who developed esophageal cancer, 10 admitted to having used the *Krameria ixina* for treatment. Recently leaf extracts from this species induced local fibrosarcomas at the injection site in all rats tested.[55] Similar results to those found for *K. ixina* have also been reported for tannin-rich *Annona muricata.*

Tannins are also found in tea, sorghum, smartweed, acacias, and oaks. For example, tannins, as well as potentially synergistic gallic acid, are high in tea, particularly in the black teas originating in India and Ceylon, in the darker purple and red varieties of sorghum (*Sorghum bicolor*), in wines, especially the more bitter and astringent reds, and in the smartweeds (*Polygonum* spp.), which are often used as folk medicines and occasionally as foods. Strong correlations exist between the use of these plants and high esophageal cancer areas in Honan Province, China, in central Asia, in Curacao, West Indies, and in the Transkei area of South Africa. In addition, sorghum (and *Solanum incanum*) accumulates nitrosamines (the nitrates reaching near toxic levels), and these may act alone or as cocarcinogens with tannin. It is interesting that sorghum, until recently, was the staple foodstuff of Curacao and a primary material for making the popular Kafir beer of the Transkei.[54] Thus we have a link between two cultures, otherwise only remotely associated, namely, a common use of sorghum and a high incidence of esophageal cancer.

The black tea preferred in Ceylon, Indonesia, India, Holland, Britain, and North America has already been noted as very rich in tannins. But according to Jacobs and Ukers[56] these potentially dangerous compounds are rendered insoluble by milk, for the casein of milk fixes the tannin and prevents its action on the mucous membrane of the mouth.

PYRROLIZIDINE ALKALOIDS

The pyrrolizidine alkaloids are found in many plants from unrelated families. Those known to be hepatocarcinogenic occur among species of *Senecio* (Asteraceae), *Amsinckia, Cynoglossum, Heliotropium* and *Trichodesma* (Boraginaceae), and *Crotalaria* (Fabaceae).[57] Rats, for example, develop chronic lesions and hepatomas even after a single dose of retrorsine extracted from South African species of *Senecio*. Others fed whole dried ground *Senecio longilobus* form a high proportion of hepatic tumors. In addition, pancreatic tumors have been found in rats given pyrrolizidine alkaloids from seeds of *Amsinckia intermedia* and dried ground leaves and stems of *Heliotropium supinum,* the latter species being used by women in Tanzania after childbirth. Finally, it appears that the very young are more susceptible than adults to these alkaloids. Lactating mothers, for example, remain unscathed after ingestion, but the suckling young suffer ill effects and may develop tumors. These data led Schoental[58] to correlate the use of folk remedies with the high incidence of tumors of the liver and pancreas in the Bantu of Africa.

CHEWING AND SMOKING PLANTS

In vast tropical and subtropical areas of the world, man has a widespread chewing habit. He chews or sucks three distinct quids: in southern Asia it is *betel,* which includes the seed of *Areca cat-*

echu, leaf of the pepper, lime, and various additions of tobacco and spices; in Iran and in the south central Soviet Republic it is *nass,* which consists of tobacco, wood ash, lime, water, and oil of cottonseed or sesame; and in Andean South America it is *coca,* which is the leaf of *Erythroxylum coca* (the source and main ingredient of cocaine), and lime.

These three quids, used in different parts of the world, have alkaloids and lime in common (betel also contains high levels of catechin tannin). Although firm conclusions regarding the causes of oral cancers among these chewing populations are difficult, it is interesting to observe that they do develop oropharyngeal and esophageal cancers at a higher rate than do most other people who do not practice these habits.[59] Lime additives appear to release the alkaloids, thus hastening the physiological effects by damaging the oral mucous membrane. Lime may also facilitate carcinogenesis by plants in other ways.[59]

Experimental data from hamsters tend to support these correlations.[60] When extracts of betel were applied topically to the mucous membranes of the animal's pouch, tumors developed in 38% of the hamsters sampled; extracts of betel and tobacco applied together resulted in tumors 78% of the time, showing that the incidence of tumors was clearly enhanced by tobacco. No tumor was found among the controls nor in the hamsters treated with tobacco extract alone, although the latter did develop leukoplakia. Autopsies typically showed squamous cell carcinomas of varying degrees of malignancy.

The complexity of establishing carcinogens and tumor-promoting agents from plant material is well characterized by the leaf of tobacco (*Nicotiana tabacum*), where more than 1200 organic compounds are known and many more remain to be characterized.[61] Many of these components are volatilized during burning, and others, including the aromatic hydrocarbons, are formed during combustion of the leaf components.

Thirteen carcinogenic hydrocarbons residing in the "tar" fractions have been isolated from tobacco or smoke condensate.[62] Even so, other carcinogens must be present in tobacco smoke; the presence of nitrosamines in smoke and of free radicals in cigarette tars may be very important, for removing a concentrate of polynuclear aromatic hydrocarbons from smoke condensate resulted in about a 50% reduction in tumorogenic activity when assayed on mouse skin.[63] The remainder has not yet been defined. Clearly, however, the particulate matter of tobacco smoke is carcinogenic to a variety of animals and tissues. Whether from cigarettes, cigars, or pipes, tobacco smoke acts as a complete carcinogen in that it can induce squamous cell cancer, with the risk of bronchogenic carcinoma increasing with the number of cigarettes smoked daily.[64]

Like quids chewed elsewhere, chewing tobacco in the United States is associated with both oral carcinoma and leukoplakia. In many cases it has been established that the tumor appears at the site where the quid is held, and conceivably the lesions are a result of continuous trauma, since they may be directly related to the chemical components of the quid.[65]

OILS, FLAVORS, AND SPICES

Croton oil, obtained from the seeds of *Croton tiglium* and well known as a powerful purgative, has no carcinogenic effect, but it can be used to augment, for example, carcinogenesis initially induced by aromatic hydrocarbons on the skin of mice. This tumor-promoting ability is affected by the diterpene esters common to many Euphorbiaceae (*Euphorbia*

cooperi, E. ingens, E. lathyrus, E. triangularis) and to the related Thymelaeaceae (*Daphne mezereum, Pimelea prostrata*).[66] According to Hecker,[67] the identification and characterization of this new group of cocarcinogens and tumor promoters are events of outstanding interest for a deeper understanding of the mechanism of tumorogenesis.

Safrole (*p*-allylyn ethylenediozybenzene) is a component of many essential oils including star anise oil (*Pimpinella anisum*), camphor oil (*Cinnamomum camphora*), mace and nutmeg (*Myristica fragrans*), Japanese wild ginger (*Asarum* sp.), California bay laurel (*Umbellularia californica*), cinnamon leaf oil (*Cinnamomum zeylanicum*), and especially sassafras oil (*Sassafras albidum*). It has been used as a flavoring agent in root beer. At concentrations of 0.5 and 1% of the diet (see refs. 68 and 64, respectively), safrole induces hepatomas in rats; casein supplements aggravate the safrole-induced adenomatosis, and biotin supplements inhibit hepatocarcinogenic activity of safrole. Citrus, turpentine, and bergamot oils have no or low activity as carcinogens.

The formation of liver tumors in rats fed red pepper (*Capsicum frutescens*) as 10% chili in their diet occurs at a higher incidence than in the control group.[70] Little is known regarding flavor and spice additives, but it should not be overlooked that prolonged exposure to even minute amounts of carcinogens may result in the development of cancers after a long latent period.

MISCELLANEOUS

The seeds of *Laburnum anagyroides* contain an antithyroid compound thiourea, which will induce adenomas and carcinomas, benign liver tumors, and malignant tumors of the eyelid and ear duct when administered in the diet of rats.[71]

The rediscovery by Redmond[16] of Sir John Hill's classic association of cancer and tobacco is appropriately titled *Tobacco and Cancer: the First Clinical Report, 1761.* Hill's discussion[16] of the mechanism of tobacco carcinogenesis is applicable today not only for this syndrome, but for the problems of the cause and origin of cancer even after more than 200 years of research.

Whether or not polypusses, which attend Snuff-takers, are absolutely caused by the custom; or whether the principles of the disorder were there before, and Snuff only irritated the parts, and hastened the mischief, I shall not pretend to determine: but even supposing the latter only to be the case, the damage is certainly more than the indulgence is worth: for who is able to say, *that the Snuff is not the absolute cause, or that he has not the seeds of such a disorder which Snuff will bring into action.* (italics added)

With respect to cancers of the nose, they are as dreadful and as fatal as any others. . . . It is evident therefore that no man should venture upon Snuff, who is not sure that he is not so far liable to a cancer: and no man can be sure of that.

DEVELOPMENT OF THERAPY

Cancer in the ancestral species of man is more than a million years old, and traces have been found in an anthropoid unearthed in Java in 1891. Bone cancer is identifiable in some mummies discovered in the Great Pyramid of Gizeh, and the famous Ebers papyrus (1500 BC) describes symptoms of cancer and primitive forms of treatment. From the Hindu epic the *Ramayana* we learn of arsenic pastes administered as long ago as 500 BC to treat cancerous growths. Hippocrates, in about 400 BC, described many forms of the disease and also employed crude caustic pastes as well as cautery for therapy.[73]

Over the centuries, treatments and remedies have varied greatly; no fewer than 3000 plant species have been used by the laiety to treat cancer.[74] Most of the early treatments had little or no effect on the disease, but perhaps they lessened suffering either physically or psychologically. Many herbal formulas were used in cancer treatment but none, as far as is known, was recorded as a cure. Early Russian healers, for example, sought only to arrest the development of the disease and to allay their patients' suffering.[75]

When grapes were in season, some healers placed their patients on massive diets of the fruit, and nothing else. Up to 15 pounds were eaten per day or whatever amount was needed to fill to absolute capacity the patient's stomach. If this routine was followed for at least 6 weeks, near cures were claimed in many cases, particularly for stomach or intestinal cancer. This is reminiscent of the Brandt modern grape diet cure, which utilizes grapes and unsweetened grape juice for several weeks followed by the addition of sour milk and raw foods.[73] The American Cancer Society has found this diet of no objective benefit for the treatment of human cancers; in fact, the high level of tannins present in certain grapes suggests a carcinogenic potential.

A treatment having even weaker foundations, but important psychological implications, was used in the court of the Roman emperor Theodosius (fourth century AD): vervain (*Verbena officinalis*) root was cut in half, with one part hung around the patient's neck and the other hung to dry over a smouldering fire. As the vervain dried, the tumor supposedly shriveled. If the patient at any time appeared to be ungrateful for the cure, however, the physician would threaten to throw the root into water, assuring the patient that as the root absorbed moisture, the tumor would return.[76]

Other plant remedies are equally historic though less bizarre. The Ebers papyrus, for example, mentions the external application of garlic (*Allium sativum*) for indurations. Hippocrates prescribed eating garlic as treatment for uterine tumors, and the Bower manuscript, dating from about AD 450 in India, recommended garlic as a cure for abdominal tumors.[77] From the National Cancer Institute central files, Hartwell[78] reported that cancer incidence in France is supposedly lowest where garlic consumption is greatest, that garlic eaters in Bulgaria do not have cancer, and that a physician in Victoria, British Columbia, related that he has successfully treated malignancies by prescribing garlic eating.

In 1957 Weisberger and Pensky[79] reported that extracts of garlic bulbs contain a powerful bactericidal agent, allylthiosulfinic allyl ester or allicin, which

is formed by the interaction of a garlic enzyme alliinase and the substrate S-ethyl L-cysteine sulfoxide. When either the enzyme or the substrate was inoculated into mice infected with a sarcoma, all animals died within 16 days; but when the enzyme was allowed to react with the substrate, followed by administration to the tumor-bearing animals, no tumor growth occurred and the animals remained alive during a 6 month observation period. To our knowledge, no further research has been conducted on the chemotherapeutic value of garlic.

Based on Indian traders' hearsay, Fell[80] reported the use of the red sap from bloodroot (*Sanguinaria canadensis,* Fig. 5-3a) for treatment of cancerous diseases by the North American Indians living along the shores of Lake Superior. On

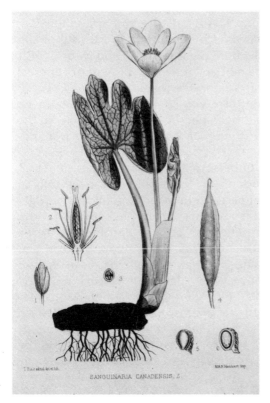

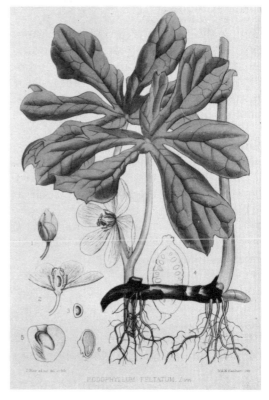

Figure 5-3a *Sanguinaria canadensis* (from R Bentley and H Trimen, *Medicinal Plants* **1**:20, 1880).

Figure 5-3b *Podophyllum peltatum* (from R Bentley and H Trimen, *Medicinal Plants* **1**: 17, 1880).

hearing of this plant, Fell developed a treatment far superior to any other, a therapy based on a paste of bloodroot extract, zinc chloride, flour, and water. The paste was smeared on a cloth or cotton and placed on the tumor daily (if healthy tissue covered the tumor, it was eroded with nitric acid). When the tumor became encrusted, incisions were made about one-half inch apart and the paste was inserted into the cuts daily. Generally within 2 to 4 weeks the disease was destroyed, with the mass falling out in 10 to 14 additional days, leaving a flat healthy sore that usually healed rapidly.

Fell's technique was perfected at the Middlesex Hospital, London, and the results of 25 cases, mostly of breast cancer, are detailed in his treatise. All cases illustrated remissions, if not cures. He compared his method with that of surgery in 1857; 8 of 10 surgical patients returned within 2 years for further treatment, only 3 of 10 returned after using his therapy. In his preface, Fell reports generally complimentary remarks from his peer group at Middlesex. This consensus is verified by Stone,[81] notwithstanding the negative note concerning the use of *Sanguinaria* by Bentley and Timen: "... it would appear that, if it produces any effect in such cases, it must be very small indeed, and that it is, therefore, practically useless for such a purpose."[82]

Prior to Fell's use, *Sanguinaria* had been widely recommended in the United States to treat warts and nasal polyps[83] and also skin cancers,[84] a folk practice extending to recent times. For centuries *Sanguinaria* has also been used as a folk remedy in Russia.[77]

These applications were first given a scientific basis by Stickl,[85] who found that the alkaloids sanguinarine and chelerythrine exerted a distinct therapeutic action on Ehrlich carcinoma in mice. Likewise, Shear et al.[86] reported that these alkaloids had a significant necrotizing effect on sarcoma 37 in mice.

A recent revival of a chemosurgical method similar to that developed by Fell[80] is being used with dramatic success against superficial carcinomas, including those of the nose and external ear. Phelan et al.[87] report a majority of patients completely healed of tumors with very few recurrences after the application of bloodroot plus zinc chloride paste.

A parallel example is found for the North American May apple (*Podophyllum peltatum,* Fig. 5-3b), the rhizome or underground stem of which was used years ago by the Penobscot Indians of Maine to treat cancer.[88] The resin from this species was recommended in an American materia medica more than 100 years ago for the treatment of cancerous tumors, polyps, and unhealthy granulations. *Podophyllum* resin, or podophyllin, was used by physicians in Mississippi and Missouri as early as 1897 and by urologists in Louisiana for the treatment of venereal warts (condyloma acuminata). Recent clinical reports[89] signify that podophyllin has become the drug of choice in the treatment of human condyloma acuminata.

Others report a destructive effect of podophyllin on different cancer cells in animals and in man.[90] Chemical investigation of this resin has revealed the presence of several lignans, the three most prevalent being podophylloxin and α and β-peltatins. Each of these lignans shows tumor-damaging activity in mice.[91] Although damage to deep-lying malignant tissues has been observed in many instances, the satisfactory use of these drugs has been complicated by their toxicity,[77] a disadvantage that may be obviated by the use of derivatives, such as epipodophyllotoxin.[92]

Thus we have two examples of crude extracts from North American plants originally used by the Indians to treat cancer. In both cases the extracts were prescribed by physicians in the nineteenth century. Today a paste containing bloodroot, which is used in conjunction with surgery to treat skin cancers, and resin from the May apple, is still the preferred therapy for venereal warts.

Constituents from many other plants are under study, and still others are now in use (see Current Therapy). Understandably, some folkloric anticancer plants remain simply as ingredients of interesting historic remedies that probably never had much therapeutic value, except perhaps a placebo effect. On the other hand, certain remedies may have contained potential carcinogens, as for example, safrole from *Sassafras,* which was one of the ingredients used in a cancer cure in Virginia (1734):

Another woeful Case, is, a Cancer, which some despairingly imagine to be incurable; tho', blessed be God, there have been some Instances of Success, by the Method hereafter mentioned. In the mean Time, it usually begins with little hard Lumps, or Swellings, in the Breast, Lip, or other glandulous Part of the Body. These afterwards break into painful Sores, which eat farther and farther, 'til at last, they reach some large Vessel, or mortal Part.

In this case, the Patient must submit, in the first Place, to have the hard Lump cut clean out, so soon as he is convinc'd it is a *Cancer.* And, for curing the Wound, he can't do better than make Use of the following *Balsam:* He must boil 6 Ounces of *Sassafras Root,* and as much *Dogwood Root,* in a *Gallon* of *Water,* 'til it be wasted to a *pint,* and having strain'd it off, must drench a *Pledget* therein, and apply it warm to the Sore, renewing it every Day; And if he will have the Patience to continue this for some Time, I can assure him, he will not be the first that has been blest with Success.

Let him drink *Sassafras Tea* every Morning, live temperately, upon light and innocent Food; and abstain entirely from strong Liquor.

The Way to prevent this Calamity, is, to be very sparing in eating Pork, to forbear all salt, and high season'd Meats, and live chiefly upon the Garden, The Orchard, and the Hen-House.[93]

No other disease has attracted such unorthodox methodology or treatment as has cancer. The best example of this is the use of Laetrile, a substance derived from an extract of apricot pits that is dispensed legally by physicians in Mexico but is illegal for use in the United States, Canada, and certain other countries.[94] Seeds (including pits?) of the common apricot (*Prunus armeniaca* or *Armeniaca vulgaris*), native to China, were used there against tumors as early as AD 502.[77] Apricot oil was also used against tumors or swellings of ulcers in England during the seventeenth century.[95] Nevertheless, even though unsubstantiated in modern therapy, these independent treatments would suggest even to the most ardent disbeliever an interesting coincidence worthy of exploration.

Laetrile therapy is based on the theory that once inside the body, the extract from apricot pits breaks down into several components including cyanide. Cyanide is released only when it comes into contact with an enzyme common to tumor cells, β-glucuronidase, at which time cyanide chokes off the tumor cells, leaving the healthy cells surrounding the growth untouched.[96] Because its use is restricted, few tests of this theory or therapy with this agent have been conducted either in animals or humans. Morrone,[97] using Laetrile, showed regression of malignant lesions in 10 cases of inoperable cancer, all with metastases. He also reported that dramatic relief from pain was associated with the treatment. Several other reports have been negative, but well-controlled experiments are lacking.[98] A test of Laetrile's effectiveness was recently announced by the Memorial Sloan-Kettering Cancer Center[99] and this is fortunate, for in the absence of such testing, debate and confusion on the issue will surely continue.[100]

Other current unproved methods of treatment include:[101] chapparral tea obtained from steeping leaves and stems of the creosote bush, *Larrea divaricata,* in hot water; CH-23, a secret remedy prepared from toxins contained in plants; Ferguson Plant Products, involving six essential plants; Krebiozen, derived from extracts of the blood of horses previously injected with a sterile extract of *Actinomyces bovis,* a bacterium causing "lumpy jaw" in cattle; KC-555, a botanical extract derived from plants grown in Asia; Nichols' escharotic method, essentially confined to the use of escharotic pastes of arsenic and/or zinc compounds; and numerous others.[102]

CURRENT THERAPY

When a growth endangers your life, remove it. What simpler concept could exist for the cure of cancer than an operation to remove the disease? As early as 2500 BC the Hindus applied this direct principle, eradicating cancerous lesions of the skin by cautery.[73] Today successful procedures range from the simple removal of small skin cancers by the same method to the most involved cancer surgery using the most refined techniques.

Either as an adjunct to surgery or cancer-combating drugs, or as a primary treatment for cancer, radiotherapy has become a necessity for approximately half of all cancer patients. Recent advances in the field of radiology allow earlier detection of cancer, and there are now improved techniques and treatments involving the use of X-ray, radioactive cobalt, linear acceleration, and radioactive elements (discussed under

Chemotherapy). The newer neutron therapy, and the use of pi-mesons (atomic particles that can be preset to explode at the precise site of a cancer, thereby destroying the malignancy without harm to surrounding tissue) are only now being used clinically, and their addition to the physician's arsenal should aid greatly in the all-out effort against cancer.[103]

CHEMOTHERAPY

The basic assumption in cancer treatment is that all cancer cells must be killed or removed to achieve cure—that is, to render the patient's life expectancy the same as a normal life expectancy. In many cases surgery and radiotherapy fail to cure, chiefly because the tumor is already disseminated. For this reason chemotherapeutic agents are sought, to reduce the patient's tumor burden so that a cure may be possible. Cures, or apparent cures, from drugs alone have been obtained for such diseases as choriocarcinoma, Burkitt's lymphoma, acute childhood lymphocytic leukemia, and Hodgkin's disease. The recent success of many drugs, often administered in combination, and frequently including at least one from plant sources, has in the past decade given the greatest new hope of recovery from this ominous disease complex.[104]

How do antineoplastic drugs work? Their efficacy is based on the unique abnormal metabolism of malignant cells. Normal tissue cells divide and differentiate according to a predetermined genetic plan, which is probably regulated by local growth-controlling substances. In tumor cells, this control system is annulled by mutation, by foreign nucleic acid of viral origin, by interference from carcinogens, or by any combination of these.

Metabolic differences between malignant and normal cells may be largely deletive (i.e., restrictive of substrate utilization) so that tumors are frequently at a natural disadvantage compared with normal cells. In addition, malignant cells are actively dividing, whereas the majority of adult tissue cells show only occasional mitoses. Thus agents active against cells at this stage have a marked role against the malignancy.

The aim of cancer chemotherapy is to eradicate all malignant cells, ideally with little or no effect on the normal cells. It is comparatively easy to kill 99% of the malignant cells, but resistant ones are nearly always present, and from these recurrences result.

Antineoplastic drugs may be classified as alkylating agents, antimetabolites, hormones, and radioactive isotopes, besides a miscellaneous group from naturally occurring sources.[105]

Alkylating agents, which include one of the first discovered cytotoxic compounds, mustine hydrochloride (Nitrogen Mustard®), are able to kill malignant cells during all phases of their cycle by combining chemically with nucleic acids. Mechlorethamine (Mustargen®) given intravenously is somewhat effective against Hodgkin's disease and may provide up to 2 months or more remission. The substance is extremely irritating, and side effects are numerous. Other commercially available alkylating agents include Thiotepa®, chlorambucil, cyclophosphamide, Triethylene-melamine®, melphalan, and busulfan; in general, these are used against Hodgkin's disease and other lymphomas, lymphocytic leukemia, and certain solid cancers.

Antimetabolites include Methotrexate®, mercaptopurine, Thioguanine®, Fluorouracil®, and cytarabine, all available commercially. These agents usually kill cells at the time of DNA synthesis in preparation for cell division, either by depriving the cell of vital substrates necessary for DNA synthesis or by being incorporated into DNA as gradulent precursors.

Hormones available commercially are prednisone, a widely used adrenal corticosteroid in compound chemotherapy; diethylstilbestrol and ethinyl estradiol, both estrogens effective in the treatment of breast carcinoma and in the carcinoma of the prostate; androgens (testosterone propionate, testosterone enanthate, testolactone) also effective in the treatment of breast cancer; and the progestagens (hydroxyprogesterone, megestrol acetate) used to treat metastatic and recurrent endometrial carcinoma.

Radioactive isotopes include:[106] iodine [131] readily taken up by the thyroid gland, where the destructive action of radiation may be effective in treating carcinoma of the thyroid; phosphorus[32] in the form of sodium phosphate, which is useful in the treatment of polycythemia vera, inhibiting the overproduction of red and white blood cells; and gold[198] used when cancer results in excessive fluid accumulation in the peritoneal cavity.

Naturally Occurring Agents

With the discovery of antineoplastic compounds from plants, cancer chemotherapy can be said to have come of age. The modern era began in 1938 when it was learned that colchicine was cytotoxic.[107] This alkaloid is obtained from the autumn crocus (*Colchicum autumnale*), and it acts by disrupting the spindle mechanism during mitosis, thereby blocking cell division. Clinical studies with colchicine have been disappointing, but compounds from other plants, such as the periwinkle *Catharanthus (Vinca) roseus* (Fig. 5-4), exhibit similar inhibitory properties (Fig.

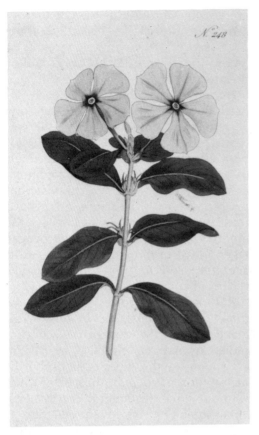

Figure 5-4 *Catharanthus* (*Vinca*) *roseus* (from *Curtis's Botanical Magazine* 7: 248, 1794).

ganulocytes, and profoundly depressed bone marrow activity in rats. From these specific observations, they studied the effects of the active leukopenic extract against leukemia cells *in vitro*. This eventually led to the isolation of vincaleukoblastine by Noble and co-workers. Meanwhile at Eli Lilly, Svoboda tested an extract of periwinkle in a routine screening program, which included tests on mice against the P-1534 leukemia, a tumor system particularly sensitive to the periwinkle alkaloids. The inhibitory action of the extract was dramatic, and Svoboda and his co-workers developed the technology that eventually led to the commercial production of vincaleukoblastine. Later work by the Lilly group culminated in the discovery of leurocristine, now considered the drug of choice for inducing remissions in childhood leukemias, usually in combination with other drugs.[109] Thus quite independently, two distinct approaches, one following a specific experimental observation and the other stemming from a broad screening program, led to similar conclusions and at last to the production and use of two drugs of plant origin, leurocristine and vincaleukoblastine.

As a postscript to this story, we should note that the National Cancer Institute in their screening program also tested extracts from periwinkle and found no antineoplastic activity. This is because the screening program of the government did not include the P-1534 leukemia, and unexpectedly, the periwinkle alkaloids were not active against the tumor systems in use at that time by the National Cancer Institute. Activity of any known drug or treatment is not univeral against this disease complex, as these results so clearly indicate; they stress, however, the necessity for multiple approaches and combination of different compounds.

The commercially available drugs from periwinkle are vincaleukoblastine sulfate

5-5)[108] and have been used with considerable success.

The story of the discovery of the antitumor value of periwinkle extracts is well worth repeating, if only to illustrate and to emphasize that chance discoveries are still made in science.

Because the plant had been cited in folk medicine as an aid in treating diabetes, periwinkle extracts were studied as part of a survey seeking oral insulin substitutes, by Noble and Beer at the University of Western Ontario, and by Svoboda at Eli Lilly in Indianapolis. Neither group could substantiate the folklore, but the Canadian investigators noted that a crude extract of this plant drastically reduced white blood cell counts, especially the

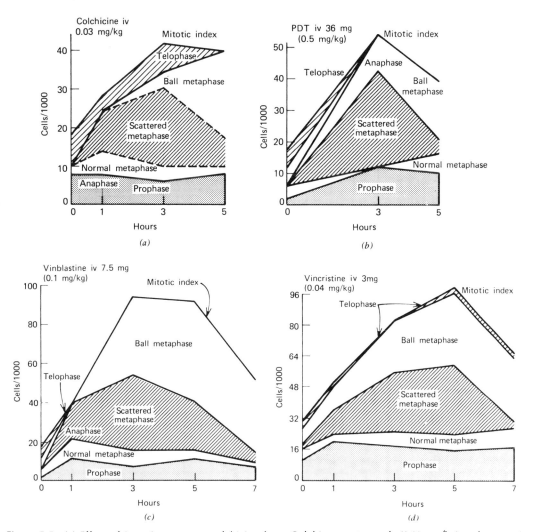

Figure 5-5 (a) Effect of 3 mg intravenous colchicine from *Colchicum autumnale* (0.03 mg/kg) on bone marrow mitotic index. (b) Effect of 36 mg intravenous podophyllotoxin from *Podophyllum peltatum* (0.5 mg/kg) on bone marrow mitotic index. (c) Effect of 7.5 mg intravenous vinblastine from *Catharanthus roseus* (0.1 mg/kg) on bone marrow mitotic index. (d) Effect of 3 mg intravenous vincristine from *Catharanthus roseus* (0.04 mg/kg) on bone marrow mitotic index. Note the high level of effects on mitotic disturbance following treatment with vinblastine and vincristine alkaloids. (Adapted from H Savel, "The metaphase-arresting plant alkaloids and cancer chemotherapy," p 189–224, in H Homburger (ed), *Progress in Experimental Tumor Research*, Volume 8, 1966. Copyrighted © by S. Karger AG, Basel, and reprinted with permission.)

(vinblastine sulfate, VLB, Velban®) and leurocristine sulfate (vincristine sulfate, VCR, Oncovin®). Although these alkaloids are very similar in chemical structure, they differ markedly in antitumor spectra and side effects. VLB is particularly useful in Hodgkin's disease and in choriocarcinoma, as well as other neoplasms, whereas VCR has its main use in treating acute leukemia in children (Table 5-1). Remission rate and cure can be spectacular (Table 5-2), although toxic side effects such as nausea, vomiting, local irritation, loss of reflexes, and so

Table 5-1 Commercially Available Cancer Chemotherapeutic Drugs of Plant Origin (1974)[110]

Drug	Species	Toxicity		Major Indications
		Acute	Delayed	
Vinblastine sulfate (Fig. 5-6) (Velban®)	*Catharanthus (Vinca) roseus*	Nausea and vomiting, local irritant	Alopecia; stomatitis; bone marrow depression; loss of reflexes	Hodgkin's disease and other lymphomas, solid tumors
Vincristine sulfate (Fig. 5-6) (Oncovin®)		Local irritant	Areflexia; peripheral neuritis; paralytic ileus; mild bone marrow depression	Acute lymphocytic leukemia, Hodgkin's disease and other tumors of childhood
Dactinomycin (Fig. 5-6) (actinomycin D; Cosmegen®)	*Streptomyces parvullus*	Nausea and vomiting, local irritant	Stomatitis; oral ulcers; diarrhea; alopecia; mental depression; bone marrow depression	Testicular carcinoma, Wilms' tumor, rhabdomyosarcoma, Ewing's and osteogenic sarcoma, and other solid tumors
Mithramycin (Fig. 5-6) (Mithracin®)	*Streptomyces plicatus*	Nausea and vomiting, hepatotoxicity	Bone marrow depression; hypocalcemia	Testicular carcinoma, trophoblastic neoplasma
Bleomycin sulfate (Blenoxame®)	*Streptomyces verticillatus*	Nausea, vomiting, fever: very toxic	Edema of hand; pulmonary fibrosis; stomatitis; alopecia	Hodgkin's disease, non-Hodgkin's lymphomas, squamous cell carcinomas in the head and neck, penis, cervicus, and vulva, testicular carcinomas
Adriamycin	*Streptomyces peucetius var. caesius*	Nausea, red urine (not hematuria)	Bone marrow depression, cardiotoxicity, alopecia; stomatitis	Soft tissue, osteogenic and miscellaneous sarcomas, Hodgkin's disease, non-Hodgkin's lymphomas, bronchogenic and breast carcinoma

Table 5-2   Prolonged Survival or Cure of Neoplastic Diseases Responding to Chemotherapy[111]

Type of Cancer	Useful Drug (often used in combination; those of plant origin in italics)	Result
Gestational choriocarcinoma tumors	*Vinblastine, Dactinomycin, Mithramycin,* Methotrexate	70% cured
Burkitt's lymphoma	*Vincristine,* Cyclophosphamide, Methotrexate, Cytosine arabinoside	50% cured
Testicular tumors	*Dactinomycin, Mithramycin,* Methothrexate, Chlorambucil	30–40% response, 2–3% cured
Wilms' tumor	*Vincristine, Dactinomycin* (+ surgery and radiotherapy)	80% cured
Acute lymphocytic leukemia	*Vincristine,* Prednisone, *Daunomycin*	99% *remission,* 50% survive after three years
Hodgkin's disease	*Vincristine,* Prednisone, Procarbazine, *Bleomycin,* nitrogen mustard	40% survive after five years

forth, necessitate close surveillance during therapy. VLB depresses the bone marrow, whereas VCR does not; similarly, VCR is neurotoxic, while VLB is not.

It is not surprising that bacteria, well known for their antibiotic properties, also produce antineoplastic agents. At least four of these derived from species of *Streptomyces* are used commercially: dactinomycin (actinomycin D), which binds directly to DNA; mithramycin, which inhibits the synthesis of RNA; bleomycin, and adriamycin. The first two antibiotics exhibit major efficacy against testicular carcinomas; but dactinomycin also acts against Wilms' tumor and Ewing's carcinoma, and mithramycin can be effective against trophoblastic neoplasms (Table 5-1). Bleomycin sulfate is effective against squamous cell carcinomas in the head and neck regions, and adriamycin against Hodgkin's disease and other lymphomas. In addition, streptozotocin is used against carcinoid tumors of the appendix and gastrointestinal tract, and

against malignant insulinoma. Undoubtedly this drug and others noted in Table 5-3 will be released soon for general medical use.

In addition, drugs under active study by the Drug Development Branch of the National Cancer Institute are classified under four categories according to trial level and activity (Table 5-4). The drugs were obtained from numerous higher plant families of wide evolutionary divergence from either temperate or tropical regions. Chemically the drugs are also very diverse, for they include alkaloids, triterpenes, lignans, quinones, diterpenes, and saponins.

Extracts of species from the Apocynaceae, Celastraceae, Magnoliales, Rutaceae, Simaroubaceae, and Thymelaeaceae are among the most active against cancer, and because of their primary importance, research for naturally occurring agents is now focusing on these taxa at the National Cancer Institute. Certain tribes of the Rubiaceae

Table 5-3 Investigational Cancer Chemotherapeutic Drugs of Bacterial Origin (1974)[110]

Drug	Species	Toxicity		Major Indications
		Acute	Delayed	
Daunorubicin (daunomycin, rubindomycin; Cerubidine®)	*Streptomyces peucetius*	Nausea, fever, red urine (not hematuria)	Bone marrow depression, cardiotoxicity, alopecia	Acute lymphocytic and granulocytic leukemia
Streptozotocin	*Streptomyces achromogenes*	Nausea, vomiting	Renal damage	Malignant insulinoma, carcinoid
Asparaginase (Elspar®) (Fig. 5-6)	*Escherichia coli*	Nausea, fever, possible anaphylactic reaction	Hepatoxicity; pancreatitis; central nervous system depression	Acute lymphocytic leukemia

are also being examined vigorously because of potentially significant antineoplastics newly discovered in that family.

To date, about 25,000 species of vascular plants have been examined at the Institute. Extracts of samples are tested against two lines, a cell culture of human nasopharynx carcinosarcoma (KB) and mouse leukemia (P-388), and against a second mouse leukemia line (L-1210) if encouraging results are obtained initially. When noteworthy remissions are found, the crude plants are fractionated to isolate their active constituents, and these are eventually used in pharmacological regimens including those for cancer patients (Table 5-4).[112]

Not all results from this survey have been encouraging. In fact, two of the largest Angiosperm families have been disappointing in their yield of active compounds. The Asteraceae principally have sesquiterpene lactone agents and pyrrolizidine alkaloids, and the Fabaceae often have highly active tannins and pyrrolizidine alkaloids, but their erratic activity and toxicity preclude further interest in them as antitumor agents for man.[113]

The following compilation, though by no means complete, is sufficiently inclusive to illustrate the active research for naturally occurring agents from among many groups of plants (see also Table 5-4). The species have been organized by major plant groups; the Angiosperms are also indicated by family, and common names and major chemotherapeutic compounds have been added when known (Fig. 5-6). General references for these agents[114] are followed by a selection of papers representing a range of families, compounds, and researchers.[115]

BACTERIA. *Actinomyces albus* var. *bruneomycin* = streptonigrin (= bruneomycin); *Streptomyces carzinostaticus* = neocarzinostatin (a protein), *S. caspitosus* = mitomycins; *S. chrisomottus* = actinomycins, *S. flocculus* = streptonigrin, *S. griseus* = toyomycin (chromomycins), *S. malayensis* = mitomalcin, *S. olivoreticuli* = olivomycins, *S. refuineus* = anthramycin (refuin), *S. rufocromogenes* = rufochromomycin, *S. showoensis* = showdomycin, *S. verticillatus* = mitomycin C and porfiriomycin, *S. spp.* = mithramycin, and *S. sp.* unidentified = sangivamycin.

FUNGI. *Amanita phalloides* = crude extract; *Aspergillus fumigatus* = fumagillin;

Boletus edulis = fruiting body extracts; *Calvatia gigantea* (giant puffball) = calvacin (a protein); *Claviceps purpurea* (ergot) = ergotamine, ergocryptine, and ergocornine; *Penicillium* spp. = mycophenolic acid; *Poria corticola* = poricin (a protein).

FERN. *Polypodium leucotomos* = saponin.

GYMNOSPERMS. *Juniperus virginiana* (juniper or red cedar) = podophyllotoxin; *Libocedrus decurrens* (incense-cedar) = deoxypodophyllotoxin; and *Taxodium*

Table 5-4   Cancer Chemotherapeutic Drugs from Higher Plants[a]

Family and Species	Active Compound	Original Source
Now or Formerly[b] in Clinical Trial		
APOCYNACEAE. *Catharanthus (Vinca) roseus*	Vinblastine sulfate, vincristine sulfate	India
ASCLEPIADACEAE. *Tylophora crebriflora[b]*	Tylocrebrine	Australia
BERBERIDACEAE. *Podophyllum emodi*	4'-Demethylepi-podophyllotoxin thenylidene glucoside	India
BIGNONIACEAE. *Tabebuia[b]* and *Tecoma[b]* spp.	Lapachol	Brazil
LILIACEAE. *Colchicum autumnale*	Demecolcine, colchicine	Europe
MENISPERMACEAE. *Stephania hernandifolia*	Tetrandrine	India
NYSSACEAE. *Camptotheca acuminata[b]*	Camptothecin	China
RANUNCULACEAE. *Thalictrum dasycarpum*	Thalicarpine	United States
RUBIACEAE. *Cephaelis ipecacuanha[b]*	Emetine	South America
RUTACEAE. *Acronychia baueri*	Acronycine	Australia
Scheduled for Clinical Trial, in or Through Pharmacology		
APOCYNACEAE		
Excavatia coccinea	Ellipticine	New Guinea
Ochrosia moorei	Ellipticine	Australia
BORAGINACEAE. *Heliotropium indicum*	Indicine *N*-oxide	India
CELASTRACEAE		
Maytenus buchananii	Maytansine	Kenya
Putterlickia verricosa	Maytansine	South Africa
Scheduled for Pharmacology		
ACERACEAE. *Acer negundo*	*Acer*-saponin	United States
CEPHALOTAXACEAE. *Cephalotaxus harringtonia*	Harringtonine, homoharringtonine	United States
FABACEAE. *Caesalpinia gilliesii*	Cesalin	United States
RUTACEAE. *Fagara macrophylla*	8-Methoxy-dihydronitidine	Nigeria
Also of Interest		
CELASTRACEAE. *Tripterygium wilfordii*	Triptolide, tripdiolide	China
SIMAROUBACEAE. *Brucea antidysenterica*	Bruceantin	Ethiopia
TAXACEAE. *Taxus brevifolia*	Taxol	United States

[a] Based on a personal communication from Dr. J. L. Hartwell, Head, Natural Products Section, National Cancer Institute, Bethesda, Maryland.
[b] Clinical trial discontinued.

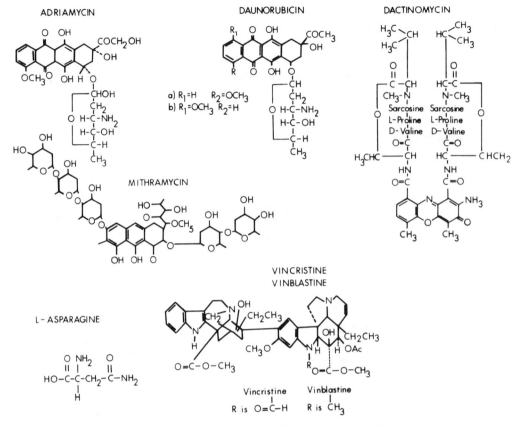

Figure 5-6   Chemical formulas of some naturally occurring chemotherapeutic agents.

distichum (bald cypress) = taxodione and taxodone.

ANGIOSPERMS

ANNONACEAE. *Annona purpurea* (custard-apple) = apomorphine alkaloids.

APOCYNACEAE. *Apocynum cannabinum* (Indian hemp) = apocannoside and cymarin (cardiac glycosides); *Bleekeria* sp. = ellipticine; *Catharanthus lanceus* (periwinkle) = leurosine; *Ochrosia elliptica* and *O. poweri* = ellipticine.

ARALIACEAE. *Panax ginseng* (ginseng) = crude root extracts (steroids?).

ARISTOLOCHIACEAE. *Aristolochia indica* (Birthwort) = aristolochic acid.

ASCLEPIADACEAE. *Asclepias curassavica* = calotropin (cardiac glycoside); *Cryptostegia grandiflora* = cardiac glycosides.

ASTERACEAE. *Balduina angustifolia* = angustibalin, rotenone, helenalin, and hispidulin; *Carduus benedictus* (plumeless thistle) = crude extract; *Elephantopus elatus* (elephant's-foot) = elephantopin and elephantin; *Eupatorium cuneifolium* (thoroughwort) = eupacunin, eupacunoxin, eupatocunin, eupatocunoxin, and eupacunolin; *E. formosanum* = eupatolide, *E. rotundifolium* = euparotin acetate and eupachlorin acetate, *E. semiserratum* = eupaserrin and deacetyleupaserrin; *Gaillardia pulchella* (blanket-flower) = gaillardin; *Gutierrezia sarothrea* (broom-snakeroot) = protein; *Liatris chapmannii* (blazing-star) = liatrin; *Senecio triangularis* (groundsel) = senecionine, senecionine-N-oxide; *Tagetes minuta* = crude extract; *Vernonia amygdalina* (ironweed) = vernodalin and vernomygdin, *V. hymenolepis* = vernolepin.

BERBERIDACEAE. *Podophyllum peltatum* (May apple) = podophyllotoxin and related lignans.

BETULACEAE (CORYLACEAE). *Alnus oregona* (alder) = betulin and lupeol.

BIGNONIACEAE. *Stereospermum suavolens* = lapachol.

BURSERACEAE. *Bursera microphylla* = burseran, *B. schlechtendalii* = lignans.

BUXACEAE. *Buxus sempervirens* (boxwood) = cycloprotobuxine.

CORNACEAE. *Cornus canadensis* (dwarf cornel) = tannin.

CUCURBITACEAE. *Brandegea bigelovii* = cucurbitacins.

ERICACEAE. *Arctostaphylos pringlei* (bearberry) = crude extracts.

EUPHORBIACEAE. *Croton macrostachys* = crotepoxide; *Jatropha gossypiifolia* and *J. macrorhiza* = jatropham; *Ricinus communis* (castor bean) = ricin.

FABACEAE. *Abrus precatorius* (rosary pea) = abrin; *Crotalaria assamica* and *C. spectabilis* (rattlebox) = monocrotaline; *Lespedeza capitata* var. *velutina* (bush-clover) = tannin.

HERNANDIACEAE. *Hernandia ovigera* = thalicarpine.

JUGLANDACEAE. *Juglans nigra* (black walnut) = ellagic acid and juglone.

LAMIACEAE. *Hyptis emoryi* = betulinic acid.

LILIACEAE (including AMARYLLIDACEAE). *Agave schottii* = saponin; *Allium sativum* (garlic) = allicin; *Colchicum autumnale, C. luteum* = colchicine; *Gloriosa superba* (African climbing lily) = colchicine; *Muscari comosum* (African onion) = bulb extract; *Narcissus tazetta* = pseudolycorine; *Paris formosana* = crude extract.

LORANTHACEAE. *Viscum album* (European mistletoe) = 11 proteins.

MAGNOLIACEAE. *Magnolia grandiflora* = parthenolide.

MELASTOMATACEAE. *Calycogonium squamulosum* = a tannin, having a partial structure of tri-O-galloyl-D-glucose.

MELIANTHACEAE. *Bersama abyssinica* = bufadienolides.

MENISPERMACEAE. *Cyclea barbata* and *C. peltata* = tetrandrine, isotetrandrine, and dimethyltetrandrine.

MYRSINACEAE. *Myrsine africana* and *Wallenia yunquensis* = myrsine-saponin.

MYRTACEAE. *Leptospermum scoparium* = ellagic acid.

NYCTAGINACEAE. *Mirabilis multiflora* (four-o'clock).

ONAGRACEAE. *Oenothera caespitosa* (evening-primrose) = gallic acid.

PAPAVERACEAE. *Sanguinaria canadensis* (bloodroot) = sanguinarine and chelerythrine.

PIPERACEAE. *Piper brachystachum, P. futokadzura,* and *P. hookeri* = crotepoxide.

POLYGONACEAE. *Rumex hymenosepalus* (dock) = a tannin that following hydrolysis yields leucodelphinidin and leucopelargonidin.

PRIMULACEAE. *Cyclamen hederifolium* and *C. persicum* = saponins.

RANUNCULACEAE. *Thalictrum minum* subsp. *elatum* and *T. revolutum* = thalicarpine, *T. rugosum* = thalidasine.

ROSACEAE. *Amelanchier utahensis* (juneberry or serviceberry) = crude extracts; *Rubus odoratus* (thimbleberry) = tannin.

RUTACEAE. *Acronychia petiolaris* = acronycine; *Fagara zanthoxyloides* = fagaronine.

SIMAROUBACEAE. *Holacantha emoryi* = holacanthone.

SOLANACEAE. *Acnistus arborescens* = withaferin A and withacnistin; *Jaborosa integrifolia* = jaborosolides; *Solanum dulcamara* (woody nightshade) = β-solamarine, *S. tripartitum* = solapalmitine and solapalmitenine; *Withania coagulans* and *W. somnifera* = withanolides.

URTICACEAE. *Boehmeria cyclindrica* (false nettle) = cryptopleurine.

ZINGIBERACEAE. *Kaempferia rotunda* = crotepoxide.

The list is noteworthy for the number of bacteria of the genus *Streptomyces* included, and for the broad array of plant families in the dicotyledons, with a strong focus on the Liliaceae among the monocotyledons. With continued exploration, particularly in the families of known ef-ficacy, new drugs should soon be available to increase the value of chemotherapeutic agents against cancer.

IMMUNOTHERAPY

Protein changes known to be induced by chemical carcinogens or oncogenic virus infections in malignant cells are referred to as tumor antigens (Fig. 5-7). The recognition and response of the immune system to these specific chemicals correspond with the patient's ability to control the development and progression of his cancer. Destruction of these malignant cells may be mediated by specific cytotoxic antibodies or sensitized phagocytic cells. As long as this mechanism functions efficiently, malignant transformations, which constantly arise, are eliminated before they can reach cell proportions where immunological control is no longer effective. However if the body produces antibodies that "block"

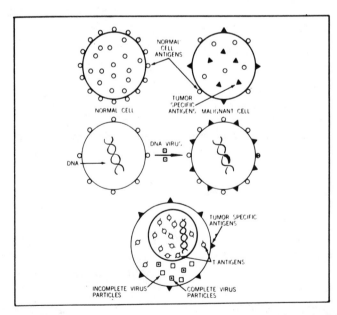

Figure 5-7   Virus induction of tumor antigens. Normal surface antigens may be reduced in malignancy; none completely missing. New tumor specific antigens may appear. (From *Scope® Monograph on Immunology*, p 33, fig 33, 1972, by permission of The Upjohn Company, Kalamazoo, Michigan.)

cytotoxic antibody activity, or if cell-mediated immunity malfunctions, malignancies can develop. Therefore the basis of immunotherapy is the utilization of techniques that can directly or indirectly induce or enhance the body's immune system to act against the cancer.[116]

Active Immunotherapy

Techniques that can assure successful active immunotherapy have yet to be developed. Problems have occurred in connection with rejection phenomena associated with the introduction of foreign histocompatibility transplantation antigens (HLA) from donor tumors, the inactivation of tumor oncogenicity without destruction of specific tumor transplantation antigens from donor and the enhancement of antigenicity of these tumor antigens. Once malignancies are understood well enough to permit the identification and isolation of specific tumor antigens with techniques that will retain or enhance their antigenicity, it is expected that this techinque will be applied once again among immunocompetent patients.

Passive Immunotherapy

Little success has been achieved by using antitumor sera from foreign species, since toxicity results from the activity of cytotoxic antibodies made by this technique to normal tissue (transplantation-HLA) antigens. Theoretically, this problem would be overcome once specific antitumor transplantation antibody could be made. Regressions of certain sarcomas and leukemias could be expected with the use of such a high titered specific antitumor antibody, which would either reverse the inhibiting effect on killer lymphocytes by circulating antigen-antibody complexes or "deblock" the effect of blocking antibodies.

Experimental evidence supports the concept that antitumor immunity is primarily in the mediated cell. In this context passive immunotherapy, using sensitized lymphoid (killer cells), could be applied to overcome the defects of cell-mediated immunity found in cancer patients. To have such optimal immunotherapeutic effect, however, transferred lymphocytes must persist in the host for a significant period of time. To circumvent the problems related to HLA-type rejection of donor lymphocytes, several techniques have been devised.

The most obvious approach is to grow the patient's own lymphocytes in bulk in tissue culture, then reinfuse them into the patient or inject them directly into his tumor deposits. Various degrees of success have been reported in attempts to further enhance their antitumor effect by exposing these cultured cells to phytohemagglutinin (PHA) derived from the kidney bean, *Phaseolus vulgaris*. The uses of other mitogens derived from plant lectins such as the pokeweed mitogen (PWM) from *Phytolacca americana*, derivatives of several species of *Wisteria* including *W. floribunda*, the jack bean Concanavalin A from *Canavalia ensiformis*, that from *Lathyrus odoratus* and other species, have yet to be included in clinical protocols (Chapter 4).

Although recent animal experiments have indicated that *in vitro* sensitization of cultured lymphocytes with tumor cells treated with mitomycin C (derived from *Streptomyces verticillatus*) is a very effective way to induce enhanced antitumor immunity, less impressive results have been obtained in limited clinical trials. Nevertheless, the utilization of this ability of mitomycin C to prevent tumor cells from forming metastases when reinfused into the patient deserves further study. Alternatively, family members of patients with sarcomas—individuals already naturally sensitized to these tumor specific antigens—could contribute lymphocytes, or these could be obtained from allogenic cancer patients who have undergone spontaneous remissions.

Although the reasons for the limited success ascribed to immunotherapy with lymphocytes sensitized by transplantation in the treatment of tumors remain obscure, this form of therapy has resulted in complete regressions of 3 to 5% of the cases so treated and partial regression in an additional 15 to 20%. Although the donor lymphocytes may be HLA incompatible and undoubtedly will be rejected in the immunocompetent patient, at least for a short vital period they are able to enhance a patient's immune system, permitting active regression to proceed.

Of considerable promise is the possible therapeutic use of informational molecules that can be extracted from sensitized lymphocytes and have the ability to induce a specific immune response in the recipient's immune effector system. Immune RNA can be produced in a xenogenic host (in this case, other than human), giving this substance decided pharmaceutical advantages over a transfer factor that must come from human sources.[116]

Nonspecific Immunotherapy

The ability of certain bacterial infections, particularly erysipelas, to enhance nonspecifically the host's immune response to other disease and malignancies has been recognized since the time of Hippocrates (460–377 BC). Once bacterial techniques, devised in the late 1800s, permitted investigators to culture the organism Streptococcus pyogenes (= S. erysipelatosus), serious research was undertaken by many workers, particularly

Dr. W. B. Coley, to further ascertain why such malignant regressions could be induced. This led him to develop Coley's toxins, consisting of mixtures of the living or heat-killed Streptococcus and of Bacillus prodigiosus; the latter, he believed, intensified the potency of the preparations. Although Coley documented several impressive regressions attributed to this therapy, less remarkable independent studies by his peers resulted in a lack of recognition of his therapy.[118]

More recently other nonspecific immune stimulators have been found to be effective in eliciting an immune response against a wide range of tumor types, including spontaneous autochthonous tumors. Aside from zymosan, oleic acid, nucleic acid, DNA digest, and vaccinia virus, the following bacteria or bacterial products found to be active are Corynebacterium parvum, Bordetella pertussis endotoxin, members of the genus Mycobacterium (including Freund's adjuvant containing M. butyricum), and most frequently the attenuated tubercle bacillus vaccine, Bacillus Calmette-Guerin. Generally those nonspecific immunologic adjuncts act similarly. The mechanism for BCG has been postulated by Rapp[119] and is illustrated in Fig. 5-8. BCG stimulates active tumor immunity by increasing the number of lymphocytes and macrophages available to participate in the immune processes only if the patient is immunologically competent and can be shown to elicit tuberculin hypersensitivity. For optimal therapeutic effect, not only must BCG come in direct contact with the tumor, the mass of the tumor cell burden in the patient must not exceed 10^9 cells or about 0.6 to 0.9 cm of tumor size. Regressions have been achieved when BCG has been injected into metastatic nodules of malignant melanoma, mycosis fungoides, and other cancers that originate on the skin, as well as deep-seated tumors such as breast

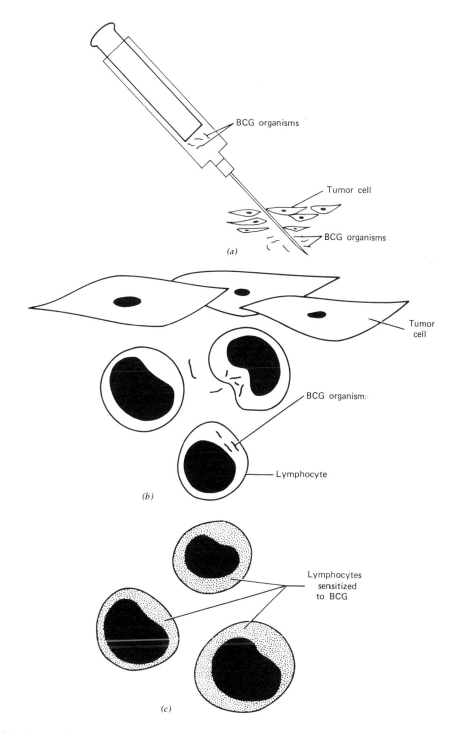

Figure 5-8 Proposed mode of action of BCG. (a) BCG injected into tumor. (b) Host responds with an inflammatory reaction that is primary lymphocytic in 3 days. (c) Lymphocytes are sensitized to BCG. (d) Lymphocytes secrete soluble mediator substances (migration inhibition factor—MIF). (e) MIF mobilizes histiocytes (wandering scavenger cells). (f) Nonselective destruction of tumor cells takes place. (g) Tumor-associated antigens are released. (h) Lymphocytes are sensitized to tumor-associated antigens. (i) Sensitized lymphocytes directly destroy tumor cells or (j) sensitized lymphocytes secrete MIF and (k) MIF attracts histiocytes, which destroy tumor cells "specifically."

139

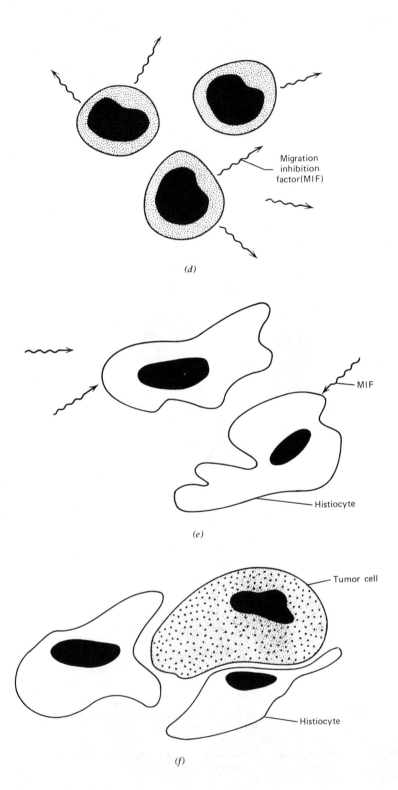

(d)

Migration inhibition factor(MIF)

MIF

Histiocyte

(e)

Tumor cell

Histiocyte

(f)

Figure 5-8 (Continued)

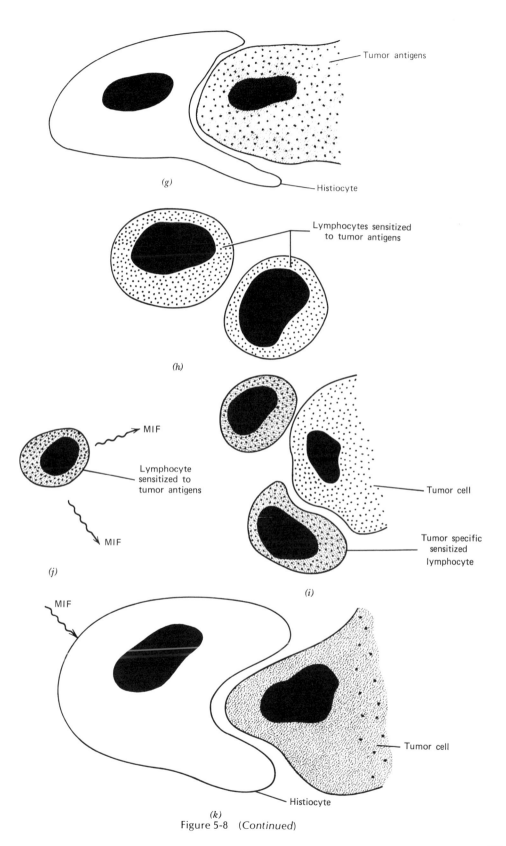

(g)

Tumor antigens

Histiocyte

(h)

Lymphocytes sensitized
to tumor antigens

(j)

MIF

Lymphocyte
sensitized to
tumor antigens

MIF

(i)

Tumor cell

Tumor specific
sensitized
lymphocyte

(k)

MIF

Tumor cell

Histiocyte

Figure 5-8   (Continued)

cancer and cancer of the thymus. It has also been used successfully in exacting remissions among children with leukemia.

Once surgery or radiotherapy has removed excess tumor mass and chemotherapy has drastically reduced the number of tumor cells, BCG alone or coupled with neuramidase, which removes tumor cell sialomucin coating, thereby increasing cell immunogenicity, may be used to complete the "mopping up" operation.[116]

LITERATURE CITED

DESCRIPTION

1. Cancer census. *Time* **15** Nov 1971: 86–87.

2. Abelson PH. 1973. Prevention of cancer. *Science* **182:** 973.

3. Silverberg E, Holleb AI. 1975. Cancer statistics, 1975—25-year cancer survey. *Ca-Cancer J Clin* **25**(1): 2–21.

4. Anderson WAD, Scotti TM. 1968. *Synopsis of Pathology.* CV Mosby, St. Louis. 957 p; Copra HC, Feller WF. 1969. Viruslike particles in human breast cancer. *Tex Rep Bio Med* **27:** 945–953; Moore DH, Charney J, Kramarsky B et al. 1971. Search for a human breast cancer virus. *Nature* **229:** 611–614; Holland JF, Frei E III (eds). 1973. *Cancer Medicine.* Lea & Febiger, Philadelphia. 2018 p; Osterkamp RW, Whitten JB. 1973. The etiology and pathogenesis of cancer. *Ca-Cancer J Clin* **23:** 28–32.

5. Ackerman LV. 1972. Some thoughts on food and cancer. *Nutrit Today* **7**(1): 2–9.

6. Allen DW, Cole P. 1972. Viruses and human cancer. *New Eng J Med* **286:** 70–82, and *Ca-Cancer J Clin* **23:** 127–136, 193–200; Culliton B. 1972. Cancer virus theories: focus of debate. *Science* **177:** 44–47; Culliton B. 1973. Cancer virus: link to disease in man reported again. *Science* **180:** 572–574.

CARCINOGENESIS

7. Temin HM. 1964. Nature of the provirus of Rous sarcoma. *Nat Cancer Inst Monogr* **17:** 557–570.

8. Huebener RJ, Todaro GJ. 1969. Oncogenes of RNA tumor viruses as determinants of cancer. *Proc Nat Acad Sci (US)* **64:** 1087–1094.

9. Temin H. 1971. The protovirus hypothesis: speculations on the significance of RNA-directed DNA synthesis for normal development and for carcinogenesis. *J Nat Cancer Inst* **46**(2): III-VII.

10. Modan B, Lilienfeld AM. 1964. Leukaemogenic affect of ionizing irradiation treatment in polycythaemia. *Lancet* **2:** 439–441.

11. Hasterlik RJ, Finkel AJ. 1965. Diseases of bones and joints associated with intoxication by radioactive substances, principally radium. *Med Clin N Am* **49:** 285–296.

12. Blum JF. 1959. *Carcinogenesis by Ultraviolet Light.* Princeton University Press, Princeton, NJ. 340 p; Harris RJC (ed). 1969. *Cellular Basis and Aetiology of the Late Somatic Effects of Ionizing Radiation.* Academic Press, New York. 359 p.

13. Twelfth Symposium on Fundamental Cancer Research. Houston, 1958. Radiation biology and cancer; a collection of papers. Austin, published for the University of Texas MD Anderson Hospital and Tumor Institute [by] University of Texas Press. 1959. 494 p.

14. Gatti RA, Good RA. 1971. Occurrence of malignancy in immunodeficiency diseases. *Cancer* **28:** 89–98.

15. Lewis WH. 1970. Extreme instability of chromosome number in *Claytonia virginica. Taxon* **19:** 180–182.

16. Hill J. 1761. *Cautions Against the Immoderate Use of Snuff,* ed 2. R. Baldwin, London; Redmond DE. 1970. Tobacco and cancer; the first clinical report, 1761. *New Eng J Med* **282:** 18–23.

17. Pott P. 1775. Chirurgical observations relative to the cancer of the scrotum. London. Reprinted in *Nat Cancer Inst Monogr* **10:** 7–13, 1963.

18. Shubik P and Hartwell J. 1957. Survey of compounds which have been tested for carcinogenic activity. Suppl 1, Washington, US Department Health, Education and Welfare, Public Health Service.

19. Rook AJ, Gresham GA, Davis RA. 1956. Squamous epithelioma possibly induced by the therapeutic application of tar. *Brit J Cancer* **10:** 17–23.

20. Boyd JT, Doll RR. 1954. Gastro-intestinal cancer and the use of liquid paraffin. *Brit J Cancer* **8:** 231–237.

21. Brookes P, Lawley PD. 1964. Reaction of some

mutagenic and carcinogenic compounds with nucleic acids. *J Cell Comp Physiol* **64** (Suppl 1): 111–128.

22. Tebbens BD, Thomas JF, Mukai M. 1956. Hydrocarbon synthesis in combustion. *AMA Arch Ind health* **13**: 561–573.

23. Miller JA. 1970. Carcinogenesis by chemicals: an overview—GHA Clowes Memorial Lecture. *Cancer Res* **30**: 559–576.

24. Graef W. 1965. The natural occurrence and significance of carcinogenic polycyclic aromatic hydrocarbons. *Med Klin Munich* **60**(15): 561–565; Graef W, Diehl H. 1966. The natural normal levels of carcinogenic polycyclic aromatic hydrocarbons and the reasons therefore. *Arch Hyg Bakterion* **50**(1–2): 49–59.

25. Blumer M. 1964. Benzyprenes on soil. *Science* **134**: 474.

26. Cramer JW, Miller JA, Miller EC. 1960. *N*-Hydroxylation: a new metabolic reaction observed in the rat with the carcinogen 2-acetylaminofluorene. *J Biol Chem* **235**: 885–888.

27. Miller JA, Miller EC. 1965. Natural and synthetic chemical carcinogens in the etiology of cancer. *Cancer Res* **25**: 1292–1304.

28. Brown RR, Price JM, Wear JB. 1955. The metabolism of tryptophan in bladder tumor patients. *Proc Am Ass Cancer Res* **2**: 7.

29. Boylant E, William K. 1969. Reaction of urethane with nucleic acids in vivo. *Biochem J* **111**: 121–127.

30. Reynolds ES. 1967. Liver parenchymal cell injury. IV. Pattern of incorporation of carbon and chlorine from carbon tetrachloride into chemical constitutents of liver in vivo. *J Pharm Exp Ther* **155**: 117–126.

31. Farber E. 1968. Ethionine carcinogenesis. *Adv Cancer Res* **7**: 383–474.

32. Weisburger JH, Preston H, Grantham PH et al. 1964. Activation and detoxification of *N*-2-fluorenylacetamide in man. *Cancer Res* **24**: 475–479.

33. Riper HJP. 1971. Chemical carcinogenesis. *New Eng J Med* **285**: 721–734.

34. Kyle RA, Pierre RV, Bayrd ED. 1970. Multiple myeloma and acute myelomonocytic leukemia. Report of four cases possibly related to melphalan. *New Eng J Med* **283**: 1121–1125.

35. Abell CW, Falk HL, Shimkin MB et al. 1965. Uracil mustard: a potent inducer of lung tumors in mice. *Science* **147**: 1433–1444.

36. Druckrey H, Kruse H, Preussmann R. 1968. Propanesultone, a potent carcinogen. *Naturwissenschaften* **55**: 449.

37. Berg JW, Burbank F. 1972. Correlations between carcinogenic trace metals in water supplies and cancer mortality. *Ann NY Acad Sci* **199**: 249–264.

38. Berg JW, Schottenfeld D, Hutter RVP et al. 1969. *Histology, Epidemiology and End Results: The Memorial Hospital Cancer Registry:* 1–117. Memorial Hospital for Cancer and Allied Diseases, New York.

39. Wagner JC, Sleggs CA, Marchand P. 1960. Diffuse pleural mesothelioma and asbestos exposure in northwestern Cape Province. *Brit J Ind Med* **17**: 260–271.

40. Selikoff IJ, Churg J, Hammond EC. 1968. Asbestos exposure, smoking and neoplasia. *JAMA* **204**: 106–112.

41. Nelson AA, Fitzhugh OG, Morris HJ et al. 1942. Neurofibromas of rat ears produced by prolonged feeding of crude ergot. *Cancer Res* **2**: 11–15.

42. Kobayashi Y, Uranguchi K, Sakal F et al. 1959. Toxicological studies on the yellowed rice by *P. islandicum* Sopp. III. Experimental verification of primary hepatic carcinoma of rats by long term feeding with the fungus-growing rice. *Proc Japan Acad* **35**: 501–506.

43. Wilson BJ, Wilson CH. 1962. Extraction and preliminary characterization of a hepatotoxic substance from cultures of *Penicillium rubrum*. *J Bacteriol* **84**: 283–290.

44. Barich LL, Schwartz J, Barich D. 1962. Oral griseofulvin: a cocarcinogenic agent to methylcholanthrene induced cutaneous tumors. *Cancer Res* **22**: 53–55; Hurst EW, Paget GE. 1963. Protoporphyrin, cirrhosis and hepatomata in the livers of mice given griseofulvin. *Brit J Dermatol* **75**: 105–112.

45. Burnside JE, Siypel WL, Forgaca J et al. 1957. A disease of swine and cattle caused by eating mouldy corn. II. Experimental production with pure cultures of molds. *Am J Vet Res* **18**: 817–824; Iongh H de, Vles RO, Pelt JG van. 1964. Milk of mammals fed on aflatoxin-containing diet. *Nature* **202**: 466–467; Spivak J. 1964. U.S. scientists look for traces of poison from mould on peanuts. *Wall Street J* 27 Apr.

46. Berg GG (ed). 1972. *Master Manual of Molds and Mycotoxins.* Farm Technology/Agri-Fieldman. Celanese Chemical Agricultural Products Group, New York.

47. Levenberg B. 1962. An aromatic diazonium compound in the mushroom *Agaricum bisporus. Biochem Biophys Acta* **63**: 212–214; Levenberg B. 1964. Isolation and structure of agaricine, a glutamyl substituted arylhydrazine

derivative from Agaricaceae. *J Biol Chem* **239:** 2267–2273.

48. Fisher JF, Mallette MF. 1961. The natural occurrence of ethionine in bacteria. *J Gen Physiol* **45:** 1–13.

49. Rose EF. 1968. The effects of soil and diet on disease. *Cancer Res* **28:** 2390–2392.

50. Whiting MG. 1963. Toxicity of cycads. *Econ Bot* **17:** 269–320.

51. Laqueur GL, Spetz M. 1968. Toxicology of cycasin. *Cancer Res* **28:** 2262–2267.

52. Acheson ED, Cowdell RH, Jolles B. 1970. Nasal cancer in the Northamptonshire boot and shoe industry. *Brit Med J* **1:** 385–393.

53. Gigoux M, Bernard P. 1969. Malignant ethmoid tumors in woodworkers. *J Med Lyon* **50:** 731–736.

54. Morton JF. 1968. Plants associated with esophageal cancer cases in Curacao. *Cancer Res* **28:** 2268–2271; Morton JF. 1970. Tentative correlations of plant usage and esophageal cancer zones. *Econ Bot* **24:** 217–226; Morton JF. 1972. Further associations of plant tannins and human cancer. *Quart J Crude Drug Res* **12**(1): 1829–1841.

55. O'Gara RW, Lee C, Morton JF. 1971. Carcinogenicity of extracts of selected plants from Curacao after oral and subcutaneous administration to rodents. *J Nat Cancer Inst* **46:** 1131–1137.

56. Jacobs MB. 1951. *The Chemistry and Technology of Food and Food Products,* Vol 2. Wiley-Interscience, New York; Ukers WR. 1935. *All About Tea,* Vol 1. *The Tea and Coffee Trade.* Trade Journal Co, New York.

57. Harris PN, Chen KK. 1970. Development of hepatic tumors in rats following ingestion of *Senecio longilobus. Cancer Res* **30:** 2881–2886; Schoental R. 1968. Toxicology and carcinogenic action of pyrrolizidine alkaloids. *Cancer Res* **28:** 2237–2246; Schoental R, Fowler ME, Coady A. 1970. Islet cell tumors of the pancreas found in rats given pyrrolizidine alkaloids from *Amsinckia intermedia* Fisch and Mey. and from *Heliotropium supinum* L. *Cancer Res* **30:** 2127–2131.

58. Schoental R. 1972. Prevention or cure? *Trop Geog Med* **24:** 194–198.

59. Dunham LJ. 1968. A geographic study of the relationship between oral cancer and plants. *Cancer Res* **28:** 2369–2371.

60. Suri K, Goldman HM, Wells H. 1971. Carcinogenic effect of a dimethyl sulphoxide extract of betel nut on the mucosa of the hamster buccal pouch. *Nature* **230:** 383–384.

61. Stedman RL. 1968. The chemical composition of tobacco and tobacco smoke. *Chem Rev* **68:** 153–207.

62. Van Duuren BL. 1968. Tobacco carcinogenesis. *Cancer Res* **28:** 2357–2362.

63. Hoffmann D, Wynder EL. 1971. A study of tobacco carcinogenesis. XI. Tumor initiators, tumor accelerators, and tumor promoting activity of condensate fractions. *Cancer* **27:** 848–864.

64. Weiss W, Boucot KR, Seidman H et al. 1972. Risk of lung cancer according to histologic type and cigarette dosage. *JAMA* **222:** 799–801.

65. Moore GE, Bissinger LL, Proehl EC. 1953. Intraoral cancer and the use of chewing tobacco. *J Am Geriatr Soc* **1:** 497–505; Rosenfeld L, Callaway J. 1963. Snuff dipper's cancer. *Am J Surg* **106:** 840–844.

66. Hecker E. 1971. Cocarcinogens from Euphorbiaceae and Thymelaeaceae, 147–155. In H Wagner, L Hörhammer (eds), *Pharmacognosy and Phytochemistry.* Springer-Verlag, Berlin, Heidelberg, and New York; Libermann C, Lazar P, Chouroulinskow E et al. 1968. Response of an active component of croton oil to short-term tests of carcinogenicity. *Nature* **217:** 563–564.

67. Hecker E 1968. Cocarcinogenic principles from the seed oil of *Croton tiglium* and from other Euphorbiaceae. *Cancer Res* **28:** 2338–2349.

68. Long EL, Nelson AA, Fitzhugh OG et al. 1963. Liver tumors produced in rats by feeding safrole. *Arch Pathol* **75:** 595–604.

69. Homburger F, Boger E. 1968. The carcinogenicity of essential oils, flavors, and species; a review. *Cancer Res* **28:** 2372–2374.

70. Hoch-Ligeti C. 1952. Naturally occurring dietary agents and their role in production of tumors. *Tex Rep Biol Med* **19:** 996–1005.

71. Fitzhugh OG, Nelson AA. 1948. Liver tumors in rats fed thiourea or thioacetamide. *Science* **108:** 626–628; Rosin A, Aungar H. 1957. Malignant tumors in the eye lids and auricular region of thiourea-treated rats. *Cancer Res* **17:** 302–305.

72. Cater DB. 1961. The carcinogenic action of carrageenin in rats. *Brit J Cancer* **15:** 607–614.

DEVELOPMENT OF THERAPY

73. Richards V. 1972. *Cancer; The Wayward Cell: Its Origins, Nature and Treatment.* University of Calif Press, Berkeley, Los Angeles, London. 308 p.

74. Hartwell JL. 1967–1971. Plant used against cancer. A survey. *Lloydia* **30:** 379–436, 1967; **31:** 71–170, 1968; **32:** 79–107, 153–205, 247–296, 1969; **33:** 97–194, 288–392, 1970; **34:** 103–160, 204–255, 310–360, 386–425, 1971; Perdue RE Jr, Hartwell JL. 1969. The search for plant sources of anticancer drugs. *Morris Arb Bull* **20:** 35–53.

75. Kourennoff PM. 1971. *Russian Folk Medicine.* Pyramid Books, New York (Translated by G St George). 287 p.

76. Butler F. 1955. *Cancer Through the Ages: The Evolution of Hope.* The Virginia Press, Fairfax. 147 p.

77. Hartwell JL. 1960. Plant remedies for cancer. *Cancer Chemother Rep* 1960 (July): 19–24.

78. Hartwell JL. 1968. Plants used against cancer: A survey. *Lloydia* **31:** 72.

79. Weisberger AS, Pansky J. 1957. Tumor-inhibiting effects derived from an active principle of garlic (*Allium sativum*). *Science* **126:** 1112–1114.

80. Fell JW. 1857. *A Treatise on Cancer, and its Treatment.* J Churchill, London. 95 p.

81. Stone WS. 1916. A review of the history of chemical therapy in cancer. *Med Rec* **90:** 628–634.

82. Bentley R, Trimen H. 1880. *Medicinal Plants,* Vol 1, plate 20. J & A Churchill, London.

83. Barton WPC. 1817. *Vegetable Materia Medica of the United States; or Medical Botany.* Vol 1. W Carey & Sons, Philadelphia; Schoepf D. 1787. *Materia Medica Americana.* JJ Palm, Erlangen, Germany. 170 p.

84. Osol A, Farrar GE Jr. 1947. *The Dispensatory of the United States of America,* ed 24. Lippincott, Philadelphia, London, Montreal. 1928 p.

85. Stickl O. 1929. Chemotherapeutische Versuche gegen das Übertraghore Mäusecarcinom. *Virchow's Arch Pathol Anat* **270:** 801–867.

86. Shear MJ, Hartwell JL, Leiter J. 1960. In JL Hartwell, Plant remedies for cancer. *Cancer Chemother Rep* 1960 (July): 19–24.

87. Phelan JT, Milgram H, Stoll H et al. 1962. The use of Mohs' chemosurgery technique in the management of superficial cancer. *Surg Gynecol Obstet* **114:** 25–30; Phelan JT, Juardo J. 1963. Chemosurgical management of carcinoma of the nose. *Surgery* **53:** 310–314; Phelan JT, Juardo J. 1963. Chemosurgical management of carcinoma of the external ear. *Surg Gynecol Obstet* **117:** 224–246.

88. Hartwell JL. 1967. Plants used against cancer. A survey. *Lloydia* **30:** 379.

89. Kaplan IW. 1942. Condylomata acuminata. *New Orleans Med Surg J* **94:** 388; Culp OS, Kaplan IW. 1944. Condylomata acuminata, two hundred cases treated with podophyllin. *Ann Surg* **120:** 251–256; Culp OS, Magid MA, Kaplan IW. 1944. Podophyllin treatment of condylomata acuminata. *J Urol* **51:** 655–659; Sullivan M, King LS. 1947. Effects of resin of *Podophyllum* on normal skin, condylomata acuminata and verrucae vulgares. *Arch Dermatol Syphilol* **56:** 30–47.

90. Belkin M. 1947. Effect of podophyllin on transplanted mouse tumors. *Fed Proc Soc Exp Biol* **6:** 308; Hartwell JL. 1947. Chemotherapy of cancer: classes of compounds under investigation and active components of podophyllin. *Cancer Res* **7:** 716–717; Ormsbee RA, Cornman I. 1947. The effect of podophyllin on tumor cells *in vitro. Cancer Res* **7:** 717.

91. Kelly MG, Hartwell JL. 1954. The biological effects and the chemical composition of podophyllin. A review. *J Nat Cancer Inst* **14:** 967–1010.

92. Broc AR, Brulé G, Cabanne F et al. 1972. Clinical screening of epipodophyllotoxin VM 26 in malignant lymphomas and solid tumors. *Brit Med J* **2:** 744–748.

93. 'Anonymous [J Tennent]. 1734. *Every Man His Own Doctor: or, The Poor Planter's Physician,* ed 2. William Parks, Williamsburg and Annapolis. Reprint edition, St Louis Medical Museum, St Louis. 56 p + index.

94. Schultz T (with B Lindeman). 1973. The victimizing of desperate cancer patients. *Today's Health* **51**(11): 28–33, 59.

95. Cole W. 1657. *Adam in Eden: or, Natures Paradise. . . .* Printed by J Streater for N Brooke, London.

96. *Kittler GD.* 1963. *Laetrile (The Anti-cancer Drug): Control for Cancer.* Paperback Library, New York. 255 p.

97. Morrone JA. 1962. Chemotherapy of inoperable cancer, preliminary reports of 10 cases treated with laetrile. *Exp Med Surg* **20:** 299–308.

98. Another "anti-cancer" drug: laetrile. *Med Letter* **5:** 55–56, 1963; Unproven methods of cancer management: laetrile. *Ca-Cancer J Clin* **22:** 245–251.

99. Culliton BJ. 1973. Sloan-Kettering: the trials of an apricot pit—1973. *Science* **182:** 1000–1003.

100. Debate over laetrile. *Time* **12** Apr 1971: 80.

101. Unproven methods of cancer management: chaparral tea. *Ca-Cancer J Clin* **20:** 112–118, 1970; CH-23. **18:** 174–175, 1968; Ferguson plant products. **22:** 113–117, 1972; Krebiozen and carcalon. **17:** 111–115, 1967; KC-555. **17:** 196–197, 1967; Nichols escharotic method. **18:** 246–

247; Nichols P. 1954. *The Value of Escharotics* (*Cancer: Its Proper Treatment*). Kingsport Press, Kingsport, Tenn. 400 p.

102. Bureau of Investigation. 1940. Some fraudulent "cancer cures." *JAMA* **115:** 1037–1038; Bureau of Investigation. 1952. Mr Hoxsey has a setback. *JAMA* **150:** 54–55; The cancer underground. *Newsweek* **17** Sept 1973: 57; Bainbridge WS. 1915. *The Cancer Problem.* Macmillan, New York. 534 p; Larrick GP. 1956. The Hoxsey cancer "cure." *Consumer Rep* **21:** 303.

CURRENT THERAPY

103. Fresh strides in attack on cancer. *US News World Rep* 17 Sept 1973: 41–42.

104. Selected papers of cancer diseases in which chemotherapeutic agents of plant origin are used: Bagley CM Jr, DeVita VT Jr, Berard CW et al. 1972. Advanced lymphosarcoma: intensive cyclical combination chemotherapy with cyclophosphamide, vincristine and prednisone. *Ann Intern Med* **76:** 227–234; Burchenal JH, Carter SK. 1972. New cancer chemotherapeutic agents. *Cancer* **30:** 1639–1646; Carbone PP. 1972. Non-Hodgkin's lymphoma: recent observations on natural history and intensive treatment. *Cancer* **30:** 1511–1516; Carter SK. 1972. Single and combination nonhormonal chemotherapy in breast cancer. *Cancer* **30:** 1543–1555; Chanes RL, Condit PT, Bottomley RH et al. 1971. Combined actinomycin D and vincristine in the treatment of patients with [lung] cancer. *Cancer* **27:** 613–617; Cole WH (ed). 1970. *Chemotherapy of Cancer.* Lea & Febiger, Philadelphia; D'Angio GJ. 1972. Management of children with Wilms' tumor. *Cancer* **30:** 1528–1533; DeVita VT, Schein PS. 1973. The use of drugs in combination for the treatment of cancer. *New Eng J Med* **288:** 998–1006; DeVita VT, Canellos GP, Moxley JH III. 1972. A decade of combination chemotherapy of advanced Hodgkin's disease. *Cancer* **30:** 1495–1504; DeVita VT Jr, Serpick AA, Carbone PP. 1970; Combination chemotherapy in the treatment of advanced Hodgkin's disease. *Ann Intern Med* **73:** 881–895; Frei E III. 1972. Prospectus for cancer chemotherapy. *Cancer* **30:** 1656–1661; Garattini S, Franchi G (eds). 1973. *Chemotherapy of Cancer Dissemination and Metastasis.* Raven Press, New York; Goldin A, Sandberg JS, Henderson ES et al. 1971. The chemotherapy of human and animal acute leukemia. *Cancer Chemother Rep* pt 1, **55**(4):

309–508; Gottlieb JA, Baker LH, Quagliana JM et al. 1972. Chemotherapy of sarcomas with a combination of adriamycin and dimethyl triazeno imidazole carboxiamide. *Cancer* **30:** 1632–1638; Husto HO, Pinkel D, Pratt CG. 1972. Treatment of clinically localized Ewing's sarcoma with radiotherapy and combination chemotherapy. *Cancer* **30:** 1522–1527; Karon M, Sullivan MP, Frei E III. 1968. Management of patients with acute leukemia. *Mod Med* **36**(9): 66–72; Knock FE. 1967. *Anticancer Agents.* Charles C Thomas, Springfield, Ill. 272 p; Krakoff IH. 1971. The present status of cancer chemotherapy. *Med Clin N Am* **55:** 683–701; Krakoff IH. 1973. Cancer chemotherapeutic agents. *Ca-Cancer J Clin* **23:** 208–219; Lewis JL Jr. 1972. Chemotherapy of gestational choriocarcinoma. *Cancer* **30:** 1517–1521; Luce JK. 1972. Chemotherapy of malignant melanoma. *Cancer* **30:** 1604–1615; MacLeod RM, Leymeyer JE. 1973. Suppression of pituitary tumor growth and function by ergot alkaloids. *Cancer Res* **33:** 849–855; Marsh JC, Mitchell MS. 1974. Chemotherapy of cancer I. Overview of clinical pharmacology *Drug Ther* **4**(1): 93–114; Simone J, Rhomes JAA, Husto HO et al. 1972. "Total therapy" studies of acute lymphocytic leukemia in children. *Cancer* **30:** 1488–1494; Ultmann JE, Nixon DD. 1969. The therapy of lymphoma. *Semin Hematol* **6:** 376–402; Ziegler JL. 1972. Chemotherapy of Burkitt's lymphoma. *Cancer* **30:** 1534–1540; Zubrod CG. 1972. The basis for progress in chemotherapy. *Cancer* **30:** 1474–1479; Therapy of common skin cancers and keratoses. *Med Let* **12**(14): 57–58, 1970; The choice of therapy in the treatment of malignancy. *Med Let* **15**(3): 9–16, 1973.

105. AMA Department of Drugs. 1973. *AMA Drug Evaluations,* ed 2. Publishing Sciences Group, Acton, Mass. 1032 p.

106. Quinn JO III. 1971. Radionucleic imaging procedures in the diagnosis of cancer. *Ca-Cancer J Clin* **21:** 292–301.

107. Dustin A-P. 1938. Nouvelles applications des poisons caryoclassiques à la pathologie expérimentale, à l'endocrinologie et à la cancerologie. *Sang* **12:** 677–697.

108. Savel H. 1966. The metaphase-arresting plant alkaloids and cancer chemotherapy, 189–224. In F Homburger (ed), *Progress in Experimental Tumor Research,* Vol 8. Hafner, New York.

109. Noble RL. 1965. Anti-cancer alkaloids of *Vinca rosea,* 61–78. In *Pharmacology of Oriental Plants.* Pergamon Press, Oxford; Symposium on vincristine, *Cancer Chemother Rep* **52**(4):

452–535, 1968; Taylor WI, Farnsworth NR (eds). 1973. *The Vinca Alkaloids*. Dekker, New York. 357 p.

110. The choice of therapy in the treatment of malignancy. *Med Lett* **15**(3): 9–16, 1973.

111. Krakoff IH. 1973. Cancer chemotherapeutic agents. *Ca-Cancer J Clin* **23**: 208–219.

112. Perdue RE Jr. 1966. World plant search. *Agric Res* **14**(11): 3–4; Perdue RE Jr, Hartwell JL. 1969. The search for plant sources of anticancer drugs. *Morris Arb Bull* **20**: 35–53.

113. Fong HHS, Bhatti W, Farnsworth NR. 1972. Antitumor activity of certain plants due to tannins. *J Pharm Sci* **61**: 1818.

114. Espenshade MA. 1969. The search for antitumor agents among the higher fungi. *Morris Arb Bull* **20**: 54–58; Farnsworth NR. 1968. The search for new anticancer drugs from natural sources. *Tile & Till* **54**(Mar): 7–9; Gregory FJ, Healy EM, Agersborg HPK Jr et al. 1966. Studies on antitumor substances produced by Basidiomycetes. *Mycologia* **58**: 80–90; Hartwell JL. 1960. Plant remedies for cancer. *Cancer Chemother Rep* 1960(July): 19–24; Jewers K, Manchanda AH, Rose HM. 1972. Naturally-occurring antitumour agents, 1–63. In GP Ellis, GB West (eds), *Progress in Medicinal Chemistry*, Vol 9. Butterworths, London; Kupchan SM. 1971. Drugs from natural products—plant sources. *Adv Chem Ser* **108**: 1–13; Kupchan SM. 1972. Recent advances in chemistry of tumor inhibitors of plant origin, 262–278. In T Swain (ed), *Plants in the Development of Modern Medicine*. Harvard University Press, Cambridge, Mass; Oliver-Bever B. 1971. Vegetable drugs for cancer therapy. *Quart J Crude Drug Res* **11**(1): 1665–1683; Perdue RE Jr, Hartwell JL. 1961. The search for plant sources of anticancer drugs. *Morris Arb Bull* **20**: 35–53; Svobada GH. 1971. Recent advances in the search for antitumor agents of plant origin, 166–200. In H Wagner, L Hörhammer (eds), *Pharmacognosy and Phytochemistry*. Springer-Verlag, Berlin, Heidelberg, and New York.

115. Cobb EM. 1972. Antineoplastic principle derived from *Carduus benedictus*. *Quart J Crude Drug Res* **12**(2): 1877–1879.

Doskotch RW, Malik MY, Hufford CD et al. 1972. Antitumor agents V: Cytotoxic cardenolides from *Cryptostegia grandiflora* (Roxb.) R Br. *J Pharm Sci* **61**: 570–573.

Espenshade MA, Griffith EW. 1961. Tumor-inhibiting Basidiomycetes. Isolation and cultivation in the laboratory. *Mycologia* **58**: 511–517.

Farnsworth NR et al.: Tin-wa M, Farnsworth NR, Fong HHS et al. 1970. Biological and phytochemical evaluation of plants. VIII. Isolation of new alkaloids from *Sanguinaria canadensis*. *Lloydia* **33**: 267–269; Farnsworth NR. 1972. Anomalous isolation of an active antitumor alkaloid from a fraction of *Catharanthus lanceus* devoid of anticancer activity. *J Pharm Sci* **61**: 1840–1841; Fong HHS, Bhatti W, Farnsworth NR. 1972. Antitumor activity of certain plants due to tannins. *J Pharm Sci* **61**: 1818; Messmer WM, Tin-wa M, Fong HHS et al. 1972. Fagaronine, a new tumor inhibitor isolated from *Fagara zanthoxyloides* Lam (Rutaceae). *J Pharm Sci* **61**: 1858; Ickes GR, Fong HHS, Schiff PL Jr et al. 1973. Antitumor activity and preliminary phytochemical examination of *Tagetes minuta* (Compositae). *J Pharm Sci* **62**: 1009–1011; Loub WD, Fong HHS, Theiner M et al. 1973. Partial characterization of antitumor tannin isolated from *Calycogonium squamulosum* (Melastomataceae). *J Pharm Sci* **62**: 149–150.

Kupchan SM et al.: Kupchan SM, Doskotch RW. 1962. Tumor inhibitors. I. Aristolochic acid, the active principle of *Aristolochia indica*. *J Med Pharm Chem* **5**: 657–659; Kupchan SM, Doskotch RW, Vanevenhoven PW. 1964. Tumor inhibitors. III. Monocrotaline, the active principle of *Crotalaria spectabilis*. *J Pharm Sci* **53**: 343–345; Kupchan SM, Hemingway JC, Knox JR. 1965. Tumor inhibitors. VII. Podophyllotoxin, the active principle of *Juniperus virginiana*. *J Pharm Sci* **54**: 659–660; Kupchan SM, Knox JR, Kelsey JE et al. 1964. Calotropin, a cytotoxic principle isolated from *Ascelpias curassavica* L. *Science* **146**: 1685–1686; Kupchan SM, Anderson WK, Billinger P et al. 1969. Tumor inhibitors. XXXIX. Active principles of *Acnistus arborescens*. Isolation and structural and spectral studies of withaferin A and withacnistin. *J Org Chem* **34**: 3858–3866; Kupchan SM, Aynehci Y, Cassady JM et al. 1969. Tumor inhibitors. XL. The isolation and structural elucidation of elephantin and elephantopin, two novel sesquiterpenoid tumor inhibitors from *Elephantopus elatus*. *J Org Chem* **34**: 3867–3875; Kupchan SM, Kelsey JE, Maruyana M et al. 1969. Tumor inhibitors. XLI. Structural elucidation of tumor-inhibitory sesquiterpene lactones from *Eupatorium rotundifolium*. *J Org Chem* **34**: 3876–3883; Kupchan SM, Hemingway RJ, Hemingway JC. 1969. Tumor inhibitors. XLIV. The isolation and characterization of hellebrigenin 3-acetate and hellebrigenin 3,5-diacetate, bufadienolide tumor inhibitors from *Bersama abyssinica*. *J Org Chem* **34**: 3894–3898; Kupchan SM, Hemingway RJ, Smith RM. 1969. Tumor inhibitors.

XLV. Crotepoxide, a novel cyclohexane diepoxide tumor inhibitor from *Croton macrostachys*. *J Org Chem* **34**: 3898–3902; Kupchan SM, Smith RM, Aynehchi Y et al. 1970. Tumor inhibitors. LVI. Cucurbitacins O, P, and Q, the cytotoxic principles of *Brandegea bigelovii*. *J Org Chem* **35**: 2891–2894; Kupchan SM, Court WA, Dailey RG Jr et al. 1972. Triptolide and tripdiolide, novel antileukemic diterpenoid triepoxides from *Tripterygium wilfordii*. *J Am Chem Soc* **94**: 7194–7195; Kupchan SM, Komoda Y, Thomas GJ et al. 1972. Maytanprine and maytanbutine, new antileukeimic ansa macrolides from *Maytenus buchanani*. *J Chem Soc Chem Commun* **1972**: 1062; Kupchan SM, Fujita T, Maruyama M et al. 1973. The isolation and structural elucidation of eupaserrin and deacetyleupaserrin, new antileukemic sesquiterpene lactone from *Eupatorium semiseratum*. *J Org Chem* **38**: 1260–1264; Kupchan SM, Davies VH, Fujita T et al. 1973. The isolation and structural elucidation of liatrin, a novel antileukemic sesquiterpene lactone from *Liatris chapmanii*. *J Org Chem* **38**: 1853–1858; Kupchan SM, Britton RW, Ziegler MF et al. 1973. Bruceantin, a new potent antileukemic simaroubolide from *Brucea antidysenterica*. *J Org Chem* **38**: 178–179; Kupchan SM, Liepa AJ, Baxter RL et al. 1973. New alkaloids and related artifacts from *Cyclea peltata*. *J Org Chem* **38**: 1846–1852.

Lee, K-D, Huemer RP. 1971. Antitumoral activity of *Panax ginseng* extracts. *Japan J Pharm* **21**: 229–302.

Lee K-H et al.: Lee, K-H, Anuforo DC, Huang E-S et al. 1972. Antitumor agents I: Angustibalin, a new cytotoxic sesquiterpene lactone from *Balduina angustifolia* (Pursh) Robins. *J Pharm Sci* **61**: 626–628; Lee K-H, Huang H-C, Huang E-S et al. 1972. Antitumor agents II: Eupatolide, a new cytotoxic principle from *Eupatorium formosanum* Hay. *J Pharm Sci* **61**: 629–631.

Li MC, Koo W-Y, Hsu K-P. 1972. Anti-neoplastic property of a crude extract from *Paris formosana*. *Nature (New Biol)* **235**: 223–224.

Lin J-Y, Tseng K-Y, Chen C-C et al. 1970. Abrin and ricin: new anti-tumour substances. *Nature* **227**: 292–293.

McDaniel PB, Cole JR. 1972. Antitumor activity of *Bursera schlechtendalii* (Burseraceae): isolation and structure determination of two new lignans. *J Pharm Sci* **61**: 1992–1994.

Nienhaus J, Stoll M, Vester F. 1970. Thymus stimulation and cancer prophylaxis by *Viscum* proteins. *Experimentia* **26**: 523–525.

Noble RL, Beer CT, Cutts JH. 1958. Role of chance observations in chemotherapy: *Vinca rosea*. *Ann NY Acad Sci* **76**: 882–894.

Perdue RE Jr et al.: Perdue RE Jr, Wall ME, Hartwell JL et al. 1968. Comparison of the activity of crude *Camptotheca acuminata* ethanolic extracts against lymphoid leukemia L-1210. *Lloydia* **31**: 229–236; Perdue RE Jr, Spetzman LA, Powell RG. 1970. *Cephalotaxus*—source of harringtonine, a promising new anticancer alkaloid. *Am Hort Mag* 1970: 19–22.

Pettit GR, Traxler PM, Pase CP. 1973. Antineoplastic agents 31. *Oenothera caespitosa*. *Lloydia* **36**: 202–203.

Sheth K et al.: Sheth K, Holad S, Wiedhopf R et al. 1972. Tumor-inhibitory agent from *Hyptis emoryi* (Labiatae). *J Pharm Sci* **61**: 1819; Sheth K, Bianchi E, Wiedhopf R et al. 1973. Antitumor agents from *Alnus oregana* (Betulaceae). *J Pharm Sci* **62**: 139–140; Wiedhopf RM, Young M, Bianchi E et al. 1973. Tumor inhibitory agent from *Magnolia grandiflora* (Magnoliaceae) I: Parthenolide. *J Pharm Sci* **62**: 345; Wiedhopf RM, Trumbull ER, Cole JR. 1973. Antitumor agents from *Jatropha macrorhiza* (Euphorbiaceae) I: Isolation and characterization of jatropham. *J Pharm Sci* **62**: 1206–1207.

Sonnet PE, Jacobson M. 1971. Tumor inhibitors II: Cytotoxic alkaloids from *Annona purpurea*. *J Pharm Sci* **60**: 1254–1256.

Svoboda GH, Poore GA, Simpson PF et al. 1966. Alkaloids of *Acronychia baueri* Schott I. *J Pharm Sci* **55**: 758–768.

116. Good RA, Fisher DW (eds). 1973. *Immunobiology*. Sinauer, Stamford, Conn. 305 p; Libassi PT. 1973. Cancer immunology, Part I. Putting the body's own defenses to work. *Lab Manage* **11**(5): 27–39, 62–63, 75; Martin DS. 1973. The necessity of combined modalities in cancer therapy. *Hosp Pract* **12**(1): 129–136; Morton DL. 1972. Immunotherapy of cancer. *Cancer* **30**: 1647–1655; Toward cancer control. *Time* 19 Mar 1973: 64–69.

117. Barker BE. 1969. Phytomitogens and lymphocyte blastogenesis. *Hemic Cells in Vitro* **4**: 64–79; Barker BE, Farnes P, Fanger H. 1965. Mitogenic activity in *Phytolacca americana* (pokeweed). *Lancet* **1**: 170; Barker BE, Farnes P, LaMarche PH. 1966. Peripheral blood plasmacytosis following systemic exposures to *Phytolacca americana* (pokeweed). *Pediatrics* **38**: 490–493; Barker BE, Farnes P. 1967. Mitogenic property of *Wistaria floribunda* seeds. *Nature* **215**: 659–660; Farnes P, Barker BE, Brownhill LE et al. 1964. Mitogenic activity in *Phytolacca americana* (pokeweed). *Lancet* **2**:

1100–1101; Douglas SD, Kamin R, Davis WC et al. 1967. Biochemical and morphological aspects of phytomitogens: jack bean, wax bean, pokeweed (PWM) and phytohemagglutinin (PHA). Third Leucocyte Culture Conference.

118. Bainbridge WS. 1915. *The Cancer Problem.* Section 10, Chapter 3, Biotherapy, 327–344. Macmillan, New York.

119. Rapp HJ. 1973. Jogging immunologic memory with BCG. *Lab Manage* **11**(5): 42–43.

Chapter 6
Nervous System

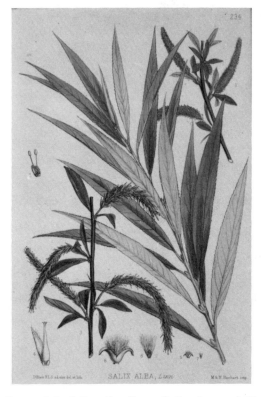

Figure 6-1 *Salix alba* (from R Bentley and H Trimen, *Medicinal Plants* 4: 234, 1880).

What is the most successful synthetic drug in the whole field of pharmaceutical chemistry? Aspirin, of course, consumed by Americans at the rate of 44 million tablets daily. In North America and elsewhere aspirin is undoubtedly the most widely used drug after alcohol and nicotine.

More than 2400 years ago, the Greeks used extracts of *Salix alba* (Fig. 6-1) and bark from several other species of willow to treat pain, as well as gout and other illnesses. Equally long ago, the North American Indians were using willow to relieve pain and to fight fever: the Houmas and Alabamas used a decoction of the roots and bark of *S. nigra* for internal consumption and for bathing to relieve fevers; the Chickasaws used the roots of *S. lucida* for headaches; and the Montagnais steeped its leaves and drank the liquid to relieve their headaches. They also made a mash of the bark, which was strapped to the forehead to relieve pain. There are many such examples to be found among the folk remedies of North American and Eurasian peoples who utilized species of willow to obtain generalized relief from aches and pains.

The effect of the willow was largely due to the activity of a glycoside, salicin, which was first isolated in the nineteenth century from numerous species of *Salix* (e.g., *S. alba, S. helix, S. pentandra, S. praecox*); the main commercial sources today are *S. fragilis* and *S. purpurea*, which are native to Europe and/or Asia.

Salicin was also obtained from the poplars (e.g., *Populus alba*, Fig. 6-2a; *P. balsamifera, P. candicans, P. nigra*). Today it is used as an antirheumatic drug. Salicin is readily hydrolyzed to saligenin, which has some use in medicine as an analgesic. Following ingestion, salicin is probably decomposed to salicylic acid, a compound originally isolated in 1839 from the flowerbuds of *Filipendula (Spiraea)* (Fig. 6-2b) *ulmaria*, the Eurasian queen-of-the-meadow (Rosaceae); a few years later it was synthesized. Salicylic acid is an active disinfectant, probably superior to phenol in its antiseptic properties. The acid is also widely used in the form of lotions and ointments in the treatment of various skin diseases, especially chronic eczemas, in which its actions are primarily keratolytic, and secondarily antibacterial and fungicidal.

Not long after its discovery in *Filipendula ulmaria*, salicylic acid in the form of its methyl ester was found to be the chief constituent of wintergreen oil obtained from *Gaultheria procumbens* leaves (Ericaceae) and of sweet birch oil from *Betula lenta* bark (Betulaceae) following hydrolysis of its precursor. Its chief use is as a rubifacient, and in former times it served as an antirheumatic.

Like methyl salicylate, salicylic acid is an antirheumatic, but when widely used in the nineteenth century, it effectively brought quick relief from other kinds of pain—neuralgia, sciatica, myalgia, and headaches—and it was certainly unsurpassed as an antipyretic. Unfortunately

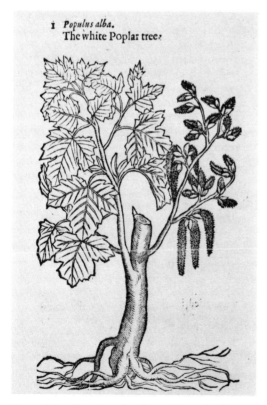

Figure 6-2a *Populus alba* (from J Gerard, *The Herball*, ed 2, 1636).

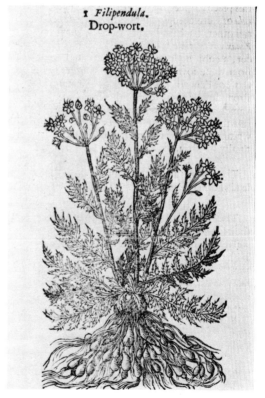

Figure 6-2b *Filipendula sp.* (from J Gerard, *The Herball*, ed 2, 1636).

the drug caused so much gastric discomfort and nausea in some users that many preferred the pain of rheumatoid arthritis to the cure. When salicylic acid was first synthesized from carbolic acid (phenol) in 1853, a number of other derivatives of this new acid were prepared, and one was acetylsalicylic acid. No one bothered with this synthetic product, however, until the Bayer Company directed its staff to find a substitute for salicylic acid that would be an even better antipyretic, antirheumatic, and analgesic agent than salicylic acid, but without unpleasant side effects. Acetylsalicylic acid was "rediscovered" in 1899, and it passed all of Bayer's requirements, being named "aspirin" from the combination of "a" for "acetyl" and the original generic name *Spiraea* = spirin, from which salicylic acid was first isolated.

Aspirin is widely used medically as (1) an *antipyretic,* facilitating the dissipation of heat through increased peripheral blood flow and sweating; (2) an *analgesic* agent, probably through its depressant action on the central nervous system; and (3) an *anti-inflammatory agent* for treatment of rheumatic fever, acute intraocular inflammation, lumbago, rheumatoid arthritis, osteoarthritis, and a host of other conditions commonly lumped together as "rheumatism."

This story, which began long ago with willow bark and yielded a compound that has served as a model for many nineteenth-century synthetic derivatives, continues into the twentieth century as we attempt to learn how these types of drugs act to relieve much of man's pain and suffering.

DESCRIPTION OF THE NERVOUS SYSTEM

By conducting impulses from receptors to appropriate effectors, the nervous system coordinates and integrates the body's many activities. The nervous system is composed of many billions of nerve cells (neurons), which conduct the impulses, and an even larger number of various supporting cells. There are two main parts: the central nervous system, consisting of the brain and spinal cord, and the peripheral nervous system, comprising the spinal and cranial nerves and the nerves associated with the autonomic nervous system. The peripheral nervous system is responsible for conducting messages from all sense organs of the body to the central nervous system, but it also includes two motor divisions: the somatic (voluntary) motor system, which activates the voluntary (skeletal) muscles, and the autonomic (involuntary) nervous system, which innervates the smooth and other involuntary muscles, such as the heart and various glands.

Between the sensory (afferent) neurons, which convey impulses from the sense organs to the brain or spinal cord, and the motor (efferent) neurons, which relay impulses from the brain or spinal cord to the muscles and other effectors of the body, there are many types of connector (internuncial) neurons located entirely within the central nervous system. A specific example illustrates how these neurons transmit impulses. When your finger touches a hot stove, a temperature receptor in the skin is stimulated and initiates an impulse in an afferent neuron. This neuron extends a process into the spinal cord, where it ends in a synapse (junction with an internuncial neuron). This neuron in turn carries the impulse to an appropriate efferent neuron, which extends from the spinal cord, and carries the impulse back to groups of muscle fibers in the forearm and hand. Contraction of the muscle fibers causes you to withdraw your finger from the hot object.

CENTRAL NERVOUS SYSTEM

The brain and the spinal cord function to correlate and integrate information. Within the brain such functions as consciousness, memory, and reason are thought to be due to the activity of the cerebral cortex, which receives and interprets all the more complex sensations—sight, sound, odor, and touch—and completely overshadows the other regions of the brain. These include the *thalamus,* which serves largely as a sensory station functioning at the subconscious level, and the *hypothalamus,* important because it contains integration centers for the autonomic or visceral functions (i.e., digestion, appetite, fear and rage) and centers that regulate the activity of the *pituitary gland,* which is the master coordinator of the endocrine organs throughout the body and utilizes the bloodstream to transport its secretory products to target areas. In addition, there is the brain stem, comprising the *midbrain, pons,* and *medulla* through which the main sensory pathways pass toward the thalamus; it contains the *reticular activating system,* responsible for maintaining wakefulness and attention (thus of importance to agents affecting sleep and wakefulness). Finally the *cerebellum* is concerned primarily with regulating motor activity and equilibrium.

Also included within the brainstem are areas containing vital reflex centers for respiration, blood pressure control (vasomotor center), vomiting, and so forth. Associated with these centers are chemosensitive cells that respond to internal changes in the body. For example, certain drugs induce vomiting by stimulating a group of chemosensitive cells that are distinct from the vomiting center, the chemoreceptor trigger zone for vomiting.

The other part of the central nervous system is the spinal cord. It serves to carry impulses to and from the brain and the periphery (in the white matter that forms the peripheral part of the cord) and to carry the synaptic connections between the sensory and motor neurons, which provide for various reflexes, and the autonomic and somatic motor neurons (which comprise the gray matter).

An important consideration in neuropharmacology is the existence of a barrier between the central nervous system and the blood system through which the drugs are distributed after absorption from the digestive tract or the site of injection. The capillaries' barrier appears to function because of the selective permeability of the cerebral vessels, which are not as easily passed by drugs: this hindrance is termed the blood-brain barrier.

Drugs may also reach the nervous system through the cerebral spinal fluid, which can serve as an alternative route.

PERIPHERAL NERVOUS SYSTEM

This peripheral nervous system is composed of two major parts, sensory and motor. The sensory system receives information from outside the body and within it and conveys the data to the central nervous system by way of afferent neurons whose cell bodies lie in sensory ganglia alongside the spinal cord or associated with certain of the cranial nerves. Then the motor system carries impulses through efferent neurons from the central nervous system to the various effector organs throughout the body. The motor system is complex and has two major parts, the somatic motor system and the autonomic nervous system.

Somatic Motor System

The somatic motor system innervates all voluntary (striated or skeletal) muscles, thus providing for voluntary movements and appropriate motor adjustments to changes in the external environment. This involves especially the muscles composing the framework of the body as distinguished from the viscera.

The cell bodies of the somatic motor neurons lie either in the anterior part of the gray matter of the spinal cord or in certain parts of the brainstem from which the cranial nerves arise. The neurons extend without interruption to the neuromuscular junction, where the transmission of the impulse to the muscle fibers is mediated by acetylcholine (Fig. 6-3).

Autonomic Nervous System

That portion of the peripheral nervous system which is concerned primarily with the involuntary, automatic, or unconscious control of the operation of the body viscera, is the autonomic nervous system. This system regulates the functions of all smooth muscles and glands throughout the body; these in turn

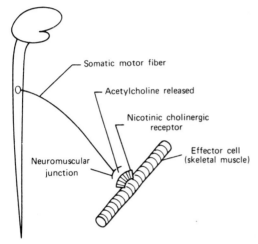

Figure 6-3   Schematic portrayal of a somatic motor nerve.

regulate the internal environment, in contrast to the external environment toward which the somatic system is directed. The cells of origin of the autonomic nervous system lie within the central nervous system.

The system has two divisions (Fig. 6-4). The parasympathetic portion is associated with cranial nerves III, VII, IX, and X and with certain of the sacral spinal nerves; of these the tenth cranial or vagus nerve is the single most important one, since it provides innervation for most of the major organs in the thorax and abdomen. Under normal or resting conditions, it serves as main adjuster of the internal environment by (Table 6-1): decreasing the size of the pupil, promoting copious salvation, reducing the cardiac output (by reducing its stroke volume and its rate), promoting blood flow to the viscera, increasing the motility of the stomach and intestines, and so forth. The parasympathetic division is characterized by the presence of long preganglionic and short postganglionic fibers, which release acetylcholine as the neurotransmitter at their terminals, that is, between the pre- and postganglionic fibers and the postganglionic fiber and the effector cell (Fig. 6-5a).

The sympathetic portion of the autonomic nervous system is associated with the thoracic and upper lumbar spinal nerves. The autonomic fibers in these nerves supply the same organs served by the parasympathetic division, but produce the opposite (or antagonistic) effect on the organs innervated. Thus pupil size is increased, secretion of saliva is reduced, stroke volume and heart rate are increased, peripheral skin and visceral blood vessels are constricted, and motility of stomach and intestinal walls is decreased. This division functions to prepare the body for rigorous activity in response, for example, to fear and rage. During severe stress it can be lifesaving, but under normal resting conditions the sympathetic division is hardly active and, provided the body is subjected to no stress, it is not essential for the maintenance of life. In contrast, to the parasympathetic division, the preganglionic fibers of the sympathetic system are short, the postganglionic fibers generally long (Fig. 6-5b), and the chemical neurotransmitter between the postganglionic fibers and the effectors is usually norepinephrine (or less commonly epinephrine and, in the case of sweat glands, acetylcholine).

It is from adrenaline that "adrenergic" has been derived. This term refers generally to the nerves that liberate norepinephrine and/or epinephrine, to the effector organs that are influenced by these agents, and to the drugs that act like norepinephrine or epinephrine.

The term "cholinergic" is analogous to "adrenergic" and refers to any fiber that liberates acetylcholine as a transmitter, to any tissue that is primarily stimulated by acetylcholine as a transmitter, and to any drug that acts in a way similar to acetylcholine.

Release of these transmitter substances is part of a complex process by which conduction of nervous impulses in one set of nerve fibers influences the activity of other nerve cells or effector organs. Nerve conduction itself is an electrical phenomenon; an electrical change occurs across the membrane of the nerve cell that is propagated along the process of the neuron. When the propagated impulse reaches the end of the nerve fiber, the information is transmitted chemically to the next cell in the chain, across the intercellular gap. Sites at which one nerve fiber contact another are called synapses, and in the autonomic nervous system, transmission across the synapse involves the release by the

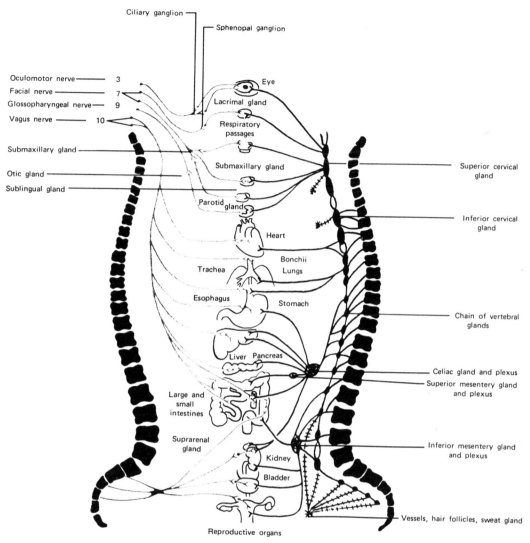

Figure 6-4 Autonomic nervous system, parasympathetic portion *left,* sympathetic portion *right.* (Adapted from JE Crouch and JR McClintic, *Human Anatomy and Physiology,* p. 567, Fig 20–26, 1971. Copyrighted © by John Wiley & Sons, Inc. and reprinted with permission.)

"presynaptic" fiber of either acetylcholine or norepinephrine.

There are two functional groups of cholinergic or acetylcholine-releasing junctions. In the first, the acetylcholine is accepted on receptors of the postsynaptic cells called "nicotinic receptors" (because of nicotinelike responses of acetylcholine). The neuromuscular junction already mentioned and also the junction between the pre- and postganglionic fibers in both the parasympathetic and sym-

pathetic divisions of the autonomic nervous system have receptors of this kind. The effects of acetylcholine at these sites, which are like the effect of nicotine or the drug lobeline, include peripheral vasoconstriction and rise in blood pressure. The action of acetylcholine on smooth muscles and glands on the other hand resembles the effect of muscarine, because these postsynaptic cells have appropriate "muscarinic receptors" (so designated because of muscarine-mushroomlike poison-

Table 6-1 Effects of Autonomic Stimulation[a]

Organ Affected	Parasympathetic Effects	Sympathetic Effects
Iris	Contraction of sphincter pupillae; pupil size decreases	Contraction of dilator pupillae; pupil size increases
Ciliary muscle	Contraction; accommodation for near vision	Relaxation; accommodation for distant vision
Lacrimal gland	Secretion	Excessive secretion
Salivary glands	Secretion of watery saliva in copious amounts	Scanty secretion of mucus—rich saliva
Respiratory system		
Conducting division	Contraction of smooth muscle; decreased diameters and volumes	Relaxation of smooth muscle; increased diameter and volumes
Respiratory division	Effect same as on conducting division	Effect same as on conducting division
Blood vessels	Constriction	Dilation
Heart		
Stroke volume	Decreased	Increased
Stroke rate	Decreased	Increased
Cardiac output and blood pressure	Decreased	Increased
Coronary vessels	Constriction	Dilation
Peripheral blood vessels		
Skeletal muscle	Constriction	Dilation
Skin	Dilation	Constriction
Visceral organs (except heart and lungs)	Dilation	Constriction
Stomach		
Wall	Increased motility	Decreased motility
Sphincters	Inhibited	Simulated
Glands	Secretion stimulated	Secretion inhibited
Intestines	Increased motility	Decreased motility
Wall		
Sphincters		
Pyloric, iliocecal	Inhibited	Stimulated
Internal anal	Inhibited	Stimulated
Liver	Promotes glycogenesis, promotes bile secretion	Promotes glycogenolysis, decreases bile secretion
Pancreas (exocrine and endocrine)	Stimulates secretion	Inhibits secretion
Spleen	Little effect	Contraction and emptying of stored blood into circulation
Adrenal medulla	Little effect	Epinephrine secretion
Urinary bladder	Stimulates wall, inhibits sphincter	Inhibits wall, stimulates sphincter
Uterus	Little effect	Inhibits motility of nonpregnant organ; stimulates pregnant
Sweat glands	Normal function	Stimulates secretion (produces "cold sweat" when combined with cutaneous vasoconstriction)

[a] Adapted with permission from JE Crouch and JR McClintic (1971)[1].

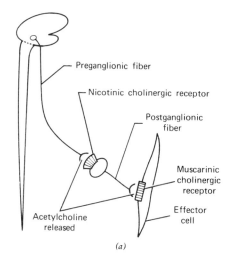

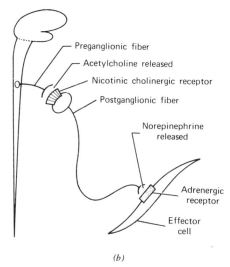

Figure 6-5 (a) Schematic portrayal of a parasympathetic nerve. (b) Schematic portrayal of a sympathetic nerve.

ing). The effect of acetylcholine and that of certain acetylcholinelike drugs such as muscarine, pilocarpine, and arecoline (from betel nuts), and the anticholinesterases (physostigmine) include a decrease in heart output; constriction of the pupil and contraction of the ciliary muscle for near vision; stimulation of secretions from sweat glands, salivary glands, mucous glands, stomach, intestine, and pancreas; increase in motility and tone of the stomach and intestine; contraction of the gallbladder and musculature of the bladder wall; relaxation of the sphincter. In addition, since most blood

vessels have muscarinic receptors, acetylcholine can produce vasodilation. All these actions can be reduced or abolished by atropine or atropinelike compounds including scopolamine (hyoscine), homatropine, and lachesine.

As atropine and similar compounds antagonize the muscarinic effect of acetylcholine by competing for the receptor sites, the sympathetic division of the autonomic system has a similar antagonistic effect on smooth muscles and glands. Thus stimulation at the adrenergic junction by release of norepinephrine, or norepinephrinelike drugs, will result in actions similar to those described for sympathetic divisional stimulation, and these are exactly the opposite effects brought about by muscarinic action—there is usually an increase in heart output, pupil dilation, blurred near vision, vasoconstriction of most blood vessels, decrease in motility and tone of the stomach and intestine, relaxation of the detrusor and contraction of sphincter muscles of the bladder, increased metabolism in the liver, inhibition of secretions of the pancreas, and stimulated secretion of the sweat glands.

Figure 6-6 illustrates the principal features of the physiology and biochemistry of a typical postganglionic adrenergic nerve terminal at this synapse with a postsynaptic cell containing the appropriate receptors. Chemical transmission is essentially the same as at cholinergic junctions, although the biochemical pathways are, of course, different. The major steps are as follows. (a) Norepinephrine (NE) is synthesized in the neuron from tyrosine, which is first hydrolyzed to give dopa, then decarboxylated to give dopamine; NE is also taken up from the circulation. (b) NE is stored in dense-cored or granular vesicles. (c) The arrival of a nerve impulse causes the release of NE from the nerve terminal; the uptake pump inactivates, by returning to the terminal, up to 60% of released NE. (d) NE diffuses to the immediate region of the receptors on the surface of the effector cell, but only about 5% reaches these sites. (e) NE combines with the receptor mechanism triggering the response, then dissociates itself from the receptor and diffuses freely into the surrounding medium. (f) NE is metabolized intraneuronally by monoamine oxidase (MAO) and extra-

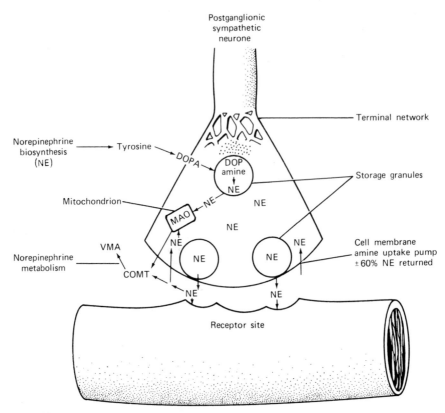

Figure 6-6   Diagrammatic representation of the principal features of the physiology and biochemistry of the postganglionic sympathetic neuron. (Adapted from WB Abrams, "The mechanisms of action of antihypertensive drugs," *Dis Chest* **55**(2):148–159, 1969. Reprinted with permission of CHEST, and the author.)

neuronally by catechol-O-methyl transferase (COMT) to produce vanillylmandelic acid (VMA); the free NE, being metabolized much more slowly than acetylcholine, therefore exerts continuing influence throughout the body.

Many drug actions may be exerted at this site.[4] Epinephrine, for example, stimulates adrenergic effects by releasing norepinephrine without in any way blocking neural transmission. As a result blood vessels constrict, the heart is stimulated, blood pressure is elevated, and nasal congestion is reduced. Thus when hypotension and shock threaten as a result of trauma, anesthesia, anaphylactic reactions, or other similar developments, peripheral vascular tone can be restored by vasoconstriction, and the

drug's strengthening and speeding effects on the heart can also restore abnormally low blood pressure. When used as a treatment of reaginic mediated (Type I) allergy, epinephrine increases the level of cAMP within the cell and thereby prevents the release of histamine and serotonin.

Acting in an opposite way, reserpine and the other *Rauvolfia* alkaloids have little effect on the norepinephrine-releasing mechanism, but they gradually deplete almost all the norepinephrine from sympathetic neurons by inhibiting the uptake of this substance by the storage granules. Thus by blocking adrenergic neurotransmission, the reserpine-type drugs reverse the effect of norepinephrine, lowering blood pressure, reducing heart output, and dilating blood vessels.

DRUGS ACTING ON THE NERVOUS SYSTEM

CENTRAL NERVOUS SYSTEM

In ever increasing numbers we suffer from anxiety, neurosis, psychopathy, drug dependence, and psychosis. It is not surprising, therefore, that the production and use of drugs that act on the central nervous system and affect the mind are expanding at an equally rapid pace.[3] Many of the drugs mentioned here will be discussed in greater detail in Section 3, Chapters 17 to 19.

Depressants

ANESTHETICS

Anesthetic drugs depress vital functions of all types of cells, but especially those of nervous tissue. General anesthetics depress the central nervous system so that all sensitivity to pain is lost and the individual suffers a lapse in consciousness. If anesthetics are applied to specific structures, such as the spinal fluid, they may block impulses transmitted by the neurons to the organs normally being innervated. When only peripheral nerve endings are involved, local anesthetics can be applied directly to the restricted area at which relief of pain is desired.

Clearly, since a great many substances are capable of inducing reversible unconsciousness, the mode of action of each cannot be specific. All anesthetics depress the utilization of oxygen by cells, and this explains in part why the brain, as the organ most abundantly supplied with blood and requiring large amounts of oxygen, is so highly susceptible to lack of oxygen and is rapidly affected by anesthetics.

Anesthetics such as thiopentone so-dium are delivered by intravenous injection, but more commonly anesthesia is by inhalation using nitrous oxide (laughing gas), halothane, and other drugs, often in combination. Preanesthetic medications to relieve pain and to decrease preoperative apprehension include morphine and morphine derivates, scopolamine, and others.

HYPNOTICS AND SEDATIVES

A hypnotic is a drug that produces sleep; a sedative is one used to relieve tension and anxiety. Hypnotics make the patient sleepy and are often used in cases of insomnia, whereas sedatives are usually given throughout the day without lowering sensory perception and alertness below safe levels.

The most commonly used hypnotics and sedatives are the barbiturates, all derivates of barbituric acid (synthesized from malonic acid and urea); all are almost insoluble in water, consequently pass readily through the blood-brain barrier. They especially depress the brain (hypothalamus first), but the duration of the depression and the intensity of the action are dependent on the drug chosen, the mode of administration, and the amount used. Other depressants include ethyl alcohol, chloral hydrate, xopium, chlorpromazine, and reserpine.

For milder cases of anxiety and tension, a number of antianxiety agents are prescribed (meprobamate—Miltown®, chlordiazepoxide—Librium®, diazepam—Valium®), but they should be taken with restraint, since they are often misused to lessen the minor stresses of everyday living.

NEUROLEPTICS (ANTIPSYCHOTICS)

The antipsychotic agents or major tranquilizers modify the symptoms of acute and chronic psychoses. The calming effect of these drugs is distinguished from that of the barbiturates and most hypnotic-sedatives in that large doses do not usually produce unconsciousness or depression of vital centers. All are synthetic compounds, of which chlorpromazine is the prototype, and they are widely used to treat psychoses (schizophrenia, senility, organic and toxic psychoses) and to a lesser extent neuroses (where antianxiety agents are preferred). Many have anticholinergic action.

ANTICONVULSANTS

By far the most common convulsive disease is epilepsy. This disorder, afflicting one in 200 individuals, is characterized by severe muscle spasms, loss of consciousness, and excessively abnormal discharges of electricity (grand mal). The nature of the factors inducing these discharges is unknown. In other types of epilepsy (e.g., petit mal), convulsions do not occur and the encephalogram exhibits alternate slow and fast waves.

Relief from convulsions is obtained by sufficient doses of barbiturates, the drug of choice being phenobarbital because of its efficient depression of motor activity, or other long-acting barbiturates such as mephobarbital and metharbital.[4] The hydantoins (phenytoin, methoin, thotoin) are also effective anticonvulsants in grand mal and prevent electrically induced seizures, though unlike phenobarbital they do not additionally prevent chemically induced seizures. Ethosuximide is used to treat petit mal.

Chorea (St. Vitus dance) in children, which is characterized by irregular spasmodic movements of the limbs and facial muscles, is treated by reserpine.

Disturbances of certain brain centers cause muscular rigidity and may impair normal movements, posture and equilibrium, and the ability to speak and write. This condition, known as Parkinson's disease, is caused by injury to basal ganglia and is a frequent sequel to "slow" virus infections, which may trigger this chronic degenerative disease.

The parkinsonian state is currently believed to reflect an imbalance between cholinergic and dopaminergic mechanisms in the central nervous system. Dopamine, which is normally present in the brain, is selectively depleted in patients with parkinsonism, resulting in a cholinergic dominance. Treatment is thus directed toward administering anticholinergic drugs and enhancing dopamine.[5] Unfortunately, dopamine does not readily penetrate the blood-brain barrier; but its immediate precursor levodopa (L-dopa) does, and this drug, originally identified in 1913 from the broad bean Vicia faba, is the most effective agent known against parkinsonism. Moderate to marked improvement is found for 50 to 90% of patients when the drug is administered for 6 months or longer. There is no reduced effectiveness with prolonged use, as occurs with all other drugs used, but side effects including gastrointestinal, cardiovascular, and psychiatric disturbances are commonplace.

Considerably less effective are the anticholinergic drugs, atropine, scopolamine, and many synthetic compounds, which are used in mild impairment or for patients not able to tolerate levodopa.

Recently Garcia et al.[6] concluded that the active pharmacological ingredient present in the purple portion of the leaves of Rhoeo spathacea (oyster plant, Commelinaceae) is dopamine; clearly this species is of potential value in combating parkinsonism.

Convulsive diseases were apparently more common in the Middle Ages than now, and epilepsy was regarded then as a manifestation of evil in the afflicted individual. Proof of the presence of such a spirit was a major convulsion, foam at the mouth, bleeding, unconsciousness, and various outcries during the attack. The best treatment of epilepsy was thought to be exorcism of the evil spirit and abandonment of the hapless victim during the convulsive stage. Thus epileptics not only had to try to live through the attacks, they were obliged to ward off those ready to burn at the stake all who harbored the devil, as epileptic witches were wont to do!

ANALGESICS

Pain-relieving drugs are called analgesics. There are several distinct types of pain, the pain of a headache, the throbbing of an abscess, the continuous pain of a broken bone, or anguish of angina pectoris and myocardial infarction. The primary aim in considering these and other kinds of pain should be to derive from the description of the distress enough information to secure relief by treating the cause.

Strong analgesics are primarily alkaloids isolated from opium, which is obtained from the latex of immature capsules of *Papaver somniferum,* or synthetics having similar properties, often referred to as opioids. Many opioids have been synthesized in an attempt to overcome certain defects of the natural alkaloids, but so far success has been limited. Morphine is the most important and abundant alkaloid of opium (3–20%); it is a strong analgesic, and it is easily absorbed when administered orally, smoked, or injected. Its effects can be observed in about 30 minutes and may last up to 12 hours.

Morphine exerts its greatest effects on the central nervous system, where it causes depression and excitation of selected centers. A depression of the cerebral cortex reduces the powers of concentration, as well as fear, anxiety, and prolonged pain, and these effects produce a great feeling of contentment. Initially the centers for vomiting, salivation, sweating, and bronchial secretion in the medulla are stimulated, but with larger doses these become depressed. Sweating is associated with vasodilation of the skin vessels, thereby giving a heat loss and a mild antipyretic (fever-reducing) effect. Among the most significant effects of morphine are depression of the respiratory and cough centers, and stimulation of the part of the parasympathetic nervous system affecting the eye, such that pupils may become very constricted. Although little is known about how morphine effects these changes, it does inhibit the hydrolysis of acetylcholine, which is a neurotransmitter in the brain; thus this inhibition may relate to the action of morphine.

Of the 25 different alkaloids isolated from *Papaver somniferum,* the other most important are codeine, narcotine, thebaine, narceine, and papaverine. Codeine is a mild analgesic, almost devoid of euphoric action, but it is much used in cough-suppressing medicines and in combination with aspirin and other weak analgesics for the relief of arthritic pain, headaches, and colds.

A second group of mild analgesics also has antipyretic action, and some have anti-inflammatory effects as well. Aspirin is the drug of choice. It is also used in the management of some rheumatic diseases because it has both analgesic and anti-inflammatory properties (p. 166).

Many plants have analgesic or numbing principles, such as *Ervatamia dichotoma* (Apocynaceae), *Boswellia serrata* (Burseraceae), and *Chrysanthemum anethifolium* (Asteraceae),[7] but none is used beyond domestic and folk medicine.

Stimulants

ANTIDEPRESSANTS

Depression is one of the most common psychiatric disorders. A number of antidepressant drugs are widely used for patients who are socially maladjusted, apathetic, and depressed.

Amphetamines, the most widely prescribed stimulants, exert a direct and powerful effect on the central nervous system, particularly in the reticular activating area of the brainstem, producing a general feeling of well-being and delaying the onset of mental and physical fatigue. Furthermore, they stimulate respiration and reduce appetite. Their action on the system is complex: they act as direct sympathomimetic drugs, as releasers of norepinephrine, and as competitive substrates for monoamine oxidase (see Fig. 6-6 and related text).

A number of other stimulants are available; the most commonly used are monoamine oxidase inhibitors (e.g., iproniazid, phenelzine, tranylcypromine) and the dibenzazepine derivates (imipramine, amitriptyline), but side effects of these synthetics are significant, and their use must be well controlled.

In decreasing strength as central nervous system stimulants, caffeine, theophylline, and theobromine all induce excitation at varying levels, but the cortex appears to be the most vulnerable site. Their main effects are to produce clear thought and to reduce drowsiness and fatigue. One or two cups of coffee is sufficient to increase the motor effects of conditioned reflexes and improve the higher functions of the brain. In addition, these alkaloids stimulate the respiratory, vagal, and vasomotor centers in the medulla.

CONVULSANTS AND ANALEPTICS

Convulsant and analeptic drugs excite and stimulate many parts of the central nervous system. Their most important actions are often on the medulla—in small doses as stimulants or analeptics; in sufficiently high doses, however, all such drugs produce generalized convulsions. As therapeutic agents, they are most effective against failure of vital functions resulting from overdoses of depressant drugs.

One of the best known convulsants is strychnine, an alkaloid obtained from the dried seeds of *Strychnos nux-vomica* and *S. ignatii* (Loganiaceae), which are native to southern Asia and Australia. A related alkaloid brucine is also extracted from these plants; it is less toxic than strychnine. Neither drug is popular in modern medical practice, but strychnine has been much used in neurologic investigations to illustrate the action of convulsant drugs because it stimulates the vasomotor and vagal centers of the medulla and has a remarkable effect in enhancing the sensations of touch, smell, hearing, and sight. Strychnine also acts on the alimentary canal: its bitter taste increases appetite, and since it stimulates intestinal action, it can be used in the treatment of constipation.

Another powerful stimulant is the sesquiterpene picrotoxin, obtained from the dried fruit of *Anamirta cocculus* (Menispermaceae), a woody climber native to southeastern Asia. It is effective in restoring respiration depressed by barbiturates or morphine and thus finds its therapeutic use as an antidote for these drugs. Picrotoxin is known to act on the spinal cord by blocking presynaptic inhibition.

A convulsant as potent as strychnine is the alkaloid bicuculline, isolated from *Corydalis cava* (Papaveraceae). It is a specific and reversible antagonist of the inhibitory action of γ-amino butyric acid

(GABA) on some central neurons. Its site of action is likely in those areas of the brain where GABA is a major transmitter.

Lobeline, from *Lobelia inflata* (Campanulaceae), is also a powerful alkaloid having actions similar to nicotine. It stimulates respiration and is used to revive patients who have taken an overdose of a narcotic.

HALLUCINOGENS

Drugs with marked ability to distort perception are discussed in Section 3. Although no regular therapeutic use is made of drugs that produce reversible toxic hallucinosis, many therapeutic substances (e.g., atropine) have this effect when taken in overdose.

PERIPHERAL NERVOUS SYSTEM: SENSORY OR AFFERENT NERVES

Local anesthetics and counterirritants are widely used to reduce peripheral pain. Counterirritant drugs are those which may be rubbed into the skin to produce a degree of irritation. Stimulation of sensory nerves gives rise to a relaxation of arterioles through the vasodilator nerve, and this in turn improves local circulation, promotes a glow or warmth, and gives relief from certain types of pain. Examples include liniments of methyl salicylate or camphor, and mustard plasters.

Local anesthetics impair conduction in nerve fibers and rapidly reduce pain, at times even in low concentrations. In higher concentrations, local anesthetics can also block somatic motor neurons and synapses and diminish the responsiveness of skeletal muscle neurons to acetylcholine. Cocaine, an alkaloid of *Erythroxylum coca,* is a well-known local anesthetic, but the most important and useful ones are synthetic substances, lignocaine, procaine, benzocaine, and others.

Somatic Nervous System

Therapeutically valuable stimulation of voluntary muscles may be brought about by inhibiting the catalytic action of cholinesterase. Excess acetylcholine at neuroskeletal junctions therefore produces a stimulatory effect.

Thus for the condition known as myasthenia gravis, in which the weakness and rapid fatigability of skeletal muscles following exercise often becomes severe enough to endanger life, neostigmine or pyridostigmine can inhibit the destruction of acetylcholine, thereby increasing its effective concentration at the motor endplate receptors. At one time physostigmine (eserine) from *Physostigma venenosum,* which also prolongs the effect of the transmission of nerve impulses to voluntary muscles by anticholinesterase action, was used to treat myasthenia gravis; but now its application is largely with the eye (Chapter 9). In addition, galanthamine obtained from *Galanthus waronowii* (Caucasian snowdrop), *Leucojum aestivum,* and *Ungernia victoris,* is used to treat myasthenia gravis in parts of Europe.

Presumably by blocking acetylcholine receptor sites at neuroskeletal junctions, drugs may be used to reversibly paralyze skeletal muscles. These relaxants include curare, a crude dried extract obtained from the bark and stems of *Strychnos castelanei, S. toxifera, S. crevauxii* (Loganiaceae), and *Chondodendron tomentosum* (Menispermaceae)—substances long used as arrow poisons by South American Indians. Curare poisoning leads to death from paralysis of the respiratory organs.

Curare varies in composition among the Indian tribes, each modifying the formula in accordance with custom, but the most important constituent of curare is the isoquinoline alkaloid D-tubocurarine obtained from *Chondodendron tomentosum*. This drug is used to secure muscle relaxation in surgery without deep anesthesia and to control convulsions of strychnine poisoning. Similar curarelike activity is exhibited by a group of alkaloids from tropical species of *Erythrina*,[9] but these are no longer used clinically.

Autonomic Nervous System[10]

A number of drugs act predominantly at the junction of the postganglionic parasympathetic neuron and smooth muscle, heart, or gland cells.

CHOLINERGIC NERVES: MUSCARINIC SITE OF ACTION

1. Effects of stimulating the neuron may be imitated by acetylcholine, cholimimetic esters (carbachol), cholimimetic alkaloids such as muscarine (from *Amanita muscaria, A. pantherina, Boletus luridus, B. satanus, Clitocybe dealbata,* and *Russula emetica*), arecoline (from *Areca catechu*), and pilocarpine (from *Pilocarpus jaborandi, P. microphyllus, P. pennatifolius, P. spicatus, P. trachylopus*), and the anticholinesterase compounds physostigmine (from *Physostigma venenosum*), and a large number of synthetics (echothiophate, malathion).

2. Other drugs antagonize or inhibit the muscarinic actions of acetylcholine by blocking the site of action: atropine ((±)-hyoscyamine), and scopolamine (hyoscine) obtained from many plants in the Solanaceae; papaverine from *Papaver somniferum*; and a new alkaloid anisodiamine (8-hydroxyatropine) from *Anisodus tanguticus* (Solanaceae) reportedly is an even better antispasmodic than atropine.[11]

These anticholinergic drugs as well as many synthetic compounds are widely used as antispasmodic and antiulcer agents in the treatment of many pathological conditions, including peptic ulcers (by decreasing vagal nerve stimulation and acid secretion); spasms of the stomach, intestine, bladder, urinary tract, and biliary and pancreatic ducts; spastic, painful menstruations; pernicious vomiting of pregnancy; excessive salivation, perspiration, and secretions of the nose, pharynx, and bronchi; fainting due to heart block; arterial spasms; threatened gangrenous conditions of the extremities; spastic constipation; bed wetting; and inflammations of the cornea and iris. All these conditions are alleviated partially or completely by the use of anticholinergic drugs.

CHOLINERGIC NERVES: NICOTINIC SITE OF ACTION

Certain drugs act predominantly at the junction of the pre- and postganglionic neurons in autonomic ganglia. They include acetylcholine stimulants like nicotine (from *Nicotiana tabacum*) and depressants including the toxin from *Clostridium botulinum*, which prevents the release of acetylcholine, and a number of synthetic compounds (hexamethonium, mecamylamine, pempidine).

ADRENERGIC NERVES

Other drugs act on the sympathetic neuron at its junction with smooth muscle or gland cells. Stimulants include norepinephrine, epinephrine (adrenaline), dopamine, isoprenaline, amphetamine, and ephedrine. Of these only ephedrine is readily available as a natural alkaloid; it is obtained from *Ephedra equisetina* and *E. sinica*, but can be made synthetically. Among the antagonists are reserpine (from *Rauvolfia* spp.) and ergotamine (from *Claviceps purpurea*), as well as a number of synthetic compounds (bretylium, guanethidine, phentolamine, propranolol).

NERVOUS SYSTEM ASSOCIATED DISEASES AND ACTIVITIES

A number of diseases are clearly the result of nervous system deficiencies, but the etiology of others has not been clearly defined. For convenience, those discussed below are considered in association with nervous system disorders; additionally, various activities associated with the mental process are included.

HYPERACTIVE CHILDREN

Hyperactivity in children, as a function of inherent temperament, immaturity, emotional disorders, or diffuse brain damage, is characterized by excessive physical activity and the inability to concentrate and learn.[12] Recently environmental factors such as artificial flavors and color additives in food have been suggested as triggering certain cases of hyperactivity in a type of allergic reaction.[13] Dextroamphetamine (Dexedrine®) is the drug of choice for hyperkinetic impulse disorders, but there are side effects: loss of appetite, sleep disturbance, and facial changes. Recently Schnackenberg[14] reported that two cups of coffee (equivalent to 200–300 mg) is sufficient to calm overactive children without the tremendous costs of typical drug therapy and the troublesome side effects. Noting that 5% of American children are affected by this condition, Schnackenberg adds that children in South America who routinely drink coffee apparently do not display problems of overactivity, for inadvertently they are being treated for the problem.

MANIC INSANITY

The best treatment by far for manic insanity is regular administration of lithium carbonate, a medication with an ancient history that has proved in recent years not only to calm the manic highs but to prevent future severe swings in mood as well.

MEMORY PROCESS

In mice, injection of strychnine produces significantly improved learning ability and facilitates the long-term and perhaps short-term store of memory.[15]

MIGRAINE

Severe headaches that tend to arise suddenly and recur may be caused by changes in the cranial blood vessels by dilation of arteries and arterioles. Ergotamine from the fungus *Claviceps purpurea* is thought to counteract vasodilation and is the drug of choice in treating acute migraine attacks. It is particularly effective in combination with caffeine, scopolamine, atropine, and hyoscyamine.[16]

MOTION SICKNESS

Those troubled by motion sickness should stay near the middle of a ship or plane, or in the front seat of a car, where linear acceleration is minimal. If symptoms persist, scopolamine may be worth trying in a single small dose.[17]

RHEUMATISM AND ARTHRITIS

"Rheumatism" describes many conditions associated with diseases of the joints, tendons, muscles, or bones; arthritis is inflammation of a joint. The most common diseases among these are rheumatoid arthritis, a joint inflammation characterized by pain and limited motion of such joints as the fingers, and osteoarthritis, in which the bone and cartilage of the joint are affected; symptoms include aches and soreness of the joints, especially following extensive physical exercise. Although the etiology of these diseases is unknown, rheumatoid arthritis is, at least in part, an immune complex disease, for it has been demonstrated that the rheumatoid factor is an autoantibody to immunoglobulin G (IgG), with which it circulates in a complex in body fluids. Deposits of these complex molecules can be observed in the inflamed arteries and joint fluids of patients with rheumatoid arthritis. Thus immunosuppressive agents such as corticosteroids, antifolates, and alkylating agents may be used in treatment, although serious adverse side effects are frequent.[18] A mild analgesic like aspirin is still the drug most widely used to treat rheumatic and arthritic diseases.

SLEEPING PILL PSYCHOSIS

Because they are widely advertised and sold without prescription, such over-the-counter sleeping pills as Compoz®, Sominex®, and Sleep-Eze® are generally considered safe. But overuse of these drugs can be dangerous and may trigger hallucinations and schizophrenic behavior. A key ingredient in many such preparations is scopolamine, and there is little doubt that this plant alkaloid is responsible for the psychotic behavior mentioned. The condition of most patients can be improved by injecting the alkaloid physostigmine.[19]

INFECTIONS

There are a variety of bacteria that cause acute suppurative (purulent) bacterial meningitis. This potentially fatal infection of the central nervous system is generally characterized by headache, vomiting, meningeal involvement, irritability, convulsions, coma, stiff neck, and bulging fontanelle. Most of the organisms responsible for this disease are found among those of the normal body flora. In this respect, enterobacteria from man's intestinal tract, especially Escherichia coli, have been most frequently isolated from spinal fluids of neonates whose mothers have developed obstetrical complications during late pregnancy or at delivery. In these cases, death may result from endotoxic shock. Meningitis usually develops later in infants born without complication, and organisms such as staphylococci and streptococci, from the skin and elsewhere, are usually involved. It is also possible for certain normal nasopharyngeal inhabitants to produce respiratory tract, sinus, and ear infections that can, on extension directly or through the blood, produce disease in the central nervous system.

Infections of Hemophilus influenzae are more common in children under 6 years of age, whereas those of Streptococcus pneumoniae may also be found in adults. Unlike these sporadic infections, those of Neisseria meningitidis transmitted by asymptomatic carriers are associated with outbreaks of epidemic proportions. Hemorrhagic pathological petechiae on the skin and systemic endotoxemia may be clinical and pathological features of this disease. Septic meningitis results from an extension of systemic infections of tularemia, brucellosis, gonorrhea, and listerosis.

Since the advent of antibiotic therapy, the mortality rate from infections has dropped dramatically. Nonetheless, therapy is successful only when diagnosis is made early. Penicillin or ampicillin are drugs of choice for meningococcal, *H. influenzae,* streptococcal, and staphylcoccal infections; kanamycin or gentamicin are usually selected for *Escherichia coli;* and gentamicin, carbenicillin, and polymyxin B are best whenever *Pseudomonas aeroginosa* is implicated.

Aseptic meningitis is a benign syndrome characterized by meningeal involvement, headache, fever, and vomiting, which may give rise to severe diseases of the nervous system such as meningoencephalitis, encephalitis, and encephalomyelitis. With certain infections, aseptic meningitis may be a primary symptom, whereas with others it is merely an extension of a disease elsewhere. Noteworthy among the latter are polio, the arthropod-borne encephalitis, tuberculosis, syphilis, leptospirosis, toxoplasmosis, torulosis, and coccidiomycosis. Therapy depends on the organism involved; specific antibiotics, which can be used for bacterial and fungal infections, are only supportive in viral disease.

HERBOLOGY

ARTHRITIS INCLUDING RHEUMATISM

Jarvis[20] prescribed a Vermont folk remedy to treat arthritis involving apple cider vinegar, honey, Lugol's solution (iodine), and Parkelp (alga) tablets, plus careful daily food selection. There is apparently no scientifically accepted basis for this treatment, and numerous others currently recommended in unorthodox medicine lack similar support.[21]

Aralia racemosa (spikenard). Cherokees and Appalachian whites took a root tea for backache, as well as for rheumatoid arthritis.

Chimaphila umbellata (spotted wintergreen). Catawbas used a medicine made from wintergreen for backache.

Gentiana catesbaei (blue gentian). Catawbas steeped the roots in hot water and applied the liquid to aching backs.

Hamamelis virginiana (witch hazel). Many American Indians prepared a liniment or decoction of boiled leaves and stems of witch hazel for external use against inflammations and aching backs.

Monarda punctata (horsemint). Catawbas mashed the green leaves and let them stand in cold water, which was drunk for relief of backaches.

Phytolacca americana (poke). Pamunkey Indians of Virginia drank a tea of boiled fruit to cure rheumatism; they also used the plant internally in treatment of chronic rheumatism.

Sanguinaria canadensis (bloodroot). A root infusion as a tea was a favorite remedy for rheumatism among the Rappahannocks and the Indians of the Mississippi River region.

CONVULSIONS, FITS, AND EPILEPSY

Datura stramonium (jimson weed). In Europe the seeds and plant extracts were used in the treatment of mania, epilepsy, melancholy, rheumatism, convulsions, and madness.

Heracleum lanatum (cow parsnip). The species was widely used by eclectic physicians to treat epilepsy.

DEPRESSANTS AND SEDATIVES

Cypripedium spp. (lady's slipper) (Fig. 6-7a). At one time lady's slippers were considered to be effective nerve sedatives and were widely used in domestic medicine to treat hysteria, neuralgia, and similar complaints. The Indians employed them to treat all nervous diseases and hysterical afflictions by allaying pain (i.e., as an anodyne), quieting the nerves, and promoting sleep.

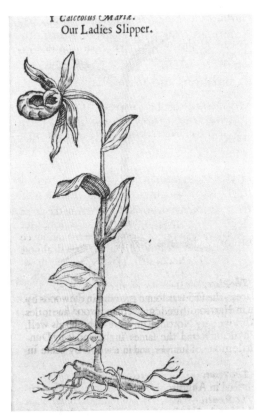

I *Calceolus Mariæ.*
Our Ladies Slipper.

Figure 6-7a   *Cypripedium calceolus* (from J Gerard,
The Herball, ed 2, 1636).

Passiflora incarnata (passion flower) (Fig.
6-7b). The passion flower was formerly
prescribed as a nerve sedative, to relieve
insomnia, and for treating certain types
of convulsions and spasmodic disorders.
It was also attributed with anodyne
properties and was used in the treatment
of various neuralgias and for epilepsy.
Now it is an ingredient in certain types of
sleeping pills.

Valeriana officinalis and *V. wallichii.* Oil
of valerian is depressing to the whole
central nervous system and is prescribed
by some physicians as a remedy for
hysteria, hypochondriasis, and nervous
unrest, as well as for insomnia and as an
anticonvulsant in epilepsy.The major
sedative principles present in *Valeriana*

species are known to be the monoterpene
valepotriotes, which are widely used in
Europe.

FEVERS

Cornus florida (dogwood). In pioneer
days country doctors prescribed a bitter
drink made by steeping dogwood flowers,
fruit, and bark in water for fevers and
chills. This treatment had been gleaned
from the many eastern American Indians,
who had long used dogwood as an antipyretic.

Eupatorium perfoliatum (boneset). Ex-
tolled for its many properties and uses
against intermittent fevers, arthritis, gout,
and epilepsy by early American physicians and the Indians, *E. perfoliatum*

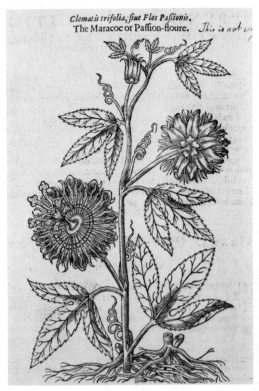

Clematis trifolia, sive Flos Passionis.
The Maracoc or Passion-floure.

Figure 6-7b   *Passiflora* sp. (from J Gerard, *The Herball,* ed 2, 1636).

was a virtual panacea and was always found in the well-regulated household. It was widely used by Confederate troops, who drank hot infusions of the plant as a febrifuge and as a substitute for quinine.

Myrica cerifera (bayberry). Choctaws of Louisiana boiled the leaves and stems in water as a decoction for fever.

Oldenlandia corymbosa. This plant is used in India as a decoction in remittent fever, such as malaria and undulant fever, and the juice is applied to palms and soles to relieve the burning sensation in fevers; it is also used against nervous depression.[22]

Salix spp. and *Populus* spp. (willow and poplar). Analgesic properties are discussed earlier in this chapter.

HEADACHES

Anemone cylindrica (long-headed anemone). Meskwakis made a tea of the roots and used it against headaches and vertigo.

Arisaema atrorubens (jack-in-the-pulpit, Indian turnip). Pawnees pulverized and dried the roots and dusted the resulting powder on the head and temples to relieve aches.

Hedeoma pulegioides (pennyroyal). Indians believed that the application of this herb to pains of any limb would bring immediate relief. A tea from this aromatic herb was used by the Onondagas as a headache medicine, and the Mescalero and Lipan Indians treated prolonged headaches by rubbing the aromatic twigs of the related *H. reverchoni* and inhaling the odor.

Symplocarpus foetidus (skunk cabbage). Micmacs crushed the leaves and inhaled the pungent oils as a headache remedy; yet an overdose of the rhizome, for example, allegedly causes nausea, vomiting, vertigo, disturbed vision, and headaches.

INSOMNIA

Mitchella repens (partridge berry). Menominees drank a tea made from the leaves to cure insomnia.

Solanum americanum (black nightshade). Rappahannocks used it as a cure for sleeplessness, steeping a few leaves in a large quantity of water and drinking the infusion.

MENTAL DISEASE

Of the 19 African plants Watt lists as remedies for mental disease, he makes particular note of *Canthium glabriflorum* root and leaf and *Capparis tomentosa* bark. He also includes other African treatments for such ills as hysteria, amnesia, and vertigo.[23]

NEURALGIA

In India, dramatic relief from trigeminal neuralgia (pain in the sensory divisions of the fifth cranial nerve distributed to the skin of the face and head, and to other areas) is obtained by prescribing an indigenous drug recipe along with isonicotinic acid hydrazide.[24] The patent drug taken in tablet form includes *Capparis moonii*, *Caesalpinia digyna*, *Withania somnifera*, *Tinospora cordifolia*, *Allium sativum*, and other species, but the specific plant or plant combinations necessary to relieve this peripheral nerve pain are unknown.

ACUPUNCTURE, ACUPRESSURE, AND HERBS

No discussion of the nervous system can end without mention of the use of needles and pressure in Chinese medicine to affect analgesia, to treat disease, and to eliminate pathologic conditions. In addition, the Chinese combine ionizing mechanisms and herbs[25] to treat "facial neuralgia" in which a brown solution made from t'u ho (*Vitis serjanifolia?*) is placed on a moist gauze under the positive pole and over the face, while the negative pole is hand-held. For treatment of trigeminal neuralgia the cation and a poultice of the herb wu-ton (black bean) are held against the face, and again the anion is held in the hand.

LITERATURE CITED

1. Crouch JE, McClintic JR. 1971. *Human Anatomy and Physiology.* Wiley, New York. 646 p.
2. Abrams WB. 1969. The mechanisms of action of antihypertensive drugs. *Dis Chest* 55: 148–159.
3. Heilbronn E, Winter A (eds). 1970. *Drugs and Cholinergic Mechanisms in the CNS.* Forsvarets Forskningsanstalt, Research Institute of National Defense, Stockholm. 577 p; Root WS, Hofmann FG (eds). 1963. *Physiological Pharmacology.* Vol 1, *The Nervous System—Part A, Central Nervous System Drugs,* 703 p; 1965. Vol 2, *The Nervous System—Part B, Central Nervous System Drugs,* 486 p; Sulser F, Sanders-Bush E. 1971. Effects of drugs on amines in the CNS. *Ann Rev Pharm* 11: 209–230.
4. Dreifuss MB, Sato S. 1972. Anticonvulsant drugs in clinical practice. *Drug Ther* 2(8): 9–11, 15–17, 20–22; Griggs WL III. 1971. Epilepsy: practical medical treatment. *Mod Treat* 8(2): 258–276.
5. Barbeau A. 1969. L-Dopa therapy in Parkinson's disease: a critical review of nine years' experience. *Can Med Ass J* 101: 791–800; Brogden RN, Speight TM, Avery GS. 1971. Levodopa: a review of the pharmacological properties and therapeutic uses with particular reference to parkinsonism. *Drugs* 2: 262–400; Calne DB, Reid JL. 1972. Antiparkinsonian drugs: pharmacological and therapeutic aspects. *Drugs* 4: 49–74; El-Yosef MK, Janowsky E, Davis JM et al. 1973. Reversal of antiparkinsonian drug toxicity by physostigmine: a controlled study. *Am J Psychiatr* 130: 141–145; Kast EC. 1967. Drug treatment of Parkinson's disease. *Mod Med* 35(20): 24–30; Yahr MD. 1972. The treatment of parkinsonism. Current concepts. *Med Clin N Am* 56: 1377–1392; Yahr MD, Duvoisin RC. 1972. Drug therapy of parkinsonism. *New Eng J Med* 287: 20–24.
6. Garcia M, Miyares C, Menendez E et al. 1971. Blockade of the antiadrenergic action of bretylium by an aqueous extract of the leaves of *Rhoeo spathacea. Can J Phys Pharm* 49: 1106–1110.
7. Doskotch RW, Beal JL. 1970. The isolation and identification of the numbing principle in *Chrysanthemum anethifolium. Lloydia* 33: 393–394; Grover N. 1965. Man and plants against pain. *Econ Bot* 19: 99–112; Kar A, Menon MK. 1969. Analgesic effect of the gum resin of *Boswellia serrata* Roxb. *Life Sci* 8(1): 1023–1028; Kupchan SM, Bright A, Macko E. 1963. Alkaloids of *Ervatamia dichotoma.* Isolation, crystallization, and pharmacological properties of coronaridine. *J Pharm Sci* 52: 598–599.
8. Dahl DS. 1973. The management of myasthenia gravis. *Drug Ther* 3(3): 51–53, 57–59.
9. *Erythrina* Symposium. 1974. *Lloydia* 37(3): 321–487, 37(4): 543–588.
10. Loggie JM, Van Maanen EF. 1972. The autonomic nervous system and some aspects of the use of autonomic drugs in children. *J Pediatr* 81: 205–216, 432–445; Root WS, Hofmann FG (eds). 1967. *Physiological Pharmacology.* Vol 3, *The Nervous System—Part C, Autonomic Nervous System Drugs.* 519 p; Vol 4, *The Nervous System—Part C, Autonomic Nervous System Drugs.* 535 p.
11. Absorption, distribution and excretion of anisodiamine. 1973. *Chin Med J* 1973(5): 59; Pharmacologic effects of anisodiamine. 58 (without authors).
12. Solomons G. 1967. Child hyperactivity: diagnosis, treatment. *Tex Med* 63: 52–57; Amphetamine-type drugs for hyperactive children. *Med Lett* 14(7): 21–23, 1972.
13. Hot dogs and hyperkinesis. *Newsweek* 9 July 1973: 57.
14. McNeely PG. 1973. Coffee may calm hyperactive children. *Nat Obs* 15 Sept: 10; Schnackenberg RC. 1973. Caffeine as a substitute for schedule II stimulants in hyperkinetic children. *Am J Psychiatr* 130: 796–798.

15. Alpern HP, Crabbe JC. 1972. Facilitation of the long-term store of memory with strychnine. *Science* **177:** 722–724; Hu JW. 1973. Strychnine and memory process. *Science* **181:** 363.

16. Lovshin LL. 1968. The treatment of migraine. *Mod Med* **36**(5): 87–91.

17. Motion sickness drugs. *Med Lett* **3**(13): 47–48, 1961.

18. Bennett JC (ed). 1971. Chronic arthritis. *Mod Treat* **8**(4): 751–858; Vaughan JH, Blomgren SE, Edgington TS. 1973. Treatment for rheumatoid arthritis. *Mod Med* **41**(3): 32–37.

19. Sleeping-pill psychosis. *Time* 4 Sept 1972: 59.

20. Jarvis, DC. 1958. *Folk Medicine, A Vermont Doctor's Guide to Good Health.* Holt, Rinehart & Winston, New York. 182 p; Jarvis DC. 1960. *Arthritis and Folk Medicine.* Holt, Rinehart & Winston, New York. 179 p.

21. Lamont-Havers RW. 1960. Misrepresentation of treatments for arthritis. *Bull Rheum Dis* **11**(1): 223–226.

22. Datta PC, Sen A. 1969. Pharmacognosy of *Oldenlandia corymbosa* Linn. *Quart J Crude Drug Res* **9**(2): 1365–1371.

23. Watt JM. 1967. African plants potentially useful in mental health. *Lloydia* **30:** 1–22.

24. Kanwar KS, Dudani IC. 1969. An indigenous drug with I.N.H. in trigeminal neuralgia—a new approach. *J Ind Dent Ass* **1969:** 209–211.

25. Ingle JI. 1973. Acupuncture, analgesia and therapy in the People's Republic of China. Presented to Annual Meeting of the American Dental Association, Houston, 29 October 1973.

Chapter 7
Heart and Circulation

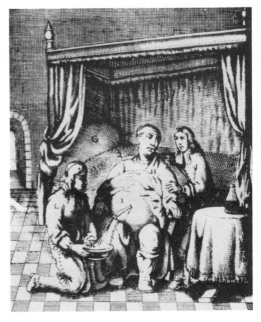

Figure 7-1 Relief of dropsy (P Barbette, 1672).

For a thousand centuries, men have suffered from a widespread malady that puffed their bodies into grotesque shapes, squeezed their lungs, and finally brought slow but inexorable death.

Steadily, as the disease progressed, a watery liquid filtered into every available space and expanded it like a balloon. Sometimes the liquid—quarts or even gallons of it—made arms and legs swell so that they were immovable. Sometimes it poured into the abdomen to form a tremendous paunch. Sometimes it waterlogged the lung cavity and thereby made it impossible for the victim to breathe unless he sat bolt upright all day and all night.

This watery sickness was *hydrops* or, more commonly, *dropsy*. After tuberculosis and the other infectious diseases, it was one of the chief causes of death. It was so ten thousand years ago, a thousand years ago, even a century ago, and, but for an almost miraculous green leaf, it might be the same today[1] (Fig. 7-1).

Cures for dropsy were numerous. Those described by Tennant in 1734 emphasized self-denial and treatment with herbal concoctions against what was then a mortal enemy.

He [Earl of Oxford] *purg'd* 2 or 3 Times, drank sparingly of *Canary* and *Water, thickened* with the *Yolk* of a *new-laid Egg*; and all his Victuals besides were cook'd with abundance of *Garlick*; and *Horse-radish*. This Method was pursued with great Constancy for 3 Months, and blest with intire Success.

The Last Instance, is an *Ancient Gentlemen,* who trusted to the Remedies of our own Country with the like happy Effect. He drank the *Decoction of Sassafras,* as soon as he got up, and chew'd the *Root* of it all the rest of the Morning, 'til Dinner; then observ'd a light, and nourishing Diet; and Drank moderately of clear sound *Cider,* wherein a *hot iron* had been plentifully quench'd.

Of these several Remedies, you may please to take your choice; or, instead of *Sassafras,* you may hold the *Seeds* of *Pellitary of Spain* in your Mouth, which will salivate the more powerfully.

The rest of the Cure must be compleated with restorative Meats, and a very short Allowance of Drink.[2]

No suggestion of a link between this fluid accumulation or edema and heart disease was possible in the early eighteenth century. How could physicians of that age guess that blood pumped from a damaged heart returns by way of the vena cava vessel at low pressure, allowing fluids to leak out of the capillaries into surrounding tissues? In addition, the kidney is prevented from functioning at the level of efficiency necessary to excrete the fluid, and the result is swollen areas of the body, great stress on the heart, and ultimately congestive heart failure.

Soon after Tennant published anonymously in 1734 and 1741 the foregoing treatments for dropsy, William Withering was born in England. He studied medicine at Edinburgh and there was influenced by some of the greatest professors in all Europe, including the distinguished botanist John Hope. Withering, however, did not like botany. Medicine, surgery, and anatomy—these had color, excitement, and practical application; but botany, he wrote his father, gave him only disagreeable ideas. This was at the age of 23, yet Withering later wrote the first complete English-language

handbook of plants in the British Isles,[3] and by discovering the use of *Digitalis,* he became one of the greatest medical botanists of all times.

Digitalis, or foxglove (Fig. 7-2), had been used by illiterate farmers and housewives in England and on the Continent for centuries. These people knew nothing about medicine, but they were wise enough to use a concoction that included *Digitalis* in treating dropsy. In Shropshire, Yorkshire, and other counties, the home remedies always contained *Digitalis* leaves, and it was Withering who had the ingenuity and imagination to select this substance as the probable active ingredient. He worked for many years observing its activity on the heart and eventually gave the world

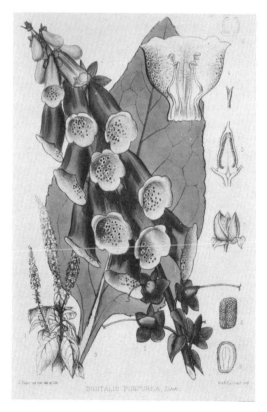

Figure 7-2 *Digitalis purpurea* (From R Bentley and H Trimen, *Medicinal Plants* **3:** 195, 1880).

his remarkable book, *An Account of the Foxglove, and Some of Its Medical Uses, with Practical Remarks on Dropsy, and Other Diseases.*[4] Today hundreds are engrossed in research on digitalis and other heart drugs. It is imperative that they succeed, because the partial conquest over dropsy and angina pectoris represents only a pitifully small part of the problem solved since Withering's time. The incurable diseases of the heart and blood vessels lead all other causes of death; they are the number one killers of modern civilization.

In the United States during 1972 more than one million people died from major cardiovascular diseases, a majority from heart attacks and strokes (Table 7-1). A meaningful comparison of death rate with that of earlier periods is difficult, but between 1940 and 1960 there was a marked increase in deaths from cardiovascular diseases among American males over 45 years of age.[5]

DESCRIPTION AND ETIOLOGY

The circulatory system (schematized in Fig. 7-3) serves many functions, but the chief one is that of obtaining oxygen in the lungs and carrying it to the cells in the various parts of the body. Within this system, the heart has but one function: to propel blood through the blood vessels of the body. It is simply an oxygen pump.

Blood enters the right atrium of the heart from the lower body by way of the inferior vena cava and from the upper body by way of the superior vena cava (Fig. 7-4). Blood is bluish as it enters the right atrium because the oxygen has been largely extracted by the body tissues. Blood pressure is low, as the heart relaxes and the right atrium fills with blood. To drive the blood from the right and left atria, the heart's "spark plug" (the sinoatrial node or normal pacemaker, a small bundle of nerve tissue in the right atrium) generates an electric wave that starts the heartbeat; the wave spreads across the atria, causing them to contract, and forcing the blood into the ventricles. The blood is thus forced through the tricuspid valve to the right ventricle. Meanwhile, part of the electric wave travels along the atrioventricular node, a connecting nerve between the atria and the ventricles. This nerve divides into two branches between the ventricles, and these in turn branch into many nerve fibrils that permeate the ventricular muscle walls. The impulse stimulates contraction, and with great force the blood is pumped into the pulmonary artery from the right ventricle at the same time that blood is forced by high systolic pressure from the left ventricle into the aorta. The contraction just described takes place when the ventricles are filled to capacity; it is synchronized, and it is normally regular in rhythm.

Returning to the sequence of circulation, the blood is pumped into the pulmonary artery through the pulmonary valve and is carried to the lungs. There it receives a fresh supply of oxygen, carbon dioxide is released, and from the lungs the blood passes to the left side of the heart to the left atrium by way of the pulmonary veins. As noted already, in coordination with the contraction of the right atrium by the pacemaker, the blood is forced through the mitral valve into the left ventricle. This thick-walled chamber then pumps the blood to the whole body by way of the aortic valve and the aorta. The blood circulates

Table 7-1 Cardiovascular Deaths in the United States During 1972[5]

Disease	Deaths	
	Total	per 100,000
Heart	752,450	361.3
Cerebrovascular	210,050	100.9
Arteriosclerosis	32,820	15.8
Hypertension	7,680	3.7
Others	25,560	12.3
Total	1,028,560	493.9

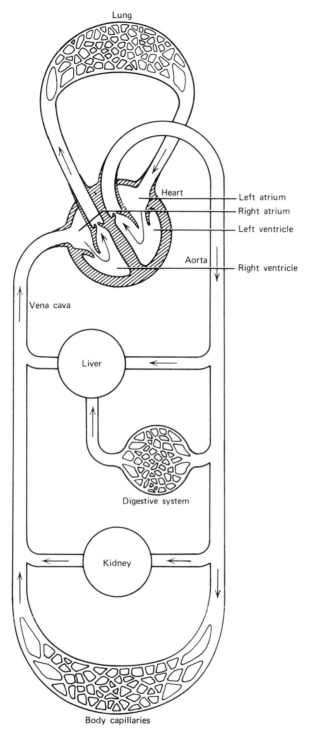

Labels on the figure:

Lung

Heart

Left atrium
Right atrium
Left ventricle

Aorta

Right ventricle

Vena cava

Liver

Digestive system

Kidney

Body capillaries

Figure 7-3   Schematic diagram of the circulatory system. (Adapted from JW Estes and PD White, "William Withering and the purple foxglove," *Scientific American* June 1965, p 112. Copyrighted © 1965 by Scientific American, Inc., and reprinted with their permission.)

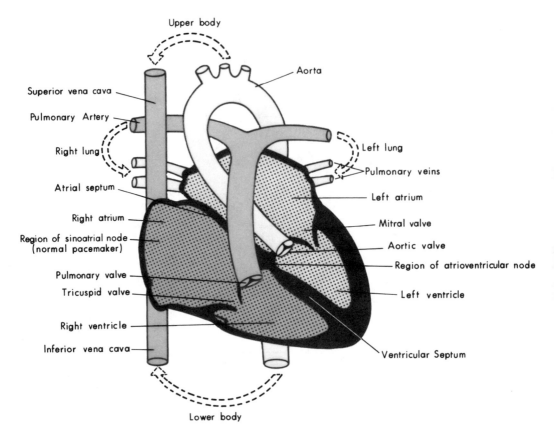

Figure 7-4 Normal heart. The arrows indicate the direction of blood flow through the four chambers and great vessels. (Adapted from the Ross Clinical Education Aid No. 7, 1970. Copyrighted © by Ross Laboratories, Columbus, Ohio, and reprinted with their permission.)

through the arteries, capillaries, and veins and eventually returns to the right side of the heart (systemic circulation), about 6 quarts of blood making a complete cycle in less than a minute.

The highest (systolic) pressure exists within the arteries when the left ventricle is ejecting the peak volume of blood into the aorta, and it is designated by measuring the height of a column of mercury in a glass tube that arterial pressure will support (e.g., a "120" reading means that the pressure in the arteries is equal to the weight of a column of mercury 120 mm high). The bottom (diastolic) pressure in the arteries is reached when the aortic valve has closed and the left ventricle is refilling. For most adults the systolic pressure lies some-

where between 100 and 140 (millimeters of mercury), and diastolic is between 60 and 90.

This is the normally functioning condition of the heart and of circulating blood. But what are the abnormalities?

CARDIAC AND CARDIOVASCULAR DISEASES

HEART ATTACK, CORONARY THROMBOSIS OR MYOCARDIAL INFARCTION

Blood supplying the heart muscle comes entirely from two coronary (heart)

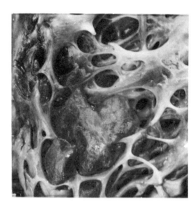

Figure 7-5 Interior view of the heart—myocardial trabeculae and thrombus. (Photograph No. 8 by L Nilsson).

arteries, both lying along the outside surface of the heart. If one of these arteries or any part of one suddenly becomes blocked (Fig. 7-5), the portion of the heart being supplied by the artery dies. The death of a portion of the heart muscle is called a heart attack, and the amount of the heart affected by the sudden occlusion will depend on the severity of this attack and will determine whether the individual dies or survives. If the heart continues to function, the dead portion is eventually walled off as new vascular tissue supplies the needed blood to adjacent areas.

ARRHYTHMIA

Arrhythmia is lack of regular heart beat due to the development in the heart muscle of new pacemakers distinct from the normal ones in the nodal tissue. These extra pacemakers often fire extra or ectopic beats, which may or may not interrupt the normal rhythm. An interruption might be at a very rapid regular rate (tachycardia); it might involve irregular, rapid twitching (fibrillation) or very rapid flapping in which only every

other atrial beat can travel through to the ventricles (atrial flutter). If the cells of the atrioventricular node lose their function and become unable to transmit an activating wave from the sinoatrial node to the ventricles, a heart block results. Life is maintained by one of the extra pacemakers, which begins setting the heart beat (regular or irregular in rhythm), but regularity not withstanding, the atria and ventricles now beat independently of each other, for there is no functional rhythmic connection.

CONGESTIVE HEART FAILURE

Congestive heart failure is the inadequate functioning of the heart as a pump, giving rise to either congestion of blood in the lungs or backup pressure of blood in the veins of the body (edema or dropsy).

ANGINA PECTORIS

Angina pectoris is an intermittent chest pain usually precipitated by exercise, emotional stress, or other factors such as exposure to cold. Anginal pains are evidence of coronary insufficiency, since the coronary arteries are so narrowed by deposits or clots that the heart cannot receive sufficient blood to support its functions during periods of greater need. Although an angina pectoris attack is a matter for serious concern, it is also a valuable warning of restricted circulation of blood.

HEART VALVE STENOSIS AND REGURGITATION

Scar tissue may form on the valves following infection, perhaps giving rise to stenosis or narrowing of the valves and regurgitation or leaking of the valves. Both conditions will cause increased back pressure into the lungs and typical left heart failure. A narrow valve opening will also result in one kind of heart murmur.

CEREBROVASCULAR STROKE

Sudden occlusions are not restricted to the coronary arteries. They may occur almost anywhere in the body, and when the arteries leading to the brain are affected, a stroke will ensue. Just as with the heart, when the blood supply to the brain is compromised by the loss of free flowing blood, the part no longer being nourished may die. Unlike the heart, which may circumvent destroyed tissue if the attack is not too great, the specialized brain part is permanently damaged and often functions are lost, producing paralysis, lack of understanding, inability to talk, and so forth. These symptoms might result from the blocking off of small cerebral vessels—a small stroke; blocking off of larger vessels results in more intense symptoms and often death.

Cerebral thrombosis results when a blood clot blocks a cerebral vessel that has been narrowed by atherosclerotic deposits.

Cerebral hemorrhage is the bleeding of a vessel into the brain.

Progressive cerebrovascular sclerosis occurs when arteries supplying the brain are progressively narrowed, resulting in chronic cerebrovascular insufficiency and giving rise to dizziness, transient paralysis, forgetfulness, and senility. Atherosclerosis is the underlying cause, either by weakening the artery walls with subsequent rupture and bleeding or by narrowing of the arteries predisposing to sudden occlusions by blood clots.

VASCULAR DISEASES

Vascular diseases involve largely or exclusively the vessels beyond the vicinity of the heart and brain.

Atherosclerosis or Arteriosclerosis (Fig. 7-6). "Hardening of the arteries" is characterized by the accumulation in the inner wall of the arteries of fatty substances that progressively decrease the size of the lumen. The fatty deposits are called atheromas and appear as raised yellowish plaques. Diseases result when bleeding around a plaque causes a clot to form, blocking the flow of blood, or when the walls weakened by such deposits eventually rupture. The rupture of an inner arterial wall results in a cerebral

NATURAL HISTORY OF ATHEROSCLEROSIS

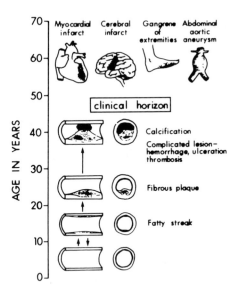

Figure 7-6 Diagrammatic concept of the pathogenesis of human atherosclerotic lesions and their clinical manifestations. (From HC McGill Jr, JC Gear and JP Strong, "Natural history of human atherosclerotic lesions," p 42, in M Sandler and GH Bourne (eds), *Atherosclerosis and its Origin*, 1963. Reprinted by permission of Academic Press, New York, and the first author.)

hemorrhage stroke; clotting causes cerebral and coronary thromboses.

Peripheral arteries. Atherosclerosis of the arteries of the legs because of vascular insufficiency will result in leg muscle pains, and gangrene of the toes, feet, and legs.

Aneurysms. A weakening of the wall of the main aorta will lead to great dilation, eventual rupture, and sudden death from hemorrhage.

Physiologic sexual impotency may occur in the male as a result of vascular insufficiency or blocking of the normal blood supply to the sexual organs.

BLOOD PRESSURE

Hypertension is characterized by abnormally high constrictive tension of muscle cells in peripheral blood vessels, especially the arterioles; usually hypertension is revealed as high blood pressure at a reading of 160/100 mm Hg.

Hypotension is characterized by abnormally low tension of muscle cells in peripheral blood vessels, which are marked by capillary permeability and fragility; the condition is revealed by abnormally low blood pressure (shock).

Many factors influence the incidence of these coronary and vascular diseases (Fig. 7-7). Some are known, others are suspected, and probably still others are unthought of. Let us look specifically at coronary artery disease, due largely to narrowing and blocking of arteries, chiefly caused by the formation of atheromas or fat masses on the living surfaces of the coronary arteries. Infiltrations of fibrous or scar tissue grow into the fatty deposits and eventually calcium is deposited in the atheroma, making a hard, chalky mass. These deposits may block the arteries themselves, and they may lead to the formation of a blood clot, which may also block the arteries (Fig. 7-5). But actual mechanisms causing atherosclerosis are obscure.[9] Recently a viral origin was hypothesized,[10] and it was suggested that atheromas are really small benign tumors.

AGE AND SEX

The older individuals become, the more likely they are to suffer from coronary artery disease. The risk of heart attack is four times greater to a man in his fifties than to one in his thirties, and greatest among men in the 50- to 60-year age group. An important difference in the sexes exists: the disease is very rare in women before menopause, although after menopause the incidence is just as great as for men. This near immunity is unexplained, but it is thought to be related in some way to the protection afforded by estrogenic secretions, which inhibit the formation of atheromas.

HEREDITY

The tendency toward coronary artery disease is in part inherited. In fact, heredity should be emphasized more than it has been. There are inherited differences in the anatomy of the coronary arteries, and the predominantly left coronary arterial pattern, for example, is correlated with greater susceptibility to coronary occlusions than the more balanced pattern, characterized by an equal flow from both left and right arteries.

HOW TO DIE OF CORONARY ARTERY DISEASE

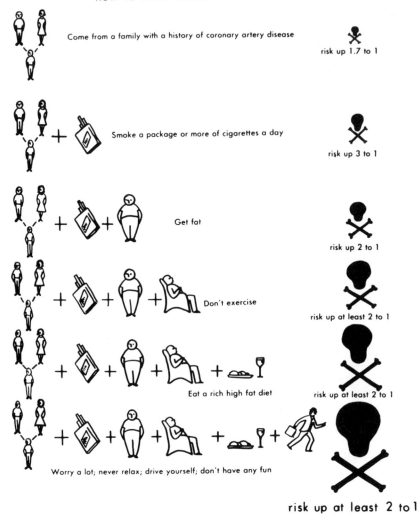

Come from a family with a history of coronary artery disease — risk up 1.7 to 1

Smoke a package or more of cigarettes a day — risk up 3 to 1

Get fat — risk up 2 to 1

Don't exercise — risk up at least 2 to 1

Eat a rich high fat diet — risk up at least 2 to 1

Worry a lot; never relax; drive yourself; don't have any fun — risk up at least 2 to 1

**Total increase in risk of death from coronary disease
from these factors about 13 to 1**

Figure 7-7   Risk factors in coronary artery disease. (From GC Griffith, "Coronary artery disease," in B Phibbs, *The Human Heart*, ed 3, 1975. Reprinted by permission of the CV Mosby Co, St. Louis, and B Phibbs.)

CIGARETTE SMOKING

The death rate from heart disease is 300% higher in cigarette smokers than in non-smokers in the United States.[11] Curiously, the effects of cigarette smoking are equivocal: the practice is not related statistically to heart disease among, for example, Japanese men who smoke heavily. Reasons for an increased risk at least among many populations include lowered ability of the lungs to exchange oxygen and carbon dioxide, toxicity from nicotine (which makes the heart beat faster and causes small arteries to narrow, thereby increasing blood pressure and the work load on the heart), and increased platelet aggregation, suggesting that the deposition of these bodies on arterial walls may lead to vascular occlusion and atherosclerosis.[12]

OBESITY

Whether obesity (10–20% above ideal weight) is a cause of atherosclerosis is questionable, but once this process has been initiated and becomes well advanced, there is little doubt that overweight adds to the work load of the heart and is therefore to be avoided.

LACK OF EXERCISE

Lack of regular daily exercise is presumably a factor in coronary disease; men engaging in heavy physical work seem to have a significantly lower death rate from coronary disease than more sedentary job holders.[13]

DIET AND HIGH BLOOD CHOLESTEROL LEVEL

Foods of high fat and sugar content should be avoided; a nutritious and balanced diet includes protein, carbohydrate, and a moderate amount of fats.

Cholesterol comes from eating food of animal origin; when ingested in the form of fat, this substance is absorbed from the intestinal tract, converted in the liver, and added to the total amount of cholesterol already circulating in the serum. When the amount of cholesterol becomes high, arteries begin to show an increase in fatty deposits. Coronary atherosclerosis is rare, for example, in individuals whose cholesterol level approximates 100–150 mg%, but where a high fat diet is common and cholesterol level reaches above 285 mg%, coronary artery disease develops in 60–70% of individuals in the population. Other fats circulating in the serum (triglyceride and phospholipid), e.g., may also be important in the development of atherosclerosis; triglyceride levels are increased in the serum by alcohol.[14]

ALCOHOL

Although patients are often advised to take a drink to relax or to dilate their coronary arteries, the potentially adverse effects of ethyl alcohol on the heart are becoming more apparent. A healthy heart, for example, can tolerate 6 ounces of liquor over a one hour period, but more than this amount rapidly weakens muscle contraction and can lead to alcoholic myocarditis.[15]

COFFEE

The risk of developing myocardial infarction is about twice as great for heavy coffee drinkers as it is for individuals who drink no coffee at all. Since there appears to be no link between heavy tea drinking and heart disease, this correlation is presumably not due to the presence of caffeine. Available evidence, however, does not justify an interpretation naming coffee as a cause of myocardial infarction.[16]

HYPERTENSION

Elevated blood pressure has long been known to speed the development of clinical coronary artery disease.

STRESS AND PERSONALITY

Stress increases serum cholesterol level, which in turn may influence coronary disease; adrenaline excreted under similar conditions is a factor in increasing blood pressure. Moreover, prolonged periods of emotional upset and pressured behavioral pattern can often be correlated with incidence of stroke.[17]

ATHEROSCLEROSIS

Atherosclerosis is closely associated with diseases that produce high serum cholesterol levels, such as low thyroid, uncontrolled diabetes, and hypercholesterolemia (an inherited tendency for high cholesterol levels).

BIRTH CONTROL PILLS

The use of oral contraceptives involves an increased risk of clotting disorders,[18] increases hypertension[19] and thrombotic strokes,[20] and sharply increases the risk of stroke when cigarette smoking is also practiced.

The list of factors associated with heart disease continues to grow and may include many more aspects of our environment, particularly those experienced beyond a certain level of moderation (Fig. 7-7). Excessive licorice (*Glycyrrhiza glabra*) ingestion, for example, can lead to cardiac dysfunction and severe hypertension.[21] Vitamin E deficiency is also implicated in heart disease, and homogenized milk may be involved in atherosclerosis and other cardiovascular diseases.[22] Even drinking water "hardness" is thought to be involved in heart disease,[23] whereas chlorine added to drinking water given to chickens, rabbits, and dogs markedly increases atherosclerosis and death rates.[24]

"Everything I enjoy in life," runs the ancient lament, "is either illegal, immoral, or fattening." A steady accretion of evidence is now beginning to suggest, unfortunately, that the old lament should bear a new addendum: "and hazardous to the heart."[25]

PREVENTION

The cardinal risk factors for coronary disease in the United States are hypercholesterolemia, hypertension, and cigarette smoking, especially when these factors are present in combination.

Changes in the living habits aimed at controlling these risk factors probably can reduce the incidence of fatal myocardial infarctions and coronary heart disease. In a seven-year study Stamler[26] modified the nutritional habits of high-risk American men, substituting diets moderate in calories, total fat, and carbohydrate, low in saturated fat, cholesterol, and simple sugars, and moderate in polyunsaturated fat. Once eating habits had been changed, cigarette smoking was reduced. Heart disease mortality rate among this group was about one-half that of the matched group not undergoing preventive care. The sudden death rate was only one-fourth as great, and total mortality was lower by 40%.

Extending the study of coronary heart disease to seven countries,[26] age-standardized average yearly incidence after five years per 10,000 men proved to be: 198 in Finland, 177 in the United States, 139 in the Netherlands, 100 in Italy, 53 in Yugoslavia, 32 in Greece, and 15–20 in Japan. Evaluation of the so-called risk factors shows that most of these dimensions cannot explain the differences in incidence between countries. Only the concentration of cholesterol in the blood proved to be the outstanding risk factor within and between national groups. As these data indicate, Japanese men have the lowest incidence of coronary heart disease of any industrialized nation; they smoke heavily and they have high blood pressure, but they eat a low cholesterol diet.

THERAPY

CARDIOTONIC DRUGS

Cardiotonic agents are primarily of value in the treatment of congestive heart failure. They increase the force of heart muscle contraction without a concomitant increase in oxygen consumption. The myocardium thus becomes a more efficient pump and is better able to meet the demands of the circulatory system.

A number of natural products have been shown to possess cardiotonic activity, particularly the cardiac glycosides. These are all complex steroids having one or more carbohydrate residues attached to position 3 of the steroid nucleus and position 17 of the nucleus substituted with an unsaturated

lactone ring. The steroid residue, after removal of the sugar(s), is referred to as the aglycone or genin (Fig. 7-8).

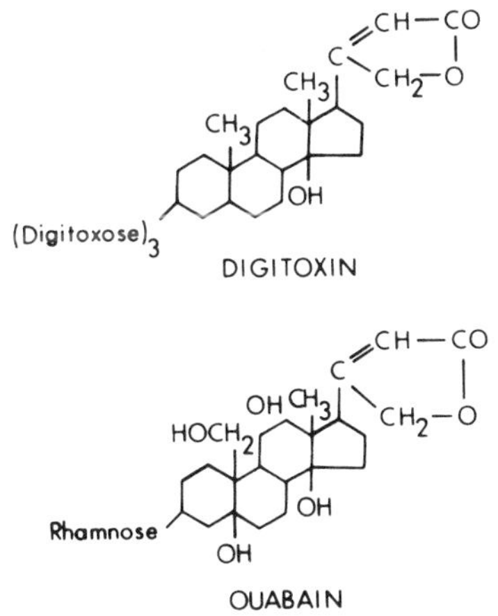

If heart failure is brought on by hypertension or atherosclerosis, *Digitalis* therapy promises the best result.[27] It increases the contractibility and improves the tone of the heart muscle, resulting in a slower but much stronger heart beat. *Digitalis* slows the wildly beating ventricles to a normal level by blocking or delaying the conduction of the electric impulse through the atrioventricular node. By increasing the heart stroke, *Digitalis* increases the amount of blood being oxygenated by the lungs, as well as the blood in general circulation, as much as 30% with each beat. Because of this improved action of the heart and the improved circulation, the drug tends to improve renal secretion (i.e., is a diuretic), to relieve edema, and to aid the cardiac muscle to compensate for mechanical defects or structural lesions. The magnitude of the need for cardiotonic therapy of this type is suggested by the estimate that more than 3 million cardiac sufferers in the United States routinely use the glycoside digoxin from *D. lanata*,[28] and this is but one of six glycosides from *Digitalis* prescribed today: *Digitalis* whole leaf, digitoxin, digoxin, lanatoside C, acetyldigitoxin, and deslanoside.

As noted in Table 7-2,[29] however, *Digitalis*-like activity is widespread in plants. An interesting illustration of this was the observation that monarch butterflies (*Danaus plexippus*) sequester cardiac glycosides from milkweeds.[30] The glycosides are quite harmless to the butterflies, but on ingestion by avian predators such as the blue jay, they act as emetics. The birds react to the vomiting by rejecting numerous subsequent monarchs on sight alone; thus a single emetic experience confers considerable immunity on the prey species. The milkweed known to

Figure 7-8 Chemical structure of digitoxin (from *Digitalis*) and of ouabain (from *Strophanthus*).

Table 7-2   Cardiac glycosides from natural products (a Partial List)

Source	Active Ingredient
PLANTS	
APOCYNACEAE	
Acokanthera schimperi wood	Ouabain (G-strophanthin)
Apocynum cannabinum (dogbane) roots	Apocannoside, cymarin
Nerium oleander (oleander) leaves	Oleandrin
Strophanthus gratus seeds	Ouabain (G-strophanthin)
S. hispidus and S. kombe seeds	K-Strophanthin
Thevetia neriifolia (exile tree), T. peruviana, and T. yecotli	Thevetin, thevetoxin
BIGNONIACEAE. Tecomella undulata bark	Tecomin
BRASSICACEAE. Cheiranthus cheiri (wallflower)	Cheiranthin
CACTACEAE. Selenicereus grandiflorus (night-blooming cereus) stems	Similar to digitalin
ANIMALS	
Bufo spp. secretory cells	Bufotoxins (bufalin)
LILIACEAE	
Convallaria majalis (lily of the valley) rhizome	Convallatoxin
Ornithogalum umbellatum (star of Bethlehem) bulbs	Convallatoxin, convalloside
Urginea maritima (white or Mediterranean squill) and U. indica (Indian squill) leaf scales of bulbs	Scillaren A and B
RANUNCULACEAE	
Adonis vernalis (pheasant's eye) rhizomes and roots	Adonitoxin, cymarin, K-strophanthin
Helleborus niger (Christmas rose) rhizomes and roots	Hellebrin
SCROPHULARIACEAE	
Digitalis lanata[a] (Grecian foxglove) leaves	Acetyldigitoxin, deslanoside, digoxin, lanatoside C
D. purpurea (purple foxglove) leaves	Digitoxin, gitaloxin, gitoxin

[a] Many other species of Digitalis possess cardiac glycosides, including D. dubia, D. ferruginea, D. grandiflora, D. lutea, D. mertonensis, D. nervosa, D. subalpina, and D. thapsi.

cause this effect is Asclepias curassavica in a family (Asclepiadaceae) closely related to and sometimes combined by taxonomists with the Apocynaceae, which possesses more genera with cardiac glycosides than any other yet known.

Therapeutic selection of the specific cardiac glycoside and dosage varies according to a patient's need and tolerance. Since the effective dose may be as high as 70% of the toxic dose, administration must be done carefully on an individual basis. Various Digitalis glycosides, all taken orally, include D. purpurea whole powdered leaf, containing a large number of glycosides of which about 30 are identified besides the medicinally important digitoxin, gitaloxin, and gitoxin. The average concentration of these three glycosides in a leaf is 0.16%. Recently, Burch[31] recommended the use of whole leaf preparations over isolated glycosides, and he suggested that the choice of a glycoside probably rests as much with the prejudice of the physician as with the effect on the patient. However detailed knowledge of a single intermediate-acting agent such as digoxin is sufficient for most clinical needs. Table 7-3 summarizes the data for the most commonly used

Table 7-3   Cardiac Glycoside Preparations[32]

Agent	Gastro-intestinal Absorption	Onset of Action[a]	Peak Effect	Average Half-Life	Average Dose Oral[b]	Average Dose Intravenous
Ouabain	Unreliable	5–10 min	30–120 min	21 hr	—	0.3–0.05 mg
Deslanoside	Unreliable	10–30 min	1–2 hr	33 hr	—	0.8 mg
Digoxin	60–85%	15–30 min	1.5–5 hr	36 hr	1.25–1.5 mg[c]	0.75–1.0 mg
Digitoxin	90–100%	25–120 min	4–12 hr	4–6 days	0.7–1.2 mg[e]	1.0 mg
Digitalis leaf	ca. 40%	—	—	4–6 days	0.8–1.2 g[c]	—

[a] For intravenous use.
[b] Divided doses over 12 to 24 hours at intervals of 6 to 8 hours,
[c] Daily oral maintenance dose: digoxin 0.25–0.5 mg, digitoxin 0.1 mg, digitalis leaf 0.1 g.

preparations, listed in order of rapidity of onset and duration of action.

Absorption from the intestine is somewhat more complete with digitoxin; but digoxin, which has the advantage of more rapid diminution of effect, is the most widely prescribed cardiotonic drug in the United States. In exceptional cases calling for large maintenance doses, where digoxin would have to be taken more than once daily, the longer acting *Digitalis* leaf or digitoxin may be preferred. In emergency cases necessitating digitalization, the fast-acting ouabain, given intravenously, is considered the drug of choice by many physicians.

Cardiac glycosides bring only temporary relief and must be administered orally during the whole course of the disease, that is, usually the life of the patient. The toxic dose lies close to the therapeutic dose, and death from *Digitalis* poisoning is usually caused by ventricular fibrillation. Side effects are numerous and include nausea, salivation, headache, fatigue, extrasystoles, and arrhythmias, as well as a synergistic toxicity with calcium.[33] Adverse reactions are found in about 20% of hospitalized patients receiving *Digitalis* preparations,[34] the incidence of toxicity being greatest among elderly persons suffering advanced heart and other diseases.[35] In cardiac infarctation, morphine may be useful in calming the patient, in stopping the pain, and in preventing descent into shock.

ANTIHYPERTENSIVE OR HYPOTENSIVE DRUGS[36]

At what point does hypertension exist, and when should treatment begin? There is no universal answer to these questions, but results of a poll involving about a half-million hypertensive patients in the United States gives some clue concerning the level at which their physicians are reacting.[37] For example, a diastolic reading of 90 was used by the largest group of physicians as indicative of hypertension, but only 6% actively treated at this level. All physicians, however, treated for hypertension at a diastolic reading of 100 or more. For the systolic pressure, 71% percent recognized hypertension at 150 to 170, and all actively treated their patients at 160 or more. Thus, when blood pressure was 160/100 mm Hg or greater, all physicians treated for hypertension.

Vascular pressure, however, is only a part of the mechanism that regulates perfusion of the body with blood, thereby becoming involved in hypertension. The condition of the heart and blood vessels is also important and these are in turn affected by, for example, heredity, age, and lipid level. In short, numerous factors must be considered before treatment is initiated. After these factors are established, the type of therapy becomes an entirely individualized matter.

"Mild" Hypertension

The synthetic chlorothiazide is useful in treating mild hypertension because it has a diuretic effect and slowly relaxes the muscles regulating the contraction of precapillary vessels. Side effects include hypokalemia (too little potassium in the blood) and hyperuricemia (excess uric acid in the blood, a potential cause of gout).

"Moderate to Severe" Hypertension

RAUVOLFIA ALKALOIDS

One of the outstanding developments in the field of natural products in recent times has been the discovery of the therapeutic properties of *Rauvolfia* alkaloids. In addition to providing useful agents for the treatment of hypertension and mental disease (see Depressants, Chapter 19), this discovery stimulated investigators the world over to reemphasize the search for medicinal plants. Clearly our use today of *Rauvolfia* derivatives was foreshadowed by the folk medicine of the Eastern peoples and the research in Asia during the 1930s by Siddiqui and Siddiqui,[38] but for some incomprehensible reason, the search it stimulated continued for only about a decade.

Rauvolfia is a genus of Afro-Asian shrubs classified in the Apocynaceae. Dried powdered roots of *R. serpentina* (Fig. 7-9), for example, yield about 50 different alkaloids. Reserpine, the alkaloid usually employed against hypertension,[39] is obtained commercially primarily from *R. vomitoria*, and to a lesser degree from four other species: *R. canescens* (also deserpidine), *R. micrantha*, *R. serpentina* (also ajmalicine, rescinnamine), and *R. tetraphylla*; reserpine has also been reported from *R. caffra*, *R. cubana*, *R. cumminsii*, *R. densiflora*, *R. heterophylla*, *R. hirsuta*, *R. indecora*, *R. lamarckii*, *R. mollis*, *R. mombasiana*, *R. natalensis*, *R. obscura*, *R. perakensis*, *R. sarapiquensis*, *R. schueli*, and *R. sellowii*, as well as *Alstonia constricta*, *Catharanthus roseus*, *Tonduzia longifolia*, *Vinca major*, and other plants. Sales of reserpine exceed $30 million annually in the United States; synthesis of the drug is possible, and semisynthetic derivates (e.g., strosingopine) are available, but synthetic reserpine is somewhat more expensive than material obtained naturally.

Reserpine and other *Rauvolfia* alkaloids act on the sympathetic nervous system by depleting almost all the neurotransmittor substance, norepinephrine, from sympathetic nerve tissue. This neural blocking results in relaxation of the vessels and output of the heart, with subsequent reduction in

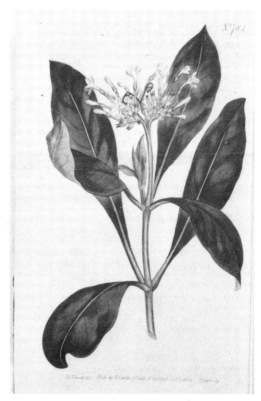

Figure 7-9 *Rauvolfia serpentina* (from *Curtis's Botanical Magazine* **20:** 784, 1804).

blood pressure. Secondarily, since these alkaloids have sedative or tranquilizing effects, their hypotensive activity may be due to a depression of the vasomotor center.[40] These findings indicate both a central depressant action and peripheral effects.

The drop in blood pressure is accompanied by a fall in body temperature and pupil constriction. Side effects of reserpine include bradycardia, fatigue, lethargy, weight gain, nightmares, and deep depressions, often accompanied by suicidal tendencies.

Rauvolfia acts synergistically with other hypotensive drugs, and in the more severe cases of hypertension it is used in combination with *Veratrum viride* or protoveratrines A and B (from *V. album*).

Guanethidine is a potent synthetic agent similar to reserpine but faster acting. In cases of *"severe" hypertension* it works by depleting or removing from the body a certain amount of adrenaline, a factor that keeps blood pressure high.

VERATRUM ALKALOIDS

Dried rhizomes and roots of *Veratrum album* (white or European hellebore: Fig. 7-10a), *V. viride* (green or American hellebore), seeds of *Schoenocaulon officinalis* (sabadilla), and other members of the Liliaceae, contain ester alkaloids that are potent hypotensive agents. Of the many steroidal alkaloids from the Liliaceae, only protoveratrines A and B are useful as medicinal agents. These

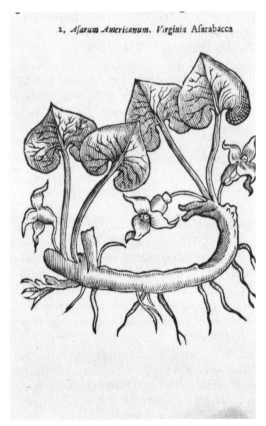

Figure 7-10b   *Asarum canadense* (from J Parkinson, *Theatrum Botanicum,* 1640).

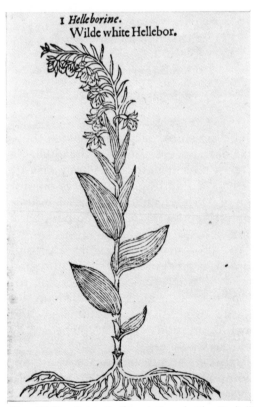

Figure 7-10a   *Epipactis* (from J Gerard, *The Herball,* 1597).

antihypertensive agents are obtained from *V. album* and must be used with caution because concomitant severe side effects occur in many individuals.

This is the only class of antihypertensive agents that acts on the afferent side of the sympathetic nervous system. These agents sensitize the afferent receptors so that a given level of pressure results in a larger amount of afferent nerve traffic. This amount of pressure is interpreted by the vasomotor centers in the brain stem as being higher than it actually is, and consequently sympathetic tone is decreased and vagal tone is increased. The result is lowering of blood pressure and bradycardia.[40] This ideal mechanism of action is not without its side effects. Since *Veratrum* alkaloids sensitize the afferent receptors for nausea and vomiting about equally, their clinical use is limited.

Drug therapy can now control about 80% of all cases of hypertension. Drugs do not cure; but their control of this disease marks a tremendous change in the outlook for patients whose inflexible fate until 1950 was a stroke, heart failure, or kidney failure. Today, just a few decades later, the ability to live a reasonably normal and healthy life reflects one of the great advances of medicine in the twentieth century.[7]

ANTIHYPOTENSIVE (HYPERTENSIVE, VASOPRESSOR) DRUGS

Therapy in hypotension and shock attempts, by raising pressure, to ensure a blood flow that will adequately perfuse tissues and sustain their nutrition. In shock this is accomplished by administration of blood or plasma volume expanders, but therapy for hypotension generally includes use of a vasoactive drug.

Many plant derivates are capable of raising blood pressure (Table 7-4). This ability may be due to constriction of blood vessels, stimulation of the heart beat, or both. But only the sympathomimetic amine, ephedrine, from *Ephedra sinica, E. distachya,* and *E. equisetina* is widely used. This adrenergic alkaloid has a pressor effect due largely to an increase in the patient's cardiac output. Ephedrine stimulates the heart and constricts resistance-capacitance vessels. It is also widely used during anesthesia, and because it may be taken orally, it is prescribed frequently for treatment of the common cold, sinusitis, hay fever, and bronchial asthma, for countering an

overdose of depressants, and for relieving especially postural hypotension.

Therapeutic doses of vasopressors like ephedrine and epinephrine (adrenaline) may cause headache, restlessness, anxiety, dizziness, and similar symptoms; convulsions and arrhythmias may result from overdoses.

One of the many vasoconstricting agents found in nature is ergonovine, from *Claviceps purpurea* (ergot), a parasitic fungus that thrives on rye and other grains. Ingestion of the contaminated grain causes burning sensations and gangrene in the extremities, as well as abortion and convulsions. Epidemics during the Middle Ages, referred to as St. Anthony's fire, were caused by ergonovine, which constricted the smaller vessels and damaged the capillary endothelium, causing peripheral gangrene, particularly of the fingers and toes, and eventually death from poisoning (see Chapter 18).

ANTIARRHYTHMIC DRUGS

In persistent cases of heart beat varying from the normal, antiarrhythmic drugs may be indicated for the management of cardiac arrhythmias. Since most such conditions are potentially dangerous, an understanding of the cardiac abnormality and its causes must precede consideration of drug therapy.

Digitalis Glycosides

Although most important in the treatment and prevention of cardiac failure, *Digitalis* glycosides are also of value in the management of certain arrhythmias, in particular, atrial tachycardia. Treatment of this disorder is aimed at converting the arrhythmia to normal rhythm or to control the ventricular rate. Digitoxin, which is slowly absorbed, is of little use in the

Table 7-4   Vasopressor Agents from Some Plants

Source	Alkaloid	Comments
Aromatic amines (sympathomimetic amines)		
Ephedra sinica, E. distachya, and *E. equisetina* whole plants	Ephedrine	Almost all analogs have been synthesized
Taxus baccata (yew) leaves *Boletus* sp. (fungus)	Ephedrine	
Phoradendron serotinum (American mistletoe)	Tyramine	
Viscum sp. (European mistletoe)		European
Acacia spp.		New Zealand
Escherichia coli, Proteus morganii, Streptococcus faecalis (bacteria)	Tyramine	Putrefied organs and "ripe" cheese
Anhalonium sp.	Tyramine	A Mexican cactus
Indolealkyl amines		
Arundo donax leaves	Gramine	
Hordeum vulgare (barley)	Gramine	
Acacia spp.	Tryptamine	
Girgensohnia dipter	Dipterin	
Arthrophytum leptocladum	Dipterin	
Bioflavonoids		
Citrus spp. fruits, *Rosa* spp. hips, black currants, etc.	Hesperidin (citrin, vitamin P)	Dried orange peel up to 8%
Aesculus hippocastanum (horsechestnut), *Humulus lupulus* (hops), *Quercus tinctoria* (oak)	Quercitrin	
Eucalyptus macrorhynchia, Fagopyrum esculentum (buckwheat), *Ruta graveolens, Sophora japonica*	Rutin	
Ergot alkaloids		
Claviceps purpurea	Ergonovine, methysergide (semisynthetic)	

management of acute arrhythmias, whereas digoxin and lanatoside C are more rapidly absorbed, producing a more rapid action and faster excretion. For extremely rapid effect either ouabain or K-strophanthin is indicated.

Cinchona Alkaloids

By chance, patients being treated for malaria with *Cinchona* bark containing quinine and other alkaloids were found to be free of arrhythmias. Subsequent inves-

tigation proved that quinine, and more importantly quinidine, from the bark of *Cinchona calisaya, C. pitayensis, Remijia pedunculata, R. purdiena,* and other species, regulated atrial fibrillation and flutter. In fact, quinidine will suppress abnormal rhythms in any chamber of the heart. The action of quinidine is similar to that of *Digitalis,* slowing conduction from atria to ventricles through the atrioventricular node. It is a cumulative drug, and if used over long periods may give rise to cinchonism (tinnitus or ringing in the ears, headache, nausea, abdominal pain, disturbed vision, skin rashes, etc.)

Cryptopinelike Alkaloids

Allocryptopine (α-fagarine) from *Fagara coca* controls atrial arrhythms and is said to be more effective than quinidine[41]; allocryptopine isomer (fagarine II) from the related *Zanthoxylum brachycanthum* has a similar action; cryptopine (another isomer) from *Papaver somniferum* (opium poppy) has a slowing action on the myocardium; protopine from *Chelidonium majus, Corydalis cava, Fumaria officinalis* (fumarine), *Macleaya cordata* (macleyine), *Papaver somniferum, Sanguinaria canadensis, Stylophorum diphyllum,* and others all belonging to the Papaveraceae or to the closely allied Fumariaceae, if segregated, have a similar effect of producing bradycardia; and corycavine and corycavamine from *Corydalis cava* also show bradycardial action. To our knowledge none of these alkaloids are used clinically as antiarrhythmic drugs.

Sparteine and Related Alkaloids

Sparteine from *Cytisus scoparius* primarily, but also found in *Chelidonium majus, Genista* spp., and *Lupinus* spp., restores normal rhythm to feeble, irregular arrhythmic myocardia. It is occasionally used as a substitute for quinidine in stubborn cases of atrial fibrillation. It also has diuretic properties. Derivatives of sparteine such as anagyrine, lupanine, and oxysparteine have similar actions.

ANTIANGINAL DRUGS[42]

Since anginal pain occurs when myocardial oxygen consumption exceeds the capacity of the coronary system to deliver oxygen, the success of any drug treat-ment depends on a favorable alteration of this metabolic balance. Lack of blood supply may be due to atherosclerosis; chest and often left shoulder pain are important symptoms of this heart disease.

Coronary vasodilators act directly but nonselectively on smooth muscles to produce relaxation without paralyzing the muscle. Following dilation of the coronary vessels, an increase in blood supply is obtained by the heart muscle.

Nitrates and nitrites are effective. When a rapid-acting derivative such as nitroglycerin is given sublingually, it is absorbed by the mucosa and has relatively direct access to the coronary circulation, where the coronary arteries appear to be particularly sensitive to dilation by the drug. Administered by this route, nitroglycerin appears in the blood in less than 2 minutes, and within 10 to 15 minutes it has largely disappeared from circulation. Amyl nitrate also acts rapidly, but is inhaled. In contradistinction to these two there are also many long-acting derivatives of nitrates and nitrites.

Papaverine, from *Papaver somniferum,* and aminophylline, now synthetically prepared from caffeine or other means, but originally obtained from tea— *Camellia sinensis*, also relax smooth muscles and are used in the treatment of angina pectoris. Their value is limited until further research proves efficacy.

Reserpine from *Rauvolfia* spp.,[43] as well as niacin and its derivates (nicotinic acid), exert direct peripheral vasodilations for treatment of, for example, Raynaud's disease.

Khellin is the aglycone of a glycoside obtained from the fruit of *Ammi visnaga* (Apiaceae), which grows in the Mediterranean region. This selective coronary vasodilator and bronchodilator has a cumulative toxicity and is no longer used in the United States.

Atropine sulfate (atropine is a racemate of L-hyoscyamine, found in *Atropa* belladonna, *Hyoscyamus niger,* and other members of the Solanaceae) is of value in the management of bradyarrhythmias after myocardial infarction. In addition, sinus bradycardia and early heart block may be corrected with atropine. When hypotension is associated with slow heart rate, the use of atropine is strongly indicated.

ANTICOAGULANT DRUGS

Anticoagulants prolong the coagulation time of blood. They may act directly by inhibition of a factor needed for coagulation or by the stimulation of an anticoagulant already present in the blood.

Heparin, a natural anticoagulant in blood, is commercially available from animal sources, especially beef lung. Like arvin, an enzyme derived from the venom of the Malayan pit viper, which directly destroys fibrinogen, heparin is a fast-acting, direct anticoagulant.

Indirect anticoagulants with a delayed effect include the vitamin K antagonists or coumarin compounds found accidentally when spoiled sweet clover (*Melilotus* spp.) eaten by cattle was observed to cause hemorrhages and often death.[44] Coumarin is a lactone widely distributed in nature: 1 to 3% in seeds of *Dipteryx* (*Coumarouna*) *odorata* and *D. oppositifolia* (Dutch and English tonka beans); it is also in *Anthoxanthum odoratum* (sweet vernal grass), *Melilotus alba* and *M. officinalis* (sweet clovers), *Asperula odorata* (sweet woodruff), *Galium triflorum* (sweet-scented bedstraw), *Trilisa odoratissima* (vanilla leaf), and other plants, including some orchids. Many derivatives and closely allied compounds are available, including dicoumarol, and warfarin sodium and potassium.

The action of the indirect anticoagulants, following oral ingestion, absorption, and metabolism in the liver, is attributable to a reduction in synthesis of prothrombin, a plasma protein produced in the liver in the presence of vitamin K and converted into thrombin in the clotting of blood.

The sensitivity of the blood clotting mechanism to oral anticoagulants is increased by factors that may interfere with vitamin K absorption or production. For example, the vitamin K normally produced by intestinal bacteria is very much reduced when any therapy regimen requires antibiotics. Thus destruction of bacterial flora may produce an increased anticoagulant effect.

Hemorrhage due to overdose of anticoagulants may be controlled quickly by the administration of vitamin K.

BLOOD COAGULATING OR HEMOSTATIC DRUGS

Production by the liver of various coagulation factors (prothrombin and others) is dependent on vitamin K (*Koagulation* vitamin). The mechanism by which vitamin K stops hemorrhage by promoting formation of these clotting factors is unknown.

Vitamin K was found originally in alfalfa and pig liver fat. It is also present in the photosynthetic portions of many other plants, especially green leafy vegetables such as spinach, kale, and tomatoes, many vegetable oils, the feces of most animals (because of vitamin K production by intestinal bacteria), and in putrefied protein. Vitamins K_1 (phytonadione) and K_3 (menadione) are available commercially.

Oral sulfonamides and broad-spectrum antibiotics may alter natural bacterial flora, reducing the availability of vitamin K, thus the body's blood clotting ability.

DIURETICS

Diuretics are chemicals that induce a net loss of extracellular fluids from the body and prevent or eliminate edema. They act by enhancing the urinary excretion of sodium and water, usually by inhibiting reabsorption of sodium in the renal tubules.

The only group of diuretics from natural products are the xanthines, and these are only occasionally effective. Caffeine (tea, coffee) is least useful as a diuretic; theobromine (chocolate, cocoa) is intermediate; and aminophylline (now all synthetic) enjoys limited clinical use. When used, the xanthines are largely indicated for the treatment of cardiac edema.

PLASMA EXTENDERS

Plasma extenders may be needed following dehydration due to diarrhea, vomiting, hemorrhage, and burning. Dextran (colloidal plasma) produced by the bacterium *Leuconostoc mesenteroides* and other organisms growing on sucrose may be used. Other water-soluble polysaccharides could serve as plasma substitutes, and the effectiveness of an aqueous extract of okra (*Abelmoschus esculentus*) has been demonstrated in dogs.

HERBOLOGY

The miraculous effects of *Digitalis* against congestive heart failure and of *Rauvolfia* against hypertension were among the great medical advances of the eighteenth and twentieth centuries. However both substances had long histories of use in domestic medicine before their rediscovery by researchers and incorporation into orthodox medical practice. Other folk remedies used to control heart and vascular diseases must await study.

Apocynum cannabinum (dogbane). Potawatomis boiled the green fruit, and the resulting decoction was drunk as a heart medicine and to combat kidney problems and dropsy. The species is now known to have *Digitalis*-like properties, and it contains the cardiac glycosides apocannoside and cymarin. Other tribes boiled the root with the hips of *Rosa* spp. to serve as a diuretic and thereby to relieve dropsy.

Asarum canadense (American wild ginger: Fig. 7-10*b*). Eastern Canadian Indians drank an infusion of this plant to relieve heart arrhythmia, and the Catawbas used it to relieve heart pains.

Asclepias spp. (milkweeds). Indians made a tea of milkweed, *Verbena* sp. (vervain) and *Populus deltoides* (cottonwood) leaves to treat dropsy. Milkweeds are now known to contain cardiac glycosides.

Crataegus tomentosa (hawthorn). Meskwakis used the unripe fruit for bladder ailments. Present work has shown that many *Crataegus* species are hypotensive and have antiarrhythmic activity.

Euonymus atropurpureus (wahoo or burning bush). A boiled decoction of the bark was used in domestic practice as a popular "heart medicine" and diuretic.

Heuchera sp. (alum root). Indians of Nevada and Utah used a root decoction to treat heart disorders.

Ilex opaca (American holly). North Carolina Indians steeped holly fruit, and the infusion was drunk as a cardiac stimulant. Currently in use in the People's Republic of China is *Ilex pubescens* root, a native Chinese holly, whose main therapeutic actions include vasodilation and increase in blood flow of the coronary arteries, in addition to hypotensive effects. Four ounces of the crude drug is taken orally each day for the treatment of coronary disease.[47]

Ipomoea leptophylla (bush morning glory). Pawnees drank an infusion as a cardiac stimulant.

Monarda sp. (horsemint). Winnebago and Dakota tribes drank an infusion of the plant as a cardiac stimulant.

Veratrum californicum (hellebore). The Thompson tribe of British Columbia drank a small quantity of the decoction for disorders of the blood.

Veratrum viride (green hellebore). Cherokees used a plant decoction to relieve body pains. The species is now known to contain ester alkaloids that are potent hypotensive agents.

Viola sp. (violet). Flambeau Ojibwas and Potawatomis made a tea of the plant to treat heart pains.

A modern use of herbs is best exemplified by traditional Chinese medicine in the treatment of thrombi or clots, which may lead to ulcers and gangrene, that block small vessels in the extremities, especially the legs. A recent report[45] described the treatment of 136 cases; 85.3% were heavy smokers and 47.1% had a history of exposure to cold. Ten different combinations of plants, involving up to 16 distinct species as decoctions and ointments, were used in therapy along with supplemental vitamin B_1 injections. The selection of roots, stems, leaves, flowers, and fruit of many diverse taxa reminds one of the elaborate recipes Withering found being used to treat dropsy in eighteenth-century England, one must assume that, as in his findings, at least one ingredient has potent curative properties. The overall average length of hospitalization was 142 days, and during this time the pulse in the affected extremities became stronger, there was a return of sensitivity to temperature, and the color of the skin improved or returned to normal. The cure rate was 54.4%; 19.1% were greatly improved, and 19.9% were improved, for a total effective rate of 93.4%. The results of treatment were followed for 1 to 6 years for 62 patients; response was excellent or good in 61.5% of patients. Only 14.5% of the cases regressed after this treatment, and the report tentatively attributed this to resumption of smoking, exposure to cold, and trauma.

What do those who return from complete cardiac arrest remember? According to recent survivors,[46] there is a feeling of peace and tranquility and even ecstasy, a sensation of floating, of moving rapidly from one location to another, and of viewing one's body from a point external to it—as many conclude, an easy, painless way to go.

INFECTIONS

Bacterial endocarditis results from actual colonization of the endocardium by infectious agents through the interstitial capillary bed beneath the endothelium and the blood within the endocardial lumen. The source of these bacteria may be a distant pyogenic infection or normal flora injected into the bloodstream in large numbers by surgical procedures.

When pyogenic organisms such as *Staphylococcus aureus* and *Streptococcus pneumoniae* are involved, acute endocarditis may result. In this case, the onset is abrupt, the illness may last up to 6 weeks, and the prognosis for cure, even with available antibiotics, is poor. Damage to normal heart tissue may be severe, and emboli arising from such infections are often septic and can give rise to suppurative complications elsewhere.

On the other hand, subacute bacterial endocarditis is more insidious, and although its duration may be prolonged, its cure is more likely, since the organisms causing it are somewhat less pathogenic and are usually members of the normal flora. Their release into the bloodstream is often due to some dental or urological procedure, and their establishment within the heart is dependent on preexisting cardiovascular disease, such as vascular heart disease (caused by rheumatic fever), congenital defects, or the presence of a valvular prosthesis. Organisms most commonly recovered from such infections are *Streptococcus sanguis, S. faecalis*, and, in heroin addicts, also *Candida parapsilosis*. Presurgical prophylaxis with either penicillin or erythromycin has been helpful in reducing the incidence of such infections among susceptible populations.

Myocarditis is an inflammatory disease of the heart muscle that can be caused by a wide spectrum of systemic disorders including those determined to be noninfectious. In most instances such involvement is incidental to another organ or system, whereas in other cases an actual myocardial tropism may exist. Therapy depends on the organism involved, and spontaneous recovery usually occurs.

Similarly, pericarditis may result from numerous conditions either as part of a systemic disease or localized in the pericardium. Inflammation, when severe, may compromise cardiac function by the accumulation of exudate or insidiously through cicatricial pericardial contraction (constrictive pericarditis). Recovery is usually spontaneous, although some patients develop myocarditis and congestive heart failure, which in rare instances may be fatal.

Septic thrombophlebitis, often associated with bacteremia, can be an infection of the cerebral, pelvic, superficial, or portal venous systems. When fibrin deposition and thrombus formation results from perivascular inflammation, or inflammation of vessel walls, bacterial invasion of the clot can occur, followed by liquefaction, fragmentation, and discharge of septic emboli. The most frequently recovered organisms are the opportunistic organisms found as resident flora of specific areas, such as staphylococci on skin and cavernous sinuses and *Bacteroides* and Gram negative bacilli in pelvic regions. Cerebral and pelvic thrombophlebitis, once fatal, can be cured by appropriate antimicrobial therapy, although complications and residual abnormalities are frequent.

Disease may also result from infection of cellular components of the blood. For example, bacteria may be found in white blood cells during infections such as tuberculosis and meningococcemia. Successful therapy of these diseases is therefore dependent on the use of such antibiotics as streptomycin and rifampin, which are capable of intracellular penetration. Infection of erythrocytes can also take place, and in Peru a fatal anemia is caused by the bacterium *Bartonella bacilliformis*. The most significant parasitic disease affecting red blood cells is, however, malaria.

Malaria results from the bite of an infected *Anopheles* mosquito carrying sporozoites of *Plasmodium* species. In the life cycle of the parasite the mosquito acts as its sexual host and man as its asexual host. These sporozoites develop in the parenchymal cells of the human liver into erythrocytic forms that invade red blood cells, multiply, and at intervals of 48 (*P. vivax, P. ovale*, and *P. falciparum*) and 72 hours (*P. malariae*) are released into the blood stream as merozoites. The merozoites may reenter additional erythrocytes and proceed through another asexual cycle of schizogony, or they may develop in the red blood cells into sexual gametocytes, which if ingested by a mosquito will mate in its stomach and develop in this invertebrate host to sporozoites.

The release of the merozoites at periodic intervals produce the characteristic malarial symptoms of fever, chills and sweating. Depending on the species of *Plasmodium*, the interval before another attack occurs may range from 12 to 60 hours. A swollen and tender liver and spleen may be apparent during periods of the attack. Anemia also becomes a significant clinical feature. Prognosis is poorer if invasion of the nervous system results, and deaths in treated cases are usually due to cerebral involvement. In other cases the gastrointestinal tract, the respiratory system, and the genitourinary tract may be involved.

Cardiac failure and spleenic rupture may also result from infection of the cardiovascular and hematopoietic systems, respectively.

Plasmodium vivax, which is widely distributed in both tropical and temperate regions, is responsible for the highest incidence of malaria. The most pathogenic, *P. falciparum,* is restricted to the tropics and subtropics. More deaths are attributable to this latter infection because of its fulminant character and its ability to produce blackwater fever, a malignant form characterized by intravascular hemolysis and hemoglobinuria.

However the development of serious debility or death is generally considered a failure of the host's immune system. Treated or not, malaria is usually self-limiting. Complete recovery may occur directly after the primary attack or after a period of time, when intervals between relapses become progressively more prolonged.

The persistence of so-called blood purifiers within present-day African and southern Asian herbalism suggests that each culture originally had numerous herbal cures for this intermittent fever. However a native Peruvian remedy for malaria was adopted enthusiastically by seventeenth-century European physicians, quickly superseding medications then available. The universal use of cinchona bark, especially *Cinchona ledgeriana,* which contained numerous antimalarial alkaloids including quinine, became inevitable.

Quinine (6-methoxy-(5-vinyl-2-quinuclidyl)-4-quinoline methanol):

and synthetic derivatives—
Mepacrine (Atabrine®) (2 methoxy-6-methylbutylamino acridine):

Chloroquine (7-chloro-4-)4'-diethylamino-1'-methylbutylamino quinoline):

Primaquine (6-methoxy-8-(4'-amino-1'-methylbutylamino quinoline):

Quinine as the bark's most active component, was prepared commercially as early as 1823. After natural sources became exhausted during the mid-nineteenth century, large plantations of cinchona were established in India and Java. Active breeding programs increased the yield of quinine from 4% to more than 13%. To keep up with the ever increasing demand, however, useful synthetic quilinone compounds were formulated starting in 1930. Among these, chloroquine [7-chloro-4-(4'-diethylamino-1'-methylbutylamino)-quinoline] has higher activity and lower toxicity, thus is preferred today. This compound has replaced quinine and an earlier synthetic mepacrine (Atabrine®) in therapy and chemoprophylaxis. Such drugs cure acute attacks by acting on the asexual plasmodia, and when used chemoprophylactically they prevent the individual from manifesting clinical symptoms. Although too toxic ·to be prescribed for the treatment of acute attacks, another synthetic quinoline, primaquine, has been successfully used as a radical treatment among relapsing cases. Considered active against exoerythrocytic forms of *Plasmodium,* primaquine induces hemolysis among individuals exhibiting a glucose-6-phosphate dehydrogenase defect in their erythrocytes. Unfortunately this genetic disorder is widespread in the tropics. Chloroquine-resistant mutants, especially of the malignant species *P. falciparum,* are increasing, and investigations to discover new antimalarial substances continue.

Prophylactic therapy is not enough to control the disease. In endemic areas, malaria mosquito eradication programs also exist. Such works include destruction of mosquito breeding grounds by water drainage, spraying with DDT and pyrethrum, and introducing large numbers of genetic strains of mosquitoes incapable of carrying the parasite. These mosquito mutants breed with local strains, and since the mutants possess translocation aberrations, the formation of progeny is prevented. It is hoped that the aberrant types that cannot carry *Plasmodium* will eventually replace the wild-type.[48]

LITERATURE CITED

1. Silverman M. 1941. *Magic in a Bottle.* Macmillan, New York. 332 p.

2. [Tennant J.] 1734. *Every Man His Own Doctor: or, The Poor Planter's Physician,* ed 2. William Parks, Williamsburg and Anapolis. 56 p. + index. Written anonymously. Reprinted edition, St Louis Medical Museum.

3. Withering W. 1776. *A Botanical Arrangement of All the Vegetables Naturally Growing in Great Britain According to the System of the Celebrated Linnaeus.*

4. Withering W. 1785. *An Account of the Foxglove, and Some of Its Medical Uses, with Practical Remarks on Dropsy, and Other Diseases.* M. Swinney, Birmingham. Reprinted in *Med Classics* 5(4): 303–443, 1937.

5. Report of Inter-Society Commission for Heart Disease Resources. *Circulation* **42** (December) 1970, revised April 1972, 44 p; Delury GE (exec ed). 1974. *The World Almanac.* p. 1018.

6. Estes JW, White PD. 1965. William Withering and the purple foxglove. *Sci Am* **212**(6): 110–119.

7. Phibbs B. 1971. *The Human Heart.* CV Mosby, St Louis. 247 p.

8. McGill HC, Geer JC, Strong JP. 1963. Natural history of human atherosclerotic lesions, 39–65, Chapter 2. In Sandler M, Bourne GH (eds), *Atherosclerosis and Its Origins.* Academic Press, New York; *Arteriosclerosis.* A report by the National Heart and Lung Institute Task Force on Arteriosclerosis. National Institutes of Health, Vol 2, June 1971 (Department of Health, Education & Welfare Publ No NIH 72-219).

9. Ross R, Glomset JA. 1973. Atherosclerosis and the arterial smooth muscle cell. *Science* **180:** 1332–1339.

10. Benditt EP, Benditt JM. 1973. Evidence for a nomoclonal origin of human atherosclerotic plaques. *Proc Nat Acad Sci (US)* **70:** 1753–1756.

11. Murphy EA, Mustard JF. 1966. Tobacco and thrombosis. *Am J Pub Health* **56:** 1061–1073; Spain DM, Bradess VA. 1970. Sudden death from coronary heart disease. *Chest* **58:** 107–110; Spain DM, Siegel H, Bradess VA. 1973. Women smokers and sudden death. *JAMA* **224:** 1005–1007.

12. Levine PH. 1973. An acute effect of cigarette smoking on platelet function. *Circulation* **48:** 619–623.

13. Paffenbarger RS Jr, Laughlin ME, Gima AS et al. 1970. Work activity of longshoreman as related to death from coronary heart disease and stroke. *New Eng J Med* **282:** 1109–1114.

14. Kannell WB, Castelli WP, Gordon T et al. 1971. Serum cholesterol, lipoproteins and the risk of coronary heart disease. *Ann Intern Med* **74:** 1–12.

15. Ellestad M (reported). 1973. Your heart and alcohol. *Parade* 24 June: 12.

16. Jick H, Slone D et al. 1972. Coffee drinking and acute myocardial infarction. *Lancet* **2:** 1278–1283.

17. Adler R, MacRithie K, Encel GL. 1971. Psychologic processes and ischemic stroke (occlusive cerebrovascular disease). I. Observations on 32 men with 35 strokes. *Psychosom Med* **33:** 1–29.

18. Oral contraceptives and thromboembolism. *Med Lett* **14**(17): 61–62, 1972.

19. Chidell MP. 1970. Oral contraceptives and blood pressure. *Practitioner* **205:** 53–64; Newton MA, Sealey JE, Ledingham JGG et al. 1968. High blood pressure and oral contraceptives. *Am J Obstet Gynec* **101:** 1037–1045; Weir RJ, Briggs E, Browning J et al. 1971. Blood-pressure in women after one year of oral contraception. *Lancet* **1:** 467–471; Zacherle BJ, Richardson JA. 1972. Irreversible renal failure secondary to hypertension induced by oral contraceptives. *Ann Intern Med* **77:** 83–85.

20. Collaborative Group. 1973. Oral contraception and increased risk of cerebral ischemia or thrombosis. *New Eng J Med* **288:** 871–878; Vessey MP. 1973. Oral contraceptives and stroke. *New Eng J Med* **288:** 906–907.

21. Conn JW, Rovner DR, Cohen EL. 1968. Licorice-induced pseudoaldosteronism. *JAMA*

205: 492–496; Koster M, David GK. 1968. Reversible severe hypertension due to licorice ingestion. *New Eng J Med* **278:** 1381–1383; Robinson HJ, Harrison FS, Nicholson JTL. 1971. Cardiac abnormalities due to licorice intoxication. *Penn Med* **74:** 51–54.

22. Zikakis JP. 1974. Homogenized milk and atherosclerosis. *Science* **183:** 472–473.

23. Correa P, Strong JP. 1972. Atherosclerosis and the geochemical environment: a critical review. *Ann NY Acad Sci* **199:** 217–228.

24. Price JM. 1971. *Coronaries, Cholesterol, Chlorine.* Pyramid Communications, New York. 92 p.

25. Maugh TH II. 1973. Coffee and heart disease: is there a link? *Science* **181:** 534–535.

26. Keys A. 1970. Coronary heart disease in seven countries. *Circulation* **41:** Suppl 1, 1–211; Stamler J. 1970. Acute myocardial infarction—progress in primary prevention. *Brit Heart J* **33** (Suppl): 145–164.

27. Chung EK. 1971. The current status of *Digitalis* therapy. *Mod Treat* **8**(3): 641–714; Fisch C, Surawicz B (eds). 1969. *Digitalis.* Grune & Stratton, New York and London. 230 p.

28. Curry JP. 1974. Some of heart drugs found ineffective. *St Louis Post-Dispatch* 9 Jan: 15D.

29. McCawley EL. 1955. Cardioactive alkaloids, 79–107. In RH Manske (ed), *The Alkaloids, Chemistry and Physiology,* Vol 5, Pharmacology. Academic Press, New York; Mosig A. 1964. Cardioactive glycosides and their investigation. *Quart J Crude Drug Res* **4**(4): 613–625 (English translation by GM Hocking, 620–625.

30. Brower LP, McEvoy PB, Williamson KL. 1972. Variation in cardiac glycoside content of monarch butterflies from natural populations in eastern North America. *Science* **177:** 426–429.

31. Burch GE. 1972. Experiments of nature: whole leaf and purified alkaloids. *Am Heart J* **83:** 845.

32. Smith TW. 1973. Drug therapy, *Digitalis* glycosides. *New Eng J Med* **288:** 719–722, 942–946.

33. Nola GT, Pope S, Harrison DC. 1970. Assessment of the synergistic relationship between serum calcium and digitalis. *Am Heart J* **79:** 499–507.

34. Proctor JD. 1973. Reducing digitalis intoxication. *Mod Med* **41**(20): 26–29.

35. Beller GAL, Smith TW, Abelmann WH et al. 1971. Digitalis intoxication. *New Eng J Med* **284:** 989–997.

36. Dustan HP, Page IH. 1970. Treatment of arterial hypertension. *Mod Med* **38**(16): 75–80;

Rauwolfia products in hypertension. *Med Lett* **1:** 70–71, 1959; *Rauwolfia* alkaloids as tranquilizing and antihypertensive agents. *Med Lett* **5:** 39–40, 1963; Grenfell RF. 1971. Drug therapy of hypertension. *S Med J* **64:** 1358–1361; Page LB, Sidd JJ. 1972. Medical management of primary hypertension. *New Eng J Med* **287:** 1910–1023; Woodson RE Jr, Youngken HW, Schlittler E et al. 1957. *Rauwolfia: Botany, Pharmacognosy, Chemistry and Pharmacology.* Little, Brown, Boston and Toronto. 149 p.

37. Page IH (ed). 1970. Over 6700 readers of *Modern Medicine* reply to questions on hypertension. *Mod Med* **38:**(16): 17–26.

38. Siddiqui S, Siddiqui RH. 1931. Chemical examination of the roots of *Rauwolfia serpentina* Benth. *J Ind Chem Soc* **8:** 667–680; 1932. The alkaloids of *Rauwolfia serpentina* Benth., part I Ajmaline series. **9:** 539–544; 1939. Part II Ajmaline series, **12:** 37–47.

39. Reis ED. 1968. The treatment of primary hypertension. *Mod Med* **36:**(6): 86–91.

40. Abrams WB. 1969. The mechanisms of action of antihypertensive drugs. *Dis Chest* **55:** 148–159.

41. Deulofeu V, Labriola R, Orfas O et al. 1945. Fagarine, a possible substitute for quinidine. *Science* **102:** 69–70.

42. Rossi GV. 1971. Antianginal drugs—a review. *Am J Pharm* **143:** 153–160.

43. Romei SG, Whalen RE, Tindall JP. 1970. Intraarterial administration of reserpine. *Arch Intern Med* **125:** 825–829.

44. Huebner CF, Link KP. 1941. Studies on the hemorrhagic sweet clover disease. VI. *J Biol Chem* **138:** 529–534; Overman RS, Stahmann MA, Huebner CF et al. 1944. XIII. *J Biol Chem* **153:** 5–24.

45. Traditional Chinese medicine in the treatment of thromboangitis obliterans. 1968. *China's Med* **1968**(1): 54–64.

46. Dobson M, Tattersfield AE, Adler MW et al. 1971. Attitudes and long-term adjustment of patients surviving cardiac arrest. *Brit Med J* **3:** 207–212; Macmillan RL, Brown KWF. 1971. Cardiac arrest remembered. *Can Med Ass J* **104:** 889–890; Stevenson I. 1971. Cardiac arrest remembered. *Can Med Ass* **105:** 689.

47. Kao, FF, Kao JJ. 1974. Tung Ch'ing, a cardiac drug. *Am J. Chin Med* **2:** 85–88.

48. Russell PF, West LS, Manwell RD, MacDonald G. 1963. *Practical Malariology.* Oxford University Press, London. 750 p.

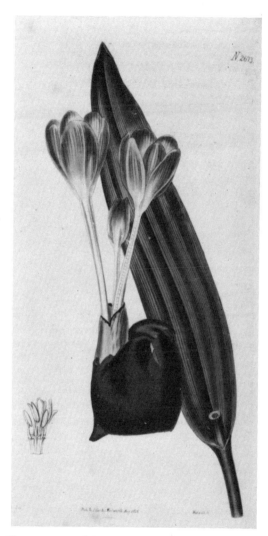

Figure 8-1 *Colchicum autumnale* (from *Curtis's Botanical Magazine* 53: 2673, 1826).

Chapter 8

Metabolism

Since the time of the ancient Greeks, seeds and corms of *Colchicum autumnale* (Autumn crocus, meadow saffron: Fig. 8-1), an autumn flowering crocus native to Europe, have been used as a specific treatment for gout. The active principle is the alkaloid colchicine, found also in *C. luteum, Gloriosa superba, Merendera persica, Androcymbium gramineum,* and other plants.

Primary gout is an inherited disease associated with high blood levels of uric acid (an end product of purine metabolism). Hyperuricemia may be due either to an abnormal production of uric acid or to a hereditary defect in the renal transport of uric acid, resulting in an increase in the uric acid pool. Uric acid is deposited in the form of monosodium urate crystals in joint tissue and in subcutaneous nodules called tophi. The associated inflammation, known as gouty arthritis, is related to the injury of leucocytes that have phagocytized these crystals, causing the release of lysosomes. Colchicine breaks the chain reaction that leads to inflammation in joints by inhibiting the phagocytic activity of leukocytes for urate crystals. Taken orally or intravenously, colchicine quickly relieves the intense pain of gout, a discomfort aptly illustrated by Fig. 8-2 and well described by Sydenham in 1683. This famous English physician, who suffered from the affliction, wrote:

He goes to Bed and sleeps well, but about Two a Clock in the Morning, is waked by the

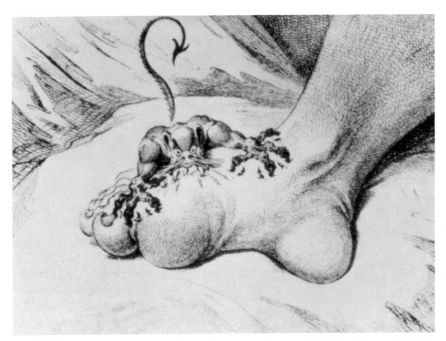

Figure 8-2   How gout feels, an eighteenth century caricature (J. Gillray lithograph, 1799).

Pain, seizing either his great Toe, the Heel, the Calf of Leg, or the Ankle; this Pain is like that of dislocated Bones, with the Sense as it were of Water almost cold, poured upon the Membranes of the Parts affected, presently shivering and shaking follow with a feverish Disposition; the Pain is first gentle, but increases by degrees (and in like manner the shivering and shaking go off), and that hourly, till towards Night it comes to its height, accompanying it self neatly according to the Variety of the Bones of the *Tarsus* and *Metatarsus,* whose Ligaments it seizes, sometimes resembling a violent stretching or tearing those Ligaments, sometimes the gnawing of a Dog, and sometimes a weight: moreover, the Part affected has such a quick and exquisite Pain, that it is not able to bear the weight of the Cloaths upon it, nor hard walking in the Chamber; and the Night is not passed over in Pain upon this Account only, but also by reason of the restless turning of the part hither and thither, and the continual Change of its Place. Nor is the tossing of the whole Body, which always accompanies the Fit, but especially at its coming, less than the continual Agitation and Pain of the tormented Member: There are a Thousand fruitless Endeavours used to ease the Pain, by changing the Place continually, whereon the Body, and the affected Members lie, yet there is not ease to be had.

This symptomatology and other aspects of metabolism including nutrition, bariatrics, and diabetes are dicussed in further detail.

NUTRITION

A well-balanced diet should contain all the essential vitamins, minerals, fats, carbohydrates, and proteins needed for body health and metabolic balance. Although a detailed treatise on nutrition is not within the scope of this book, a brief outline is provided as a means of reference.

PROTEINS

Proteins, complex chains of amino acids, are supplied in our diet chiefly by animal proteins—meat, milk, cheese, and eggs—and to a lesser degree by plants such as legumes and nuts. Protein requirements vary, with children, pregnant and lactating women, and men undergoing strenuous exercise requiring larger amounts. A fully developed man requires approximately 70 g daily. Beyond infancy, a child requires about 10% of his caloric* intake in protein, or approximately 40 g for a preschool child. During pregnancy, particularly in the second and third trimesters, a woman should increase her intake by 20 g and by 40 g during lactation. If provided for accordingly, the developing child, after weaning, should be ensured of normal skeletal and muscular growth, brain development, and future learning capacity. Protein deficiency, especially during the first year of life, has been associated with decreased brain development and lowered IQ.[3] A condition common among African native populations is called "kwashiorkor." The word means "the deposed baby" in Ga, or more literally "when baby is bumped off mother's back." In such a society, when nursing is cut off, usually because of an imminent delivery, the child may receive an inadequate supplement of protein through lack of attention, because of tribal taboos, or due to the fear that meat will make him sick, and often malnutrition develops.

Problems of protein inadequacy may also develop during disease. The alcoholic represents the most common problem of this sort because he relies for his major caloric intake on alcohol, and may additionally have an impaired hepatic protein synthesis. Protein requirements increase and must be accommodated therapeutically in individuals who have suffered extensive burns and in those having

cancer, intestinal parasitism, or protein wastage in intestinal disease (malabsorption or hastened peristalsis) and in nephrosis.

FATS

Complex compounds of fatty acids are used by the body as a source of energy and are provided for in our diet by animal fat and vegetable oils that when metabolized supply 9 cal/g. Although ingestion of certain lipids may predispose one to atherosclerosis, other lipids are essential to the health of our cells and tissues. Certain fats serve as precursors for prostaglandins, which are required for a number of physiological functions. Hyperlipidemias may result from a number of causes, as illustrated in Table 8-1.[4] Any diet normally used to control the abnormally high cholesterol and triglyceride levels associated with coronary disease dramatically reduces the amount of saturated fatty acids consumed. Such a reduction in the ratio of saturated to unsaturated fats lowers the levels of these compounds. When diet alone fails, lipoproteinemic drugs, such as cholestyramine, and large oral doses of nicotinic acid, have been found somewhat more beneficial than clofibrate and D-thyroxine used alone or in combination.[5]

CARBOHYDRATES

Carbohydrates are complex compounds made of sugars. They are the body's main source of energy, and if not stored as muscle or liver glycogen, they are converted to fat for future use. Any plant material eaten supplies us with carbohydrate, although starchy vegetables are highest in concentration. When metabolized, they yield 4 cal/g and are

---

* calorie is the heat required to raise the temperature of 1 g of water 1°C (from 15 to 16°C). The energy value of food and human energy requirements are expressed as caloric equivalents.

Table 8-1 The Five Types of Primary Hyperlipoproteinemia[a]

Feature	Type I	Type II	Type III	Type IV	Type V
Incidence	Very rare	Common	Relatively uncommon	Common	Uncommon
Appearance of plasma	Cream layer over clear infranate on standing	Clear	Clear, cloudy, or milky	Slightly turbid to cloudy with standing	Cream layer over turbid infranate on standing
Cholesterol	Normal or elevated	Elevated	Elevated	Normal or elevated	Elevated
Triglyceride	Markedly elevated	Normal	Usually elevated	Elevated	Elevated to markedly elevated
Clinical presentation	Lipemia retinalis, eruptive xanthomas, hepatosplenomegaly, abdominal pain	Xanthelasma, tendon, and tuberous xanthomas; juvenile corneal arcus; accelerated atherosclerosis	Xanthoma planum, eruptive tuberous, and tendon xanthomas; acceleratherosclerosis of coronary and peripheral vessels	Accelerated coronary vessel disease, abnormal glucose tolerance, hyperuricemia	Lipemia retinalis, eruptive xanthomas, hepatosplenomegaly, abdominal pain, hyperglycemia, hyperuricemia
Origin; possible mechanism	Genetic recessive; deficiency in lipoprotein lipase	When genetic, dominant, sporadic; decreased catabolism of β-lipoprotein	When genetic, recessive; sporadic?	When genetic, dominant, sporadic; excessive endogenous glyceride synthesis or deficient glyceride clearance?	Probably genetic sporadic
Age of detection	Early childhood	Early childhood	Adulthood (over age 20)	Adulthood	Early adulthood
Conditions to be excluded	Dysgammaglobulinemia, diabetes, pancreatitis?	Dietary cholesterol excess, porphyria, myxedema, myeloma, nephrosis, obstructive liver disease	Myxedema, dysgammaglobulinemia	Diabetes, glycogen storage disease, nephrotic syndrome, pregnancy, Werner's syndrome	Myeloma and macroglobulinemia, insulin-dependent diabetes, diabetes mellitus, nephrosis, alcoholism, pancreatitis

necessary to provide daily energy requirements for growth and metabolism. Nevertheless, overconsumption of carbohydrates is the primary cause of overweight and obesity. Under normal conditions, the number of calories derived directly from them should be one-half the total daily intake.

VITAMINS

Vitamins are usually diverse and complex organic compounds that regulate metabolism. Except for those which are fat soluble, vitamins are not stored in the body and must be provided through the daily diet. Vitamin K and most B vitamins may be synthesized by resident intestinal bacteria, given the appropriate precursors; vitamin D is formed by the action of ultraviolet light on the skin. Table 8-2 lists the common sources of vitamins and the cause and result of specific dietary insufficiencies.[6]

The taking of daily vitamin supplements by individuals who eat a normal, balanced diet is frankly redundant. Yet millions subscribe to this practice in fear that because of their cooking methods, or use of refined foods, they are not receiving nutritionally adequate amounts of vitamins and minerals. The idea persists in spite of available information to the effect that with reasonable care, the activity of most vitamins can be retained during preparation. Moreover, vitamin deficiencies are unlikely to occur if the diet contains a liberal amount of fresh meat, vegetables, and dairy products, along with lesser amounts of refined foods. Others make a fetish out of using "natural" products to ensure that they are obtaining vitamins in a natural form, although no difference has been demonstrated between the biological activity of vitamins produced synthetically and those found in foods.

Little has been made of the fact that many vitamins are not found in food as such but are readily synthesized by resident intestinal bacteria.

Few are aware of the danger of overdosage, and only recently have warnings appeared in the lay literature regarding the serious side effects, and even deaths, that can result from the overuse of certain vitamins.[7] In rare instances these phenomena have occurred accidentally when little has been known concerning toxic levels; but more frequently they are attributable to indiscriminate use, without evidence of therapeutic value. In this respect, a psychosis mimicking a brain tumor was recently induced through excessive doses of vitamin A, prescribed for a skin affliction.[8] Withdrawal of the vitamin supplement cured the psychosis, although the skin condition remained the same. Overdosage of vitamin D has even led to death through blockage of the liver and kidneys by calcium and phosphorus redisposed from bone to soft tissue.[6]

Similarly, the promotion of huge doses of vitamin C for prophylaxis and treatment of colds has been based on information derived from uncontrolled or inadequately controlled studies. Present information indicates that prophylactic use is unfounded, and prolonged overdosages may result in serious side effects. Acidification of urine, for example, can cause the precipitation of urate, oxalate, or cystine stones in the urinary tract and also produce false positive tests for glycosuria. In addition, large doses can interfere with the effects of warfarin and can precipitate crises in patients with sickle cell anemia.[9] A recent double-blind trial has indicated, however, that therapeutic doses administered during a cold may decrease its duration. Clinical trials alone cannot completely explain the vitamin's effect on colds, and studies are necessary to indicate whether it acts

Table 8-2   Vitamins Important to Man[6]

Fat-Soluble Vitamins			
Vitamin	Common Source	Stored in Body	Importance
A_1 (retinol), A_2 (dehydroretinol)	Butter, eggs, carotene, and cryptoxanthin in plants; fish oils	Hepatic and Kuppfer cells	Chemistry of vision (aldehyde form); synthesis of mucopolysaccharides of mucus
D (calciferol)	Eggs, milk, liver oils, 7-dehydrocholesterol in skin converted to D on exposure to sunlight (ultraviolet)	Liver, skin, brain, other organs	Absorption and utilization of Ca and P; activation of alkaline phosphatase
E (α-tocopherol)	Widely in food; green vegetables, wheat germ, vegetable oils	Fat	Physiological antioxidant; protects vitamin A and carotene from oxidative destruction in presence of unsaturated fats; participates in specific enzyme systems
K (menadione)	Widely in food; green vegetables, tomatoes, orange peel	If at all, in liver	Synthesis of prothrombin in liver for normal clotting of blood

Water-Soluble Vitamins		
Vitamin	Common Source	Importance
B-Complex B_1 (thiamine)	Yeast, meat, whole grains, eggs, milk, green vegetables	Coenzyme in the oxidative decarboxylation of α-keto acids

Deficiency		Excess	
Due to	Symptoms	Due to	Symptoms
Diet; obstructive jaundice	Night blindness; xerophthalmia; decrease in activity of osteoblasts and odontoblasts and reduced growth of bones and teeth; increased cornification (scaly skin); impaired immunity; obstructive atelectasis, bronchiectasis, and pneumonia in children	Therapeutic overdose	Accelerate bone growth; induced psychosis; in infants, painful subcutaneous swellings, hyperirritability, limitation of motion
Diet; obstructive jaundice; pancreatic disease; celiac disease; hypoparathyroidism; pregnancy; steatorrhea	Demineralization of bone, no mineralization in children = rickets; weak bones, defective teeth; tetany; osteomalacia (adult rickets)	Therapeutic overdose; 50,000 units after few weeks to 6 months; high doses (300,000–500,000 units daily)	Toxicity; anorexia; thirst; urinary urgency; vomiting; diarrhea; mobilization of Ca and P from bone to soft tissue; dangerous calcification of renal parenchyma
Not known	Not well defined—maybe fibrositis, progressive muscular dystrophy	Not known definitely	Large doses well tolerated; may mobilize P, causing bone decalcification
Prothrombin deficiency	Abnormal bleeding	Adults: nontoxic; premature infants: with 10 mg dose	Adults: large doses well tolerated. Premature infants; fatal hemolytic anemia

Deficiency		Excess	
Due to	Symptoms	Due to	Symptoms
Alcoholism; diet faddism in United States and Europe; decorticated rice diet in Far East	Beri-beri, characterized by accumulation of pyruvic acid and lactic acids in blood and brain and impairment of cardiovascular, nervous, and gastrointestinal functions. *Mild.* fatigue, lassitude, headache, poor concentration, insomnia, personality changes, paresthesias, dyspnea. *Acute.* cardiovascular collapse, death. *Wet*	Parenteral injection	Rare toxicity, sensitization

Table 8-2. (Continued)

	Water-Soluble Vitamins	
Vitamin	Common Source	Importance
B$_2$ (riboflavin)	Yeast, liver kidney, cheese, eggs, ham, milk, beef, spinach	In a phosphorylated form, an essential component of the flavoprotein coenzymes FMN and FAD, which are involved in the removal of hydrogen from metabolites; acts as H acceptors from the nicotinamide-containing hydrogen carriers DPNH and TPNH in the H transport system.
B$_x$ (niacin, nicotinamide)	Yeast, beef, lamb, salmon, peanuts, whole grains, soybeans, spinach; synthesized from tryptophan	Essential part of enzyme system concerned with hydrogen transport (oxidation) in cells. Functional group of coenzymes, DPN and TPN, which act in series with flavoprotein enzymes as H donors and acceptors.
B$_6$ (pyridoxine, pyridoxol)	Liver, yeast	Phosphorylated pyridoxal is prosthetic group for enzymes that remove carboxyl groups from amino acids, transfer amino groups, remove sulfhydryl

Deficiency		Excess	
Due to	Symptoms	Due to	Symptoms
	form. edema and cardiovascular symptoms. *Dry form.* peripheral neuritis, paralysis, atrophy of muscles. *Pseudoencephalitis. Mixed symptoms.*		
Achlorhydria (permits inactivation), gastrointestinal disturbances preventing absorption, associated with pellagra	*Mild.* photophobia, conjunctivitis, mild cheilosis. *Severe.* conjunctivitis, severe cheilosis (skin cracks at edge of mouth), glossitis (magenta tongue), sharklike skin. *Arboflavinosis.* lip, tongue, and eye lesions; desquamation of lips, ulceration, and cheilosis; vascularization of cornea, blepharospasm, increased lacrimation; photophobia; changes in iris pigment; disturbances in vision; magenta glossitis; seborrheic lesions of nose, cheeks, chin, earlobes, canthi of eyes; frequent involvement of vulva, scrotum	Nontoxic	Yellow urine
Poverty; chronic alcoholism; fad dieting; fever; hyperthyroidism; pregnancy; stress; skin lesions incited by sunlight or heat friction	*Pellagra* (endemic to United States, Spain, Rumania, Italy). *Mild.* similar to thiamine deficiency. *Severe.* dermatitis, diarrhea, dementia. *Skin.* first lesions on tongue, mouth, vagina; prominent exposed areas—vesiculation and bullas formation. *Nervous system.* tremors, numbness, paralysis, insanity		Intravenous transient flushing
Unsupplemented infant formula; pregnancy; transfused familial hypochromic, microcytic anemia; isoniazid treatment; altered tryptophan metabolism	Retardation, convulsions; nausea, vomiting, anemia, peripheral neuritis	Intramuscular injection	Pain

Table 8-2. (Continued)

	Water-Soluble Vitamins	
Vitamin	Common Source	Importance
		groups; conversion of tryptophan to nicotinamide moiety of NAD and NADP, utilization of essential fatty acids; involved in production of GABA, synthesis of pyrrole ring of heme molecule
B_{12} (cobalamin, cyanocobalamin)	Liver, kidney, milk products	Participates in nucleic acid synthesis. Precursor of purine, inosinic acid; coenzyme in propionic acid metabolism; biosynthesis of methyl groups from glycine, serine, formate, and in transmethylation reactions
Biotin	Widely distributed: kidney, yeast; bacterial synthesis in intestine	CO_2 fixation, carboxylation; synthesis of fatty acids
Folic acid (pteroylglutamic acid)	Liver, kidney, yeast; intestinal bacterial synthesis	Nucleoprotein synthesis; necessary in mitosis
Pantothenic acid	Widely found in nature: liver, kidney, yeast, wheat, bran, peas; synthesized by intestinal bacteria	Cellular metabolism, particularly acetyl transfer
C (ascorbic acid)	Citrus fruits, berries, greens, cabbages, peppers	Not well understood, likely in H transport, metabolism of aromatic amino acids; activity of adrenal cortex and metabolism of cortical hormones, required for reticulum formation by osteoblasts; promotes healing; may shorten duration of colds

Deficiency		Excess	
Due to	Symptoms	Due to	Symptoms
Impairment of absorption due to lack of intrinsic factor; fish tapeworm infestation; abnormal growth of intestinal bacteria causing intestinal stasis; intestinal malabsorption; sprue steatorrhea, regional enteritis	Pernicious anemia		Not known
Excessive raw egg white ingestion creates biotin complex that prevents its absorption from gastrointestinal tract	Rare: exfoliative dermatitis, conjunctivitis		No toxicity
Treatment of leukemic patient with antagonist; malabsorption due to gastrointestinal disease; alcoholism	Megaloblastic anemia		No toxicity known
Malnutrition associated with prison camps	Burning feet		No toxicity known
Dietary insufficiency	*Scurvy.* Inability to lay down bone reticulum; hemorrhagic manifestations; delayed healing, edema, loosening teeth, gingivitis; generates secondary anemia, swollen joints, weakness, separation of the epiphyses of long bones and enlargement of costochondral junction of infants	Overdose	Diarrhea, urinary tract stones, affects activity of certain drugs like warfarin and produces sickle cell crises, acidifies urine causing false negative readings of glycosuria

by accelerating the repair of injured tissues, affecting viral replication, or increasing the cells' potential to produce interferon.[10]

When carefully administered, therapeutic doses of vitamins are very useful for specific conditions other than the treatment of frank vitamin deficiency. For example, the prophylactic use of multivitamins is warranted in pregnancy and to treat alcoholism or when broad spectrum antibiotic therapy may have temporarily destroyed the vitamin-producing bacterial population of the gut. More specifically, prophylactic therapy with pyridoxol (a B$_6$ vitamer) has been found useful in preventing peripheral neuritis associated with concurrent isoniazid therapy, inhibition of endogenous heme synthesis among patients who have received multiple transfusions, and to a lesser extent, to treat morning sickness during pregnancy. Similarly, it is possible to use vitamins involved in blood formation in the treatment of certain anemias, examples are vitamin B$_{12}$ in pernicious anemia, folic acid in macrocytic anemia of pregnancy or infancy, and folic acid and ascorbic acid in cases of megaloblastic anemias of pregnancy or infancy associated with disorders of folic acid synthesis.

Fat-soluble vitamins are often given alone or in combination to prevent deficiencies, since impairment of fat metabolism can directly affect either the absorption or utilization of these compounds. Prophylactic therapy is also indicated when obstructive jaundice prevents the normal flow of bile, which normally aids in absorption of carotene, the vitamin A precursor, or when cirrhosis and hepatocellular diseases prevent its storage in the liver. Vitamin D is recommended for persons who are not exposed to adequate sunlight, or for the elderly, in addition to those who have conditions related to impairment of fat metabolism, such as obstructive jaundice, pancreatitis, celiac disease, steatorrhea, or in hypoparathyroidism. Low prothrombin levels associated with vitamin K deficiency develop when the microorganisms necessary for its synthesis are absent from the gut, particularly in the newborn, after antibiotic therapy, or when liver damage prevents the conversion of K to prothrombin. Vitamin K is therefore prescribed prophylactically to mothers for help in blood clotting prior to delivery and to infants at birth. It is also used to counteract overdosages of anticoagulants dicoumarol and Tromexan® and to treat thromboembolic phenomena. On the other hand, the therapeutic or prophylactic value of vitamin E remains an area of active controversy. Its therapeutic usefulness has been based only on uncontrolled trials, clinical impressions, or extrapolations from animal studies; nevertheless, it is used to treat habitual abortion, sterility, coronary, cerebral and peripheral vascular disease, muscular dystrophy, nocturnal leg cramps, retardation of aging, and impotence, and to speed healing of wounds, burns, and periodontal disease.[11]

BARIATRICS

Why in a society such as ours, so abundantly supplied with foodstuffs, do diet faddism and vitamin cultism reach a high level? In part, the educational system is to blame. Few school systems require courses in health and nutrition and even contribute to the establishment of poor eating habits by allowing snacks high in calories and low in nutritional value to be readily available. It is easy to see why so many teenagers, through lack of proper knowledge, present nutritional crises because of their dietary habits. Nowadays, few schools would even consider offering as an alternative to the usual stodgy, high carbohydrate meal, a low calorie, nutritionally balanced lunch for the child who requires it. In the same light, school systems in communities that also support breakfast programs would do well to promote appropriate educational programs to parents, which would help families to upgrade their nutritional habits.[12]

What is especially shocking is that few medical schools offer courses that adequately prepare the practitioner to handle competently the complexities of nutritional imbalance and obesity seen in the average practice.[13] This void has allowed a number of physicians, with little experimental evidence to back up their claims, to promote metabolically unsound and even dangerous regimens in the name of weight control. In this respect, pregnant women especially should avoid diets that promote ketosis, which could have an adverse effect on the child. Similarly, such dieting can produce an excess of free fatty acids, which can in turn induce cardiac arrhythmias in individuals with cerebrovascular and coronary artery disease.[14] Unfortunately it is assumed that knowledge of nutrition, like knowledge about sex, is acquired automatically. Not only does everyone become a self-appointed nutritionist, but each is easy prey to anyone, regardless of credentials, who glibly promotes a panacea to health through a special diet or vitamin.

WEIGHT GAIN

Overweight undoubtedly constitutes the greatest single health hazard in the United States today. One-tenth to one-quarter of the population is overweight to some extent, and millions more are unhappy about their girth. Obesity is certainly a factor in shortening the life span and in the incidence of diabetes, cholelithiasis, hypertension, gallbladder disease, and vascular disorders including atherosclerosis.[15] Orthopedic problems, too, occur with appreciably higher frequency in the obese.[16]

That obesity is due to an excess of caloric intake over metabolic need is accepted by nearly everyone. It is not clear in many cases, however, whether this excess is derived from overeating alone or whether other physical and metabolic factors are involved. Contrary to popular belief, endocrine disorders[17] and brain tumors or damage only rarely cause increased appetite or decreased metabolic rates. Since heredity determines both body size and metabolic rate, these genetic factors, compounded with detrimental eating habits, certainly account for obesity in some individuals.[18] Moreover, an excess number of adipose cells persists in many formerly obese individuals who have lost much weight, suggesting a possible mechanism whereby this type of person has difficulty in staying thinner. Furthermore, research has indicated that overfeeding in early childhood can increase the number of adipose cells, although no precise recommendation for infant feeding to prevent later obesity has been forthcoming. A fat child may, therefore, be predisposed to a weight problem for the rest of his or her life (Fig. 8-3).[14,19]

Appetite is to some extent controlled by habit, which is established in childhood and tends to carry over into adult life. There is a natural tendency to gain weight as one becomes older, for metabolic demands decrease and physical activity lessens. Also, the eating habits developed through the increased appetite of pregnancy and nursing may become a natural part of the dietary regimen.

Weight gain associated with withdrawal from cigarette smoking is linked both to the loss of nicotine as an appetite depressant and the substitution of food

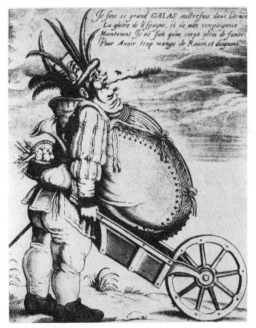

Figure 8-3 The epitome of obesity: a seventeenth century French woodcut caricature of the Spanish general Galas. Housed in the Cabinet des Estampes, Paris.

for oral gratification. In other instances neuroses are responsible, when self-gratification is the basis of excessive intake of calories. Weight control cannot be achieved in any of these cases unless a complete change of eating habits is accomplished.[20]

An endless variety of weight reducing methods have been tried: diet, drugs, hormones, hypnosis and other types of psychotherapy, as well as mechanical and electrical devices for the removal of local accumulations of fat. Yet none has been found to be universally successful. Although temporary weight loss can be achieved through crash diets low in calories or compounded of unusual mixtures of food, and auxiliary maintenance diets offer a means to hold weight down, few individuals adhere to such rigid diets and most eventually regain the weight that was lost.[21] This weight rebound or "yo-yo" phenomenon may happen throughout life unless a pattern of food

intake is established that equals the unique metabolic and energy requirements of the individual involved. With regard to group therapy and nutritional education, such organizations as TOPS (Take Off Pounds Sensibly) and Weight Watchers have been helpful to those seeking to achieve and maintain their weight goals.

Reliance on pills rather than diet is seldom successful, for the medication does not result in a permanent change of dietary habits. The appetite depressants may be initially valuable in reducing caloric intake, but tolerance, irritability, sleeplessness, toxic psychosis, and addiction often develop. Phenmetrazine (Preludin®) and diethylpropion (Tenuate®, Tepanil®), both amphetamine congeners,[22] are popularly prescribed for weight loss; but wide abuse of amphetamines leads to serious drug problems, as discussed elsewhere. Recently the Bureau of Narcotics and Dangerous Drugs (BNDD) placed these and related substances on the controlled substances list.[23]

Thyroid extract has been found both safe and helpful only in the rare obese individual who is hypothyroid. Although diuretics can achieve a dramatic temporary weight loss, their use is justified only for the brief period during dieting when water retention has produced a temporary plateau in weight loss.

In India, as early as 3000 BC, the Caraka Samhits described the use of certain plants for the treatment of obesity. Trivedi and Mann[24] believe that these plants contain drugs that correct the malfunctioning of glands and cure obesity due to auxiliary causes. Specifically, *Holoptelea integrifolia* (Ulmaceae) and *Iris versicolor* (Iridaceae) apparently possess the ability to increase the rate of fat catabolism. Other plants were listed, but their uses were not clear: *Saussurea lappa, Curcuma longa, Berberis aristata, Acorus calamus, Aconitum hetero-*

phyllum, Picrorhiza kurroa, and *Plumbago zeylanica.*

West Africans use the cola nut (*Cola acuminata, C. nitida*), with its high amount of caffeine, as a stimulant and as an appetite depressant. The nut is frequently chewed during religious or mourning fasts to abate hunger, and it is sold everywhere in marketplaces.

In North America, both Indians and early settlers used tobacco smoking to suppress their appetites.[25] In addition, a tea made from the fruit of the bearberry or kinnikinick (*Arctostaphylos uva-ursi*) was used by the Indians for weight control.[26]

In a society that constantly bombards us with tasty, high caloric inducements, easy to prepare and "quick in energy," it is not surprising to find a growing industry designed to counteract such potentiators of obesity.

Saccharin, which is 300 times sweeter than sugar, is the most widely used and accepted sugar substitute. However it has recently been shown to incite bladder tumors in animals when administered in large doses,[27] and for this reason limits on its use have been established by the Food and Drug Administration (FDA). In addition, saccharin has been moved from the list of food additives recognized as safe to the interim regulated additives list.

Presently, an intense search is underway to discover a commercially feasible replacement for synthetic sweeteners. Many candidates are under investigation, including certain flavonoids, synthetic dipeptides, and naturally occurring sweet substances having little or no caloric value. The latter have been isolated from such common plants as grapefruit, licorice, and pine, as well as from diverse species occurring in Africa and Paraguay (Table 8-3). However problems still exist relating to their cultivation, or to extraction, synthesis, or stability of the active compounds. In spite of their ability to sweeten, which is from 50 to 3000 times

greater than that of sucrose, the sweetness may be different and associated with either a persistent sweet aftertaste or a menthol, licorice, or bitter flavor. Also, with the exception of glycyrrhizin from licorice, which has a wide range of biological activity, little is known of their other biological or toxic properties (Table 8-3).

A variety of plants also yield certain taste-modifying compounds that have the ability to enhance the sweetening properties of food stuffs as described in Table 8-4. Some of these are commercially available, and FDA approval has been obtained for the use of chlorogenic acid, cymarin, and maltol.[28]

WEIGHT LOSS

Although the causes of obesity are obvious, those associated with weight loss are not as easily understood. If history does not reveal a faddist diet or inability or unwillingness to purchase sufficient food, physical or emotional states may be the cause. For example, anorexia nervosa (nervous loss of appetite) is well known to the psychiatrist. Also easily recognized and treated is loss of weight from an elevated metabolism, as in thyrotoxicosis or fever, or through caloric waste in the glycosuria of a diabetic. Treatment is therefore an individual matter, although supplemental vitamins and minerals in addition to an increase in the balanced diet of carbohydrates is usually prescribed.[29]

California Indians used decoctions of the Oregon grape *Mahonia aquifolium* to stimulate appetite.

DIABETES MELLITUS

One characteristic symptom of a metabolic disorder known as diabetes mellitus is loss of weight despite an exceedingly

Table 8-3 Sugar Substitutes[24]

Chemical Group	Substitute	Source	Sweetness Relative to Sugar	Remarks on Use
Dipeptide	L-aspartyl-1-phenylalanine methyl ester CH_2COOH CH_2—⬡ H_2NCHCO-NH-CHCOOCH$_3$	Synthetic	160 ×	Unstable in acidic solutions; sweetness lost during storage, hot processing of food
Protein	Monellin	African *Dioscoreophyllum cumminsii* berries (serendipity)	3000 ×	Sweetness lost within a day at 20°C storage; may become putrefied
Protein	Thaumatin	West African seeds of *Thaumatococcus daniellii*	750 ×	Slight licorice aftertaste, heat labile
Monoterpene	Perillartine OH H—C=N	*Perilla frutescens*, essential oil (an α-syn-oxime derivative)	200 ×	Toxicity not known; used in Japan to sweeten tobacco
Diterpene	Diastereoisomeric diterpene acids	*Pinus* resin	1600–2000 ×	Toxic effects not known
Diterpene glycoside	Stevioside	Leaves of shrub *Stevia rebaudiana* (yerba dulce) from Paraguay; not easily cultivated, scarce in wild	300 ×	Toxicity not known; used in Paraguay for treatment of diabetes

Type	Compound	Structure	Source	Sweetness	Comments
Triterpene glycoside	Glycyrrhizin (ammoniated)		Roots of *Glycyrrhiza glabra* (licorice)	50 ×; 100 ×	Flavoring limits use; used also as demulcent; expectorant; possesses wide range of useful and toxic biological properties
Flavonoids	Naringin		*Citrus paradisi* (grapefruit), commercially abundant	1000 ×	Long-lasting sweetness, which is slow to develop; aftertaste, menthol-type cooling or licoricelike
	Neohesperidin (dihydrochalcone)		*Citrus grandis* (Seville oranges), commercially rare; chalcone derivatives to neohesperidin (dihydrochalcone)		Acid stable
Steroid saponin	Osladin		Rhizomes of *Polypodium vulgare* (low yield)	300 ×	Toxicity not studied

215

Table 8-4 Taste-Modifying Sugar Substitutes[24]

Chemical Group	Substitute	Source	Mode of Action	Remarks on Use
Glycoprotein	Miraculin	West African tree fruit, *Synsepalum dulcificum* = miraculous berry (extraction difficult)	Modifies taste of sour foods and mineral and organic acids	Persistent sweet taste for 1–2 hours
Gymnemic acids (related to triterpine acids)	Gymnemic acids	Leaves of *Gymnema sylvestre*	Obtunds the taste for bitter and sweet substances, not for astringent or pungent substances	
Caffeoylquinic acids	Chlorogenic acid, cynarin	*Cynara scolymus* (artichoke)	Sweetens solutions of different taste qualities, solvent in water	Persistent sweet for 4–5 minutes; FDA approved
Pyrone	Maltol (3-hydroxyl-2-methyl-4-pyrone)	Larch bark, pine needles, chicory (*Cichorium intybus*), roasted malt	Flavoring to bread and cakes, intensify flavor of sugar 30–300 ×	FDA approved

good appetite. This is due to the depletion from the cells of fat and protein to fulfill the cellular energy requirement not supplied by a properly functioning glucose metabolism. Often accompanying this symptom is a characteristic breath odor, the result of excessive ketones in the blood formed through partial breakdown of fatty acids in the liver. Such excessive formation of acetoacetic and β-hydroxybutyric acids may also result in ketonuria. Glucose may also be found in the urine as a result of exceedingly high blood sugar. Hyperglycemia results from lack of insulin, which promotes the transfer of glucose from the tissue fluids into fat and muscle cells and fibroblasts. Such an abnormaltiy exists when β cells in the pancreas are unable to produce insulin; then glucose is not transmitted to insulin-dependent cells, and depletion of liver glycogen and decrease in uptake of glucose from the blood ensue.

Heredity and obesity are very important predisposing causes of diabetes, although inflammatory and degenerative lesions of the pancreas resulting from pancreatitis, carcinoma, arteriosclerosis, and hemochromatosis account for a small number of cases. Symptoms can vary widely, and a large number of patients with hyperglycemia manifest no symptoms whatsoever. Weakness, weight loss, increased thirst and urination, diabetic neuritis, failure of vision, impotence, itching of the skin, and furunculosis are all common manifestations of this disease.

Treatment of uncomplicated diabetes is usually an individualized problem and, depending on the severity of the symptoms, may involve diet control alone, diet and use of orally active antidiabetic agents, or diet and one or more injections per day of insulin. Insulin is replacement therapy only, and does not cure or prevent the pathologic condition. Its use can, however, often prevent the causes of diabetic death related to arteriosclerosis, hypertension, nephritis, superficial ulcers and infections, gangrene of the extremities, and gallstones.

Insulin is prepared commercially from extracts of beef and swine pancreases. All the oral antidiabetic drugs are prepared synthetically. The sulfonylureas, which are derivatives of sulfanilamide, stimulate the pancreas to produce insulin and affect hepatic enzymes so that glycogen deposition is increased. Moreover, the diguanidines increase glucose utilization by the tissues and tissue glycolysis and decrease hepatic glucose output without glycogen storage.

There are many hypoglycemic plants known through folklore, but their introduction into modern therapy awaits the discovery of an animal test system that closely parallels the pathological course of diabetes in humans. Such potential oral hypoglycemic agents as the cyclopropanoid amino acids and hypoglycins A and B, derived from the unripe fruit of the West Indian tree *Blighia sapida,* are too toxic for use as insulin substitutes. Moreover, their action differs from that of insulin in that they appear to act as antimetabolites capable of blocking the pathway of oxidation of fatty acids. This depletion of liver glycogen subsequently induces hypoglycemia. Other folklore remedies, such as tea made from Queen Anne's lace (*Daucus carota*) or from periwinkle *Catharanthus* (*Vinca*) *roseus,* which have allegedly been used successfully to maintain low blood sugar levels in humans, have no effect on diabetes artificially induced in animals. Tea from *C. roseus* has been used in South Africa, Nepal, Australia, South Vietnam, and the Philippines, and the proprietary products Covinca® and Vinculin® are still marketed as oral insulin substitutes in some of these countries. Although hypoglycemic activity cannot be established from crude extracts, two purified alkaloids, vindolinine dihydro-choloride and leurosine sulfate, have a high degree of hypoglycemic activity. Follow-up studies are warranted for these alkaloids from C. *roseus* and also those from *Tecoma stans*, which could serve as models for new prototypes of hypoglycemic agents. The latter alkaloids, tecomine and tecostanine, were isolated from leaves of various species of *Tecoma*, used by Mexican natives for the control of diabetes. More than 200 species could be added to a folklore list of insulin substitutes, including many common plants such as immature bean pods, olive leaves, potatoes, wheat, celery, blackberry leaves, sugar beet, and the leaves and roots of banana. The following compilation, based largely on the efforts of Farnsworth and Segelman,[30] illustrates the diversity of plants showing experimental hypoglycemic activity.

FERN ALLY. *Lycopodium clavatum* (running clubmoss).

GYMNOSPERM. *Taxus cuspidata* (spreading yew).

ANGIOSPERMS

ANACARDIACEAE. *Anacardium occidentale* (cashew); *Rhus typhina* (staghorn sumac).

APIACEAE. *Apium graveolens* (celery); *Coriandrum sativum* (coriander); *Daucus carota* (carrot, Queen Anne's lace: Fig. 8-4a).

APOCYNACEAE. *Rauvolfia serpentina* (snakeroot).

ARALIACEAE. *Oplopanax horridum* (devil's club); *Panax ginseng* (ginseng).

ARECACEAE. *Cocos nucifera* (coconut).

ASTERACEAE. *Arctium lappa* (burdock); *Artemisia vulgaris* (mugwort); *Erigeron canadensis* (horseweed); *Eupatorium purpureum* (joe-pye weed); *Helianthus annuus* (sunflower), *H. tuberosus* (Je-

rusalem artichoke); *Lactuca sativa* (lettuce); *Taraxacum officinale* (dandelion).

BRASSICACEAE. *Brassica oleracea* (cabbage), *B. rapa* (turnip).

CACTACEAE. *Lophophora williamsii* (peyote).

CARICACEAE. *Carica papaya* (papaya).

CHENOPODIACEAE. *Spinacia oleracea* (spinach).

CONVOLVULACEAE. *Ipomoea batatas* (sweet potato).

CUCURBITACEAE. *Momordica charantia* (wild cucumber).

ERICACEAE. *Chimaphila umbellata* (spotted wintergreen); *Vaccinium oxycoccus* (cranberry).

EUPHORBIACEAE. *Euphorbia pilulifera* (pill-bearing spurge).

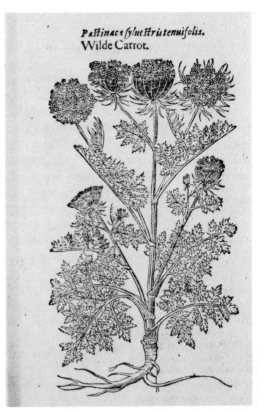

Figure 8-4a *Daucus carota* (from J Gerard, *The Herball* 1597).

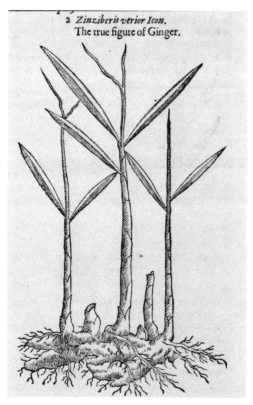

2 *Zinziberis verior Icon.*
The true figure of Ginger.

Figure 8-4b   *Zingiber officinale* (from J Gerard, *The Herball,* 1597).

FABACEAE. *Cassia occidentalis* (senna); *Lupinus albus* (lupine); *Pisum sativum* (pea); *Trigonella foenum-graecum* (fenugreek).

GERANIACEAE. *Geranium maculatum* (wild cranes bill).

LAMIACEAE. *Lycopus virginicus* (bugleweed).

LILIACEAE. *Allium cepa* (onion), *A. sativum* (garlic); *Convallaria majalis* (lily-of-the-valley); *Polygonatum officinale* (Solomon's-seal).

LOGANIACEAE. *Gelsemium sempervirens* (yellow jasmine).

LYTHRACEAE. *Lagerstroemia speciosa* (queen crape myrtle).

MUSACEAE. *Musa sapientum* (banana).

MYRTACEAE. *Pimenta officinalis* (allspice).

OLEACEAE. *Olea europaea* (olive).

PAPAVERACEAE. *Chelidonium majus* (celandine poppy).

POACEAE. *Avena sativa* (oats); *Hordeum vulgare* (barley); *Zea mays* (corn).

RANUNCULACEAE. *Cimicifuga racemosa* (black cohosh); *Hydrastis canadensis* (golden seal).

SOLANACEAE. *Capsicum frutescens* (red pepper); *Nicotiana tabacum* (tobacco).

ZINGIBERACEAE. *Zingiber officinale* (ginger: Fig. 8-4b).

GOUT

As already described, colchicine obtained principally from *Colchicum autumnale* is the drug of choice in acute attacks of gouty arthritis. Once pain and inflammation have subsided, therapy should be directed toward preventing future attacks by control of abnormal uric acid metabolism. Foods high in purine content, such as sweetbreads, sardines, brains, kidneys, liver, anchovies, and meat extracts, should be avoided, and a treatment using probenecid, which enhances uric acid excretion, and/or allopurinol, which impedes uric acid synthesis, may be followed.[31] Thus gout can now be controlled most effectively with modern chemotherapy: acute attacks can be terminated with colchicine and their recurrence prevented by various synthetic drugs.

It is worth noting that *Prunus avium* fruit (common or sweet cherry), containing keracyanin, has successfully maintained normal uric acid levels in gouty patients[32] before the introduction of a synthetic maintenance therapy.

LITERATURE CITED

1. Copeman WSC. 1964. *A Short History of the Gout and the Rheumatic Diseases.* University

of California Press, Berkeley and Los Angeles. 236 p; Copeman WS. 1970. Historic aspects of gout. *Clin Orthop* **71:** 14–22.

2. Pechey J. 1717. *The Whole Works of that Excellent Practical Physician, Dr. Sydenham,* ed 7. M. Wellington, London. *In* JH Talbott. 1970. *A Biographic History of Medicine,* 125–128. Grune and Stratton, New York.

3. Coursin WE. 1970. Relationship of nutrition to mental growth and development. *Mod Med* **38**(24): 81–84.

4. Levy RI, Fredrickson DS. 1970. The current status of hypolipidemic drugs. *Postgrad Med* **47:** 130–136.

5. Charman RC, Matthews LB, Braeuler C. 1972. Nicotinic acid in the treatment of hypercholesterolemia. *Angiology* **20:** 29–35.

6. *Vitamin Manual.* 1965. Upjohn, Kalamazoo, Mich. 88 + index.

7. Stricter controls on vitamins. *US News World Rep* 13 Aug 1973: 83.

8. Do-it-yourself psychosis. *Newsweek* 17 July 1972: 4, 44.

9. Vitamin C—Were the trials well controlled and are large doses safe? *Med Lett* **13:** 46–48, 1971.

10. Vindicating vitamin C. *Newsweek* 21 Jan 1974: 56.

11. Ehrlich HP, Tarver H, Hunt TK. 1972. Inhibitory effects of vitamin E on collagen synthesis and wound repair. *Ann Surg* **175:** 235–240; Vitamin E. *Med Lett* **13:** 97–98, 1971; Vitamin E and teeth. *Mod Med* **41**(3): 119, 1973.

12. Smith RE. 1970. Breakfast and breakfast cereals: where do they fit? *Mod Med* **38**(24): 109–112; White PL. 1970. Nutrition in an affluent society. *Mod Med* **38**(64): 71–73.

13. Kampmeier RH. 1970. Responsibility of the physician for nutritional health. *Mod Med* **38**(24): 74–80.

14. Dr. Atkins' Diet Revolution. *Med Lett* **15:** 41–42.

15. Connor WE. 1970. Diet and coronary heart disease. *Mod Med* **38**(24): 85–88.

16. Nelson RA, Anderson LR, Gastineau CF et al. 1973. Physiology and natural history of obesity. *JAMA* **223:** 627–630.

17. Martin MM, Martin A. 1973. Obesity, hyperinsulinism and diabetes mellitus in childhood. *J Pediatr* **82:** 192–201.

18. Penick SB, Filion R, Fox S et al. 1971. Behavior modification in the treatment of obesity. *Psychosom Med* **33:** 49–55.

19. The treatment of obesity. *Med Lett* **13:** 61–63, 1971.

20. Fineberg SK. 1972. The realities of obesity and fad diets. *Nutr Today* **7**(4): 23–26.

21. Itallie TB, Hashim SA. 1970. Obesity in an age of caloric anxiety. *Mod Med* **38**(24): 89–96; Vieth I. 1971. Beware of foods when you are not hungry. *Mod Med* **39**(2): 214–216; Calories do count. *Med Lett* **4:** 24, 1962; The perils of eating, American style. *Time* 18 Dec 1972: 68–76.

22. Preludin. *Med Lett* **2:** 31–32, 1960.

23. Six diet pills placed on US control list. *St Louis Post-Dispatch* 15 June 1973: 10A.

24. Trivedi VP, Mann AS. 1972. Vegetable drugs regulating fat metabolism in Caraka (*Lekhaniya dravyas*). *Quart J Crude Drug Res* **12**(4): 1988–1999.

25. Meyer C. 1973. *American Folk Medicine.* Thomas Y. Crowell, New York. 296 p.

26. Scully V. 1970. *A Treasury of American Indian Herbs.* Crown, New York. 306 p.

27. Ban on saccharin for food additive use is seen as possibility. *Chem Eng News* **50**(6): 5.

28. Farnsworth NR. 1973. Current status of sugar substitutes. *Cosmet Perfum* **88**(July): 27–35; Inglett GE, May JF. 1968. Tropical plants with unusual taste properties. *Econ Bot* **22:** 326–331.

29. Butterworth CE. 1970. Correcting malnutrition: practical therapeutic approaches. *Mod Med* **38**(24): 97–102.

30. Farnsworth NR, Segelman AB. 1971. Hypoglycemic plants. *Tile & Till* **57**(Sept): 52–55.

31. Zyloprin and other drugs in the management of gout. *Med Lett* **8:** 98–99, 1966.

32. Blau LW. 1950. Cherry diet control for gout and arthritis. *Tex Rep Biol Med* **8:** 309–311.

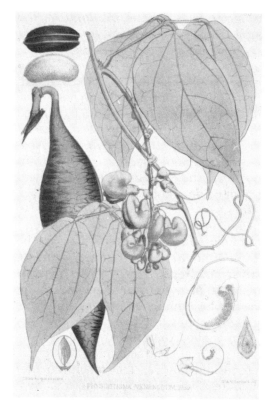

Figure 9-1 *Physostigma venenosum* (from R Bentley and H Trimen, *Medicinal Plants* **2:** 80, 1880).

Chapter 9

Special Sensory Organs: Eye and Ear

The Efik of the eastern region of Nigeria believe that calabar beans (*Physostigma venenosum,* Fabaceae: Fig. 9-1) possess the power to reveal and destroy witchcraft. A suspected "witch" is given a drink made from eight of the beans, ground up and added to water. If he is guilty, his mouth shakes and mucus comes from his nose. His innocence is proved if he lifts his right hand and then regurgitates. If the poison continues to affect the suspect after he has established his innocence, he is given a concoction of excrement mixed in water that has been used to wash the external genitalia of a female. When a person dies from the ordeal the usual procedure is to remove the eyes and throw the body into the forest.[1]

This vivid description of the poison ordeal custom would probably not be reported today, for Nigerian law forbids the use of the calabar bean and possession entails fine and imprisonment. Even so, its use in sorcery dies hard: some Efik keep one bean in their coin purse or with their cache of coins, to prevent witches from "drinking" their money.[1]

The tales spun around the use of the ordeal poison in the drawing rooms of Europe, and the nineteenth century zeal of missionaries to eliminate the practice, all served to focus attention on this otherwise obscure botanical species of limited distribution in western Africa. Early toxicologic studies in Scotland led to the isolation of physostigmine (eserine), an indole alkaloid that usually causes death from paralytic asphyxia. Recent research has shown that the alkaloid, a reversible inhibitor of the cholinesterases, can thereby prolong and exaggerate the effects of acetylcholine. The changes in the body functions produced by injecting physostigmine are very similar to those which would occur from simultaneous stimulation of all the parasympathetic nerves—contraction of the pupil, constriction of the bronchi, increased contraction of the intestinal musculature, and so forth (Chapter 6). The ability to contract the pupil led to the use of this substance in treating glaucoma, the leading cause of blindness in adults.

EYE

Several drugs of natural plant origin are important in ophthalmology because of their ability to open and close the pupil; thus they are used in treating glaucoma and to provide anti-infective and anti-inflammatory action.

The iris (colored portion of the eye) is a thin, muscular diaphragm that has at its center a circular aperture, the pupil, and lies in front of the lens. The muscle fibers of the iris are of two types: circular (sphincter) fibers, which following contraction give rise to pupil constriction, and radiating (dilator) fibers, which have an opposite effect when contraction occurs and cause the pupil to dilate. The circular fibers are controlled by parasympathetic nerves, the radiating fibers by sympathetic nerves. Correlated with this action of the iris is the accommodation or focusing that takes place in the lens. On contraction, the ciliary muscle, innervated by parasympathetic nerves, reduces the tension on the fibers of the suspensory ligament that supports the lens, thus regulating the curvature of the lens. When sphincter fibers of the iris contract, the pupil is small (miosis), and when the ciliary muscles contract, causing the suspensory ligament of the lens to relax and the lens to thicken, the eye is focused with sharp near vision (Fig. 9-2a). When radial fibers dominate, the pupil is dilated (mydriasis), and when the ciliary muscles are paralyzed, thus allowing the suspensory ligament to constrict and the lens to narrow, the eye is unfocused with sharp distant vision and blurred near vision (Fig. 9-2b).

Cholinergic and anticholinergic agents may be used to alter this mechanism. The cholinergic or miotic drugs stimulate parasympathetic effector cells directly (i.e., are parasympathomimetics) or indirectly by inhibiting cholinesterase, the enzyme that destroys acetylcholine. When applied topically to the eye, these agents cause contraction of the pupil, refocusing, and a fall in intraocular pressure. Since the goal in the treatment of glaucoma is to reduce this pressure sufficiently to prevent damage to the optic nerve and retina, miotic drugs, together with surgery, are used for treatment.

In the treatment of glaucoma[2] the alkaloid pilocarpine, derived from leaflets of *Pilocarpus jaborandi, P. microphyllus,* or *P. pinnatifolium* (Rutaceae, shrubs native to Brazil), acts directly on cholinergic receptor sites, thus mimicking the action of acetylcholine. Intraocular pressure is thereby reduced, and despite its short-term action, pilocarpine is the standard drug used for initial and maintenance therapy in certain kinds of primary glaucoma.

A second short-acting agent of this type is physostigmine, obtained from the

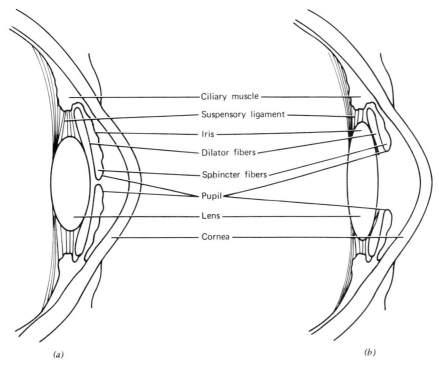

Figure 9-2 Schematic longitudinal view of the front of the eye. (a) Cholinergic effect. (b) Anticholinergic effect.

calabar bean, which acts indirectly by inhibiting cholinesterase; it too may be used for the treatment of primary glaucoma, but it is not as well tolerated as pilocarpine and may cause local irritation and allergic reactions. Neostigmine, one of the better known synthetic analogs, is less effective than physostigmine.

There are a number of long-acting anticholinesterase agents (demecarium, isoflurophate); all are synthetic, and because of their toxicity they are generally used only when short-term miotics have failed.

Anticholinergic drugs, when applied topically to the eye, paralyze accommodation and dilate the pupil (mydriasis) (Fig. 9-2b). They are used primarily in the treatment of some (secondary) glaucomas, as an aid in refraction, and for other diagnostic purposes. Among the most successful are the tropane alkaloids

atropine and scopolamine (hyoscine), derived originally from several solanaceous plants: *Atropa belladonna, Duboisia myoporoides,* and *D. leichardtii* leaves yield atropine, which is formed from hyoscyamine during the process of extraction. Atropine is also available synthetically but costs much more than that extracted naturally. *Datura fastuosa* and *D. metel* are abundant sources of scopolamine. A number of synthetic derivatives (homatropine, eucatropine) are also used, but atropine is a potent, long-acting anticholinergic drug and enjoys the widest use in ophthalmia.

When cocaine (*Erythroxylum coca*) is applied to the eye it produces mydriasis, vasoconstriction, and other effects, and may also reduce intraocular pressure. It is often used in combination with atropine and epinephrine, another mydriatic drug.[3]

INFECTIONS

Most eye infections are preferentially treated by topical applications of medicaments, since the intensive systemic therapy required for severe or intraocular disease can increase the risk of adverse reactions. Topical therapy allows clinicians to use antibiotics that are rarely if ever used systemically, because there is no risk of developing resistant bacterial mutants that could initiate infections elsewhere in the body. Among those used alone or in combination are the polypeptide antibiotics derived from species of *Bacillus,* such as polymyxin B (*B. polymyxa*), bacitracin (*B. subtilis*), and gramicidin (*B. brevis*), as well as the aminoglycoside neomycin sulfate from *Streptomyces fradiae.* Care must be taken in selecting the antibiotic for treatment, since the penicillins, streptomycin, neomycin, and some sulfonamides have the ability to sensitize potentially allergic individuals. On the other hand, chloramphenicol, erythromycin, or the tetracyclines have a low sensitizing potential. Depending on the peculiar antibiotic susceptibility of the organism involved, external eye infections such as staphylococcal blepharoconjunctivitis may be treated with neomycin, corneal ulcers with polymyxin B or Loridine®, intraocular infection with a variety of systemic antibiotics, and chlamydial eye infections, with some degree of success, by combination therapy of tetracycline and sulfadiazine. Bacitracin ointment may also be used as an alternative to silver nitrate in prophylactic chemotherapy of gonorrheal ophthalmia neonatorum.

HERBOLOGY

North American folklore describes the use of many decoctions of roots, leaves, and flowers as eyewashes or poultices to treat sore or bruised eyes.

Achillea spp. (yarrow) leaves and flowers. A decoction was used by the Blackfoot as an eyewash.

Argemone intermedia (prickly poppy) sap, *Maclura pomifera* (Osage orange) root, or *Salix* spp. (willow) stem ash. Comanches used a decoction of any one of these for the treatment of sore eyes.

Hydrastis canadensis (golden seal) roots. Featured prominently by midwest Indians and early European settlers, one teaspoon of dried roots was steeped in about one cup of water, cooled, and applied to the inflamed eye; used either alone or in combination with *Hamamelis virginiana* (witch hazel) and *Heuchera* sp. (alum root).

Linum spp. (flaxseed) seeds. Used in domestic medicine to remove foreign material from the eye, a seed is moistened and placed under the eyelid, the eye is closed for a few moments, and the material in the eye sticks to the seed and can be removed with it.

Monotropa uniflora (Indian pipe) stems. As a domestic remedy in the nineteenth century, the juices were squeezed directly on inflamed eyes.

Prosopis spp. (mesquite) leaves. Indians in the southwestern United States and in Mexico applied them to irritated conjunctiva.

Saponaria officinalis (soapwort) roots, *Hydrastis canadensis* (golden seal) roots, *Ulmus fulva* (slippery elm) bark, or *Hyssopus officinalis* (hyssop) leaves. Decoctions of any one of these were widely used as poultices to remove discoloration around black or bruised eyes.

EAR

INFECTIONS

External ear infections are treated with topical antibiotics such as the polymyxins and neomycin, in addition to the tetracyclines, the sulfonamides, chloramphenicol, gentamicin, nitrofurazone, and nystatin. Systemic therapy is necessary only when cellulitis involves the external meatus or auricle, or when pain cannot be controlled by local medicaments. It is noteworthy that a 5% aqueous solution of acetic acid (vinegar), by lowering the pH, will prevent the growth of most external ear pathogens. Simple irrigation of an ear with dilute ethyl alcohol (10–20%) in hypertonic saline or hydroalcoholic solutions has been found equally useful in removing the water causing swimmer's ear or external otitis.

Infections of the external or middle ear are usually of mixed microbial origin, although predominantly streptococcal and staphylococcal, and they require broad-spectrum antibiotic therapy. Final selection of the antibiotic should not be made, however, until the culture has revealed the identity of the organisms involved, since some (e.g., *Pseudomonas* and *Proteus*) may be refractory to such broad-spectrum antibiotics as tetracycline.

HERBOLOGY

Achillea spp. (yarrow) plant. Winnebagos steeped whole yarrow and poured liquid into aching ears.

Asarum canadense (wild ginger) roots. Meskwakis steeped crushed roots and poured the liquid directly into the ear; wild ginger owes its activity to aristolochic acid, which is known to have antimicrobial properties.

Polygala alba (white milkwort) roots. Sioux scraped the roots, boiled them, and poured the liquid into aching ears. *Polygala* species contain saponins and methyl salicylate: the former is now known to have anti-inflammatory properties, and methyl salicylate is similar to oil of wintergreen and is readily absorbed through the skin.

LITERATURE CITED

1. Holmstedt B. 1972. The ordeal bean of Old Calabar: the pageant of *Physostigma venenosum* in medicine, 303–360. In T Swain (ed), *Plants in the Development of Modern Medicine*. Harvard University Press, Cambridge, Mass; Simmons DC. 1956. Efik divination, ordeals and omens. *Sw J Anthropol* **12:** 223–228.

2. Willetts GS, Hopkins DJ. 1972. Systemic therapeutic agents and glaucoma. *Practitioner* **209:** 27–34.

3. Ing HR. 1955. Mydriatic alkaloids, 243–263. In RHF Manske (ed), *The Alkaloids, Chemistry and Physiology*, Vol 5, *Pharmacology*. Academic Press, New York.

Chapter **10**

Oral Hygiene

Man has been preoccupied with his teeth throughout the ages. In some cultures teeth dyed shiny black by various plant products were as sexually appealing as the pearly white teeth promoted in today's advertisements. Certainly the adage "cleanliness is next to godliness" could have been derived from Muhammed, who said that "the Siwak (chewing stick) is an implement for the cleansing of teeth and a pleasure to God."[1]

The oral cavity contains the teeth and its supporting structures, the gums (gingiva), surrounded by the periodontium and alveolar bone of the jaw. The roof of the mouth is known as the hard palate, and posterior to this the soft palate; these and the inner tissues of the cheek are lined with oral mucosa. The tongue (having taste buds on its surface) is a muscle that aids in talking and swallowing. We acquire our first set of teeth during the first year of life, and begin to lose them, prior to replacement with the permanent set, from 6 years of age onward.

CARIES

Childhood is the time when the teeth are most susceptible to the infection of the tooth structure known as caries. The incidence is highest between 5 and 15 years of age and drops off dramatically thereafter as we become immune to the organisms that cause tooth decay. These organisms, primarily certain species of *Streptococcus* (*S. mutans*: Fig. 10-1, *S. faecalis, S. salivarius, S. sanguis*), adhere to the tooth surfaces by their extracellular insoluble glucans (large polymers of glucose) and cell wall components. They are especially likely to stick to areas of the tooth already covered with a microscopic layer of protein known as calculus, which has been precipitated on the tooth surface by the action of bacterial enzymes on saliva. They accumulate on these areas and form large colonies that develop and mature, becoming a mixture of many organisms, some establishing symbiotic relationships. These colonies on the tooth surface are known as plaque.

If plaque contains cariogenic organisms, caries may develop. These organisms are able to colonize the tooth surface and utilize sugars from our diet, particularly sucrose, to produce acid. When the pH drops below 5.5 at the tooth surface, the calcium phosphate in the apatite of the enamel surface dissolves. (It has been postulated that the organisms utilize the extracted phos-phates to buffer the acid environment, which is toxic to them.) The organisms invade the tooth along the dentinal tubules, and since they possess potent proteolytic enzymes and/or chelating agents, they eventually are able to break down the protein of the enamel matrix. If the disease goes unchecked, the pulp (center of the tooth, which is vascularized and contains nerves) may also be affected (pulpitis), causing pain. If the root area is invaded, causing abscesses, the infection may spread throughout the body. In this manner, the tooth may eventually be destroyed (Fig. 10-2).

Different organisms predominate in various types of caries. Those occurring on the smooth surface of the lingual, buccal, and interproximal regions are usually initiated by oral streptococci, particularly strains of *S. mutans*. The lesion starts as a small area of decalcification, then extends in a conelike fashion into the deeper layers of the tooth; this procedure is similar to the mechanism just described. The appearance of deep dentinal caries, which also involve species of lactobacilli, differs in that the lesion is small, almost pinpoint at the sur-

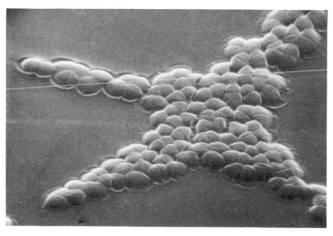

Figure 10-1 Scanning electron micrograph of *Streptococcus mutans* surrounded by extracellular polysaccharide (×5600).

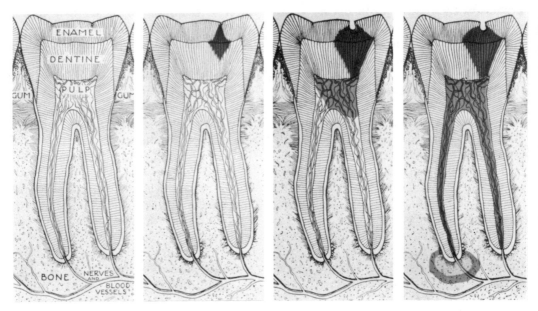

Figure 10-2 Development of carious lesion. (a) Normal tooth. (b) Initial enamel infection and dissolution. (c) Extension of infection into pulp. (d) Extension of infection through pulp to root creating a periapical abscess. Courtesy American Dental Association and Chicago Dental Association Society, *Exhibit for Dentistry at a Century for Progress,* International Exposition, Chicago 1933–1934, Figs. 4, 7 and 11.

face, and is larger in the interior of the tooth (implosive form). In addition to *Streptococcus,* organisms of *Actinomyces, Rothia* (Fig. 10-3), and *Arthrobacter* predominate in caries of both root and crevicular areas. Root caries seems to be a disease peculiar to adults rather than children, and the condition is initiated at the gingival margin, where the tooth and gum come together. Caries found within the crevicular or biting surfaces of the tooth are thought to be initiated by impaction of food; therefore the organisms responsible for these lesions do not have to have plaque-forming ability. The mechanisms involved in deep dentinal and root caries are not well understood but should become clearer once the particular characteristics of the organisms involved are known.

Caries is not inevitable and can be prevented. This is especially important in countries where refined foods and sugars are abundantly supplied in the diet.

It is now generally accepted that at a concentration of 1 ppm, fluoride in the water supply not only strengthens the apatite of teeth by increasing the rate of maturation of the enamel surface but reduces enamel solubility, favors formation of hydroxy-apatite crystal structure during dissolution and remineralization of enamel, and exerts an effect on the growth of the organisms or their cariogenic potential by blocking bacterial enzymes. This element and other ions found in water, food, and plants may therefore help prevent caries.[2]

Epidemiological studies have shown that the incidence of caries is low in areas where strontium, molybdenum, boron, and lithium have been found in the water supply or soil, and higher in areas where selenium, beryllium, copper, and lead are abundant. Although the mode of action of these elements is not as well defined as that of fluoride, molybdenum apparently acts in reducing acid production of bacteria and strontium affects the crystal structure of enamel.[2]

Aside from the water supply, these anticariogenic ions may concentrate in certain genetic varieties of plants if they are grown in soils plentiful in the elements. The concentration of fluoride may also differ depending on the season of harvest of the plant; for example, fluoride concentrations are higher in green teas harvested in Taiwan in the spring than in the summer months. Unlike the black teas, the green, spring teas can supply enough natural fluoride for caries prevention, if consumed in quantities of from 3 to 10 cups per day.[3]

Potherbs, such as southern greens, can absorb fluoride, lithium, molybdenum, and strontium through the cooking water. Reduction of enamel solubility can also be achieved through buffering action and complexing of calcium by the phytates (organic phosphates), orthophosphates, pyrophosphates, and polyphenols found in unrefined cereals or by the inorganic phosphates added to breakfast cereals.[4]

In countries where preventive programs are actively underway, children are regularly surveyed and topical fluoride and/or sealants are applied to their teeth. The use of fluoride-containing toothpastes is also promoted to prevent the development of caries. When lesions do occur, they are arrested through regular excavation and restorative procedures, since a carious juvenile tooth, left unattended, could lead to extension of the infection to the adult tooth underlying it. As an adjunct to this, programs of instruction on oral hygiene are carried out by dentists or schools.

TOOTH CLEANING

Various methods of tooth cleaning have been devised to retain oral hygiene. The practice of using the toothbrush and toothpaste originates from populations who once cleaned their teeth by using equivalents of toothbrushes (chewing sticks) or such forms of mechanical plaque removers as chewing gum or

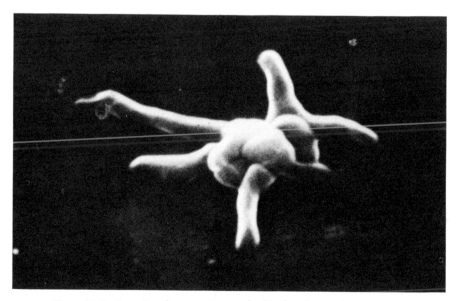

Figure 10-3 Scanning electron micrograph of *Rothia dentocariosa* (x19,055).

bark. Some cultures preferred abrasive powders prepared from dried parts of plants.

Chewing Sticks

In vast parts of the world where tooth-brushing is uncommon, the practice of tooth cleaning by chewing sticks has been known since antiquity. The precise method for use of these implements was recorded by the Babylonians in 5000 BC, and the fashion ultimately spread throughout the Greek and Roman empires and elsewhere. In China sticks were fashioned into ornate toothpicks, and the counterpart to the modern toothbrush was devised by the Chinese in the fifteenth century.[1,5]

The use of chewing sticks persists today among many African and southern Asian communities as well as in isolated areas of tropical America and the southern United States, particularly in Appalachia and the Ozarks. This practice was unknown among American Indian populations, who cleaned their teeth with fibrous plant materials (quids), sinews, bones, and toothpicks,[6] and it is interesting to speculate how the chewing stick habit was introduced. Our clue comes from the early nineteenth-century writings of Barton:

The wood of the Cornus florida (Dogwood) is much used by Dentists, in the insertion of artificial teeth and the young branches stripped of their bark, and rubbed with their ends against the teeth, render them extremely white. The creole negroes who inhabit Norfolk in Virginia, in great numbers, are in the constant practice of substituting the Dogwood twigs, for a West India shrub in cleansing their teeth. The striking whiteness of these, which I have frequently observed, is a proof of the efficacy of the practice. The application of the juice of these twigs to the gums, is also useful in preserving them hard and sound.[7]

Users who often prefer chewing sticks to modern toothbrushing techniques attribute their dental health to the traditional practice. It is noteworthy that caries rates are often very low among such users, in spite of the high carbohydrate diets they normally consume and the lack of exposure to modern dental procedures or prophylactic regimens.[8]

The plants used are very carefully selected for such properties as foaminess, hardness, or bitterness, and certain species are more popular than others. A great number have related medicinal properties that may be antibacterial, anti-neoplastic, anti-sickle cell, or analgesic. Moreover, extracts from many of these plants are also used to treat inflammations, mucocutaneous lesions of various kinds, and eye infections (Table 10-1). Fashioned from roots, twigs, or wood into sticks about 8 inches long and finger width, the implements are readily obtained in many parts of Africa in marketplaces, bundled and ready for use (Fig. 10-4). Elsewhere, if the plant is common, the material is collected when needed.

The stick is first washed, then gnawed on the tip to macerate it so that the end is frayed and brushlike. The teeth are brushed very thoroughly, and care is taken to clean both the inside and the outside of the tooth surfaces (Fig. 10-5). Usually this procedure takes from 5 to 10 minutes and often, the stick is sucked for several hours after brushing is completed. It is not uncommon to see individuals going about their chores with the remainder of a chewing stick in the mouth.

Examination after such an exercise reveals teeth with little or no remaining plaque and gums that are usually pink and firm. A transient gum inflammation is only rarely apparent and occurs more often with certain species such as Massularia. Because dental surveys have yet to

Table 10-1 Chewing Sticks for Cleaning Teeth

Order, Family, and Species	Source	Locality Used	Used as/Treatment of	Remarks
DICOTYLEDONS				
Phylogenetic group 1				
Annonales				
LAURACEAE				
Sassafras albidum	Twig without bark	Appalachia, United States	Antiseptic; disinfect root canals; flavoring; tonic	Contains safrole (a carcinogen)
Berberidales				
MENISPERMACEAE				
Penianthus zenkeri	Twig and root	West Africa	Aphrodisiac; evacuant; swollen limbs; wounds	
Sphenocentrum jollyanum	Root	West Africa	Aphrodisiac; cough; wounds	
Tiliacora dielsiana	Stem	West Africa		
Phylogenetic Group 2				
Hamamelidales				
HAMAMELIDACEAE				
Liquidambar styraciflua	Twig	Eastern United States, Mexico		
Fagales				
BETULACEAE				
Alnus glutinosa	Inner bark	England	Inflamed gums, toothache	
Betula lenta	Twig	Southeastern United States		
B. lutea	Twig	Southeastern United States		Twig soaked in water or whiskey (Appalachia)
Phylogenetic Group 3				
Chenopodiales				
AMARANTHACEAE				
Achyranthes aspera	Branch	Arabia, Panama	Seeds emetic; branch used for hydrophobia and snake bite; roots for scorpion stings	
Aerva tomentosa	Root	Red Sea area		

Table 10-1 (Continued)

Order, Family, and Species	Source	Locality Used	Used as/Treatment of	Remarks
Phylogenetic Group 4				
Theales				
CLUSIACEAE				
Allanblackia floribunda	Root	West Africa	Analgesic; dysentery; toothache	
Garcinia afzelii	Twig	West Africa	Aphrodisiac; dysentery	
G. kola[a]	Root	West Africa	Aphrodisiac; evacuant; dysentery; headache; malignant tumors; respiratory ailments; wounds	Tannin, reducing sugar, antidote for *Strophanthus gratus* poisoning
G. mangostana	Twig	West Africa	Dysentery	Ambisiasin; tannin
G. mannii	Root, stem	Ghana	Diuretic	
Pentadesma butyracea	Root	West Africa	Vermifuge; diarrhea	
DIPTEROCARPACEAE				
Monotes expansa	Twig	Liberia		
LECYTHIDACEAE				
Napoleona leonensis	Twig	West Africa	Asthma; cough	Saponins; often toxic
N. vogelii	Bark	West Africa	Febrifuge	
Ericales				
ERICACEAE				
Gaultheria procumbens	Root	United States	Antirheumatic; analgesic; dysentery; toothache	Methyl salicylate; root chewed 6 weeks each spring by young people prevents toothache
Ebenales				
SAPOTACEAE				
Synsepalum dulcificum	Twig	West Africa		Sweetener
EBENACEAE				
Diospyros barteri	Stem	West Africa		Antibacterial activity; alkaloid scopolin, tannin, saponin, naphthoquinones (most species of *Diospyros*)

	Part	Location	Use	Comments
D. elliotii	Twig	West Africa		
D. heudelotii	Twig	Sierra Leone		
D. loureiriana	Root	South Africa		
D. lycioides[a]	Stem	Zambia		
D. tricolor	Root	West Africa	Anticariogenic	Red dye; antibiotic
Euclea fruticosa	Root	Kenya		Diosquinone Black dye from roots; twigs make lips and mouth very red (cosmetic)
E. multiflora	Root	Tanzania	Vermifuge	Tannin
Phylogenetic Group 5 **Cistales** FLACOURTIACEAE				
Casearia barteri	Stem	West Africa		
VIOLACEAE				
Rinorea subintegrifolia	Stem	West Africa	Ophthalmia	
PASSIFLORACEAE				
Androsiphonia adenostegia	Twig	Liberia		
Smeathmannia pubescens	Twig	Liberia	Toothache	Wood hard
Salicales SALICACEAE				
Populus spp.	Twig	Southeastern United States		
Capparidales CAPPARIDACEAE				
Maerua crassifolia	Twig	West Africa		High calcium content
Phylogenetic Group 6 **Malvales** TILIACEAE				
Glyphaea brevis	Twig	West Africa	Evacuant; diarrhea; fever; respiratory ailments; wounds	
STERCULIACEAE				
Grewia mollis	Bark and leaf	West Africa	Evacuant; fever; wounds	
Cola laurifolia	Twig	West Africa	Dysentery	
Nesogordonia papaverifera	Twig	West Africa		

Table 10-1 (Continued)

Order, Family, and Species	Source	Locality Used	Used as/Treatment of	Remarks
Waltheria indica	Root	Ghana	Cough; dysentery; fever; external hemorrhage; ophthalmia; wounds	Tannin; mucilage; sugar
MALVACEAE				
Hibiscus rosa-sinensis	Stem	Ghana		Fiber
Euphorbiales				
EUPHORBIACEAE				
Alchornea cordifolia	Root and stem	West Africa	Evacuant; dysentery; leprosy; ophthalmia; oral wounds; venereal disease; fever; diuretic; respiratory ailments; skin infections; toothache	Tannin
Antidesma venosum	Twig	Northern Nigeria	Evacuant; itch; vermifuge	Fruit edible
Cleidion gabonicum	Twig	Ghana		
Drypetes floribunda	Stem	West Africa		Wood very hard and sweet
Jatropha curcas	Stem	India	Purgative	Tannin, foamy, manufacture soap, curcin; lather mixed with salt to clean teeth
Mallotus oppositifolium		West Africa	Aphrodisiac; headache; vermifuge; wounds	
Phyllanthus engleri	Fruit	Tanzania	Constipation; cough; stomachic	
P. muellerianus	Twig, bark peeled	Nigeria		
P. reticulatus	Twig	South Africa	Diuretic	Sweet, fibrous
Tetrorchidium didymostemon	Stem	South Africa	Evacuant; fever	Wood soft
DICHAPETALACEAE				
Dichapetalum guineese	Stem	West Africa	Jaundice	

Rhamnales

RHAMNACEAE				
Gouania lupuloides	Stem	Tropical America	Heal and harden gums; dried powdered stems made into dentrifices	Toothwash ingredient in Jamaica
G. polygama	Twig	Honduras		Lathers on chewing
Lasiodiscus mildbraedii	Stem	West Africa		Wood hard
Phylogenetic Group 7				
Rosales				
ROSACEAE				
Parinari curatellifolia	Twig	West Africa	Antimalarial; blood tonic; cardiac stimulant; eye lotion; respiratory ailments	Tannin, wood hard
Potentilla rubra	Root	Mexico		
CONNARACEAE				
Agelaea obliqua	Fruit	West Africa		
A. trifolia	Stem	Southern Nigeria		
Castanola paradoxa	Stem	West Africa		
FABACEAE: CAESALPINIOIDEAE				
Burkea africana	Twig	Ghana, Northern Nigeria	Dysentery; fish poison; headache; septic sores	Tannin
Cassia auriculata	Twig	India	Aphrodisiac; diuretic; dysentery; evacuant; fever; leprosy; venereal disease; vermifuge	
C. sieberiana	Root	Sierra Leone		
Desmodium lasiocarpum	Twig			
Griffonia (Bandeiraea) simplicifolia	Stem	West Africa	Aphrodisiac; evacuant; soft chancre	
Daniellia oliverae	Twig	Ghana	Evacuant; itch; mouthwash; venereal disease	Resin, volatile oil
Dialium guineense	Twig	West Africa	Evacuant; fever; ophthalmia; sore throat; tumor	
Humboldtia laurifolia	Twig	Ceylon		
Hymenostegia afzelii	Twig	West Africa	Cough; piles	
Mezoneuron sp.	Twig	Liberia		

Table 10-1 (Continued)

Order, Family, and Species	Source	Locality Used	Used as/Treatment of	Remarks
Piliostigma reticulatum	Root and twig	Tropical Africa		
P. thonningii	Root and twig	Tropical Africa	Dysentery; evacuant; fever; infections; leprosy; respiratory ailments; snake bite; toothache	Tannin
Pongamia pinnata	Twig	Ceylon	Skin disease	Pongam oil; manufacture of soap
Tamarindus indica	Twig	West Africa	Dysentery; evacuant; fever; leprosy; ophthalmia; oral infections; respiratory ailments; wounds	Tannin
FABACEAE: FABOIDEAE				
Abrus schimperi	Stem	East Africa	Aphrodisiac; irregular menstruation; scorpion bite	Abrin
Baphia nitida	Stem	West Africa	Evacuant; dysentery; ringworm; venereal disease	Red dye isosantaline
Eriosema griseum	Stem	West Africa	Fish poisons	
Lonchocarpus sp.	Stem	West Africa	Insecticide	
Milletia thonningii	Stem, bark peeled	Nigeria		Sweet taste
FABACEAE: MIMOSOIDEAE				
Acacia modesta	Twig	Pakistan		
A. nilotica (incl. *A. arabica*)	Twig	Tropical Africa, Pakistan	Dysentery; leprosy; oral wounds; trachoma; toothache; venereal disease	Anthraquinones
A. pinnata	Stem	Tropical Africa	Aphrodisiac; evacuant	Anthraquinones
	Twig and root	India		

236

Phylogenetic Group 8

Myrtales

COMBRETACEAE

	Part	Location	Uses	Compounds
Anogeissus leiocarpus, A. schimperi	Root	Tropical Africa	Vermifuge	
Guiera senegalensis	Root and stem	West Africa	Diuretic; dysentery; poultice	Alkaloids; tannin
Terminalia glaucescens	Root	West Africa	Evacuant; cough; evacuant; venereal disease; wounds	

MYRTACEAE

Eugenia coronata	Twig	Ghana	Dysentery	
Syzygium guineense subsp. *huillense*	Twig	Zambia		

Phylogenetic Group 9

Polygales

POLYGALACEAE

Carpolobia alba	Stem	West Africa	Aphrodisiac; evacuant	
C. lutea	Stem	West Africa	Evacuant; fever; headache; leprosy; snake bite; venereal disease; wounds	

Rutales

RUTACEAE

Aegle marmelos	Twig	India, Pakistan	Dysentery	
Citrus aurantifolia	Twig	West Africa	Dysentery; fever; headache; ophthalmia; oral infections; vermifuge; vomiting	Volatile oil
Clausena anisata	Stem	Kenya, West Africa, South Africa	Evacuant; headache; liniment; respiratory ailments	
Fagara chalybaea	Twig	South Africa	Gargle; emetic; swelling	
F. deremensis	Twig	South Africa	Stomach ache	
F. zanthoxyloides	Stem	West Africa	Anticariogenic; evacuant; dysentery; fever; edema; ophthalmia; toothache; ulcers; vermifuge; venereal disease; anti-sickle cell factor	Atarine isoquinoline with bacterial action; resin irritant; essential oil

237

Table 10-1 (Continued)

Order, Family, and Species	Source	Locality Used	Used as/Treatment of	Remarks
Glycosmis pentaphylla	Stem	India	Fever; liver ailments; intestinal worms; skin diseases	
Teclea verdoorniana	Twig	West Africa	Cough; ophthalmia	Bitter hard wood
Zanthoxylum alatum	Wood and bark	India		
Z. senegalense	Stem	West Africa	Antirheumatic	
MELIACEAE Azadirachta indica[a]	Twig	Asian subcontinent	Antipyretic; antiseptic; febrifuge; insecticide; skin diseases; tonic	Bark with bitter alkaloid margosine; fruit with toxic alkaloid azaridine; leaves insect repellant; Neem toothpaste
Carapa procera	Twig	West Africa	Evacuant; fever; ophthalmia; skin infections; vermifuge	Bark contains carapin and tulukunin; wood bitter and hard; soap manufacture
ANACARDIACEAE Mangifera indica	Twig and leaf	Panama, India	Astringent; bronchitis; catarrh, internal hemorrhage; toothache	
Rhus cotinus	Twig	Tanzania	Gargle; mouthwash	Tannin, volatile oil; no bactericidal action
R. glabra Sorindeia wooneckei	Twig Stem	American Ozarks Nigeria	Anticariogenic	Sweet flavor
SAPINDACEAE Allophylus africanus	Root and twig	West Africa	Diuretic; gastritis; hookworm; venereal disease	
Lecaniodiscus cupanioides	Stem	West Africa	Burns; fever; sores	
Paullinia pinnata	Root	Tropical Africa	Aphrodisiac; dysentery; diuretic; leprosy; jaundice; oral wounds; snake bite	

Taxon	Part used	Location	Uses	Notes
Juglandales				
JUGLANDACEAE				
Juglans regia	Stem bark	Pakistan		
Phylogenetic Group 10				
Santalales				
OLACACEAE				
Coula edulis		West Africa	Anemia; dysentery; evacuant; skin infections	
Olax gambecolia	Twig	West Africa		
O. subscarpioidea	Twig	West Africa		Root with saponin
Oleales				
SALVADORACEAE				
Salvadora oleoides	Twig	East Africa to Western India		
S. persica[a]	Twig	East Africa and Western India	Diuretic; gastritis; hookworm; venereal disease	Sarakan toothpaste
OLEACEAE				
Ligustrum medium	Stem	Japan (Ainu)		Used as chopsticks
Cornales				
CORNACEAE				
Cornus florida	Twig without bark	Eastern United States	Astringent; colic; emetic; febrifuge	Very hard wood; bitter
Phylogenetic Group 11				
Gentianales				
LOGANIACEAE				
Strychnos afzelii	Stem	West Africa	Evacuant; bad breath; plugging teeth	
RUBIACEAE				
Adina microcepala	Twig	Tropical Africa	Oral infections	Hard wood; alkaloid mitra-phylline
Aulaocalyx jasminiflora	Twig	West Africa		
Coffea ebractealata	Stem	West Africa		
Craterispermum caudatum	Stem	West Africa		
C. laurinum	Stem	Tanzania	Aphrodisiac; fever; vermifuge	

Table 10-1 (Continued)

Order, Family, and Species	Source	Locality Used	Used as/Treatment of	Remarks
Massularia acuminata	Stem	Southern Nigeria	Aphrodisiac; dysentery; anticariogenic; evacuant, lumbago; ophthalmia	
Mussaenda afzelii	Calyx lobe	West Africa	Cough; mouthwash; ophthalmia	Tannin
M. erythrophylla	Root	Tropical Africa	Appetizer; cough; mental problems	
Oxyanthus speciosus[a]	Plant	Tropical Africa	Fever	
O. tenuis	Twig	Tropical Africa		Juice makes skin black
Psychotria suboliqua		West Africa		
P. vogeliana	Stem	Tropical Africa	Analgesic; emetic; fever; filariasis; dysentery	
Rothmannia longiflora		Tropical Africa		
APOCYNACEAE				
Landolphia owariensis		Tropical Africa	Vermifuge	
ASCLEPIADACEAE				
Gongronema latifolium	Stem	Sierra Leone	Colic	
Bignoniales				
BIGNONIACEAE				
Stereospermum kunthianum	Stem	West Africa	Dysentery; evacuant; respiratory ailments; venereal disease; wounds	
Newbouldia laevis	Twig	Nigeria	Bark chewed and swallowed for stomach pains; diarrhea; toothache	
Lamiales				
BORAGINACEAE				
Ehretia thonningiana	Stem	Tropical Africa	Evacuant; dysentery; fever; tetanus	
VERBENACEAE				
Vitex simplicifolia	Stem	Northern Nigeria	Fever; skin infections; toothache	

Asterales			
ASTERACEAE			
Vernonia amygdalina	Roasted root, stem	West Africa	Appetizer; diuretic; evacuant; fever; respiratory; skin infections
V. colorata	Stem	West Africa	Fever
MONOCOTYLEDONS			
Phylogenetic Group 15			
Liliales			
VELLOZIACEAE			
Vellozia equisetoides	Small stem	Tanzania	Asthma

[a] Considered a favorite.

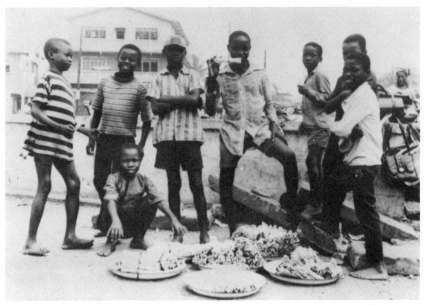

Figure 10-4   Chewing sticks for sale in a Nigerian marketplace (Courtesy C Okolie).

correlate chewing stick use with dental health, it is now not possible to ascertain what impact their use has on a population. The fact remains that in countries where such use is popular caries rates are low, and teeth are retained for longer periods of time.

Chewing sticks used for tooth cleaning are arranged in Table 10-1 by a phylogenetic scheme largely following Thorne[9]

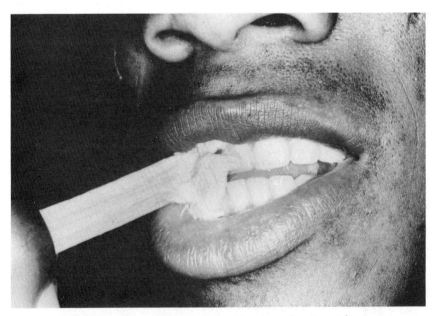

Figure 10-5   Using nature's toothbrush—a chewing stick.

(see Fig. 2-2 and Appendix I). If we accept such a grouping, a number of species concentrations come to have special importance. For example, among the flowering plants, chewing sticks are almost exclusively from dicotyledons with significant numbers among five phylogenetic groupings: group 4, Theales-Ebenales, particularly of *Garcinia* (four spp.) and *Diospyros* (six spp.); group 6, Malvales-Euphorbiales-Rhamnales including nine genera in the Euphorbiaceae; group 7, Rosales, predominantly among the Fabaceae (e.g., *Acacia,* with three spp.); group 9, several important families in the Rutales, particularly the Rutaceae, Anacardiaceae, and Meliaceae; and group 11, a large number of species among the Rubiaceae.

A number of properties, common to these families and genera, may relate to the efficacy of chewing sticks. Thus the Theales-Ebenales grouping is noteworthy for the high fluoride concentrations among certain genera such as *Camellia*[3]; moreover, the widely used genus *Diospyros* produces secondary metabolites having antineoplastic properties,[10] and a 10% infusion of the bark is antibacterial.[11] The compounds having these properties are unknown, yet their activity might well reflect the value placed on them in many African communities.

Among the sixth and seventh phylogenetic groups, the Euphorbiaceae and Fabaceae often possess high concentrations of tannins and resins. The potential protection these compounds provide for the teeth is perhaps reflected by the practice of blackening the teeth with bark from *Antidesma* sp. (Euphorbiaceae) in the Philippines, while peoples of northern Nigeria use twigs of *A. venosum* as toothbrushes.

The Rutaceae possess many alkaloids, resins, and essential oils. *Fagara* species, which are widely used as chewing sticks,

contain the alkaloid artarine; this isoquinoline is related to berberine and has bactericidal, trypanocidal, and antimalarial actions[11] and may also possess anti-sickle cell properties.[12] Moreover, extracts from *F. macrophylla* are scheduled for pharmacological trial in the cancer chemotherapeutic drug program of the (U.S.) National Institutes of Health (Chapter 5). Species of the related genus *Zanthoxylum* are also used as chewing sticks in West Africa, Pakistan, and India. Both genera are prescribed in folk medicine of tropical Africa (*Fagara,* six spp.) and eastern North America (*Zanthoxylum,* two spp.) for treatment of toothache.

The Rubiaceae also contain many alkaloids, and the numerous kinds of sticks used from this large tropical family (best known for coffee and quinine alkaloids) may possess anticariogenic properties.[13]

Some species among certain closely related genera or families are used as chewing sticks throughout their distributions. Thus twigs of the genus *Rhus* in the Anacardiaceae are used in Tanzania and in the Ozarks. In the same family twigs and leaves of *Mangifera* are used in Panama for similar purposes. Likewise, in the Rhamnaceae, several species of *Gouania* are used in tropical America, and *Lasiodiscus* is utilized throughout West Africa.

Many of these plants possess antibacterial properties and high amounts of fluoride or silicon,[14] and this may account, at least in part, for the low caries rate seen among their users. Preliminary studies[13] indicate that certain species used in Africa and the Ozarks have antibacterial properties and can reduce the growth rate and production of acid in cultures of cariogenic bacterial species. In this respect, *Diospyros tricolor,* which had the highest fluoride content of all chewing sticks tested, produced an activity directly attributable to the high content of this ion: it reduced acid production without affecting the rate of growth of cariogenic bacteria. On the other hand, an extract of *Rhus glabra* produced an opposite effect. Both *Massularia acuminata* and *Fagara zanthoxyloides* exerted the greatest anticariogenic effects by affecting both acid production and growth, whereas little activity was noted among species of *Azadirachta, Garcinia,* and *Betula.* Nevertheless, the active ingredients have yet to be identified.

Chewing Sponges

Chewing sponges are a popular means of tooth cleaning in Ghana and are prepared from certain plants and vines, such as *Acacia pennata, Hibiscus rostellatus,* and *Lasianthera africana,* which grow in the Cape Coast region. After branches or vines are harvested from the forest in meter lengths, the bark is removed by scorching and the sticks are beaten on rocks until the interior fibers are released. These are washed, formed into strawlike sponges about 5 inches in diameter, and allowed to dry. Such material is available in market places in Ghana. Throughout West Africa similar sponges are also prepared for body washing, but the use of a tooth-cleaning sponge seems to be more popular in Ghana.

To clean the teeth a bite-sized portion of the sponge is placed in the mouth and vigorously chewed for up to 20 to 30 minutes. This activity produces foam, stimulates the saliva flow, and promotes frequent expectoration. Following this, the sponge is then taken in the fingers and rubbed over the teeth and gums. Throughout this procedure water is used to rinse out the mouth. Usually those that clean with the chewing sponge prefer it to the chewing stick, although its efficacy as a tooth cleaner has yet to be proved.

The use of another West African species, *Termanilia glaucescens,* produces no apparent adverse clinical effect; water extracts have been found to have antibacterial activity.[13]

The vine *Gouania lupuloides,* known throughout West Indies as either the "chaw stick" or the "bon bois," is used in a similar manner, but it is chewed as picked, without elaborate preparation. In this way, pieces of the stem are used both for tooth cleaning, and also to heal and harden the gums.

Tooth-cleaning Fruit

The use of certain fruits for cleaning the teeth is a popular habit among African children of Ghana and Sierra Leone. Both *Agelaea obliqua* and *Cnestis ferruginea* are used for this purpose. *Cnestis* has an especially attractive fruit that grows in bunches on this small shrub. The bright red berries are strawberry shaped, quite pubescent and release a very refreshing, citrus-flavored astringent substance when bitten.

In Ghana, herbalists have used these species and others of the Connaraceae for the treatment of infections, including those of the oral cavity. When alcoholic extracts of some of these genera were tested for their antibacterial activity, inhibitory properties were present in all species tested except those of *Agelaea.*[13]

Toothpicks

Toothpicks made from various willows (*Salix alba, S. jessoensis*) and poplars (*Populus* spp.) are commonly used to remove food impacted between teeth. Fruiting pedicels of *Ammi visnaga* (Apiaceae) serve as toothpicks in Egypt.

Periodontists occasionally prescribe the use of Stim-U-Dents, a triangular piece of wood made from balsa (*Ochroma lagopus,* Bombacaceae), flavored with peppermint, and colored orange. Stim-U-Dents are dispensed on some commercial airlines for after meal cleaning.

Dentrifices

The abrasive substances in most commercially available toothpastes are now largely of inorganic origin, but when toothpastes are unavailable natural abrasives are widely used (Table 10-2). Frequently users also attribute gum-strengthening and tooth-whitening properties to these natural products.

Occasionally a mixture of several plants has been used. Thus in eastern North America the early settlers combined equal amounts of the pulverized barks of *Alnus glutinosa* (black alder), *Myrica*

pensylvanica (bayberry), and *Quercus velutina* (black oak), to which was added one part *Asarum canadense* (American wild ginger) powdered rhizome. Applied as a powder or a decoction, using the finger or a brush, the mixture was said to prevent tooth decay. An infusion of the cortex of *Caesalpinia pulcherrima* (Fabaceae) is applied to the teeth for cleaning by the natives of Nicaragua. Likewise, *Gaultheria procumbens* (wintergreen) roots were chewed for 6 weeks each spring by youngsters to prevent caries.

Commercial toothpastes incorporate hydrophilic colloidal binders to stabilize the formulation and to prevent the separation of solid and liquid phases during storage. These binders, which form

Table 10-2 Abrasive Dentifrices of Natural Origin

Family and Species	Common Name	Locality Used	Plant Material
ANACARDIACEAE			
Lannea grandis		India	Powdered bark
ARACEAE			
Acorus calamus	Sweet flag	Europe and North America	Powdered root
BURSERACEAE			
Commiphora myrrha	Common myrrh tree	Near East	Powdered gum-resin
COMBRETACEAE			
Myrobalanifera sp.		India	Powdered fruit
FABACEAE			
Peltophorum pterocarpum	Soga	Southeast Asia	Powdered bark
KRAMERIACEAE			
Krameria triandra		Bolivia, Peru	Powdered root
LESSONIACEAE (ALGAE)			
Macrocystis pyrifera	Brown alga	[Commercial]	Sodium algenate thickener
POLYGONACEAE			
Rumex crispus	Yellow dock	North America	Powdered root
RHAMNACEAE			
Gouania lupuloides	Toothbrush tree	Central America	Powdered stem
RUBIACEAE			
Cinchona officinalis	Peruvian bark	Europe and North America	Powdered bark
VITACEAE			
Vitis vinifera	European grape	England	Ashes of burned branches

viscous liquid phases by emulsifying droplets or absorbing water, include gum arabic (*Acacia senegal* and other related African species), gum karaya (*Cochlospermum gossypium* and others, *Sterculia tragacantha*, *S. urens*, *S. villosa*), gum tragacanth (*Astragalus gummifera*, *A. prolixus*) and the mucilages from red algae (carrageenan or Irish moss from *Chondrus crispus* and *Gigartina mamillosa*), and brown algae (algin from *Laminaria digitata*, *L. saccharina*, *Macrocystis pyrifera*, and *Nereocystis luetkeana*).

The characteristic flavor of each toothpaste is obtained from several blended components. Among these are the ketone volatile oils extracted from spearmint (*Mentha cardiaca*, *M. spicata*), caraway (*Carum carvi*), and orris root (*Iris germanica*—no longer used because of its allergic potential); the alcohol volatile oil from peppermint (*Mentha piperita*); the aldehyde volatile oils from cinnamon (*Cinnamomum zeylanicum*) and sweet orange, bitter orange, lemon (*Citrus* spp.); phenol volatile oils from cloves (*Eugenia caryophyllus*), thyme (*Thymus vulgaris*), pimenta (*Pimenta officinalis*); phenolic ether volatile oils from anise (*Pimpinella anisum*), nutmeg (*Myristica fragrans*) and sassafras (*Sassafras albidum*); oxide volatile oil from eucalyptus (*Eucalyptus globulus*); and the ester volatile oil from wintergreen (*Gaultheria procumbens*). It is noteworthy that several of these genera found in Africa and North America have been selected as chewing sticks by black populations.

Of special note are the plants from which some commercial toothpastes are made. For example, Sarakan® (Sarakan Ltd., Beckenham, U.K.) incorporates stem and/or root material of *Salvadora persica*. From east Africa through the Sudan and Arabia to western India, this species has long been known as the toothbrush tree[14] and arak.[1] Its use as a chewing·stick or

siwak was documented in the Arabian *Muwashsha* written in AD 900.

The choice of *S. persica* as a dentifrice and chewing stick is attributed to the plant's chemical constituents and anatomical structure, for a nineteenth-century analysis showed that root bark contains 27.06% ash, large amounts of chlorine, and trimethylamine, an alkaloid, and a resin. In addition, Farooqui and Srivastava[14] found silica, sulfur, and vitamin C, but negligible quantities of tannins and saponins. They believe that some of these components are useful in tooth cleaning. For example, the high chloride content would impart dentifrice properties to aid in removing tartar and other stains from the teeth; the silica by its mechanical action should be helpful in tooth whitening, and the resin may form a coat over the enamel, to protect against tooth decay. Moreover, the presence of trimethylamine may have a stimulatory effect on the gingiva, and vitamin C may help in healing spongy and bleeding gums. Bactericidal properties have been attributed to the species having many sulfur compounds.

Anatomically, *S. persica* is well suited to its role as a toothbrush. The large amounts of intraxylary phloem and the widely spaced, thick-walled fibers in the pericycle of the root allow the spongy wood to be easily crushed by the teeth, and softened, if dry, with water. The xylem contains numerous thick-walled vessels and fibers, characteristic of many chewing sticks. These cells produce the fiberlike quality of wood.

A widely used species in the subcontinent of Asia, from which other dentifrices are made (Neem Toothpaste, Calcutta Chemical Co. Ltd., Calcutta and Nimodent toothpowder, Hamdard Co., Karachi, Pakistan), is *Azadirachta indica* or neem tree (Meliaceae: Fig. 10-6). As with Sarakan®, the formulation of the

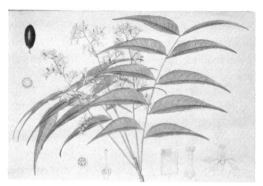

Figure 10-6 *Azadirachta indica* (from R Bentley and H Trimen, *Medicinal Plants* **1**: 62, 1880).

toothpaste and powder is not known, although according to the packaging, fluoride is added along with an extract of the plant. Neem oil, extracted from the seeds, is known to have anti-inflammatory and healing properties and is used especially to treat skin infections. In limited trials carried out in our clinic and elsewhere[15] the toothpaste's possible usefulness in the treatment of gingivitis has been demonstrated. One other commercial product containing plant extracts is known: *Gouania lupuloides* (Rhamnaceae) is used in Jamaica in a mouthwash known as Chew-Dent.

Cleaning Gums

North American Indians and early settlers chewed the gum from *Silphium* spp. (rosinweed) to clean the teeth and keep them white. Similarly, gum from *Myroxylon balsamum* (balsam of Peru) continues to be chewed by the Indians of South America to keep their teeth clean and to tighten and sooth them as well; gum exudate from the trunk of *Croton xalapensis* is likewise used in Mexico for cleaning teeth. Among Bedouin women chewing gum arabic (*Acacia senegal*) is preferred over the use of the siwak (*Salvadora persica*).

TOOTHACHE

Until fairly modern times, caries and accompanying toothache was considered a form of worm infestation (Fig. 10-7) and cures found throughout the world's folk medicine reflected this notion.[1] Reference to this belief was first found in an ancient papyrus dating circa 1200–1100 BC, but ancient Assyrian, Indian, and Aztec[16] works alluded to the same idea. In Babylon toothache was supposed to be caused by a demon that was identified with a worm, as quoted from a text of the time:

After Anu (had created the Heavens),
The heavens created the earth,
The earth created the rivers,
The rivers created the canals,
The canals created the marsh,
The marsh created the worm,
Then came the worm weeping before
  Shamash;
Before Ea came her tears:
"What wilt thou give me for my food?
What wilt thou give me as mine to destroy?"
I will give thee ripe figs and soft pomegranates."
"Me! What are these ripe figs and soft pomegranates
Lift me up, between the teeth and the jawbone set me,
That I may destroy the blood of the teeth,
And ruin their strength,
Grasp the prong and seize the root."

Therefore treatment in China utilized the anthelmintic properties of santonin, and a typical fourteenth-century prescription from the British Isles reads as follows:[17]

Si vermes corrodent dentes—Take the seed of henbane [*Hyoscyamus niger*] and the seed of leeks [*Allium porrum*] and recheles (incense) and do these three things upon a hot glowing tile stone; and make a pipe into the teeth and it shall slay the worms and do away the ache.

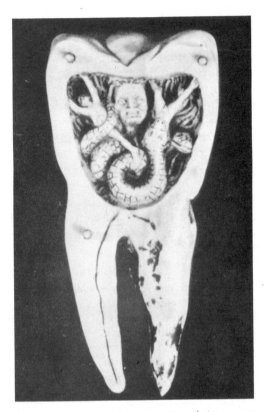

Figure 10-7 Eighteenth century French ivory carving showing the tooth worm (from VM DuMont, *Bildgeschichte der Zahnheilkunde*, Schamberg, Cologne, 1962).

A wide variety of plants, specifically those with analgesic or counterirritant properties, have been used throughout the world to treat toothache. No subculture, from peasants to royalty,[18] is without a seemingly exhaustive list of remedies; many, but by no means all, are listed in Table 10-3.

Many plants found in phylogenetic group 9 are used as toothache remedies. Most notable are members of the genus *Fagara* (Rutaceae): either bark or leaf is chewed for relief, or a decoction is prepared to rinse out the mouth. The citruslike oils found in these plants undoubtedly act as counterirritants, as do other volatile oils so commonly used to treat toothache. Among other groups, the largest number of genera used now or in the past to treat aching teeth are in the families Euphorbiaceae, from which latex is carefully placed in the hollow of carious teeth for relief, Fabaceae, from which gargles and mouthwashes using bark rich in tannins are popular, and Asteraceae, from which some plant parts are chewed and act as local anesthetics.

Toothache is a continuing discomfort to man, but the following quotation from a New England physician practicing in 1677 illustrates how relief could be obtained:

Take a Litle Pece of opium as big as a great pinnes head & put it into the hollow place of the Akeing Tooth & it will give pleasant Ease,

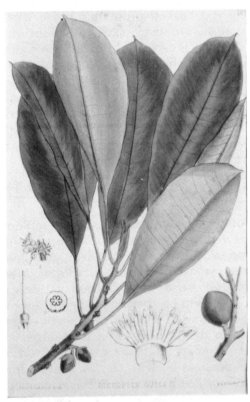

Figure 10-8 *Palaquium gutta* (from R Bentley and H Trimen, *Medicinal Plants* 3: 167, 1880).

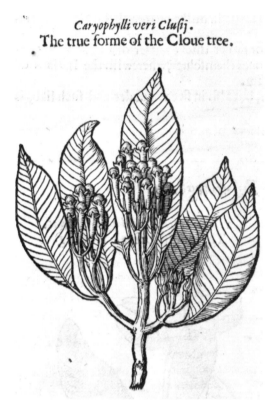

Caryophylli veri Cluſij .
The true forme of the Cloue tree.

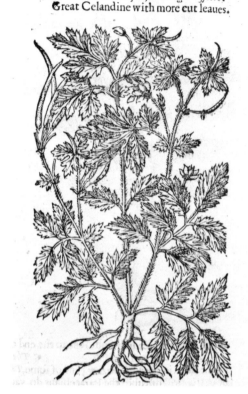

‡ 2 *Chelidonium majus folio magis diſſecto.*
Great Celandine with more cut leaues.

Figure 10-9a *Eugenia caryophyllus* (from J Gerard, *The Herball,* ed 2, 1636).

Figure 10-9b *Chelidonium majus* (from J Gerard, *The Herball,* ed 2, 1636).

often tryed by me upon many People and never fayled.[19]

RESTORATIVE MATERIALS

Latex called gutta percha from numerous sapotaceous trees such as *Palaquium ahernianum* (Philippines), *P. gutta* (Malaya: Fig. 10-8), *P. leiocarpon* (Borneo), *P. maingayi* (Malacca), *P. obovatum* (Malaya), *P. oxleyanum* (Malaya), *Payena leerii* (Burma), *P. obscura* (Malaya), *Sideroxylon attenuatum* (India, Philippines), and *S. kaernbachianum* (New Guinea) is used as a temporary filling for prepared tooth cavities. Its value in

dentistry is related to the ability to harden without becoming brittle on exposure to air; it must be softened by heat before using.

Mastic, the resin from the inner bark of *Pistacia lentiscus* (pistachio tree) was favored by the Turkish people for temporary fillings.

Eugenol, which is the main constituent of clove oil (*Eugenia caryophyllus*: Fig. 10-9a), is mixed with zinc oxide and used as the temporary filling to disinfect root canals from which the pulp has been removed during endodontic treatment prior to permanent restoration of the tooth.[1]

Table 10-3 Plants Used to Relieve Toothache

Order, Family, and Species	Common Name	Locality Used	Procedure
GYMNOSPERMS			
CUPRESSACEAE			
Cupressus arizonica	Arizona cyprus	Southwestern United States	Leaves pounded
PINACEAE			
Thuja plicata	Western red cedar	Northwestern United States	Buds chewed
ANGIOSPERMS:			
DICOTYLEDONS			
Phylogenetic Group 1			
Annonales			
ILLICIACEAE			
Illicium anisatum	Japanese star anise	China	Seed
MAGNOLIACEAE			
Liriodendron tulipifera	Tulip tree	Southern United States	Warm root bark decoction applied to infected teeth
ANNONACEAE			
Annona senegalensis	Wild custard apple	West Africa	Bark infusion as mouthwash
Xylopia macrantha		Panama	Plant used
MYRISTICACEAE			
Myristica fragrans	Nutmeg	Europe, North America	Nutmeg oil on cotton into carious teeth
LAURACEAE			
Cinnamomum spp.		Europe, North America	Cinnamon oil on cotton into carious teeth (see also with *Casuarina equisetifolia* and *Nepeta cataria*)
Persea americana	Avocado	Philippines	Piece of seed or decocation into carious teeth
Sassafras albidum	Sassafras	Eastern United States	Commercial dental poultice includes *Sassafras* root, *Capsicum*, and *Humulus* (hops) plus benzocaine and hydroxyquinoline sulfate; see also *Nepeta* (Lamiaceae)
PIPERACEAE			
Piper alegreanum		Brazil	Decoction of roots, stems, and leaves
P. darienense		Panama	Fruit very effective
P. sp.		Brazil	Stem anesthetizes area
Pothomorphe peltata		Brazil	Leaves on swollen area
P. umbellata		Panama	Leaves
Berberidales			
MENISPERMACEAE			
Tinomiscium tonkinense	Var kan	North Vietnam	Juice from plant

250

Table 10-3 (Continued)

Order, Family, and Species	Common Name	Locality Used	Procedure
RANUNCULACEAE			
Ranunculus hietus		New Zealand	Plant
BERBERIDACEAE			
Mahonia ganpinnensis		China	Plant
PAPAVERACEAE			
Bocconia frutescens		Panama	Latex
Chelidonium majus	Celandine poppy	England	Decoction of plant or juice gargled
Dicentra formosa	Bleeding heart	Northwestern United States	Root chewed
Papaver somniferum	Opium poppy	Europe	Opium powder into carious teeth
Sanguinaria canadensis	Bloodroot	Eastern North America	Root applied to carious teeth
Phylogenetic Group 2			
Hamamelidales			
HAMAMELIDACEAE			
Liquidambar styraciflua	Sweet gum	United States and Mexico	Gum applied to cheek
Casuarinales			
CASUARINACEAE			
Casuarina equisetifolia	Swamp oak	Panama	Fruit mixed with powdered nutmeg
Fagales			
FAGACEAE			
Fagus ferruginea	American beech	Eastern North America	Cotton soaked in creosote and placed into carious teeth
BETULACEAE			
Alnus glutinosa	Black alder	England	Inner bark as mouthwash
Phylogenetic Group 3			
Chenopodiales			
PHYTOLACCACEAE			
Petiveria alliacea	Guinea hen weed	Panama	Root chewed
AIZOACEAE			
Galenia africana		South Africa	Plant chewed
Sceletium tortuosum		South Africa	Leaf chewed (narcotic?)
AMARANTHACEAE			
Aerva sp.		Philippines	Fruit
Polygonales			
POLYGONACEAE			
Polygonum bistorta	Bistort	England	Root mixed equally with *Anacyclus pyrethrum* (Asteraceae) and alum, beaten into paste with honey, and placed into carious teeth or held between teeth

Table 10-3 (Continued)

Order, Family, and Species	Common Name	Locality Used	Procedure
Phylogenetic Group 4			
Theales			
CLUSIACEAE			
Allanblackia floribunda	Tallow tree	Central African Republic, Chad, Congo Republic, Gabon	Bark decoction
Clusia utilis		Guatemala	Fruit juice soaked in cotton, placed in tooth
Ebenales			
EBENACEAE			
Euclea natalensis		South Africa	Powdered root
E. udulata		South Africa	Root
STYRACACEAE			
Styrax benzoin		Europe, North America	Tincture of benzoin containing benzoresin soaked on cotton and pressed into carious teeth
Primulales			
MYRSINACEAE			
Myrsine australis		New Zealand	Leaf infusion
THEOPHRASTACEAE			
Jacquinia macrocarpa		Cuba	Cortex
PRIMULACEAE			
Anagallis arvensis	Pimpernel	England	Plant juices as gargle
Plumbaginales			
PLUMBAGINACEAE			
Plumbago europaea	Common plumbago	England	Root or bruised seeds into carious teeth
Phylogenetic Group 5			
Cistales			
FLACOURTIACEAE			
Paropsia brazzaeana		South Africa	Root infusion as gargle
PASSIFLORACEAE			
Smeathmannia pubescens		Liberia	Bark from twigs
CARICACEAE			
Carica papaya	Papaya	Samoa	Inner bark for sore teeth
Capparidales			
BRASSICACEAE			
Brassica nigra	Black mustard	England	Seeds chewed
MORINGACEAE			
Moringa oleifera	Horseradish tree	Panama	Bark
Phylogenetic Group 6			
Malvales			
BOMBACACEAE			
Bombax ellipticum		Central America	Bark or root decoction; hardening of gums
Urticales			
ULMACEAE			
Chaetacme aristata		South Africa	Powdered root

Table 10-3   (Continued)

Order, Family, and Species	Common Name	Locality Used	Procedure
MORACEAE			
Chlorophora tinctoria		Brazil	Milky juice
Ficus barclayana		Fiji	Ripe fruit into carious teeth
F. retusa		China	Powdered small roots mixed with salt
URTICACEAE			
Fleurya lanceolata		Tanzania	Leaf juice as mouthwash
Obetia pinnatifida		Tanzania	Leaf juice as mouthwash
Euphorbiales			
EUPHORBIACEAE			
Alchornea cordifolia	Christmas bush	West Africa	Hot root pith into carious teeth
Bischofia javanica		Samoa	Root
Breynia fruticosa		Indochina	
B. sp.		Solomon Islands	Leaf macerated in water and placed in mouth
Croton alanosanus		Mexico	Resin
C. xalapensis		Guatemala	
Euphorbia antiquorum		India	Plant juice
E. gorgonis		South Africa	Latex
E. pugniformis		South Africa	Latex into carious teeth
E. thymifolia	Golondrina	Central America	Cotton soaked in latex
E. tirucalli		India	Latex
Ricinus communis	Castor bean	South Africa	Root paste into carious teeth; root boiled twice with corn stalks, then smeared on teeth and gums
Synadenium cupulare		South Africa	Latex in carious teeth
THYMELAEACEAE			
Dirca palustris	Leatherwood	Eastern North America	Inner bark masticated
Lasiosiphon capitatus		Basutoland	Poultice of plant to jaw
L. meisnerianum		South Africa	Plant chewed; powdered root into carious teeth
Rhamnales			
RHAMNACEAE			
Krugiodendron ferreum	Black ironwood	Mexico	Bark and root
Zizyphus endlichii		Mexico	Bark
Phylogenetic Group 7			
Rosales			
ROSACEAE			
Potentilla reptans	Cinquefoil	England	Root boiled in vinegar and decoction held in mouth
Rubus spectabilis	Salmonberry	Northwestern United States	Bark pounded and placed in teeth

Table 10-3 (Continued)

Order, Family, and Species	Common Name	Locality Used	Procedure
FABACEAE			
Acacia catechu	Catechu	India	Wood and bark
A. nilotica		Ghana	Fruit decoction with ginger as mouthwash
Caesalpinia crista		Panama	Plant used
Daniellia oliveri		West Africa	Leaf and bark decoction as mouthwash
Dialium guineense		Ghana, Ivory Coast	Bark decoction as mouthwash
Dichrostachys cinerea		South Africa	
Indigofera cf. *patens*		South Africa	Powdered root into carious teeth
Intsia bijuga		Fiji	
Lysiloma watsoni			Bark chewed
Mimosa pigra		Panama	Decoction of leafy stem as mouthwash
Parkia africana	African locust	Gambia	Bark
Piliostigma thonningii		Ghana	Warm infusion of bark and leaves
		Sudan	Leaf decoction as gargle
Psoralea corylifolia	Ku-tzü	India to Southeastern Asia	Root into carious teeth
Pterocarpus marsupium	Vengai padauk	India	Gum from incised bark
Sarothamnus scoparium	Broom	England	Oil or water obtained from heated green twigs
DROSERACEAE			
Drosera sp.	Sundew	Mexico	Plant decoction
Phylogenetic Group 8			
Myrtales			
COMBRETACEAE			
Combretum hypotilinum		West Africa	Gum
MYRTACEAE			
Decaspermum coriandri		Solomon Islands	Fruit placed against teeth
Eugenia caryophyllus	Clove tree	Europe, India, North America	Cotton soaked in clove oil and placed into carious teeth; active ingredient (eugenol) has local anesthetic action; a favorite remedy (see also *Nepetia cataria*)
Melaleuca cajuputi	Cajuput	Europe, North America, Malaysia, Australia	Cotton soaked in cajeput oil and placed into carious teeth
Psidium guajava	Guava	Panama	Leaves chewed
MELASTOMATACEAE			
Osbeckia crinita	Dok ka san	Vietnam	Dried leaf decoction
Tibouchina longifolia		El Salvador	Plant decoction held in mouth

Table 10-3 (Continued)

Order, Family, and Species	Common Name	Locality Used	Procedure
Phylogenetic Group 9			
Geraniales			
ZYGOPHYLLACEAE			
Kallstroemia grandiflora	Caltrop	North America	Leaves chewed
Polygalales			
POLYGALACEAE			
Securidaca longipedunculata		South Africa	Root chewed
Rutales			
RUTACEAE			
Citrus sinensis	Sweet orange	Panama	Fruit peelings
Clausena anisata		West Africa	Roots and leaves
Fagara capensis		South Africa	Bark
F. humilis		South Africa	Leaf
F. magaliesmontana		South Africa	Bark
F. olitoria		Tanzania	Bark decoction to rinse out carious teeth
F. rubescens	Bolongo	Tropical Africa	Bark decoction
F. xanthoxyloides	Candlewood	Ghana	Root bark boiled with *Capsicum* peppers in rice water and thin corn starch and held in mouth while hot as long as possible
Murraya exotica		Panama	Twigs chewed
Ruta graveolens	Common rue	South Africa	Bruised leaf into carious teeth
Toddalia aculeata	Wild orange tree	South Africa	Leaf chewed or leaf poultice into carious teeth or against teeth
Zanthoxylum americanum	Northern prickly ash, toothache tree	Eastern North America	Bark or mashed bark into or around carious teeth
Z. clava-herculis	Southern prickly ash, toothache tree	Eastern North America	Bark or mashed bark into or around carious teeth
BURSERACEAE			
Bursera penicillata		Mexico	Resin
ANACARDIACEAE			
Mangifera indica	Mango	Panama	Bark
Pistacia lentiscus	Pistachio	Europe, North America	Resin mastic soaked in cotton and placed into carious teeth
Spondias dulcis	Otaheite apple	Fiji	Bark decoction
SAPINDACEAE			
Dodonaea viscosa	Switchsorrel	Panama	Leaves chewed
Myricales			
MYRICACEAE			
Comptonia aspleniifolia	Sweet fern	North America	Boiled leaves as poultice against cheek

255

Table 10-3 (Continued)

Order, Family, and Species	Common Name	Locality Used	Procedure
Phylogenetic Group 10			
Santalales			
CELASTRACEAE			
Celastrus richii		Fiji	Leaves chewed
OLACACEAE			
Ximenia americana	Tallow wood	Panama	Root chewed
Cornales			
VITACEAE			
Cissus rotundifolia		Tanzania	Root
ARALIACEAE			
Hedera helix	English ivy	England	Gum into carious teeth
APIACEAE			
Angelica archangelica	Angelica	England	Plant juice into carious teeth; angelica oil used in dental preparations
Berula thunbergii		South Africa	Root chewed or held in mouth
Hydrocotyle bonariensis		Peru	Root
Peucedanum officinale	Hog's fennel	England	Plant juice mixed in wine, into carious teeth
Sium thunbergii	Water parsnip	South Africa (Cape)	Root
Phylogenetic Group 11			
Gentianales			
RUBIACEAE			
Calycosia petiolata		Fiji	Bark
Cephalanthus occidentalis	Buttonbush	Eastern North America	Bark chewed
Galium bungei			Heated leaves and stem placed between teeth
Morinda citrifolia		Samoa	Root
APOCYNACEAE			
Carissa edulis		Guyana	Leaf poultice
Thevetia peruviana	Trumpet flower	Panama, Yucatan	Latex soaked in cotton
Voacanga africana		West Africa	Latex into carious teeth
ASCLEPIADACEAE			
Secamone sp.		Philippines	Fruit heated, pounded with a little salt and applied to carious teeth
Bignoniales			
SCROPHULARIACEAE			
Conobea scoparioides		Colombia	Plant placed into carious teeth
Stemodia parviflora		Costa Rica	Plant
PLANTAGINACEAE			
Plantago media	Plantain	Russia	Small root placed in ear on side of aching teeth

Table 10-3 (Continued)

Order, Family, and Species	Common Name	Locality Used	Procedure
P. major	Plantain	Europe	Fibrous strands from petiole for carious teeth if placed in the *ear* of affected side
ACANTHACEAE			
Barleria prionitis		South Africa	Root decoction as mouthwash
		Java	Leaves chewed
B. procumbens		South Africa	Paste from fresh leaves applied
Solanales			
SOLANACEAE			
Hyoscyamus muticus		Middle East and North Africa (Bedouins)	Plant smoked
H. niger	Black henbane	England	Seed[17]
H. reticulatus		India	Seed
Nicotiana tabacum	Tobacco	England	Leaves crushed and placed into carious teeth or cotton soaked in leaf decoction and placed around carious teeth
Solanum indicum		India	Vapor of burning seed or root
S. panduraeforme		Basutoland	Root
CONVOLVULACEAE			
Convolvulus bidentatus		South Africa	Root
Lamiales			
VERBENACEAE			
Lippia pringlei		Mexico	Sap
Vitex simplicifolia		Ivory Coast	Bark decoction
LAMIACEAE			
Melissa officinalis	Common balm	England	Leaves steeped in wine and used as mouthwash
Nepeta cataria	Catnip	American Ozarks	Catnip + ground cloves *Eugenia caryophyllata* (Myrtaceae) in equal parts + one-half the amount of sassafras bark *Sassafras albidum* (Lauraceae)—stir in a small amount of water to moisten, and apply as poultice to aching teeth
Origanum majorana	Sweet marjoram	Europe, North America	Marjoram oil soaked in cotton and into carious teeth
O. vulgare	Marjoram	Europe	Plant
Salvia occidentalis		Panama	Plant

Table 10-3   (Continued)

Order, Family, and Species	Common Name	Locality Used	Procedure
S. officinalis	Garden sage	England	Plant decoction with wine gargled
		Russia	Plant decoction with hot water flushing the affected side of the mouth
Campanulales			
CAMPANULACEAE			
Platycodon grandiflorum		China	
Asterales			
ASTERACEAE			
Achillea lanulosa	Yarrow	Nevada	Green leaves chewed
A. millefolium	Yarrow	Eastern North America	Fresh leaves chewed
Anacyclus officinarum		England	Plant juice as mouthwash and as tincture
A. pyrethrum	Pellitory		See *Polygonum bistorta*
Artemisia afra		South Africa	Fresh tip of plant inserted into carious teeth
Crassocephalum subscandens		Tanzania	Leaf
Gaillardia aristata		Montana	Root chewed, acting as anesthetic
Hymenopappus lugens		Southwestern United States (Hopi Indians)	Root
Microglossa oblongifolia		Tanzania	Leaf
Salmea eupatoria		Mexico	Roots chewed to deaden pain
S. scandens		Panama	Plant chewed; root acts as anesthetic
Solidago sp.	Goldenrod	American Ozarks	Root into carious teeth
Spilanthes acmella	Akarkara	Pantropics	Flower tincture
S. mauritiana		South Africa	Flowers chewed or moistened; powdered leaves into carious teeth
S. ocymifolia		Panama	Root chewed
Tarchonanthus camphoratus	Hottentot tobacoo	South Africa	Plant
Verbesina pinnatifida		Mexico	Root boiled
MONOCOTYLEDONS			
Phylogenetic Group 13			
Arales			
ARACEAE			
Acorus calamus	Sweet flag	Europe, North America	Rootstock
Scindapsus sp.		Oceania	Stem chewed
Arecales			
ARECACEAE			
Cocos nucifera	Coco palm	Panama	Resin extracted by eating inner husk of coconut

Table 10-3   (Continued)

Order, Family, and Species	Common Name	Locality Used	Procedure
Phylogenetic Group 14			
Commelinales			
CYPERACEAE			
Cyperus cyperoides		Philippines	Seed infusion
Zingiberales			
MUSACEAE			
Musa paradisiaca subsp. *sapientum*	Banana	Panama, South Africa	Juice from junction of "branch with stem"
ZINGIBERACEAE			
Alpinia officinarum	Galangol		Rhizome shavings around aching teeth
Kaempferia galanga		China	Galanga rhizome; also used for purulent gums
Phylogenetic Group 15			
Liliales			
LILIACEAE			
Agave americana	Century plant	India	Root and leaf gum
Allium sativum	Garlic	Europe, North America	Bulb against gum
Asparagus officinalis	Asparagus	England	Root decoction mixed with wine
Smilax sp.		New Guinea	Macerated bark from base of stem applied to teeth
Veratum viride	White hellebore	Eastern North America	Root powder into carious teeth
IRIDACEAE			
Iris missouriensis	Wild iris	Western North America	Pulped raw rhizome
Orchidales			
ORCHIDACEAE			
Cremastra wallichiana	Hakkuri	Japan (Ainu)	Root chewed and expectorated; the sticky sap clings to teeth

TOOTH EXTRACTION

Normally teeth are extracted surgically, but according to folklore they may be removed readily if treated with certain plant materials. At one time in England, for example, the powder from dried roots of the celandine poppy (*Chelidonium majus*: Fig. 10-9*b*) was placed on aching hollow or whole teeth, to effect removal. In Panama the Indians place the latex from *Chlorophora tinctoria* (Moraceae) or *Hura crepitans* (Euphorbiaceae) on ailing teeth, to cause them to fall out. Likewise in western Africa, seed oil from *Ximenia americana* (Olacaceae) is placed in carious teeth prior to extraction in order to facilitate removal, and powdered root or bark obtained from *Acacia pennata* (Fabaceae) and soaked in palm wine is dipped in cotton for plugging carious teeth, to promote ease of extraction. From these few examples, it is apparent that the area of herbal extractors requires study.

PERIODONTAL DISEASE

The greatest loss of teeth in adults is caused by periodontal disease, which is the progressive destruction of the supporting structures of the teeth: the gingiva, periodontium, and alveolar bone. This disease, like caries, is dependent on accumulations of plaque. Although the mechanisms are not clear, it is initiated after subgingival plaque appears. The organism present can directly initiate inflammation, induce hypersensitivity (allergic) reactions, and further destroy the tissue by releasing potent enzymes such as collagenases, chondroitin sulfatases, and various other proteolytic enzymes. Its etiology remains obscure because several types of organisms, including species of *Actinomyces,* spirochetes, and *Bacteroides,* must be present in combination before the syndrome can be induced in gnotobiotic animals.

Gingival bleeding is the predominant symptom of the milder form of periodontal disease, whereas as the condition progresses, pain, inflammation, and loosening of the teeth become more apparent. Treatment, which depends on the severity, involves removal of plaque and debridement of the diseased area. Preventive methods include frequent scaling (professional cleaning) to remove accumulations of plaque and calculus, and the use of a water pulsating apparatus and dental floss to aid in removal of food and plaque that may have become impacted between the teeth.

A related disorder, acute necrotizing ulcerative gingivitis (ANUG, or trench mouth), is characterized by acute inflammation of the gums. This condition usually precipitates suddenly in young adults who are under some form of stress and practice poor oral hygiene. It is not clear whether the disease is transmissible; however oral *Bacteroides* species and spirochetes have been implicated. Treatment is similar to that for periodontal disease.

Folk medicine is rich with plant-derived products used to treat periodontal disease. Decoctions of roots or bark as mouthwashes are frequently employed to restore and strengthen gums or to cure inflammatory and infectious processes. A representative sample is provided in Table 10-4.

Various commercial mouthwashes are available for halitosis, or to sweeten the

Table 10-4   Plants Used to Treat Periodontal Disease

Family and Species	Common Name	Locality Used	Plant Material and Principal Activity
ANACARDIACEAE			
Pistacia lentiscus	Pistachio tree	Turkey	Mastic for hardening gums
Rhus virens	Lambrisco	Mexico	Plant good for gums and teeth
APIACEAE			
Heracleum maximum	Cow parsnip	Eastern North America	Dried powdered roots on gums to relieve discomfort
ARALIACEAE			
Panax ginseng	Ginseng	Eastern Europe (experimental study)	Extract applied topically into the alveolar recesses

Table 10-4   (Continued)

Family and Species	Common Name	Locality Used	Plant Material and Principal Activity
ASTERACEAE			
Solidago vergaurea	European goldenrod	England	Plant decoction helps fasten loose teeth
Spilanthes mauritiana			Flowers chewed for pyorrhea
BIGNONIACEAE			
Tecomaria capensis		South Africa	Powdered bark rubbed around teeth for bleeding gums
BURSERACEAE			
Commiphora myrrha	Common myrrh tree	Near East	Resin used for spongy gums
EUPHORBIACEAE			
Acalypha phleoides		Mexico	Plant decoction as mouthwash for sore gums and loose teeth
Fluggea virosa		Philippines	Decoction of boiled roots for curing gums
Jatropha dioica		Mexico	Tea for tightening teeth
FABACEAE			
Mimosa palmeri		Mexico	Bark chewed to harden gums
Piliostigma thonningii		Central Africa	Concentrated bark infusion as mouthwash for gum inflammation
GERANIACEAE			
Geranium maculatum	Wild cranesbill	Eastern North America	Root infusion for sore gums and pyorrhea
LILIACEAE			
Allium sativum	Garlic	Europe	For loose teeth
MELIACEAE			
Aglaia sp.		Philippines	Bark chewed for loose teeth
MYRICACEAE			
Myrica cerifera	Southern wax myrtle	Southern United States	Root bark decoction for spongy gums
POLYGONACEAE			
Eriogonum atrorubens		Mexico	Root (astringent) chewed for gums
RHAMNACEAE			
Gouania lupuloides	Toothbrush tree	Tropical Africa	Stem for healing and hardening gums
ROSACEAE			
Fragaria vesca	Strawberry	England	Root and leaves lotions and gargles for fastening loose teeth
SOLANACEAE			
Solanum merkeri		Tanzania	Root for swollen gums
SYMPLOCACEAE			
Symplocos racemosa		India	Bark decoction for gargle in bleeding gums

breath generally; most contain plant derivatives similar to the flavorings added to toothpaste. Because certain oral bacteria can develop resistance to components of these and other substances in mouthwashes, it is advisable to vary them frequently. Also, the gum-resin or myrrh from various species of *Commiphora* is employed widely as an astringent.

Although mouthwashes from noncommercial sources are normally used by indigenous peoples to combat periodontal disease and caries, a number serve strictly as breath sweeteners, namely, the mastic from *Pistacia lentiscus,* chewed by Oriental women, chamomile tea (*Matricaria chamomilla*), employed as a rinse for bad breath principally in Europe, and a leaf decoction of *Mussaenda afzelii* recommended in Liberia as a mouthwash for children.

ORAL INFECTIONS

CANDIASIS (MONILIASIS, THRUSH, CANDIDOSIS)

Although *Candida albicans* and related yeast-like species are found as normal oral inhabitants, their numbers are usually low due to competition with other organisms. Under unique conditions that upset this balance, they are able to increase their numbers dramatically and initiate disease. For example, thrush, a generalized infection characterized by pseudomembranes on the oral mucosal surfaces and tongue, usually occurs in early infancy before natural immunity develops. Similarly, when antibiotic therapy reduces the normal inhibiting bacterial flora or ill-fitting dentures increase the total acidogenic flora, *Candida* species (Fig. 10-10) can proliferate and cause adult thrush, perleche (infection of the corners of the mouth), penicillin sore-

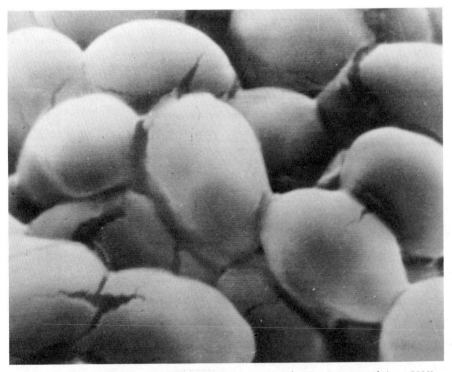

Figure 10-10   *Candida albicans* within a colony, scanning electron micrograph (ca. ×5000).

tongue, diarrhea, and anal pruritis. Although the reasons are not clear, a *Candida*-associated gingivitis may also develop among young adult females who suffer from thrush.

Treatment usually includes use of such antifungal antibiotics as nystatin (Mycostatin®) from *Streptomyces noursei* or amphotericin B from *S. nodosus*. To prevent overgrowth of *Candida* spp. during antibiotic therapy, the antifungal agents are often administered prophylactically along with broad-spectrum antibiotics. These drugs when given orally or topically are devoid of toxicity and only rarely produce mild transitory symptoms such as nausea, vomiting, or diarrhea.

The effectiveness of therapy with yoghurt (a sour-tasting milk culture containing various species of *Lactobacillus* including *L. bulgaricus,* living cultures in pill form of *L. acidophilus* [Bacid®—USV] or a mixed culture of *L. acidophilus* and *L. bulgaricus* [Lactinex®—Hynson, Westcott & Dunning]) has yet to be determined by controlled trials, but it is promoted for various oral and intestinal disorders and is also prescribed during broad-spectrum antibiotic therapy. It is believed by many that these organisms help restore the normal balance of the oral flora lost by antibiotic therapy or because of loose dentures. In this respect, physicians frequently use yoghurt for treating antibiotic diarrhea, and pruritis and oral ulcerations. Yoghurt therapy for denture sore mouth produced by *Candida* has also been successful.

Thrush was treated by the North American Indians with mouthwashes prepared from either the boiled bark of persimmon (*Diospyros virginiana*) or the root of the winter grape (*Vitis vulpina*) (Table 10-5). When introduced by settlers, the gums or resins of myrrh (*Commiphora myrrha*) were combined with tinctures of raspberry leaves and used to rinse the mouth two or three times a day. Elsewhere, the Hawaiians prescribed poultices or gargles made from *Euphorbia hirta* and the Melanese gargled with decoctions from the lime, *Citrus aurantifolia.*

HERPETIC GINGIVOSTOMATITIS (COLD SORES, RECURRENT HERPES, FEVER BLISTERS)

Infection of the oral mucosa or lips with herpesvirus (type I) can produce a primary self-limiting disease characterized by vesicular eruptions, scattered throughout the mouth and oropharynx, and recurring in some patients in a milder form thereafter. Such recurrent episodes are often predisposed by stress, endocrine disorders including menses, fever, and other infections.

Specific treatments with antiviral drugs such as 5-iodo-2′-deoxyuridine (IDU) or similar derivatives have not been as successful with oral infections as those with the eye (keratoconjunctivitis).

Early settlers applied the resin or gum of sweet gum (*Liquidambar styraciflua,* Hamamelidaceae) to alleviate the pain and inflammation of such lesions.

APHTHOUS STOMATITIS (CANKER SORES)

There are two distinct forms of recurrent oral ulcers (ROU): one is mild, the other severe and scarring. Both are characterized by the development on the oral mucosa of round or oval lesions with grayish or grayish-yellow covering of necrotic slough or serofibrinous exudate; intensely raw, red tissue may appear around the base. The lesion is larger and deeper in the more severe form and may be associated with mandibular lymphadenopathy. Recurrent episodes are predisposed by trauma, stress, chemical irritants (e.g., aspirin), and various foods containing essential oils, and citric or acetic acid. The L-form of *Streptococcus sanguis* has been implicated, and the severity of the lesion is associated with increasing degrees of autoimmunity.

Therapy with antibiotics or corticosteroids has produced little permanent improvement. Topical applications of a cream containing an-

Table 10-5   Plants and Plant Extracts for Treatment of Oral Infections

Family and Species	Common Name	Locality Used	Plant Material and Principal Activity
AIZOACEAE *Carpobrotus acinaciforme*		South Africa	Boiled fruit and leaf juices for sore mouth
ANACARDIACEAE *Rhus glabra*	Smooth sumac	North America	Root bark decoction for aphthous and mercurial sore mouth and other mucous membrane infections (e.g., venereal disease)
ASTERACEAE *Spilanthes mauritiana*		South Africa	Plant rubbed on lips and gums of child suffering from sore mouth
BURSERACEAE *Commiphora myrrha*	Common myrrh tree	Near East	Gum-resin tincture for ulcerated sore mouth
CORNACEAE *Cornus florida*	Dogwood	Eastern North America	Bark decoction for sore mouth
EBENACEAE *Diospyros virginiana*	Persimmon	Eastern North America	Boiled bark decoction for sore lips and mouth of babies
EUPHORBIACEAE *Euphorbia hirta*		Hawaii	Gargle and poultice for thrush
Hymenocardia acida		South Africa	Ashed roots for mouth infections
Sapium ellipticum		Central Africa	Bark decoction as mouthwash for scurvy
FABACEAE *Vicia faba*	Broad bean	North America	Ground dried beans for sore mouth
FAGACEAE *Quercus alba*	White oak	North America	Bark decoction for sore lips and mouth
PINACEAE *Pseudotsuga taxifolia*	Douglas fir	Washington State	Bud tips chewed for mouth sores
POLYPODIACEAE *Pellaea calomelanus*	Cliff-brake fern	South Africa	Rhizome decoction for boils and mouth cankers
RANUNCULACEAE *Coptis groenlandica*	Goldthread	Eastern North America	Roots chewed for mouth sores
Hydrastis canadensis	Golden seal	Eastern North America	Roots chewed for mouth sores

Table 10-5   (Continued)

Family and Species	Common Name	Locality Used	Plant Material and Principal Activity
ROSACEAE			
Fragaria vesca	Strawberry	England	Fruit juice for mouth ulcers, root or leaf decoctions as lotions or gargles for ulcers and sore mouths
RUBIACEAE			
Psychotria sp.		Solomon Islands	Sap decoction for sore mouth
RUTACEAE			
Citrus aurantifolia	Sour orange	Malaya	Leaf decoction as mouthwash or gargle for thrush (and sore throat)
Fagara capensis		South Africa	Root decoction as mouthwash for aphthae in children
SOLANACEAE			
Solanum verbascifolium		Solomon Islands	Leaf decoction as wash for sore mouth

tibiotics, such as neomycin and gramicin with triamcinolone acetonide, are prescribed. Abstinence from use of toothpastes, chewing gums, etc., that contain flavoring agents like peppermint and cinnamon have also often prevented recurrences.

ACTINOMYCOSIS AND OTHER BACTERIAL INFECTIONS CAUSING CELLULITIS AND OSTEOMYELITIS

Trauma through extraction or injury may allow certain of the oral *Actinomyces* to initiate a chronic, suppurative, or granulomatous lesion frequently localized in the cervicofacial region. The condition spreads slowly through the contiguous tissues and forms multiple outward draining sinuses, discharging distinctive bacterial colonies called sulfur granules. Penicillin or its synthetic derivatives are the drugs of choice.

Cellulitis and osteomyelitis, with accompanying draining sinuses and swollen facial tissues, may also result from infection with oral anaerobic streptococci and staphylococci present in tooth abscesses or diseased gums. Choice of the appropriate antibiotic depends on the organism identified and its antibiotic sensitivity. Penicillin and its synthetic derivatives, erythromycin and tetracycline, are frequently used in therapy.

SYSTEMIC INFECTIONS WITH ORAL MANIFESTATIONS

Oral lesions or symptoms, including some that are pathodiagnostic, are associated with diseases producing clinical symptoms elsewhere in the body. Among these are the bacterial infections causing syphilis, gonorrhea, tuberculosis, actinomycosis, plague, glanders, diphtheria, leprosy, sporotrichosis, and lymphogranuloma venereum; the viral infections causing varicella–zoster (chicken pox–shingles), infectious mononucleosis–Burkitt's lymphoma–nasopharyngeal carcinoma, foot and mouth disease, herpangina, hand–foot and mouth disease, acute nodular pharyngitis, vesicular stomatitis, rabies, measles, rubella, influenza, common cold, and mumps; the fungal infections causing histoplasmosis, South American blastomycosis, coccidiomycosis; and the parasitic diseases of leishmaniasis, gonglyonema, and trichinosis.

Specific antibiotic therapy is used for bacterial and fungal infections, surgery or chemotherapeutic agents for the parasitic diseases, and supportive therapy, where possible, for viral infections.[20]

CHEWING GUMS

The chewing of gum based on chicle—the latex usually obtained from the stem of *Achras zapota* (sapodilla) for ordinary chewing gum or from *Mimusops balata* for "bubble gum"—is a North American habit often viewed disparagingly by those who do not chew. It is quite clear, however, that indigenous populations throughout the world have long practiced the chewing of latex, gum, and resin (Table 10-6). This is particularly striking when one realizes that plant exudates from the Anacardiaceae, Apocynaceae, Asclepiadaceae, Asteraceae, Euphorbiaceae, Moraceae, and Sapotaceae, to note the most commonly

used families, are often quite bitter, unlike commercially available gum that is flavored with mint, sugar, and other plant products to improve taste and flavor.

Gum chewing has been considered to be a contributory factor to caries, and for many years a number of sugarless gums have been suggested as alternative to those containing sucrose. Recent clinical trials indicate, however, that no difference exists between sugarless types and gums made with sugar. Recent animal studies have shown that sorbitol and mannitol contained in the sugarless gums were just as effective in inducing caries as sucrose.[21] Moreover, chewing of gum regardless of sugar content was found to decrease dramatically the amount of plaque formed by gum users, compared to individuals who did not chew.

TOOTH COLORING

Everywhere in Southeast Asia and Polynesia tooth coloring was used by indigenous populations to indicate sexual maturity or marriage. Yap natives of the Caroline Islands considered black teeth a sort of love fetish and did the blackening

Table 10-6　Chewing Gums

Family and Species	Common Name	Locality Used	Plant Part Chewed
ANACARDIACEAE			
Pistacia mutica	Turk terebinth, pistachio	Iran	Gum (Bombay mastic)
Schinus molle	Brazil pepper-tree	Brazil	Gum (American mastic) from trunk
APOCYNACEAE			
Apocynum cannabinum	Indian hemp	North America	Latex
Couma guatemalensis		Central America	Latex
C. macrocarpa		Brazil	Latex
Dyera costulata	Jelutong	Malaya	Substitute for chicle
Stemmadenia galeottiana		Mexico	Latex

Table 10-6   (Continued)

Family and Species	Common Name	Locality Used	Plant Part Chewed
ARAUCARIACEAE			
Agathis australis	Kauri	New Zealand	Resin (kauri gum)
ASCLEPIADACEAE			
Asclepias eriocarpa	Woollypod milkweed	California	Latex
Asclepiodophora decumbens	Spider antelope horn	Nevada, Utah	Latex
ASTERACEAE			
Actinella biennis		New Mexico	Root bark
Agoseris villosa		British Columbia	Stem latex
Chrysothamnus nauseosus	Rabbit bush	Western North America	Gum
C. viscidiflorus	Rabbit bush	Nevada, Utah	Roots
Echinops viscosus		Greece	Gum
Encelia farinosa	White brittlebush	Arizona	Gum
Hymenopappus filifolius		New Mexico	Root
Lygodesmia juncea	Rush skeleton weed	Missouri valley	Juice
Silphium laciniatum	Rosinweed	Eastern North America	Resin
COMBRETACEAE			
Combretum lecananthum		West Africa	Various colored gums
EUPHORBIACEAE			
Euphorbia lorifera	Koka	Hawaii	Latex
E. marginata	Snow-on-the-mountain	New Mexico	Latex
E. tetragona		South Africa	Latex
E. triangularis		South Africa	Latex
MORACEAE			
Artocarpus cumingiana		Philippines	Latex (anubing gum)
Browallia utile		Panama and elsewhere	Latex
Ficus platyphylla	Broadleaf fig	Africa	Dried latex
RUTACEAE			
Melicope ternata		New Zealand	Gum
SAPOTACEAE			
Achras zapota	Sapodilla	Central America	Dried latex from stems (chicle), which is the base of chewing gum widely used commercially
Bumelia laetevirens		Mexico	Fruit produces chicle
B. lanuginosa	Woolly buckthorn	New Mexico	Ground bark[a]
Manilkara bidentata	Balata tree	Central and South America	Latex, substitute for chicle
Mimusops balata		West Indies, South America	Dried latex (balata), like chicle and used commercially for "bubble gum"
M. darienensis		Panama	Balata gum, source of chicle
Sideroxylon glabrescens		Malaysia	Latex?

[a] Ground bark is also the source of a mucilaginous substance that hardens quickly on exposure (like gutta percha?).

when ready for mating, as did the Malays and Japanese as part of premarital ritual. In the Philippines, ashes from the burned bark of *Antidesma* spp. (Euphorbiaceae) and the bark of *Poederia foetida* (Rubiaceae) were used; stems of *Agrostistachys borneensis* (Euphorbiaceae) served the same purpose for the Dyaks of Singhi in Malaysia; the juice of *Homonoia riparia* (Euphorbiaceae) was used in Java, and the wood tar of *Melastoma malabathrium* (Melastomataceae) by natives of Singapore. Most populations preferred to have their teeth black and shiny, but natives of New Britain and Madagascar dyed alternate teeth and even put designs on some. Elsewhere, mutilation of teeth accompanied this practice. For example, the Orang Mamma of Sumatra were known to file the crowns of their teeth to the gums at the age of puberty and varnish the stumps and other teeth with the juice of a fig. Not all tooth blackening was related to the acquisition of sex appeal: the Tonkin natives blackened theirs because of an aversion for teeth colored the same as the pig or dog. Many formulas were used to acquire the black color, and herbs alone, or in combination with iron-containing soils, were employed in New Guinea and among the Tinguians of Luzon.[1] Moreover, teeth are blackened throughout Asia wherever betelnut (*Areca catechu*) chewing is common.

Formulations of iron and herbal mixtures were also the basis of *Ohaguro* or the *honorable tooth black* of Japan. In ancient Japan the art was developed to such an extent that the Chinese of AD 25 referred to Japan as the "country of the black-teethed people." Use of *Ohaguro* varied over the ages and was adopted by royalty, warriors, and peasants alike. Until 100 years ago, long after the practice had become unpopular among men, women still blackened their teeth as a sign of marriage, much as we use the wedding ring.

The initial dying took place over a 3 day period, and thereafter repainting was carried out as needed to keep a glossy black appearance. Generally young married women applied *Ohaguro* daily; whereas older women used it only when they went out. Even black dentures were available to those who had lost their teeth. Black teeth were taken as a sign of fidelity and were considered beautiful until European distaste for their appearance became known.[22]

It was commonly believed by those who practiced *Ohaguro* that blackening preserved the teeth and prevented toothache. Scientific verification showed that *Ohaguro*-treated teeth indeed were resistant both to acid etching and demineralization.[23] The latter effect was attributed to the iron in the stain, which was chelated by the oral acids of gluconic, glutamic, and lactic, rather than the calcium on the teeth they overlayed.

Furthermore, the tannin in the solution has a powerful sterilizing and stringent effect, and the ferrous ion coagulates the protein and stabilizes the calcium phosphate of the teeth, thus preventing the carious process from starting.[24] Several formulas now available describe mixing an acidified iron solution (iron acetate) referred to as o'kane, tessho (iron juice) or dashingane (extracted metal) with a tannic acid solution extracted from the acorns of *Quercus cyclophora*, coconut (*Cocos nucifera*), Chinese nutgalls (*Quercus* spp.), or snake gourd juice (*Luffa petola*). One such solution consisted of well-boiled tea, to which were added nails or chipped iron heated until red hot, sugar, yeast, sake, and confections made from starch. This was allowed to age in a cool place in a tightly stoppered bottle for several months, until it turned a brownish black and yielded an unpleasant odor due to ferric hydroxide, ferrous carbonate, and ferric sulfate. It was assumed that the staining solution of ferric tannate was formed on mixing with the tannic acid solution.

Tooth blackening was by no means restricted to the Far East and was also found among several Indian tribes of Central and South America. The Citara of Colombia chewed *Schradera marginalis* (Rubiaceae) to preserve their teeth; both the Putumayo and Caquetá Indians of Colombia and Peru used *Neea parviflora* (Nyctaginaceae); and the Peruvians also used *Manettia divaricata* (Rubiaceae) for this purpose. The practice was common among the Ghaymas of Guyana, the Guijiros, the inhabitants of Cuman, and the Choco Indians of Panama. Furthermore, extracts of cochineal from insects were used by the Nahu Indians of Central America to impart a dark purple cast to the teeth.

On the African continent red coloring is preferred by the few tribes who subscribe to the habit of tooth staining. It is known only to the natives of Bornu (Nigeria), the Adamawa, the Wanuamwezi, and the Moroccans. Although other parts of *Hexalobus senegalensis* (Annonaceae) are used as expectorants and to treat diarrhea, its fruits are effective for dying teeth. Furthermore, the Hausa women, and a few other tribes, chew the cola nut (*Cola acuminata* and others) much as the Malays chew betel nut. Twigs from the plant are also popular chewing sticks.

In India, the Hindus of Gujarat dye their teeth before marriage with the resin from *Ficus religiosa* (peepul tree), infected with an insect belonging to the genus *Coccus*. This bright red resin is boiled until it becomes plastic, then soaked in cotton balls. The teeth are pretreated with tamarind and lemon to cause a superficial decalcination of the enamel before the dye-soaked balls are applied. A decoction of the twigs of *Rubia cordifolia* (Indian madder) is then administered to the teeth as a fixative. Teeth so stained keep their color for 20 years or longer.[1]

LITERATURE CITED

1. Kanner L. 1928. *Folklore of the Teeth.* Macmillan, New York. 316 p.

2. Losee FL, Adkins BL. 1969. A study of the mineral environment of caries-resistant navy recruits. *Caries Res* 3: 23–31; Losee FL, Bibby, BG. 1970. Caries inhibition by trace elements other than fluorine. *NY State Dent J* 36: 15–19.

3. Kao PC, Li HG. 1968. The fluoride content of Taiwan tea. *Chin Med J* 15: 119–123.

4. Role of human food stuffs in caries: proceedings of a workshop conference. 1970. *J Dent Res* 49: 1191–1351.

5. History of the toothbrush and its uses. Part one: ancient history. 1970. *Dent Health* 2: 37.

6. Molnar S. 1972. Tooth wear and culture: a survey of tooth functions among some prehistoric populations. *Curr Anthropol* 13: 511–526.

7. Barton WPC. 1817. *Vegetable Materia Medica of the United States; or Medical Botany* 1: 55–56.

8. MacGregor AB. 1963. Increasing caries incidence and changing diet in Ghana. *Int Dent J* 13: 516–522.

9. Thorne RF. 1968. Synopsis of a putatively phylogenetic classification of the flowering plants. *Aliso* 6: 57–66.

10. Thomas RH. 1971. *Naturally Occurring Quinones*, ed 2. Academic Press, New York.

11. Irvine FR. 1961. *Woody Plants of Ghana.* Oxford University Press, London.

12. Sofowora EA, Isaacs WA. 1971. Reverse of sickling and crenation of erythrocytes by root extract of *Fagara zanthoxyloides*. *Lloydia* 34: 383–385.

13. Elvin-Lewis M, Keudell K, Lewis WH et al. 1974. Anti-cariogenic potential of chewing-sticks. *J Dent Res* 53: 277; Buadu CY, Boakye-Yiadom SM. 1973. The antibacterial activity of some Ghanaian chewing sticks. *Ghana Pharm J* 1: 150–151; El-Said F, Fadulu SO, Kuye JO et al. 1971. Native cures in Nigeria. II. The antimicrobial properties of the buffered extracts of chewing sticks. *Lloydia* 34: 172–174. Boakye-Yiodom K and Konning GH 1975. Incidence of

antibacterial activity in the Connaraceae. *Planta Med* **28:** 397–400; Manley JL, Limongelli WA and Williams AC. 1975. The Chewing Stick. *J Prev Dent* **2:** 7–9.

14. Farooqui MIH, Srivastava JG. 1968. The toothbrush tree (*Salvadora persica*). *Quart J Crude Drug Res* **8**(4): 1297–1299.

15. Rathje R. 1971. Influence of Neem tree extracts on inflammatory changes of the gingiva. *Quintessenz* **22:** 25.

16. Leonard PG. 1972. The dental art of ancient Mexico. *CAL* (Cert Akers Lab), Coe Laboratories, Chicago, **36**(1): 6–9.

17. Townend BR. 1968. Dental folklore, Part I. *Dent Mag Oral Top* **85:** 157–158; Part 2. **85:** 199–202.

18. Lavine BH. 1967. Elizabethan toothache: a case history. *JADA* **74:** 1286–1290.

19. Endecott Z. 1677. *Synopsis Medicinae or A Compendium of Galenical and Chymical Physick.* Introduction and annotation by GF Dow, Salem, Mass (1914). 33 p.

20. Elvin-Lewis M. 1973. Role of microbiology in oral diagnosis, Ch 9, 90–109. In L Cohen (ed), *Oral Diagnosis and Treatment Planning.* Charles C Thomas, Springfield, Ill.

21. Navia JM, Lopez H, Fischer JS. 1974. Caries promoting of sucrose substitutes in foods: manitol, xylitol and sorbitol. *J Dent Res* **53:** 207.

22. Casal UA. 1966. Japanese cosmetics and teeth-blackening. *Trans Asiat Soc Japan,* series 3, **9:** 5–27.

23. Ai S, Ishikawa T, Seino A. 1965. "Ohaguro" traditional tooth staining custom in Japan. *Int Dent J* **15:** 426–441.

24. Yaamaga R, Nakayama M. 1973. Can "tooth black" defeat the toothache demon? *Dent Survey* **49:** 70–71.

Chapter 11

Gastrointestinal Tract

From the time of Babylon down through to-day's television commercials, the farce has been perpetuated that constipation is a disease in itself rather than a symptom of either bad diet or too much dependence on habit-forming laxatives. Today, colonic mills trap the unwary with the quackery that these clogged bowels press against the heart, squeeze the liver, and poison the blood. There is no great danger in all this unless the unfortunate is suffering from some progressive disease which might be arrested by good medical treatment. Otherwise, the patient is simply drained of both this money and those chemicals in the intestines which made digestion possible.[1]

Ancient Egyptians, who thought that all disease came from food, believed that a purge was needed three times a month. Castor oil (*Ricinus communis*) mixed with beer was their standard laxative. Among the Greeks and Romans, *Aloe barbadensis* was a highly regarded laxative, and both Dioscorides and Celsus recommended its use in that application. However a much more conservative approach was taught by Hippocrates, who prescribed purgative medicines only sparingly in acute diseases and not without proper circumspection.

Laxative makers had their heyday in England during the seventeenth and eighteenth centuries when purging was as common as eating and drinking. The English meal, three times daily, consisted of several kinds of meat, heavy pastry, and wine enough to wash it all down. Little roughage was available in this diet, for vegetables were eaten only by the poor and by animals. As a consequence, fortnightly purging was considered necessary for maintaining good health. Purges were often carried out in apothecary shops; groans from customers undergoing this bimonthly ritual were readily heard from the back rooms of every apothecary in London (Fig. 11-1).

This preoccupation with the bowels has persisted until the present time, although the laxative abuse syndrome is on the wane. Nevertheless, some 700 purgatives are available for purchase in the United States alone, and gastrointestinal disease accounts for about 10% of all illness, as well as 10% of general practitioner consultations, 8.5% of prescriptions, and 8.3% of the cost of inpatient treatment. It is responsible for 8.8% of days of certified incapacity to work and 10% of all deaths.[2]

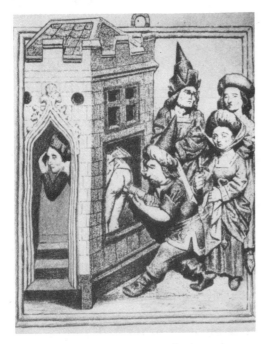

Figure 11-1 Administration of an enema: an apothocary's sign of the fifteenth century.

Relief of gastrointestinal disorders emphasizing natural products in current medical use and those employed widely in domestic medicine now and in the past are discussed under several headings: gastric antacids, indigestion, digestive stimulation, antispasmodics, emetics, antiemetics, purgatives, antidiarrheal agents, infectious diarrheas, liver, anthelmintics, amebicides, hemorrhoids, and carminatives.

GASTRIC ANTACIDS

Excessive secretion of gastric hydrochloric acid or hyperacidity can lead to ulcerations of the stomach and duodenum. Common neutralizing agents for excessive acid may be prescribed: sodium bicarbonate, calcium carbonate, and magnesium hydroxide (milk of magnesia) are a few examples. A natural remedy used by North American Indians was hops (*Humulus lupulus*); the Ojibwas made a tea of the inflorescences, which supposedly acted like sodium bicarbonate on the system, increasing urination and reducing acidity.

INDIGESTION

Upset digestion (dyspepsia, heartburn) is a subjective sensation of discomfort associated with food intake. It may be the result of poor eating habits, it may have a nervous origin, or it may be due to a disease in the gastrointestinal tract. Usually the discomfort centers around a burning or tight feeling in the chest, belching, and a cramped or bloated sensation in any part of the abdomen. If indigestion is due to poor eating habits, the condition usually can be corrected by eating in a more leisurely fashion, chewing food well, and following a blander diet. Nervous indigestion usually responds to mild sedatives and antispasmodic drugs. Antacids and carminatives also should alleviate these distresses.

A number of plants have been used in domestic and folk medicine to relieve indigestion. A few examples are:

BETULACEAE

Alnus rubra (red alder) of western North America and *A. rugosa* (hazel alder) of eastern North America. Barks used by Indians to relieve indigestion, as tonics and alternatives, and in large doses as emetics.

COMBRETACEAE

Terminalia bellirica dried fruit (bahera) is used in India for stomach disorders including indigestion.

ROSACEAE

Rubus macropetalus (dewberry). Tea made from dewberry leaves has been used for general stomach troubles by Indians in western Washington.

SAXIFRAGACEAE

Hydrangea arborescens (smooth hydrangea) and *H. quercifolia* (oak-leaved hydrangea). Roots were used in treating dyspepsia by American pioneers.

DIGESTIVE STIMULATION

A number of principles stimulate the appetite. Usually these stomachics are bitter tonics that increase pancreatic secretion by stimulating the gastric mucous membrane. Such tonics are usually supplemented with vitamins for geriatric patients, and the improved digestive and metabolic functions often result in better appetites.

Numerous plant extracts can be grouped under appetite stimulants. They seem to be particularly common in the Gentianaceae, where bitter principles are widespread. These and others include:

APIACEAE

Carum carvi (caraway). Fruit is a mild stomachic, and caraway oil often is used to correct nausea and griping.

ARACEAE

Acorus calamus (sweet flag). Roots possess aromatic bitters that are used as stomachics and tonics.

ARALIACEAE

Panax quinquefolium (American ginseng). Roots are said to stimulate the appetite.

ARECACEAE

Sabal palmetto from the southeastern United States and West Indies. Berries were credited by the Indians with marked ability to improve the digestion.

ARISTOLOCHIACEAE

Aristolochia serpentaria (Virginia snakeroot) and *A. reticulata* (Texas snakeroot). Rhizomes and roots contain a bitter principle; moderate doses act as gastric stimulants and may also aid dyspepsia.

BRASSICACEAE

Brassica juncea, B. nigra, and *Sinapis alba* (mustards). Powdered seeds act as stimulants to gastric mucosa and increase pancreatic secretions.

CANNABACEAE

Humulus lupulus (hops: Fig. 11-2a). Glandular hairs of inflorescences possess bitter components serving as stomachics and tonics (also give aroma and flavor to beer).

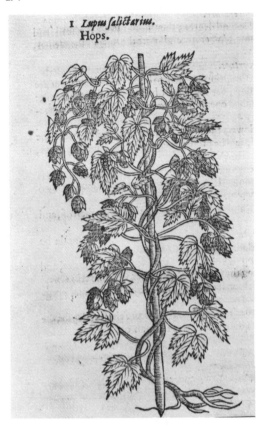

Figure 11-2a *Humulus lupulus* (from J Gerard, *The Herball*, ed 2, 1636).

RANUNCULACEAE

Coptis groenlandica (goldthread). Promotes digestion, aids dyspepsia, and strengthens the viscera; the bitter principle is said to be a good substitute for that found in *Gentiana* and *Quassia*.

RUBIACEAE

Cinchona spp. (Quinine). Bark is used as a bitter and stomachic; in small doses it is a mild irritant and stimulant of the gastric mucosa.

SCROPHULARIACEAE

Picrorhiza kurroa. Rhizome improves appetite and stimulates gastric secretions; used in India as a substitute for *Gentiana*.

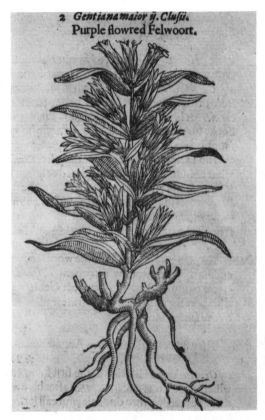

Figure 11-2b *Gentiana* sp. (from J Gerard, *The Herball*, 1597).

GENTIANACEAE

Gentiana catesbaei, G. lutea, G. macrophylla, G. punctata, and *G. purpurea.* Dried rhizomes and roots all produce bitters, perhaps at one time the most popular of all digestive stimulants (Fig. 11-2b). An overdose usually results in nausea and vomiting.

Menyanthes trifoliata (buckbean). The whole plant is bitter and acts as a stomachic and tonic (once considered a panacea in Germany).

Sabatia angularis (American centaury). Contains a bitter principle, erythrocentaurin, which promotes appetite and digestion.

SIMAROUBACEAE

Quassia amara (Surinam quassia) from the American tropics. Became popular in Europe in the mid-eighteenth century; the bitter component is from the powdered stem, a useful remedy when appetite fails.

ANTISPASMODICS

Spasms of the stomach, intestine, and also of the circulatory system and heart, are often due to excessive amounts of acetylcholine and, therefore, excessive nervous impulses. Anticholinergic drugs mediate nerve impulses when they block the action of acetylcholine by displacing it from receptor sites (Chapter 6). Excessive activity of the parasympathetic system can thus be decreased by anticholinergic compounds that exert their activity on gastric hyperacidity and on involuntary muscles.

PEPTIC ULCERS

Gastric or duodenal ulcer, collectively known as peptic ulcer, nearly always occurs in the pyloric region of the stomach or the first inch of the small intestine.

The vagal nerve is involved in the stimulation of gastric secretion: excess stimulation results in hypersecretion of gastric juice rich in hydrochloric acid, thus produces conditions favorable to the formation of peptic ulcers. Anticholinergic drugs can block excessive secretion of gastric hydrochloric acid.

Until 1965, however, there was no drug available to assist in healing the ulcer once developed; rest in bed, no smoking, and bland diets were the only forms of therapy. Now two derivates of *Glycyrrhiza glabra* root (common licorice native to Eurasia), carbenoxolone sodium and

deglycyrrhizinized licorice, can on the average reduce the size of an ulcer by 70 to 90% after one month of treatment (Fig. 11-3). Healing occurs in patients who are not confined to bed, and many who continue to work during the treatment. Undesirable side effects have been reported—edema in 20% of patients and cardiac problems in those eating excessive licorice—but benefits derived from the use of licorice extracts in the treatment of gastric ulcers far outweigh these undesirable effects.[3]

Folk remedies have long included licorice for the treatment of indigestion; in seventeenth-century Europe it was believed to be capable of clearing inflamed stomachs.

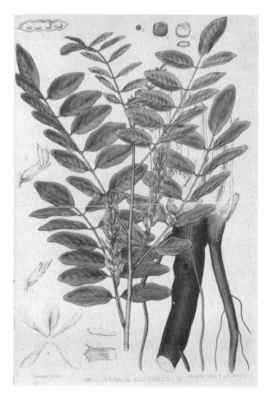

Figure 11-3 *Glycyrrhiza glabra* (from R Bentley and H Trimen, *Medicinal Plants* 2: 74, 1880).

INVOLUNTARY MUSCLES

Severe spasms of the muscles of abdominal organs cause pinching and spasmodic pain. Anticholinergic drugs can be used to correct griping abdominal pain, often called colic, and other symptoms, including spasms of the stomach and intestines, spastic constipation, spasms of the bladder and urinary tract due to inflammation, pernicious vomiting of pregnancy, spasms of the biliary and pancreatic ducts, and excessive salivation, perspiration, and secretions of the nose, pharynx, and bronchi. In addition, fainting due to heart block, arterial spasms, gangrenous conditions due to damaged and constricted blood vessels, and other important circulatory problems can be remedied by antispasmodic drugs.

The most important antispasmodics are: atropine—obtained from *Atropa belladonna, Hyoscyamus muticus, H. niger, Duboisia leichardtii, D. myoporoides,* and other solanaceous species, or produced synthetically; scopolamine (hyoscine)—which is particularly abundant in *Datura fastuosa, D. metel, D. inoxia, D. meteloides, Scopolia carniolica,* and *S. japonica,* and is usually prepared from material after the removal of hyoscyamine; and papaverine—the principal benzylisoquinoline derivative of the opium alkaloids from *Papaver somniferum.*

Without benefit of these drugs, however, spasms of the gut were treated with a number of remedies found efficacious by our North American Indians and early settlers. A number are given below.

CAPRIFOLIACEAE

Viburnum prunifolium (black haw) and *V. rufidulum* (southern black haw). Roots were used by the Catawba Indians to make a tea administered for stomach troubles. The Menominees used the inner bark of *V. acerifolium* (maple-leaved viburnum) for a tea drunk to treat cramps and colic.

GENTIANACEAE

Gentiana catesbaei and roots of other species of gentian were used by the Catawbas to stop pains in the stomach; they drank a hot or cold decoction or chewed roots.

LAMIACEAE

Mentha piperita (peppermint). Dried leaves and flowering tops were used to relieve spasmodic pains of the stomach and bowels.
Nepeta cataria (catnip). Dried leaves and flowering tops were used as a hot infusion to relieve infantile colic.

LILIACEAE

Aletris farinosa (star grass) was used by the Catawbas to relieve colic.

RANUNCULACEAE

Hydrastis canadensis (golden seal). Root infusions were used by eastern North American Indians and settlers to treat liver and stomach ailments.
Xanthorhiza simplicissima (shrub yellowroot). Roots were boiled by the Catawbas of eastern North America for treating ulcerated stomachs; or a piece of the green or dried root was chewed to relieve stomach pains. Early white settlers also made a bitter tea of the roots to treat stomach disorders as well as sore throats.

SALICACEAE

Salix humilis (small pussy willow). Roots were used by the Menominee Indians for treatment of spasmodic colic.

ZYGOPHYLLACEAE

Larrea mexicana (greasewood, creosote bush). Branches were boiled by the Pimas and Maricopas of the southwestern United States to extract the gum, which was then drunk as a hot decoction to relieve stomach trouble or to treat diarrhea.

EMETICS

As a therapeutic procedure, emesis has suffered a decline in popularity during the past century. Its use now is restricted to two main areas of treatment: ridding the stomach of irritant and poisonous substances, and using the unpleasantness of vomiting in aversion therapy in, for example, the treatment of alcoholism.

Emetic responses are mediated by way of reflex arcs, which pass through the vomiting center located in the medulla oblongata. The response is usually obtained by stimulating the vomiting center through the visceral afferent nerves by irritating gastric tissues or the back of the throat, by stimulating the chemoreceptor trigger zone by drugs, or by combining the two approaches.

Emesis is of particular value in young children for the treatment of acute poisoning. Gastric lavage (washing out of the stomach) may also be used, although the use of a small-bore tube in the young may not allow the passage of seeds, tablets, and so on, which would be readily evacuated by use of larger tubes in adults. A number of home remedies to obtain rapid vomiting are important to consider: mustard powder in warm water is an unpleasant but efficient emetic, and a strong solution of salt in warm water is also effective. If these fail, in about 15 minutes stimulate the back of the throat with a spoon handle or toothbrush. At any time ipecac syrup may be administered as 1 tablespoon (15 ml) in a large glass of orange juice and repeated if necessary after 20 minutes; however if emesis does not occur after the second dose, the ipecac should be recovered with gastric lavage. Apomorphine is very effective in the rapid production of vomiting, but it must be injected and can be used safely only in the hospital.[4]

Folk medicine is rampant with extracts from plants widely used to induce vomiting, but a small sample shows that many are very poisonous in moderate to large doses, and therefore should never be employed carelessly. Members of the Rubiaceae containing emetine and cephaeline are among the most numerous and most common plants used today as emetics. The list includes:

APOCYNÁCEAE

Apocynum androsaemifolium (wild ipecac). Root is emetic in large doses; in small amounts it is a tonic. The cardiotonic action of this plant is probably responsible for the toxicity associated with emesis and as such its use should be avoided.

AQUIFOLIACEAE

Ilex vomitoria (yaupon). Leaves have been used by Indians of the southeastern United States to promote vomiting, or when diluted, as a stimulating tea. (The plant contains caffeine.)

ASTERACEAE

Anthemis cotula (dog chamomile). A plant decoction in large doses has been used in North America as an emetic, in small amounts as a gentle tonic.

Cirsium arvense (Canada thistle). Root is an emetic and alterative.

Eupatorium perfoliatum (boneset). Dried leaves and flowering tops are popular North American home remedy emetics.

Matricaria chamomilla (chamomile). Dried flower heads are emetic in large doses.

BRASSICACEAE

Brassica juncea (Chinese mustard), *B. nigra* (common black mustard), and *Sinapis alba* (white mustard). Seeds produce mustard powder that is useful as a home remedy emetic for children; mustard is especially valuable in treating narcotic poisoning.

CAMPANULACEAE

Lobelia inflata (Indian tobacco). Dried leaves and flowering tops were used by eastern North American Indians as a speedy and severe emetic and purgative; but if not emitted, the remedy itself would cause death.

EUPHORBIACEAE

Euphorbia ipecacuanha (ipecac spurge). Root bark is a North American emetic and also purgative.

FABACEAE

Pterocarpus santalinus of tropical Asia has long been used as an emetic.

LILIACEAE

Veratrum album (Europe) and *V. viride* (eastern North America). Rhizomes are emetics, but margins of safety are small among the false hellebores. These plants contain cardiac glycosides.

LOGANIACEAE

Gelsemium sempervirens (yellow jessamine). Roots possess strong toxic alkaloids (gelsemoidine, sempervirine); this eastern American species is poisonous, and the margin of safety when used as an emetic is small.

PAPAVERACEAE

Besides apomorphine derived from morphine (*Papaver somniferum*), *Sanguinaria canadensis* (bloodroot) root is also an emetic, producing nausea and vomiting when administered in large doses.

PHYTOLACCACEAE

Phytolacca americana (poke). Dried root is a powerful emetic, and often in the nineteenth century it was combined with ipecac or *Lobelia* to cause emesis. Its use should be avoided (Chapter 4).

ROSACEAE

Gillenia stipulata (American ipecac). Root is emetic; in small doses it is used as a tonic.

Physocarpus capitatus (ninebark). Young twigs (peeled of bark) were used as emetics by the Indians of the Pacific Northwest.

RUBIACEAE

Cephaelis acuminata or *C. ipecacuanha* (Fig. 11-4) (ipecac or ipecacuahna). Dried rhizomes and roots are widely used in a syrup as emetics, particularly for children. The species are native to Brazil and are

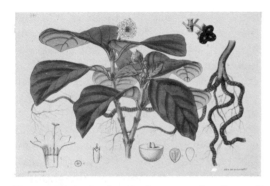

Figure 11-4 *Cephaelis ipecacuanha* (from R Bentley and H Trimen, *Medicinal Plants* **2:** 145, 1880).

cultivated elsewhere in the tropics. Their emetic value appears to reside in the alkaloids emetine and cephaeline. Other species of South American Rubiaceae also containing these alkaloids in their roots include *Bothriospora corymbosa, Caperonia decorticans, Ferdinandusa elliptica, Remijia amazonica,* and *Tocoyena longiflora;* the stem bark of *Hillia illustris* also has the alkaloids. They are often substituted for ipecac. Adulterants include *Borreria brasiliensis* and *Psychotria emetica,* but their roots possess few if any alkaloids causing emesis.

SIMAROUBACEAE

Picrasma excelsa (Jamaica quassia) and *Quassia amara* (Surinam quassia), both native to the New World tropics. Powdered stem wood is an effective simple bitter; but in larger doses it is capable of sufficiently irritating the stomach to produce vomiting.

THYMELAEACEAE

Dirca palustris (leatherwood). Bark is a powerful emetic from eastern North America.

ZYGOPHYLLACEAE

Guaiacum officinale (lignum sactum) and *G. sanctum* (lignum vitae). Resins cause nausea.

ANTIEMETICS

Vomiting is a common symptom having many causes inside and outside the gastrointestinal tract. In most cases the most appropriate course is treatment of the cause—for example, relief of intestinal obstruction (see use of plants in traditional Chinese medicine[5]) or correction of electrolyte and fluid balance. At other times, however, this is not possible and treatment must be symptomatic.

One of the most direct ways to prevent vomiting is to inhibit the hyperactivity of the vomiting center by using anticholinergic drugs. Thus atropine, hyoscyamine, and scopolamine (from several solanaceous genera), and their synthetic analogs, alleviate vomiting whatever its cause and also afford good protection against motion sickness. The widespread anticholinergic effects of these drugs, however, make them unsuitable for prolonged use as antiemetics because side effects may be troublesome. Antihistamines such as dramamine or hydramine have mild antiemetic effects and are widely used, although they too produce anticholinergic action when employed in high dosage. Two synthetic groups of compounds having powerful inhibiting action on the chemoreceptor trigger zone are the phenothiazines (chlorpromazine, piperazine) and orthopramides (metoclopramide). When administered intravenously, the orthopramides exert their effects on the stomach within 3 minutes and are very useful when vomiting has already started.[6]

To prevent or check vomiting, often with a settling and soothing effect on the stomach, the following domestic or Indian remedies may be of value.

ARISTOLOCHIACEAE

Aristolochia serpentina (Virginia snakeroot). Rhizomes and roots were used by the Indians of eastern North America to check vomiting.

MYRTACEAE

Eugenia caryophyllus (clove tree). Clove powder (dried flower buds) is used to relieve nausea and vomiting, to correct flatulence, and to excite a languid digestion.

LAMIACEAE

Mentha piperita (peppermint). The herb is used to treat nausea.

Monarda punctata (horsemint). The herb stimulates diaphoresis, and thus relieves nausea.

ROSACEAE

Rubus spp. (blackberry and thimbleberry). Indians from Vancouver Island, British Columbia, peeled roots and stems, boiled them, and drank the liquid to arrest vomiting.

PURGATIVES

Desire to purge the system of noxious products and to relieve constipation has resulted in one of the oldest practices of medicine and of self-medication. Until a few years ago ritual purgation of children and the obsessional catharsis of adults were still commonplace, but now such ritualism has virtually disappeared. Purgative drugs should be used only in response to clear indication; mere satisfaction of an individual's psychological need for a daily bowel action is not an indication for purgation. Purgative habituation is far easier to prevent than it is to cure.

Purgative drugs, in which we include all cathartics, laxatives, and aperients, may be divided into three main groups: bulk purgatives, lubricants, and irritants.

1. *Bulk purgatives.* These drugs increase the volume of intestinal contents and, by stretching the wall of the intestine, encourage the normal reflex activity of the bowel. Indigestible plant materials, such as agar and seeds of *Plantago psyllium*, absorb water in the intestine and swell, thereby increasing fecal bulk and stimulating normal peri-

stalsis. Their effect is usually produced overnight.

2. *Lubricant purgatives.* These drugs act by softening and lubricating the feces. Mineral oil (liquid paraffin) is a good example.

3. *Irritant purgatives.* Substances that have a local irritant effect on the intestinal wall are grouped in this category. Some drugs act on the sensory nerve endings in the mucosa of the bowel wall; other purgatives are absorbed from the small intestine and are carried by circulation to act on the nerves of the large intestine, thus stimulating motor propulsion. The anthraquinones from the bark of *Rhamnus purshiana* (cascara) and dried leaflets of *Cassia senna* (senna) produce examples of the latter type of colonic stimulation. These compounds bring about their action in 6 to 8 hours.

The term constipation implies that defecation is infrequent and that there is a retention of feces in the colon. Usually a retention after 72 hours indicates abnormality that may be due to functional bowel disturbances (e.g., spastic colon), organic gastrointestinal diseases caused by intestinal obstruction or acute appendicitis, or mechanical causes (e.g., fecal impaction). Often constipation is functional in origin and responds to simple changes in diet and bowel hygiene. Thus the individual should be encouraged to establish regular hours of eating and sleeping; he should take regular exercise, and a bland low-residue diet is indicated to aid in resting the colon. Warm olive oil enemas may also be useful in establishing regular bowel habit.[7]

Even though the habit of taking regular purgatives simply to produce a daily bowel action is condemned and is on the decrease, this wisdom has not been characteristic of Western civilization in the past, nor is it found in less urbanized societies throughout much of the world. All cultures maintain their purgatives, and seemingly most flowering plant families produce sufficient compounds, such as irritant oils and resins, to oblige this purging instinct in man. The partial list that follows is far from complete, but it serves to illustrate the many diverse plants found in both temperate and tropical areas that have contributed purgatives. Among the most notable, though often dangerous, families are the Convolvulaceae (morning glory), Cucurbitaceae (gourd), Euphorbiaceae (spurge), Fabaceae (pea), Polygonaceae (buckwheat), and Rhamnaceae (buckthorn).

APIACEAE

Oenanthe sarmentosa (water parsley). Roots are pounded and used as a potent laxative by the Indians of the Pacific Northwest.

BERBERIDACEAE

Podophyllum emodi (northern India) and *P. peltatum* (May apple of eastern North America). Irritant resins from these plants often are used to treat chronic constipation, but an overdose of resin (as little as 5 grains) can cause death.

CAPRIFOLIACEAE

Sambucus glauca (blue elderberry). Bark decoction is used by Indians of the Pacific Northwest.

CLUSIACEAE

Garcinia hanburyi, G. lanessonii, and *G. morella.* Resinous bark exudates are drastic purgatives of southeastern Asia, causing additionally nausea, vomiting, griping, and fatalities when taken in large doses.

CONVOLVULACEAE

Ipomoea species from many parts of the world are used as purgatives. These include *I. altissima* roots (Brazil), *I. hederacea* seeds roasted (India), *I. orizabensis* roots dried (Mexico), *I. palmatopinnata* roots dried (South America), *I. pes-caprae* seeds (pantropical), *I. (Exogonium) purga* roots dried (Jalap of Mexico introduced into Europe in the seventeenth century), and *I. turpethum* dried roots (tropical Asia and Australia). Often the active resins are mixed for greater efficacy.

CORNACEAE

Cornus pubescens (dogwood). Bark decoctions are used by Indians of the Pacific Northwest.

CUCURBITACEAE

Bryonia africana (bryony), *B. alba, B. americana,* and *B. dioica.* Dried roots contain an active irritant purgative, but the remedy is little used because of the danger of serious or fatal poisoning.

Citrullus colocynthis (bitter gourd). Dried pulp of the unripe fruit of this Afro-Asian species is a violent purgative, but because of the danger of poisoning it is little used.

Ecballium elaterium (wild cucumber). Fruit of Mediterranean origin contains the resin elaterin, a powerful hydragogue purgative.

EUPHORBIACEAE

Croton species are among the most drastic and irritant purgatives, but they are little used today because of the danger. Among these are *C. caudatus* roots (tropical Asia), *C. echinocarpus* bark (Brazil), *C. oblongifolius* seeds (tropical Asia), and *C. tiglium* seeds (purging croton of tropical Asia and cultivated), from which croton oil, the most drastic of all purgatives, is extracted. Death can result from the ingestion of only 20 drops of croton oil, which is also a co-carcinogen.

Jatropha curcas (purging nut). Seeds and extracted curcas oil are both powerful purgatives.

Mallotus philippinensis (Asia and Australia). The source of kamala powder, obtained from the glandular hairs of fruit, is used as a purgative in India.

Ricinus communis (castor bean: Fig. 11-5a). Pantropical and cultivated, this plant is the source of castor oil obtained from seeds. The taste is disagreeable, and the viscid oil is difficult to administer and thus castor oil is little used today after a long and offensive (though effective) history!

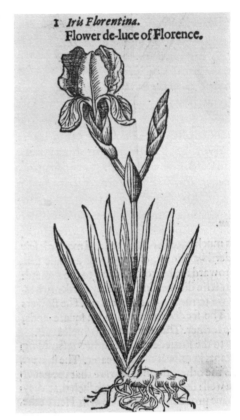

Figure 11-5b *Iris florentina* (from J Gerard, *The Herball,* 1597).

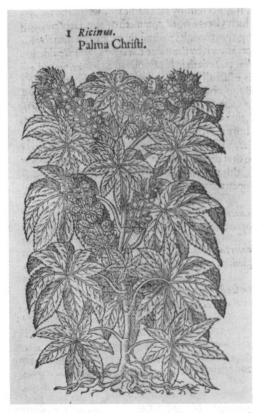

Figure 11-5a *Ricinus communis* (from J Gerard, *The Herball,* ed 2, 1636).

FABACEAE

Cassia species (senna) yield a purgative that was introduced into European medicine in the ninth or tenth century by the Arabs. Its native use antedates historic record. Purgative action is due to anthraquinones (emodin being the most important derivate), whose chief effect is to speed the passage of the colonic contents. Most species of *Cassia* probably act only on the large intestine; the better known include C. *absus* seeds (India), C. *alata* roots (Guatemala), C. *angustifolia* dried leaflets (tinnevelly senna, widely cultivated as a source of senna), C. *fistula* pulp or dried fruit (purging cassia) of pantropical cultivation and widely used medically, C. *javanica* bark (Indonesia),

C. marilandica leaflets (eastern United States), *C. moschata* leaflets (Colombia), *C. senna* dried leaflets (Alexandria senna from Egypt and cultivated, is a source of commercial senna), and *C. sophera* leaflets, bark and seeds (pantropical). Extracts from a number of these species (e.g., *C. absus* and *C. sophera*) are also used as anthelmintics.

Tamarindus indica (tamarind). Fruit pulp is used in laxatives.

IRIDACEAE

Iris florentina (Fig. 11-5*b*), *I. germanica*, and *I. pallida*, largely European, from the rhizomes of which orris root is obtained, have purgative as well as emetic properties. This is a feature of all *Iris* rhizomes tested; for example *I. versicolor* (blue flag) of eastern North America, having an acrid resin and essential oil, has been used as a purgative.

LILIACEAE

Aloe barbadensis, A. ferox, and *A. perryi*. Juice of leaves yield emodin, which acts chiefly on the large intestine. The ancients knew of the purgative action of aloes, for the plants were cultivated on the island of Socotra in the time of Alexander the Great. Action can be violent, and aloes are used today in combination with less drastic purgatives or antispasmodic drugs.

LINACEAE

Linum catharticum (purging flax) plant and *L. usitatissimum* (flaxseed) seeds. The first is of Eurasian origin, yielding a purgative decoction; the second yields linseed oil or seeds used as laxatives.

MYRTACEAE

Pimenta officinalis (pimenta oil). The oil is used as an adjuvant to purgatives; it is especially of value in cases accompanied by much flatulence.

OLEACEAE

Olea europaea (olive oil: Fig. 11-6a). The nutritious and mildly laxative oil may be used in milder cases of chronic constipation.

PLANTAGINACEAE

Plantago ovata and *P. psyllium*. Seeds absorb water and act as purgatives.

POLYGONACEAE

The family contains many anthraquinone drugs that possess purgative properties (aloe-emodin, emodin, physcion), as well

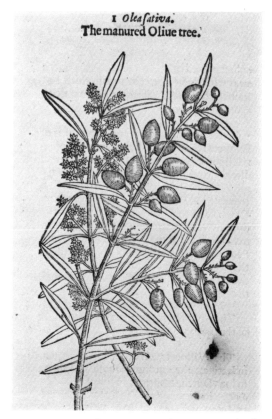

Figure 11-6a *Olea europaea* (from J Gerard, *The Herball,* ed 2, 1636).

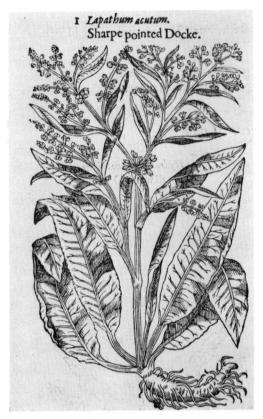

Figure 11-6b *Rumex longifolius* (from J Gerard, *The Herball*, 1597).

as astringent compounds (glucogallin, gallic acid, catechin).

Polygonum aviculare, mild astringent; *P. cuspidatum,* laxative; *P. cuspidatum,* laxative; *P. dumetorum,* laxative.

Rheum species (rhubarb). Many Asian species possess laxative properties, but because of astringent compounds (tannins), they may also be constipating (e.g., *R. officinale, R. palmatum, R. rhaponticum*). The stewed leaf stalks of *R. hybridum* are widely used as food, but the rhizomes contain laxative anthraquinones; the leafblades, however, are poisonous.

Rumex crispus (curled dock: Fig. 11-6b). Roots are used as a laxative in Europe as well as a tonic and an alterative; *R. ne-*

palensis roots in the Himalayas represent a laxative substitute for rhubarb; and *R. obtusifolius* (bitter dock) of temperate Eurasia has roots that are mildly laxative and astringent.

RHAMNACEAE

Rhamnus catharticus (buckthorn of Eurasia and North Africa). Purgative berries contain rhamnin and rhamnetin; now largely replaced by cascara. *R. frangula* (alder buckthorn), the bark containing a glucoside frangulin, has long been used as a home remedy for constipation and for "cleaning the blood." *R. japonica* bark and fruit are employed as laxatives. Bark of *R. purshiana* (cascara buckthorn), found on the North American Pacific coast, contains anthraquinone purgatives having an effect on the colon similar to that of senna; this is a widely used laxative today in the form of a liquid extract or as tablets prepared from a dry extract.

SCROPHULARIACEAE

Veronicastrum virginicum (culver's-root). Rhizomes and roots: the Seneca Indians made a tea for use as a purgative.

Very few synthetic compounds are pharmacologically superior purgatives to those obtained from plant materials; in fact the synthetic analogs usually act too drastically and may cause serious kidney damage. An exception is the readily manufactured phenolphthalein, one of the most successful laxatives, which apparently has no damaging effect on the kidney.

ANTIDIARRHEAL AGENTS

Diarrhea, an increase in the fluidity and frequency of stools, is one of the most common disorders of man. Fortunately in many cases the disorder is short-lived or responds well to a number of well-tried remedies. The causes of diarrhea are numerous: acute diarrhea results from bacterial and viral enteritis, food and toxin poisoning, chemical poisoning, and gastrointestinal allergy; chronic diarrhea is caused by chronic intestinal infections, immunologic and metabolic abnormalities, environmental factors, and the malabsorption syndrome (bilious and pancreatic disorders, genetic abnormalities, etc.). Whenever possible, the cause should be eliminated or controlled.

A number of options exist in treating diarrhea. If symptomatic relief is elected, the number of bowel actions may be reduced by administering a drug (opium derivatives, particularly morphine as paregoric; anticholinergic drugs like atropine), or harmful substances in the bowel may be neutralized by using absorbents (pectin found in raw apples and citrus fruit rinds) and astringents. Alternatively, the cause of diarrhea may be treated by administering an antibiotic or antiamebic drug or by replacing abnormal losses of water, electrolytes, protein, and blood.[8]

To restore the normal intestinal flora following administration of antibacterial drugs, which often results in diarrhea, *Lactobacillus* cultures (*L. acidophilus, L. bulgaricus*) are available for oral therapy (Bacid® or Lactinex®), or yoghurt may be eaten.

Higher plant families such as the Fabaceae and Rosaceae possess great astringent properties because of the presence of abundant tannins. Many species of these families were widely used in folk medicine to counter diarrhea and dysentery. Prolonged use of any antidiarrheal agent is discouraged, and since tannins are also suspected of carcinogenic activity (Chapter 5), their frequent internal use should be avoided.

GYMNOSPERM

Juniperus virginiana (red cedar). Berrylike fruit is used by Indians of North America against dysentery.

ANGIOSPERMS

APOCYNACEAE

Alstonia scholaris (chhatim). Bark is considered very efficacious in India against chronic diarrhea.

Vinca minor (perennial periwinkle). Leaves are a bitter astringent and are used against dysentery and hemorrhoids.

CACTACEAE

Opuntia fulgida (cholla). Roots are chewed for treatment of diarrhea.

EBENACEAE

Diospyros virginiana (persimmon). Bark is used as an astringent and also a tonic.

ERICACEAE

Vaccinium arboreum (sparkleberry). Fruit and root bark are used to treat dysentery.

FABACEAE

Pterocarpus indicus and *P. marsupium* (Malabar kino) produce kino, a juice obtained from the tree trunks and containing kinotannic acid, which is dried. At one time kino was widely administered in the treatment of diarrhea, often in combination with opium. A number of other plants exude gum and are used as kino substitutes, namely, *Pterocarpus erinaceus* (from Africa), *Butea monosperma* or Bengal kino, *Parkia insignis* (from Burma), and *Xylia xylocarpa* (from Burma).

FAGACEAE

Quercus alba (white oak) bark containing about 10% tannin, *Q. infectoria* (dyer's

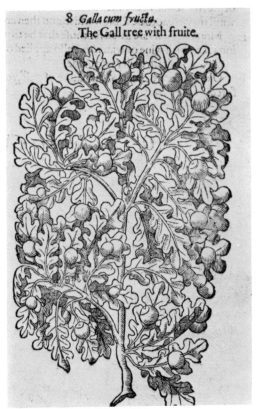

Figure 11-7a *Quercus* sp. with galls (from J Gerard, *The Herball,* 1597).

oak) nutgalls (Fig. 11-7a), *Q. lyrata* (water white oak) bark, and other species are rich in tannins and have significant astringent action. Indians of North America used them widely against dysentery, as did settlers during the nineteenth century.

GERANIACEAE

Geranium maculatum (American cranesbill) was boiled by eastern North American Indians, and the resulting astringent tea was used against dysentery.

KRAMERIACEAE

Krameria argentea and *K. triandra* (Peruvian krameria). Roots, source of rhatany, are active astringents and for-

merly were used extensively in the treatment of chronic diarrhea.

LAMIACEAE

Pycnanthemum flexuosum (dysentery weed) was popular at one time in the southeastern United States for treating diarrhea and other bowel complaints.

LAURACEAE

Aniba coto from Bolivia is the source of coto bark, which abolishes diarrhea with an action similar to that of codeine.

LILIACEAE

Aletris farinosa (star grass). Leaves were used by the Catawbas to make an antidiarrheal tea.

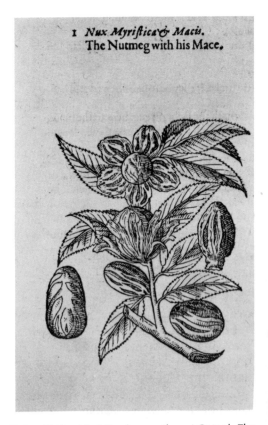

Figure 11-7b *Myristica fragans* (from J Gerard, *The Herball,* 1597).

MYRICACEAE

Comptonia peregrina (sweet-fern). Leaves and flowering tops were boiled to make a tea popularly employed until recent times in domestic treatment of diarrhea in eastern North America.

MYRISTICACEAE

Myristica fragrans (nutmeg: Fig. 11-7b). Powdered seeds and mace were used as a domestic medicine to treat diarrhea.

MYRTACEAE

Angophora lanceolata and *Eucalyptus rostrata* from Australia produce an astringent gum, a substitute for kino.

PLUMBAGINACEAE

Limonium carolinianum (sea lavender) is a powerful astringent, used in eastern North America against diarrhea and dysentery in the nineteenth century.

POLYGALACEAE

Polygala senega (seneca). The whole plant was boiled, and the liquid was used by the Nishinams to treat diarrhea.

POLYGONACEAE

Coccoloba uvifera (sea-grape). Bark extract, called Jamaica kino, is a powerful astringent and is used in tropical America to treat diarrhea.

ROSACEAE

Agrimonia eupatoria (common agrimony). The plant produces a mild astringent and is used to treat diarrhea as well as liver ailments.

Fragaria spp. (strawberry). A tea made from the plant is used to counter diarrhea by the Indians of western Washington.

Holodiscus discolor (ocean spray). A flower decoction is used for treating diarrhea by the Indians of western Washington.

Malus diversifolia (crab apple). Bark is peeled from the tree, soaked in water, and drunk to treat dysentery by the Indians of western Washington. Apples and pears also supply the carbohydrate pectin, which is an important absorbent in controlling diarrhea.

Rubus spp. (blackberry, raspberry). Root decoctions were a widespread North American Indian remedy against dysentery.

Spiraea douglasii and *S. tomentosa*. Fruit decoctions were used by North American Indians and by practitioners of domestic medicine as powerful astringents against chronic diarrhea.

RUBIACEAE

Cephaelis acuminata and *C. ipecacuanha* (ipecac). Rhizomes and roots were for centuries the standard treatment for amebic dysentery; now they are largely used as emetics.

Uncaria gambir (Bengal gambir). Leaves and twigs release an astringent extract employed to treat diarrhea in tropical Asia; *U. guianensis* is similarly used in Guyana.

RUTACEAE

Aegle marmelos (bel). The fruit, having mucilage and pectin, is useful against chronic diarrhea and dysentery (India).

Citrus spp. Fruit rind, which supplies pectin, may be used to control diarrhea.

SAXIFRAGACEAE

Heuchera americana (alum root) and other species. All parts of the plant, but especially the root, release a powerful astringent useful against diarrhea.

INFECTIOUS DIARRHEA

Gastroenteritis—inflammation of stomach and intestines—is characterized by abdominal distress, nausea, vomiting, and diarrhea and is caused by a variety of infectious and toxic agents. Many outbreaks are of viral origin, but those produced by bacteria are either intoxications resulting from the ingestion of food contaminated with bacterial toxic products (see Chapter 2) or infections resulting from the ingestion of viable bacteria. Among the latter are the enteropathogenic strains of *Escherichia coli* associated with infantile diarrhea and *Vibrio parahemolyticus*, causing Japanese raw-fish enteritis. One of the major causes of food poisoning is *Clostridium perfringens* and its toxins; *C. perfringens* strain type F can produce a rare but more fatal type, enteritis necroticans. Other outbreaks of food poisoning have implicated *Bacillus cereus* and species of *Proteus*, *Klebsiella*, *Providencia* (*Paracolon*), *Citrobacter*, *Pseudomonas*, *Enterobacter*, and *Actinomyces*.

When there is suppression of gut flora due to antibiotic therapy, overgrowth of organisms, such as *Staphylococcus aureus*, or even *Candida albicans*, *Streptococcus faecalis*, *Pseudomonas aeroginosa*, and *Proteus mirabilis*, can result in enterocolitis or infection of the bowel wall. This potentially severe infection is characterized by diarrhea, inflammation, ulcerations, and even pseudomembrane formation. Enterocolitis may also be a manifestation of *Salmonella*, cholera, and *Shigella* infections.

Enteritis caused by *Salmonella* species, particularly *S. typhimurium*, is characterized by inflammation of intestinal mucosa, lymphoid follicle enlargement with possible accompanying necrosis, and enlargement of mesenteric nodes. Extension into the peripheral blood supply may result in a bacteremia with metastases forming elsewhere.

Treatment is usually supportive. When prompt correction of dehydration and electrolyte disturbances is required, paregoric, diphenoxylate hydrochloride combined with atropine sulfate, codeine, and small doses of morphine, are used to relieve abdominal cramps and diarrhea. However antibiotic therapy in *Salmonella* infections has been found to induce resistant mutants and actually prolong the duration of the organism's excretion.

Whereas large amounts of *Salmonella* may be required to initiate enteritis, man is very susceptible to infection with *Shigella* species, which cause an intestinal infection known as bacillary dysentery, characterized by fever, diarrhea, and a bloody, mucous-filled stool. Unlike *Salmonella*, *Shigella* species are not invasive. The disease is self-limiting, although supportive electrolytic balance may be necessary if dehydration is severe.

Cholera, a nonexudative form of acute diarrheal disease, is characterized by severe bloody diarrhea and dehydration due to the choleragen endotoxin associated with the etiologic agent, *Vibrio cholerae*. This endotoxin stimulates a prolonged increase in capillary permeability, inducing a basic lesion in the jejunal microcirculation with striking water and ion fluxes. Prognosis is excellent with current electrolyte replacement therapy, which involves infusing the patient with an alkaline saline solution in order to rehydrate him and to correct his acidosis. Once hydration has been achieved, tetracycline is used to reduce the number of organisms shed in the stool, and homeostasis is maintained by infusing these solutions at a rate to match the measured stool volume by adding potassium chloride to the fluid or administering potassium orally.

LIVER

In addition to aiding in digestion, the largest gland of the body serves as a filter and clearing station for purifying blood, as a storage place for food (particularly sugar and vitamins), as a producer of various kinds of protein and antibodies, and as a remover of waste. Associated with the liver is the gallbladder, which stores bile. This substance is released into the intestine when a fatty meal is ingested; the bile acids digest fat; and the bile salts help absorb fat and fat-soluble vitamins.

One of the best examples of a basic herbal tenet is the doctrine of signatures, which originated in China and spread throughout Europe during the Middle Ages. The theory holds that for every ailment there is a specific plant remedy, the clue existing in the plant's shape, color, taste, and other properties. No better examples of the doctrine exist than those related to liver complaints—that the trilobed leaf of *Hepatica* (pertaining to the liver) *nobilis* of the Ranunculaceae (Fig. 11-8) would cure all liver and bileous difficulties, as would the thallus of liverworts, a primitive group of nonvascular plants allied to mosses; the Houma Indians, moreover, boiled a handful of roots from *Solidago nemoralis* (goldenrod) for a tea to cure "yellow jaundice," suggesting that to them color was thought to be the "signature." Of course, there is no known or even suspected value of these plants in treating diseases originating with the liver.

Other plants, however, are supposed to aid in afflictions of the liver. Physicians of the nineteenth century used dandelion roots (*Taraxacum officinale*) to treat chronic diseases of the liver, and recently a naturopath wrote that there is "abundant evidence to show that the common dandelion supplies substances to the liver that the organ can utilize to enable it to perform its duties effectively. Moreover, it does this in a natural manner, without forcing chemical changes or producing undesirable side effects."[9] A craze in nineteenth-century England was the domestic use of *Euonymus europaeus* for "liver afflictions." A few of the plants used by North American Indians are *Rumex verticillatus* (swamp dock) for jaundice, *Salix lucida* (red willow) for removing bile from the stomach, and *Zanthoxylum clava-herculis* (toothache tree) for obstructions of the liver. Fruit from *Emblica officinalis* in the Euphorbiaceae, which is very rich in vitamin C, is considered a good liver tonic in India.

For numerous recipes "to relieve distress" of the liver, read those accumulated by Meyer,[10] noting in particular how often the use of dandelion appears in seemingly disparate sources.

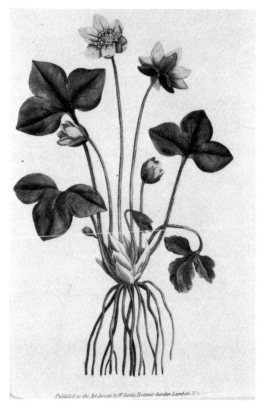

Figure 11-8 *Hepatica nobilis* (from *Curtis's Botanical Magazine* **1:** 10, 1787).

ANTHELMINTICS

Most of the worms that affect man live unobtrusively in the intestine and do little to impair the health of their host. Symptoms and signs usually appear only in cases of heavy infection, but these can be quite common among people living in warm humid areas.

The commoner helminths, with an indication of the most effective drugs administered for treatment, are round-worms or trematodes (*Ascaris* by piper-azines, *Trichinella* by prednisone, *Trichuris* or whipworms and *Strongyloides* by thiabandazole, hookworms by tetra-chloroethylene, *Enterobius* or pinworms by bacitracin); tapeworms or cestodes (*Taenia* spp. by niclosamide or dichlorophen); and trematodes or flukes (schistosomiasis by antimony). An anthelmintic drug must have a wide margin of safety between its toxicity to the worm and its toxic side effect on the host. Anthelmintic properties of many naturally occurring products have been known since the beginning of civilization and are still widely used today. To be effective they should be orally active, produce results in a single dose, and be cheap. Often the use of these drugs is followed by a purge.[11]

Either by reducing intestinal flora, which may serve as food for certain worms, or by direct toxic action on the worm, chemotherapeutic agents are administered widely today to rid the host of helminth parasites. These and various synthetics have lessened the need for ex-tracts from vascular plants, but many such plants are still in common use in domestic medicine in tropical areas where they are readily available and inexpensive. Examples are:

FERNS

Dryopteris filix-mas (European male fern) and *D. marginalis* (marginal fern). Rhizomes and stipes contain an oleoresin that paralyzes the voluntary muscles of the intestine as well as the analogous contractile tissue of the tapeworm; al-though it does not kill the parasite, the paralyzed worms are readily washed out of the gut by an active purge.

ANGIOSPERMS
ARECACEAE

Areca catechu (betelnut palm). Powdered nut is a well-known anthelmintic in Asia, especially against roundworms and tape-worms.

Cocos nucifera (coconut or coco palm). Coconut milk is used in Mexico as an anthelmintic. Its astringent roots are simi-larly employed in Indonesia.

ASTERACEAE

Artemisia cina (levant wormseed) from Russia and *A. maritima* (Fig. 11-9a) from Eurasia contain santonin in unexpanded floral heads (a rich source of this com-pound), which is very efficient in its ac-tion on roundworms.

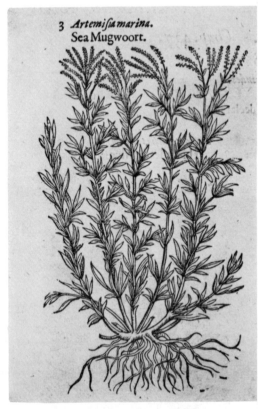

Figure 11-9a *Artemisia maritima* (from J Gerard, *The Herball*, 1597).

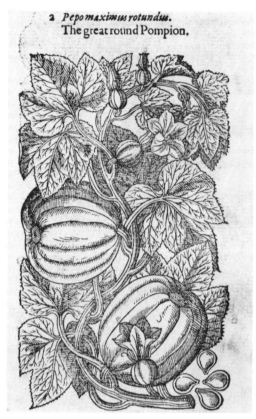

a Pepo maximus rotundus.
The great round Pompion.

Figure 11-9b   *Cucurbita pepo* (from J Gerard, *The Herball*, 1597).

Centratherum anthelminticum seeds (fresh and dried) are used in India against threadworm infections.

Matricaria chamomilla (chamomile). Dried floral heads were used against worm infections, especially in Germany.

Sphaeranthus indicus is used in India as an anthelmintic.

CAPPARIDACEAE

Polanisia graveolens (clammyweed). Root and whole plant decoctions are active anthelmintics.

CHENOPODIACEAE

Oil of wormwood is extracted from *Chenopodium ambrosioides* var. an-

thelminticum (wormwood). It is widely used against roundworms, hookworms, and intestinal amebae in tropical America, although the therapeutic dose is close to minimum toxic levels and death may result from such undesirable side effects as hyperemia of the central nervous system, convulsions, cardiac, and respiratory abnormalities.

CUCURBITACEAE

Cucurbita pepo (pumpkin: Fig. 11-9b). Seeds, as a tea, are used as a home remedy against worms.

EUPHORBIACEAE

Croton macrostachys. Leaf juice functions as an anthelmintic in Ethiopia.

Mallotus philippinensis (kamala tree). Glandular hairs from fruits yield a dye called kamala powder, which has long been used against tapeworms in India.

FABACEAE

Butea monosperma (flame of the forest). Seeds are used in India against roundworms and tapeworms.

LAMIACEAE

Thymus vulgaris (common thyme). Extracts contain an essential oil that eliminates hookworms, but there is only a small margin of safety in its use.

LOGANIACEAE

Spigelia marilandica (wormgrass). Roots were used by the Cherokees and other Indians in the eastern United States for treatment of worms, a practice adopted by orthodox medicine in the nineteenth century. Other active members of this genus include *S. anthelmia* (South America and West Indies), *S. flemmingiana* (Brazil), and *S. glabrata* (Brazil).

MORACEAE

Ficus glabrata and *F. laurifolia* (figs). The proteolytic enzyme ficin, which digests living *Ascaris* and *Trichuris* while being well tolerated and nontoxic to man when taken internally, occurs in the latex. It is widely used by the natives of South America and Panama.

MYRSINACEAE

Embelia tsjeriam-cottam. Dried fruit is used mainly in India to kill tapeworms.

PAPAVERACEAE

Dicentra formosa (wild bleeding heart). Root decoction has been used against worms by Indians in the Pacific northwest.

AMEBICIDES

Amebiasis is an infection from the ameba *Entamoeba histolytica,* which causes dysentery and liver abscesses in man. The disease may be mild and chronic or acute and fulminant, progressing rapidly to peritonitis and death in the absence of specific therapy. Since the turn of the century, emetine from *Cephaelis ipecacuanha* (ipecac) has been successfully used to treat amebic dysentery, and in 1959 its analog dehydroemetine (less toxic on the heart muscle) was introduced. Chloroquine and antibiotics such as paromomycin also have direct amebicidal action; tetracycline and erythromycin indirectly affect amebic survival by modifying the intestinal flora necessary for the existence of the organisms.[12]

Besides *Chenopodium ambrosioides* var. *anthelminticum* noted under Anthelmintics, the following plants are found in use in domestic medicine.

APOCYNACEAE

Holarrhena antidysenterica (tellicherry bark). Bark extracts are used in India to treat amebic dysentery.

CARICACEAE

Carica papaya (papaya). Latex is employed as an amebicide in Central America.

SIMAROUBACEAE

Brucea javanica and *B. sumatrana.* Seed extracts are used to treat amebic dysentery in southeastern Asia.
Simarouba amara. Bark is used as an amebicide.

HEMORRHOIDS

Hemorrhoids or piles are swellings caused by the abnormal dilation of veins of the anus or rectum. They may be located within the anal canal, or they may protrude from the anal opening. Often hemorrhoids become inflamed; ulceration and bleeding are common symptoms, and the condition may be complicated by itching and mucus leakage. The pain may become excruciating, especially during defecation.

Treatment of hemorrhoids consists of obtaining easy bowel movements augmented by the use of astringents, lotions, and ointments. Most are suppositories that combine a local anesthetic, emollients, and sometimes a corticosteroid. A number of plants particularly strong in astringent properties are used in domestic and orthodox medicine for symptomatic relief. Examples are:

ANACARDIACEAE

Rhus glabra and other species of sumac (Fig. 11-10a). Leaves or seeds are said to

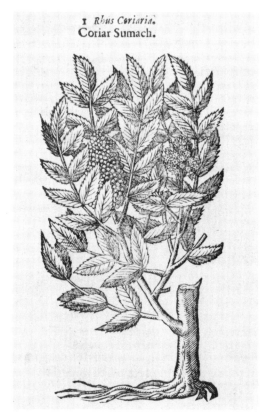

Figure 11-10a *Rhus coriaria* (from J Gerard, *The Herball,* ed 2, 1636).

source of copaiba, an oleoresin obtained from trunks of trees for use against wounds including hemorrhoids; also efficacious in treating chronic diarrhea.

FAGACEAE

Quercus infectoria (dyer's oak). Nutgall ointment is employed for its astringent effect in the treatment of hemorrhoids. In the past, Iroquois and Penobscot Indians boiled the bark of *Q. alba* and drank the liquid for bleeding hemorrhoids.

HAMAMELIDACEAE

Hamamelis virginiana (witch hazel). Leaves have astringent properties (tannins), and an extract made from them is

shrink hemorrhoids and to stop all bleeding. Sumac decoctions were widely used externally and internally during the nineteenth century in eastern North America.

ASTERACEAE

Anaphalis margaritacea (pearly everlasting). A decoction, which is mildly astringent, was a treatment for hemorrhoids employed by Indians and settlers in eastern North America.

Serretula tinctoria (centaury). Root and whole plants were used to treat hemorrhoids and wounds in general.

FABACEAE

Copaifera officinalis, C. reticulata, and other species from South America are the

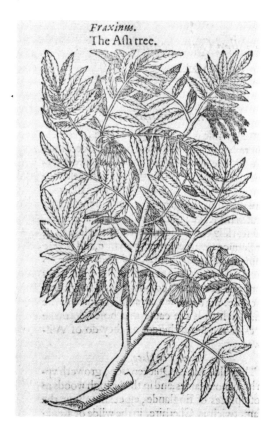

Figure 11-10b *Fraxinus excelsior* (from J Gerard, *The Herball,* 1597).

used in suppositories. Eastern North American Indians also used topical applications of the bark against hemorrhoids.

OLEACEAE

Fraxinus americana (white ash). Bark of this and other species of *Fraxinus* (Fig. 11-10*b*) was used in eastern North America for treatment of hemorrhoids in the nineteenth century and perhaps earlier.

RUBIACEAE

Quinine from *Cinchona* spp. has been used as a hardening agent in the treatment of varicose veins and hemorrhoids.

SIMOURABACEAE

Brucea javanica and *B. sumatrana* seeds have been employed for centuries from China to India for treating hemorrhoids, as well as chronic dysentery, diarrhea, and amebiasis.

CARMINATIVES

Of all the minor disorders that afflict the lower intestinal tract, perhaps none has been the source of so much folklore, low humor, and social embarrassment as flatulence—excessive gas in the stomach or intestine. To aid in the release of gas, thus relieving flatulent colic and griping, the use of a carminative is sometimes necessary. Often these are aromatic oils of plant origin—for example, members of the Apiaceae (umbel family) and Lamiaceae (mint family) as listed below—or they may be commercial preparations containing mixtures of silica gel and dimethylpolysiloxanes (simethicone). A domestic recipe to remove both gas and headache contains a mixture of cream of

tartar, sugar, water, and vinegar, to which baking soda is added.

APIACEAE

Anethum graveolens (dill). A seed decoction is widely used in the treatment of flatulent colic.

Foeniculum vulgare (fennel). Fennel oil from the fruit is widely used in domestic medicine as a carminative and to prevent colic in infants.

Pimpinella anisum (anise). Seeds are used in home remedies as a carminative.

ARACEAE

Acorus calamus (sweet flag). Rhizomes are used to relieve flatulent colic.

LAMIACEAE

Hedeoma pulegioides (American pennyroyal). Dried leaves and flowering tops have long been used as a decoction for flatulence as well as for their stimulant properties.

Mentha piperita (peppermint) and *M. spicata* (spearmint). Dried plants or oil extracts possess carminative properties.

Monarda fistulosa (wild bergamot) and *M. punctata* (horsemint) are commonly employed in domestic medicine as carminatives.

Rosmarinus officinalis (rosemary). Rosemary oil, extracted from fresh flowering tops, is used in combination with other aromatic oils as a carminative. It is also a home remedy in teas for relief of nervous headaches.

ZINGIBERACEAE

Zingiber officinale (ginger). Rhizomes are widely utilized as carminatives and stimulants.

No greater problem with flatulence

exists than for the eaters of beans (*Phaseolus vulgaris*). Recent research exposed the reason for the distressing behavior of beans in the intestinal tract.[13] The presence of complex sugars (oligosaccharides) triggers the creation of the major component of the gas produced in wind-breaking, which is nothing more complex than methane. Ordinarily, when a bean germinates, it secretes the enzyme galactosidase, which breaks down oligosaccharides. Researchers have now developed an enzyme causing this break down to occur whenever the bean is digested; thus, without oligosaccharides, the noxious gases of flatulence will be eliminated from the digestive tract. Soon bean eaters will be at peace with their neighbors!

LITERATURE CITED

1. Mathison RR. 1958. *The Eternal Search*. GP Putnam's Sons, New York. 381 p.

2. Unruly guts. *Lancet* **2:** 960–961, 1972.

3. Sircus W. 1972. Progress report: carbenoxolone sodium. *Gut* **13:** 816–824.

4. Tattersall RN. 1971. Emetics. *Practitioner* **206:** 111–113.

5. Acute intestinal obstruction treated by traditional Chinese methods. 1967. *China's Med* **9:** 690–694.

6. Cockel R. 1971. Anti-emetics. *Practitioner* **206:** 56–63.

7. Cooke WT. 1961. Laxatives and purgatives. *Practitioner* **206:**77–80.

8. Phillips SF. 1972. Diarrhea: a current view of the pathophysiology. *Gastroenterology* **63:** 495–510; Read AE. 1971. Anti-diarrheal agents. *Practitioner* **206:** 69–76.

9. Powell EFW. 1972. *About Dandelions*. Thorsons Publishers, London. 63 p.

10. Meyer C. 1973. *American Folk Medicine*. Thomas Y Crowell, New York. 296 p.

11. Cole ACE. 1971. Anthelmintics. *Practitioner* **206:** 20–25.

12. Seaton DR. 1971. Amoebicides. *Practitioner* **206:** 16–19.

13. A farewell to flatulence. *Newsweek* 9 July 1973: 69.

Chapter 12
Respiratory System

Spanish Herbal Cigarettes when smoked emit an agreeable and fragrant odor, are soothing and pleasant, and leave no objectionable after-effect upon the palate. They are quite free from all ingredients of an injurious or undesirable character, and in cases of Coughs, Colds, Bronchitis, Asthma, and Pulmonary Complaints, generally they will be found of the greatest value and benefit.

So stated a certificate of analysis on a nineteenth century box of cigarettes sold by the Spanish Cigarette Company of London and New York recommending smoking for relief of symptoms antagonized, if not initiated, by tobacco smoking. Of tobacco none would advertise that "the fumes of this plant afford instantaneous relief from afflictions of the respiratory passages," but this was the appeal for the sale of *Datura stramonium* (Solanaceae: Fig. 12-1a), commonly known as jimson weed, thorn apple, or stramonium, the major component of these herbal cigarettes.

This weed is widely distributed on all continents and is particularly common in North America in pastures, waste and cultivated grounds, along roadsides, and in rocky, open habitats. It has a number of interesting properties directly related to the possession of tropane alkaloids, hyoscyamine, scopolamine, and traces of atropine. The chief toxic symptoms appearing on smoking or ingesting large amounts of stramonium are those of atro-

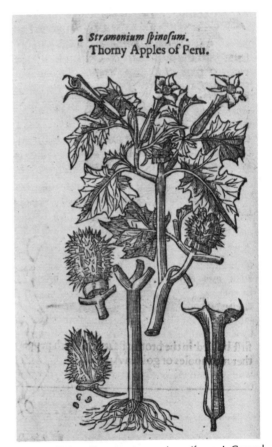

Figure 12-1a *Datura stramonium* (from J Gerard, *The Herball,* ed 2, 1636).

pine poisoning: dilated pupils, impaired vision, dryness of the skin and absence of secretions, extreme thirst, hallucinations (Chapter 18), high temperature, skin rash like that of scarlet fever, convulsions, and ultimately loss of consciousness. In small doses, atropine and the other anticholinergic alkaloids inhibit saliva production, sweating, and bronchial secretions, dilate the bronchi, and abolish vagal action. By smoking stramonium and thereby absorbing small amounts of atropine alkaloids, perhaps some symptomatic relief could be obtained, for such drugs are known to stop the secretions of the respiratory passages; but what of the dangerous side effects of even mild toxicity (i.e., the initiation of impaired vision, rise in temperature, skin rashes, and the be-

ginnings of hallucinations)? This was an interesting nineteenth century medication nonetheless.

Smoking for relief of asthma is not restricted to *Datura stramonium*. Leaves of *D. metel* and *D. fastuosa* are used in cigarettes today in various parts of the tropics, and they undoubtedly give some symptomatic relief. Other plants, such as *Verbascum thapsus* (mullein: Fig. 12-1b), have also been smoked for pulmonary ailments. A nineteenth century home remedy included dried flowers or roots of mullein used as cigarettes for asthmatics. This medication was learned from the Mohegan and Penobscot Indians, who smoked dried, often powdered, leaves, and the Menominees who smoked roots of mullein to obtain relief from pulmonary diseases.

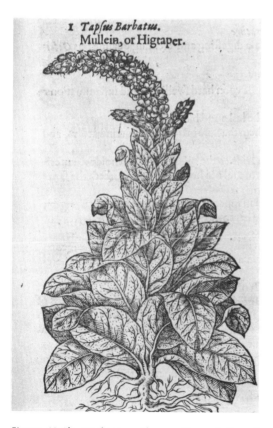

Figure 12-1b *Verbascum thapsus* (from J Gerard, *The Herball,* 1597).

BRONCHODILATORS

Bronchodilators relax the smooth muscles of the bronchioles (Fig. 12-2), the small bronchial tubes in the lungs that lead to the air cells, thereby diminishing generalized peripheral airway obstruction. They thus assist patients with bronchial asthma and those with chronic obstructive lung diseases, bronchitis (inflammation of the bronchial tubes), and emphysema (enlarged air spaces in the lungs, making breathing difficult). The narrowing of the airways in bronchial asthma is due to contraction of the smooth muscles of the bronchi, edema of their walls, and the retention of viscid bronchial secretions. In chronic obstructive lung diseases, distortion and narrowing of the peripheral bronchial airways result from repeated occurrences of bronchial infection, along with excess bronchial secretion and marked hypertrophy of mucous-producing glands.

There are two chief types of bronchodilator drugs: adrenergic agents and

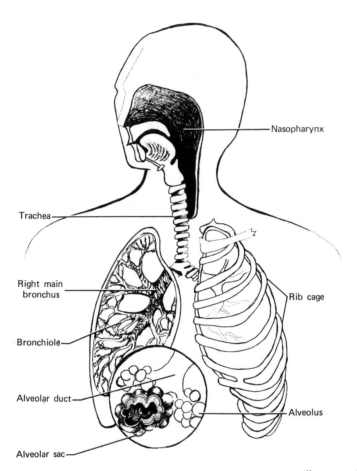

Figure 12-2   Diagrammatic representation of the respiratory system; inset illustrates alveolar sacs.

those derived from theophylline. The adrenergic drugs, which increase the volume and diameter of the bronchial smooth muscles by relaxing them, include norepinephrine, epinephrine (adrenaline), isoprenaline, and ephedrine. Ephedrine is now obtained synthetically, but it may be extracted from its original sources, *Ephedra equisetina* and *E. sinica* (Gymnosperms in the family Ephedraceae).

The second type of bronchodilator includes the theophylline derivates (originally isolated from tea, *Camellia sinensis*), which act directly on the bronchial muscle to relieve obstructions, increase

coronary blood flow, and stimulate respiration centrally. Examples are aminophylline (especially useful in treating emphysema), oxtriphylline, and theophylline monoethanolamine. In severe and persistent cases, corticosteroid therapy may be indicated. A discussion of allergic respiratory diseases appears in Chapter 3.

HERBOLOGY

Plants trusted in domestic and aboriginal medicine as efficacious for respiratory disease were often used with no great specificity; many in fact appear to have been considered panaceas. Thus in certain instances the plants given below are listed arbitrarily with regard to their presumed activity.

GYMNOSPERMS

Ephedra gerardiana (Ephedraceae). Dried stems have long been used in northern India and Pakistan to relieve bronchial asthma. Very probably this species possesses an adrenergic drug similar to ephedrine, a compound extracted from other species of *Ephedra* and, as we noted, used as a bronchodilator in orthodox medicine.

ANGIOSPERMS

ASCLEPIADACEAE

Tylophora indica root infusion is specific for asthma and bronchitis in India; it apparently also has emetic properties and is sometimes used as a substitute for ipecac syrup as an expectorant. Like most members of this family, *T. indica* is toxic and should be used with extreme caution.

ASTERACEAE

Saussurea lappa (costus) of Kashmir and neighboring areas. Root extracts reportedly relax involuntary muscles, and this property is supposedly responsible for relief gained in instances of bronchial asthma and coughs.

CAMPANULACEAE

Lobelia inflata (Indian tobacco) and to a lesser extent *L. cardinalis* (cardinalflower) and *L. siphilitica* (great lobelia), all native to eastern North America, contain the tropane alkaloid lobeline and the pungent volatile oil lobelianin. The species were widely used in the nineteenth century and were considered the most valuable of our indigenous species medically because of diaphoretic, speedy catarrh expectorant, and bronchial mucolytic properties. In Europe lobeline was considered efficacious against chronic bronchitis and asthma. The Indians smoked the leaves and thereby, so it was said, obtained relief from their respiratory difficulties.

Lobelia nicotianaefolia (wild tobacco). Whole plant is used in India to treat bronchitis and asthma.

EUPHORBIACEAE

Euphorbia hirta relaxes the bronchioles but apparently has a depressant action on general respiration and the heart. The entire dried plant is used.

FABACEAE

Glycyrrhiza glabra (licorice). Dried roots and underground stems, used as a decoction or chewed, reportedly relieve bronchitis, sore throats, and coughs.

LAMIACEAE

Monarda fistulosa (wild bergamot or horsemint) contains volatile oils, among them bergamot oil. The Ojibwas boiled dried plants and inhaled the fumes to treat catarrh and general bronchial afflictions.

SCROPHULARIACEAE

Verbascum thapsus (mullein). Employing techniques learned from the native population, pioneers of North America smoked the leaves of mullein to relieve asthma and bronchitis; the Creeks boiled roots and drank the decoction to treat coughs; the Menominees smoked the root to relieve pulmonary disease; the

Mohegans smoked the leaves to aid their asthma and sore throats; the Potawatomis also smoked dried leaves for their asthma and inhaled the fumes of a smoke smudge made from the leaves to alleviate catarrh.

SOLANACEAE

Datura stramonium and other species containing hyoscyamine, atropine, and so on, as noted, have been widely used in treating bronchitis and asthma.

ZINGIBERACEAE

Alpinia galanga (greater galangal). Dried rhizomes, containing the volatile oil essence d'Amali, is used in northern India to treat respiratory complaints particularly of children; bronchial catarrh is specifically mentioned.

Recent results of treating chronic bronchitis in the People's Republic of China using *Rhododendron anthopogonoides* (Ericaceae) extracts containing anthorhododendrin by oral and aerosol therapy are very encouraging. For example, oral treatment of 100 patients for 20 days proved effective in 93% of cases, of which 58% could be described as excellent. During the course of treatment, sputum decreased in 91% of the cases, cough in 85%, and asthmatic symptoms in 58.1%. Aerosol therapy was equally effective.[1]

In traditional Chinese folk medicine, cough and other pulmonary diseases are effectively treated by *Ardisia japonica, A. hortorum* (Myrsinaceae), and *Bergenia sibirica* (Saxifragaceae). The major antitussive constituent is bergenin, and recent studies suggest that the active expectorant ingredient in *A. japonica* may be a flavonoid. Recent research with experimental animals indicates that *A. japonica* and bergenin are effective and safe in the treatment of chronic bronchitis.[2]

EXPECTORANTS AND MUCOLYTIC AGENTS

Many individuals who suffer from respiratory disease find it difficult to clear the chest of sputum. A number of substances are used to aid them. The expectorants are administered orally to stimulate patients to cough, thereby relieving their chest congestion. Many of these are also emetics. Others, the inhalants, are mucolytic agents that act to render the sputum less viscid so that it can be expectorated more readily.

Among the expectorants known to have irritating or stimulating effects are ipecac syrup (*Cephaelis ipecacuanha*), which is especially effective if mixed with cherry or raspberry syrups, which purportedly have soothing actions on irritated throat membranes; the terpenoid volatile oils such as cineol from *Eucalyptus,* wormseed, and rosemary; pinene from pine, juniper, and other Gymnosperms; and terpin hydrate synthesized from geraniol (extracted from *Pelargonium odoratissimum*). A third type of expectorant is creosote obtained from the American beech (*Fagus ferruginea*) and other sources. Creosote is a mixture of phenolic compounds, among which guaiacol and creosol are of value in loosening mucus. At one time guaiacol was widely thought to help cure tuberculosis.

Among the mucolytic inhalant agents, whose actions include increasing the respiratory fluid volume by drawing more water into the bronchial secretions, hence diluting the mucus and reducing its viscosity, are glycerin, cysteine compounds, and a new compound bromhexine, a synthetic derived from the quinoline alkaloid vasicine. Unlike other mucolytic compounds, bromhexine has been shown to have specific action on some of the components of sputum. Vasicine was originally extracted from plant sources, but since clinical trials of the new synthetic in Great Britain have been encouraging,[3] it appears that another drug has entered modern medicine after a long and successful history of use as an expectorant by the herbalists of India.

As an adjunct to other forms of treatment, adequate humidification may prove of great therapeutic value.

HERBOLOGY

GYMNOSPERM

Pinus roxburghii, containing oil of turpentine, is used in northern India in small doses as a stimulant expectorant and also to treat chronic bronchitis.

ANGIOSPERMS

ACANTHACEAE

Adhatoda vasica. Leaves of the Malabar nut tree, either dried or fresh, are prescribed as a mucolytic agent in Asia.

APOCYNACEAE

Apocynum androsaemifolium (spreading dogbane or wild ipecac) and *A. cannabinum* (hemp dogbane) were officially recognized in the nineteenth century as diaphoretics and expectorants; they also have emetic, cathartic, and diuretic properties. However, their action may be that of toxicity directly related to their cardiotonic activity. The pioneers were said to have learned the use of these plants from the Indians.

ARACEAE

The Potawatomis sniffed the powdered root of *Acorus calamus* (sweet flag) to treat catarrh; other Indians chewed the root to stop coughs. Dried and powdered roots of *Symplocarpus foetidus* (skunk cabbage) are supposed to give significant relief to the aged from asthma and catarrh when all other remedies fail.

EUPHORBIACEAE

Acalypha indica, containing the alkaloid acalyphine in the whole plant, has expectorant and emetic properties similar to ipecac. It also possesses a cyanogenic glycoside and is poisonous.

Euphorbia corollata and *E. ipecacuanha* (ipecac spurge). Roots were used in small doses in nineteenth century domestic medicine for diaphoresis and as expectorants; in large doses they are emetic.

HYDROPHYLLACEAE

Eriodictyon californicum (yerba santa). Dried leaves have been used in powdered form as a stimulating expectorant. The Indians of the southwestern United States and Mexico have long employed the leaves for lung afflictions—dry leaves were chewed or smoked, and a tea was made from them for internal use.

ANTITUSSIVE AGENTS

Cough is a natural reflex to help clear the respiratory system of secretions and foreign materials. Antitussive (anticough) agents are sometimes needed to suppress coughing to facilitate rest and sleep, and to reduce irritation of the respiratory tract.

Acting centrally by depressing the cough reflex of the central nervous system, codeine—and to some extent other opium alkaloids—are probably the most widely used compounds. They are used in cough syrups with or without the active principles of a number of volatile oils like menthol (peppermint oil) and eucalyptol. In addition, these oils may be found in cough drops, lozenges, and inhalers for use in soothing sore and irritated throats and reducing coughing.

HERBOLOGY

A number of plants have been used to stop coughing and also to soothe sore throats; others may be found under Cold Remedies.

ANACARDIACEAE

Rhus glabra (sumac). Root bark was used in the nineteenth century as a gargle for sore throats.

ARALIACEAE

Aralia nudicaulis (wild sarsaparilla). Boiled and powdered roots were used by the Ojibwas as a cough remedy; likewise the Penobscots used the powdered roots, but they combined them with *Acorus calamus* (sweet flag) roots to make their cough medicine.

Aralia racemosa (spikenard). Roots, alone or mixed with the bark of *Pinus strobus* (white pine), formed the basis of a popular nineteenth century cough syrup.

FABACEAE

Prosopis julifora (mesquite). Pima Indians boiled the juice, poured it over the bark, and drank the hot tea for sore throats.

MYRTACEAE

Syzygium cumini. Bark is very astringent, and a decoction is used in India to treat sore throats, bronchitis, and asthma.

RANUNCULACEAE

Xanthorhiza simplicissima (shrub yellowroot). Tea made from roots was commonly used by the pioneers of the southern Appalachian Mountains to treat sore throats and colds.

ROSACEAE

Prunus serotina (wild black cherry) and *P. virginiana* (choke cherry). The Ojibwas treated coughs and colds with tea from the bark.

SOLANACEAE

Solanum surattense. Dried root was used in India to treat asthma and coughs; the fruit is said to help sore throats.

INFECTIONS

UPPER RESPIRATORY

More than 90% of upper respiratory tract infections are nonbacterial, and because of their viral etiology they resist antibiotic therapy. Treatment is primarily symptomatic and is directed against relieving sinus and chest congestion, coughing, sneezing, and malaise. Preventive measures are limited to the use of vaccines against specific serotypes of influenza and adenoviruses. Although vitamin C is promoted as a cold preventive, it has been found to do no more than shorten the duration of certain colds, rather than prevent them (Chapter 8, references 9, 10).

The vast number of viral serotypes [rhinovirus (1–80); coronavirus (1–20); adenovirus 3, 4, 17, 21] responsible for the common cold accounts for the frequency of this illness. Coldlike symptoms may also be due to viruses that usually cause more severe respiratory and other infections, such as the myxoviruses, parainfluenza (1–4), influenza (1–3), and respiratory syncytial (1), and the enteroviruses, poliovirus (1–3), echovirus (11, 20, 25), and coxsackievirus (A21, B4, B5). Similar symptoms may also be caused by *Mycoplasma pneumoniae*, *Coxiella burnetii*, and *Chlamydia psittaci*.

SINUSITIS

Bacterial infection of the paranasal sinuses may result from species of *Streptococcus* and *Staphylococcus* that normally reside in the oropharynx. Such infections occur following viral rhinitis, or more rarely from traveling in a poorly pressurized aeroplane or diving while swimming. Whereas maxillary sinus infection usually results through extension of pulp infections in teeth in the upper jaw, infection may also occur after extraction.

Treatment includes the administration of analgesics for pain (codeine, morphine), vasoconstrictors (phenylephrine or ephedrine) to promote drainage, and specific antibiotics (penicillin, erythromycin) to arrest the infection.

PHARYNGITIS

Sore throat or inflammatory disease of the pharynx may be caused by a number of viruses, bacteria, and fungi. Typical lesions are pathodiagnostic of viral diseases such as gingivostomatitis (herpesvirus I) and herpangina (coxsackievirus types A2, 4, 5, 6, 8, and 10). Exudative pharyngitis is common with infectious mononucleosis (Epstein-Barr virus) and adenovirus infection. Furthermore, sore throat may also be a symptom of poliovirus infection.

Streptococcus pyogenes (Lancefield type A), the most common cause of bacterial pharyngitis, produces an exudative (pus) infection in the lymphoid tissue of the pharynx. "Strep throat" and acute tonsillitis are often accompanied by symptoms of fever, swollen lymph nodes (adenitis), headache, chills, and muscle pains. Scarlet fever may also result from strains producing an erythrogenic toxin. In rare instances extension of infection can cause otitis media, mastoiditis, and pneumonia; and if the organisms are disseminated by the bloodstream, they can infect the bone and nervous system (meningitis) as well. After a latent period of a few days or weeks, a few patients also develop an adverse immune reaction to streptococcal components, which

then produce rheumatic fever or glomerulonephritis. Rheumatic fever is characterized by painful swollen joints, fever, myocarditis, rash on the trunk and inner aspects of the thighs and upper arms (erythema marginatum), and rheumatic nodules over the elbows, knees, hands, and ankles. Salicylates (aspirin) and glycosteroids have been found to suppress the acute febrile and exudative manifestation of rheumatic fever but cannot prevent cardiac damage.

Persistent use for several decades notwithstanding, penicillin is still the drug of choice. It is also administered prophylactically to prevent recurrences among patients with rheumatic heart disease. Routine bacterial culturing of school children with sore throat and prompt treatment of those with *Streptococcus pyogenes* has dramatically reduced the incidence of both acute infections and the sequelae.

Pharyngitis may also result from infection with *Streptococcus pneumoniae* and *Staphylococcus aureus,* which normally reside in the nasopharynx. Therapy in such cases depends on the specific antibiotic sensitivity of the organism involved. Another normal oral inhabitant, the yeast *Candida albicans,* can produce a membraneous pharyngitis that is treated with either mycostatin or fungiozone.

Before the development of a specific toxoid immunization, diphtheria infection from *Corynebacterium diphtheriae* was a major cause of infantile death throughout the world. Accompanying the pharyngitis and intoxication, membrane formation with possible airway obstruction, cough, pain, and cervical lymphadenopathy (swollen lymph glands), can occur. Treatment includes administration of antitoxin and use of penicillin G or erythromycin. To eliminate the carrier state in the convalescent patient, erythromycin therapy and surgical removal of the adenoids and tonsils has been found useful.

EPIGLOTTITIS, LARYNGITIS, AND LARYNGOTRACHEOBRONCHITIS

Inflammatory infections of the epiglottis, larynx, and laryngotracheobronchial region are collectively known as croup. Myxoviruses (parainfluenza, respiratory syncytial, and influenza) have been implicated, as have *Corynebacterium diphtheriae, Streptococcus pneumoniae, Hemophilus influenzae,* and *Bordetella pertussis.*

To relieve congestion, humidification (cold moist air) is recommended; if respiratory distress is detected, oxygen therapy should be used to prevent cyanosis. When bacterial etiology is known, the specific antibiotic should be administered promptly. In this regard, ampicillin and chloramphenicol are useful with *H. influenzae.* As a result of the widespread use of the killed bacterial vaccine of *B. pertussis,* whooping cough, with its characteristic thick ropy sputum and endotoxemia, is rare. When indicated, however, erythromycin and tetracycline are effective. Therapy for *C. diphtheriae* has been described above.

PRIMARY BRONCHOPNEUMONIA (INTERSTITIAL PNEUMONIA)

Primary bronchopneumonia is characterized by its insidious nature and lack of definitive clinical manifestations. Infections by certain viruses, and by *Mycoplasma pneumoniae, Coxiella burnetti, Chlamydia psittaci,* and the parasite *Pneumocystis carinii,* produce an interstitial inflammation of the parenchyma resulting in exudate that collects in the interalveolar septa. Parainfluenza and respiratory syncytial virus infections are more common in children; otherwise disease in both children and adults may be caused by influenza viruses, adenoviruses, variola (smallpox), varicella (chickenpox), and measles virus. In natural or induced immunodeficiency states, infections of cytomegalovirus and *Pneumocystis carinii* are more common. With *Mycoplasma, Coxiella,* and *Chlamydia* infections, tetracyclines and chloramphenicol have been found useful. Although not generally used, prophylactic therapy has been successful with Amantadine HCl for influenza A2 infections and the synthetic isoquinolines UK 2371 and UK 2054 for influenza B infections. Amantadine is not viricidal; it acts by blocking

or slowing down the penetration of virus into host cells. Similarly, isoquinolines are thought to interfere with viral neuramidase, therefore preventing the virus from attaching to cell surfaces.

LOBAR PNEUMONIA

Clinical manifestations of infection of the lung parenchyma include cough, pleural pain, pulmonary consolidation, fever, chills, malaise, and at times jaundice and cyanosis.

Bacteria that normally inhabit the nasopharynx and have the potential to incite disease in the compromised host are able to produce lobar pneumonia. Infection with *Streptococcus pneumoniae* serotypes is typified by an explosive onset, massive lung involvement, rusty sputum, short duration, and rapid resolution. *Hemophilus influenzae* pneumonia is indistinguishable from pneumococcal pneumonia, but it is more common in children than adults. Disease produced by *Staphylococcus aureus* is a necrotizing process leading to abscess formation, as is that of *Klebsiella pneumoniae,* which is further characterized by the production of a viscid, stringy sputum related to the organism's capsule. Streptococcal pneumonia is an infrequent sequela to scarlet fever or streptococcal pharyngitis. The appearance of the exudate is also pathodiagnostic, and the activity of bacterial enzymes is responsible for this thin, serous or serosanguinous, pleural fluid. Pneumonia may also result from inhalation of virulent bacterial species, such as those causing tularemia (*Francisella tularensis*), anthrax (*Bacillus anthracis*), plague (*Yersinia pestis*), tuberculosis (*Mycobacterium tuberculosis*), and in histoplasmosis the fungal spores of *Histoplasma capsulatum.*

The choice of specific antibiotics is important to the resolution of these infections: penicillin G, methicillin, and oxacillin are used to treat pneumococcal and staphylococcal pneumonia, while gentamicin and cephalothin are administered for *Klebsiella* pneumonia. Treatment of other pneumonias depends on the specific antibiotic susceptibility of the isolate.

EOSINOPHILIC PNEUMONIA

The appearance of eosinophils in sputa from patients exhibiting general symptoms of pneumonia usually indicates infection with the fungus *Aspergillus,* infestation with the lung flukes (*Paragonimus* spp.), and migration through the lungs of the roundworms *Ascaris lumbricoides, Dirofilaria,* or larva of the dog tapeworm.

CHRONIC GRANULOMATOUS AND CAVITY LUNG DISEASE

Mycotic infections usually result from inhalation of fungal spores of the saprophytic dimorphic soil-inhabiting *Coccidioides immitis, Histoplasma capsulatum, Blastomyces dermatitidis,* or yeast cells of *Cryptococcus neoformans.* They usually initiate an acute, self-limiting pneumonitis, indistinguishable from those produced by bacteria and viruses. Only infrequently does the chronic form develop, with its slow insidious course of suppurative and granulomatous lesions. When pulmonary cavitation occurs, infection of adjacent pleural tissues is possible. Dissemination by way of the bloodstream also results in the development of metastatic abscesses or granulomas in any organ including the skin, and especially with *C. neoformans,* the meninges. In the tissue phase, these fungi are not contagious. Inhalation of *Aspergillus fumigatus* mycelia can cause asthmatic attacks in hyposensitized persons or produce bronchial plugs and atelectasis in patients with bronchitis and bronchiectasis; a fatal, disseminating form of pneumonia sometimes occurs in patients who are taking cytotoxic and immunosuppressant drugs.

Chronic lung infections can also be elicited by members of the bacterial order Actinomycetales. It has yet to be firmly established whether the pathogenic species of *Actinomyces* and *Nocardia* are of exogenous or endogenous origin. Species of these genera have been found not only in the soil but as part of the normal oral flora, where they have been implicated in caries and periodontal disease. In rare instances they can produce chronic destructive abscess of connective tissue, including the lungs. Similarly, most species of *Mycobacterium* causing pulmonary infections are of human (*M. tuberculosis*) or animal (*M. bovis, M. avium*) origin, although "atypical" species that may also be saprophytic have been implicated to a greater (*M. kansasii, M. intracelluare*) or lesser (*M. scrofulaceum, M. fortuitum, M. chelonei, M. xenopi*) degree.

The disease known as tuberculosis or consumption has been an important cause of death in many parts of the world. Clinically, primary infection usually goes unnoticed, and after a few weeks the minute lesions in the lung or draining lymph node become inactive and calcification takes place. Viable organisms may remain in a latent state and, if activated, can produce a pulmonary disease having a chronic, variable, and often asymptomatic course with exacerbations and remission. Depending on the degree of lung involvement, diagnostic symptoms may not become apparent until the disease is in the advanced stages. The symptoms are fatigue, fever, cough, hoarseness, chest pain, and bloody sputum. Dissemination elsewhere in the body may occur, although extrapulmonary tuberculosis is much less common than the pulmonary disease.

After primary infection, the delayed hypersensitivity that develops can be detected by skin testing using a crude extract from tubercle bacilli known as tuberculin or a more refined product, the purified protein derivative (PPD). With the advent of successful chemotherapy, relatively few young adults in the United States are skin reactive. Among these populations, skin testing can be used as a screening device and X-rays reserved for confirming active disease. Since therapy must be carried out over a period of several months, several antibiotics in combination are often administered simultaneously to prevent the appearance of resistant mutants. For several years a combination of streptomycin, para-aminosalicylate (PAS), and isoniazid (INH) has been used. Alternatively, when allergy or resistance to the primary drugs arises, injection of kanomycin, capreomycin, or viomycin, or oral administration of cycloserine, ethionamide, and pyrinozinamide is possible. Ethambutol is now replacing PAS as a companion to INH. Furthermore, a new drug rifampin, which is relatively nontoxic and is well absorbed when administered orally with INH, may prove to be the most effective antituberculosis regimen available.

Although not commonly employed in this country, vaccination with live attenuated strains of BCG are widespread. Because the immunogenicity of these BCG strains varies, most American physicians prefer to treat the patient chemotherapeutically as soon as tuberculin conversion is detected. This is the recommended practice even within high risk populations, such as hospital personnel, as vaccination also elicits tuberculin hypersensitivity and skin testing can then not be used as a screening device to detect infection.

A chronic granulomatous pneumonitis known as meliodosis results from contact with infected horses with glanders (*Pseudomonas mallei*) or, in the Far East, from the saprophyte *Pseudomonas pseudomallei*. In its primary pneumonic form, cavitation and calcification resemble tuberculosis; if hematogenous spread occurs, however, multiple abscess formation, especially in the bone or soft tissue, results. Therapy incorporates surgical drainage of abscesses and administration of tetracycline, sulfonamides, and chloramphenicol.

In parts of Africa, South America, and the Far East, ingestion of infected freshwater crabs and crayfish can result in a chronic pulmonary infection with adult hermaphroditic flukes of *Paragonimus westermani, P. africanus, P. skrjabini,* and *P. heterotremus.* When cerebral lesions occur, as in 25% of these cases, persistent epilepsy may result. Fatalities are rare, however, and lesions spontaneously resolve in 5 to 10 years. Bithional, a 2,2'-thio-bis-(4,6)-dichlorophenol, is used for treatment.

HERBOLOGY (LARGELY COLD REMEDIES)

GYMNOSPERMS

Abies balsamea (balsam fir). Balsam pitch was considered one of the most valuable

aboriginal remedies: it was given in infusions for colds, coughs, asthma, and consumption. The Pillager Indians used the needles in a "sweat bath" and also placed them on live coals and inhaled the fumes for colds.

Juniperus virginiana (juniper or red cedar). The Dakotas, Omahas, Poncas, and Pawnees burned the twigs and inhaled the smoke for colds and also used them in vapor baths; a decoction of the boiled cones and leaves was used by the Plains tribes for treating coughs.

Tsuga canadensis (hemlock). The Menominees and Micmacs made a tea of the inner bark for treating pains and colds, the Penobscots steeped twigs in water and used the tea to treat colds, and the Potawatomis brewed a tea from the leaves to induce copious sweating, thus breaking their colds.

Many other Gymnosperms were used as teas or inhalants to relieve cold symptoms. Volatile oils common to most of them are probably the efficacious principles.

ANGIOSPERMS

ARACEAE

Acorus calamus (sweet flag: Fig. 12-3a). Indians chewed the root, drank a decoction, or inhaled smoke from the root in an attempt to relieve cold symptoms.

ASTERACEAE

Achillea millefolium (yarrow: Fig. 12-3b). The Micmacs used this plant as a "sweat herb" to cure colds. It was boiled for one hour and taken in warm milk.

CUCURBITACEAE

Momordica charantia (wild balsam apple). Whole fruit nearing maturity is pickled in whisky containing generous amounts of rock sugar; the mixture is

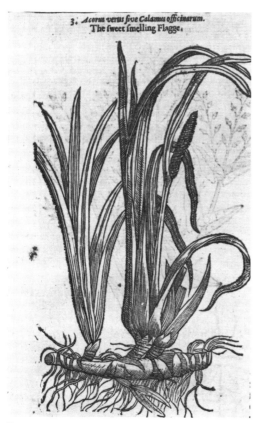

Figure 12-3a *Acorus calamus* (from J Parkinson, *Theatrum Botanicum,* 1640).

used like cough syrup as a domestic remedy against colds and sore throats in Missouri and other parts of the Ozark plateau.

BETULACEAE

Betula occidentalis (western red birch). Decoction of the inner bark was used by the western Indians for treating colds, coughs, and other pulmonary ailments; "cones" of *B. pumila* were heated over coals by the Pillager Indians to make an incense for catarrh patients.

LAMIACEAE

Hedeoma pulegioides (American pennyroyal). Dried flowers and tops contain the volatile oil ketone pulegone, and tea

made from them is supposed to promote perspiration for relief of colds. The Catawbas boiled the plant and used the extract as a cold remedy, a procedure also followed by the Plains Indians, using *H. hispida.*

Marrubium vulgare (horehound). Tea from the whole plant has long been used in domestic medicine as a cure for coughs, sore throats, and colds, and also as an expectorant. Horehound flavored candy is available today.

Nepeta cataria (catnip). Tea has been used by the inhabitants of the southern Appalachian region as a cold remedy since the eighteenth century.

Many other species of Lamiaceae are also indicated for cold treatment, un-

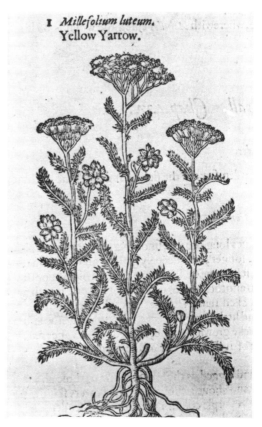

Figure 12-3b *Achillea millefolium* (from J Gerard, *The Herball,* 1597).

doubtedly because of the presence of numerous volatile oils.

SALICACEAE

Populus balsamifera (balsam poplar) and *P. candicans* (balm of Gilead). Salve was made with winter (resinous) buds from these plants boiled in mutton or bear tallow. The Menominees and the Pillager Ojibwas rubbed the ointment on the nostrils or put it up the nose, allowing the balsamic vapors to course through the respiratory passages to relieve congestion from colds, cattarh, and bronchitis.

SCROPHULARIACEAE

Verbascum thapsus (mullein). Flowers were used by the early white settlers in North America as a treatment for tuberculosis.

SOLANACEAE

Withania somnifera. Dried roots are considered useful in treating consumption in India. Antibiotic and antibacterial activity of the roots and leaves has been shown experimentally.

LITERATURE CITED

1. Anthorhododendrin in the treatment of chronic bronchitis. 1973. *Chin Med J* **158** (12).

2. Experimental studies on *Ardisia japonica* in treatment of chronic bronchitis. 1973. *Chin Med J* **158** (12), 157.

3. Gent M, Knowlson PA, Prince FJ. 1969. Effect of bromhexine on ventilatory capacity in patients with a variety of chest diseases. *Lancet* **2:** 1094–1096; Hamilton WFD, Palmer KNV, Gent M. 1970. Expectorant action of bromhexine in chronic obstructive bronchitis. *Brit Med J* **3:** 260–261.

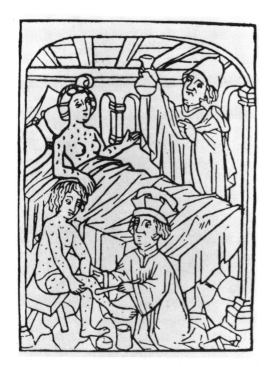

Figure 13-1a The earliest known portrayal of syphilis, showing typical skin lesions of the secondary stage (title page from B Steber's *Syphilis*, 1497 or 1498.)

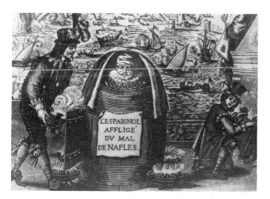

Figure 13-1b A Renaissance treatment of syphilis—the sweat bath.

Chapter 13

Urogenital System

Coincidental with Columbus's discovery of the New World, there arose in Europe toward the end of the fifteenth century an epidemic caused by a new crippler. This was the French disease, the Spanish disease (depending on your nationality), or more commonly in the medical literature of the day, the Great Pox. We call it syphilis, and we have learned that the disease is caused by the bacterium *Treponema pallidum*; but our ancestors knew nothing about this strange malady in 1494 (Fig. 13-1a).

Syphilis first appeared in Naples, where French and Spanish troops fought for control of the boot of Italy. Venereal sores were found among many of the same Spanish warriors who had served with Columbus a year earlier. Before long the French captured Naples and replaced the Spanish in rollicks with the ladies of that fair city; but within a year all the soldiers returned home, and the Spanish-French disease spread throughout Italy and France to Switzerland, Holland, Germany, and even Scotland and Russia. By 1500 it was epidemic throughout the known world.

A fierce debate waged on the origin of syphilis. Sailors with Columbus could certainly have contracted such a disease from the Carib natives of the West Indies, who were essentially immune to its virulence and have transported it to a civilization where natural immunity did not

309

exist. Still it is debatable whether its spread could have been initiated by a few sailors in so short a time. Alternately, syphilis could have been in Europe, suddenly mutating into a virulent, highly contagious form. A very mild, non-venereal infection of *T. pallidum,* known as bejel, exists among the Bedouins today.

Regardless of the origin of syphilis, its effect on Europe was devastating. Everyone and everything was to blame. Jupiter, Mars, and Saturn had been in rare conjunction, said astrologers, and syphilis was the result. The noted Spanish physician Ruy Diaz de Isla blamed cabbage. The German clergy of the day considered that it was caused by the sin of blasphemy: soldiers and sailors swore the most, they contended, hence they were most afflicted with the disease. Maximilian I was convinced by this logic, and issued an edict that all children with lesions be punished for swearing!

Few physicians treated syphilis. It begins in one of the most degrading and ignoble places of the body, wrote a medical leader, and should be ignored. Cures were few. Suicides became so commonplace that not since the time of the Greeks and Romans had so many taken their own lives. A temporary ray of hope was introduced with lignum vitae (*Guaiacum sanctum,* Zygophyllaceae) and lignum sanctum (*G. officinale*), native to tropical America; a broth made from the bark was taken for 14 days, and a bark foam was rubbed on the chancres. But interest soon faded, for the lignum vitae miracle bark, the penicillin of its time, cured few. Earthworm plasters were tried. After that, a devastating month in a hot oven with great amounts of mercury and little food was guaranteed to kill or cure (Fig. 13-1*b*). Many, of course, died from suffocation and heart failure; fewer were cured.

Superstitions were rampant and new remedies continued to appear.[1] By the middle of the sixteenth century, however, the ravages of syphilis had slowed and physicians declared that the malady had settled down. Rather, it had settled in. Men over 40 were stunted and dull. There were more madmen, more deaths from heart disease, and more men walking with the jerky gait of locomotor ataxia.

And since the disease did not go away, something or somebody had to be blamed for these tragic blights. The Roman Catholic Church blamed it on the sin of fornication when the goal was not procreation but pleasure. The Calvinists, too, attacked the syphilitics; all were publicly shamed and outcast. The belief that syphilis was a punishment by God became so commonplace that those infected feared to seek cure, and the disease continued unchecked.

North America was not immune to the thinking of the time. Syphilis was first reported in the Boston area around the middle of the seventeenth century, and a New England physician exhibiting the Puritan ethic declared it due to immoderate intercourse—a display of passion during the sex act clearly caused syphilitic infections. All vehemently denied an origin in America as claimed by Europeans; instead it had all been started by the pope!

Little progress could be made in the atmosphere created by these dogmatic pronouncements based on emotion and prejudice. By 1750, however, a London physician placed on the market small bags that rendered the male organ safe against infection. Dubbed "English frock coats" by the French, they were manufactured from the blind gut of the lamb, washed, dried, and made pliable by rubbing between the palms of the hand with bran and a little almond oil. The inventor-physician thought he was a benefactor of mankind, but Dr. Condon had not reckoned on the clergy. He was soon denounced from the pulpits for adding this new and sordid instrument of sin to an already sinful world. His torments became so violent that the good doctor found it necessary to adopt an alias, but his name, corrupted slightly to condom, lives on.

THE URINARY SYSTEM

The kidneys are bean-shaped, reddish organs that lie retroperitoneally on either side of the vertebral column in the posterior part of the abdomen. Large excretory ducts called ureters lead from each kidney into a common bladder, which collects urine until it is voided through the single urethra. Separate in the female, the urethra also serves to discharge semen in the male.

Within the kidney, a series of tubules acts to filter the blood and remove from it metabolic waters and excess material by the process of urine formation and excretion. By monitoring acid-base balance, osmotic relationships, and the content of organic and inorganic solutes, the kidney regulates the composition and physical properties of the blood.

Urine, colored yellow by urobilinogen, a breakdown product of hemoglobin, is more hypertonic than plasma and somewhat more acid; it consists of urea, uric acid, creatinine, ammonia, and hydrogen and potassium ions. Reabsorption of sodium ion by proximal tubules is dependent on the amounts of aldosterone secreted by the adrenals and calcium by parathyroid hormones. Under certain pathologic conditions such as diabetes mellitus, glucose, which is normally completely reabsorbed during the filtration process, may be found along with other metabolites such as ketone bodies, acetone, and β-hydroxybutyric acid. Just as protein (albuminuria) may also be found under abnormal metabolic conditions, urea can increase in the blood when its concentration is at a level permitting some to pass out of the tubules by simple diffusion. The appearance of microscopic casts in urine sediment is further evidence of renal lesions. The lesions maintain the shape of the kidney tubes where they were formed and are made up of epithelial cells, pus, and blood or hyaline (clear) material. Inorganic material such as oxalates and ascorbic acid crystals may also develop into large bizarre forms and accumulate in the kidney or bladder, where as kidney stones they can produce intense pain and must be removed by surgery.

The kidney also acts to control the volume of body fluids through the mediation of an antidiuretic hormone released from the pituitary. Therefore the volume of urine varies inversely with the amount of hormone secreted, which in turn depends on the amount of solute concentration of the blood reaching the hypothalamus. Excess fluid intake is compensated by decreasing the amount of water reabsorbed during filtration and increasing the amount absorbed when there is depletion of water through excessive sweating, vomiting, and diarrhea. Diuretics act both by decreasing the active removal of sodium ion from the filtrate, allowing it to remain osmotically active, and by decreasing the amount of water passing through the walls of the collecting tubules that are returning water to the body.

For the filtration process to function normally, regular blood pressure must be maintained. This is ensured by the excretion of renin by the kidney; this substance acts on plasma substrate and converts it to angiotensin, an active plasma enzyme. As an active vasoconstrictor, this enzyme can narrow arterioles throughout the body and raise the blood pressure, thereby assuring the continuance of high blood pressure to the kidney. When renin production is not diminished, chronic high blood pressure may result. Further regulatory activity can be demonstrated by noting that this enzyme also affects the adrenal cortex, which secretes the aldosterone necessary for reabsorption of sodium by the kidney tubules.

In rheumatic fever the hydrolization of sialic acid by enzymes of *Streptococcus pyogenes* in the basement membrane of the glomerular capsule results in the formation of antigenic proteins. Further basement membrane injury occurs through the action of specific antibodies to these proteins, allowing cells and more protein to leak into the filtrate.

Edema also occurs because the osmotically active protein molecules are diminished in the blood, leading to failure to return water to the system.

DIURETICS

Diuretics (see above) are chemicals that induce a net loss of fluid from the body by the urinary tract. They are used to eliminate excess liquid and toxic products from the tissues and the vascular system.

Of the many groups of diuretics (osmotic diuretics, mercurial compounds, carbonic anhydrase inhibitors, thiazides), only the xanthines (purine bases) are derived from natural sources. Coffee and tea have long been known to influence the flow of urine, but the xanthine caffeine is only weakly diuretic. About three times as active is theophylline, originally extracted from tea; the compound used today, aminophylline, is entirely synthetic, however, and is especially useful clinically. The diuretic action of theobromine, extracted from the hull of the cocoa bean (*Theobroma cacao*), occupies an intermediate position between caffeine and theophylline.

Many plants are known to exert diuretic effects (remember that the action of many, such as *Apocynum*, *Convallaria*, and *Urginea* is basically cardiotonic). The following species are noteworthy (the plant part used appears in parentheses).

FERN ALLIES

EQUISETACEAE. *Equisetum arvense* (plant), *E. robustum* (plant).

GYMNOSPERM

CUPRESSACEAE. *Callitris arborea* (gum).

ANGIOSPERMS

AIZOACEAE. *Trianthema portulacastrum* (leaves).

ACANTHACEAE. *Acanthus spinosus* (plant), *Hygrophila auriculata* (root, seed).

ALISMACEAE. *Alisma plantago* (plant).

APIACEAE. *Ammi visnaga* (fruit), *A. majus* (fruit: Fig. 13-2a), *Eryngium yuccifolium* (plant).

APOCYNACEAE. *Apocynum cannabinum* (plant).

ASTERACEAE. *Blumea lacera* (plant), *Gaillardia pinnatifida* (plant), *Hypochoeris scarzonerae* (plant), *Tagetes multifida* (plant).

ASCLEPIADACEAE. *Cynanchium vincetoxicum* (plant), *Hemidesmus indicus* (plant).

BEGONIACEAE. *Begonia cucullata* (plant), *B. sanguinea* (plant).

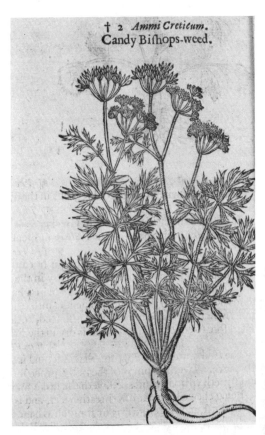

Figure 13-2a *Ammi majus* (from J Gerard, *The Herball*, ed 2, 1636).

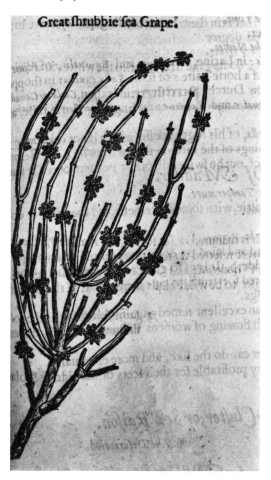

Great shrubbie sea Grape.

Figure 13-2b   *Ephedra fragilis* (from J Gerard, *The Herball*, ed 2, 1636).

CONVOLVULACEAE. *Calystegia soldanella* (plant).
CYPERACEAE. *Carex arenaria* (plant), C. *hirta* (plant).
EUPHORBIACEAE. *Acalypha evrardii* (flower, leaf).
FABACEAE. *Glycyrrhiza glabra* (root), *Psoralea corylifolia* (seed), *Rafnia perfoliata* (leaf).
LILIACEAE. *Chamaelirium luteum* (root), *Convallaria majalis* (rhizome, root), *Urginea indica* (bulb).
LAMIACEAE. *Collinsonia canadensis* (rhizome, root).

LOGANIACEAE. *Buddleja americana* (bark, leaf, root), B. *marrubiifolia* (plant).
MALVACEAE. *Abutilon indicum* (bark, root).
NYCTAGINACEAE. *Boerhaavia diffusa* (plant).
ORCHIDACEAE. *Spiranthes diuretica* (plant).
PORTULACACEAE. *Claytonia sibirica* (plant).
RANUNCULACEAE. *Anemone pulsatilla* (plant), *Clematis biondiana* (plant), C. *gouriana* (plant), C. *vitalba* (plant).
ROSACEAE. *Alchemilla arvensis* (plant).
RUBIACEAE. *Coffea arabica* (fruit).
SANTALACEAE. *Santalum album* (oil).
SCROPHULARIACEAE. *Bacopa monnieri* (plant), *Curanga fel-terrae* (leaf), *Rehmannia lutea* (plant).
SOLANACEAE. *Lycium halimifolium* (plant), *Solanum surattense* (root), *Withania somnifera* (root).
URTICACEAE. *Laportea meyeniana* (leaf, root), *Urtica dioica* (plant).
ZINGIBERACEAE. *Costus spicatus* (sap).
ZYGOPHYLLACEAE. *Tribulus terrestris* (fruit).

ANTIDIURETIC

Tea made from *Chimaphila umbellata* (spotted wintergreen of the North Temperate zone, Ericaceae) retards the excretion of urine.

INFECTIONS

Infections of the urethra and bladder (cystitis), often occurring together, can be caused by numerous microorganisms that normally inhabit the gut or adjacent skin and mucous membranes. Those most commonly isolated are *Escherichia coli*, *Klebsiella* species, and *Proteus* species, although urine may also yield the yeast *Candida albicans* in diabetics, ova in patients with *Schistosoma hematobium* cystitis, and adenoviruses in those with hemorrhagic cystitis. Mixed infections are not uncommon after instrumentation; and urethral infections with *Neisseria gonorrhoeae, Mycoplasma hominis, Trichomonas vaginalis,* and *Chlamydia* species also develop through venereal contact. In men, extension to the prostate is a further source of recurrent urinary disease, whereas women, especially during pregnancy, are more likely to develop acute pyelonephritis. The incidence of pyelonephritis is also higher among hypertensive patients; the disease has also been shown to induce this symptom. The blood is another source of kidney infection, but to a much less serious degree.

Symptoms of dysuria (pain on urination), frequency, urgency and bacteriuria are hallmarks of these diseases, which are also accompanied by fever, perineal and low back pain in prostatitis, and chills, fever, and costovertebral-angle pain in pyelonephritis. In the absence of obstruction, patients may recover spontaneously from urethritis or cystitis. However surgery is used to correct anatomical problems related to retention of bladder urine, and bladder lavage with antibiotics is used to eradicate additional bacteria. Most urinary tract infections not acquired in a hospital, where antibiotic-resistant mutants abound, are successfully treated with penicillin V and by administration of vitamin C, which lowers the urine pH. Therapy of chronic prostatitis is somewhat more difficult, because diffusion of antibiotics into prostatic fluid is often impaired. To ensure that the life-threatening complication of bacteremia from pyelonephritis does not result, careful selection of the antibiotic regimen is a requisite, and surveillance for recurrent infection must be carried out for at least 6 months thereafter.

Infections of the female genital tract can be predisposed by mechanical, venereal, or hormonal factors. Vulvovaginitis is extremely painful and is accompanied by such symptoms as local heat, edema, discharge, severe dyspareunia, all rendering coitus impossible as well as producing pain during defecation and urination. Among the many organisms, *Trichomonas vaginalis, Hemophilus vaginalis,* and *Candida albicans* have been frequently

implicated, as well as herpesvirus II. Ectoparasites, such as lice, scabies, and pinworms, may also be involved.

Extension to the cervix can occur with any of these bacteria or viruses, and also with *Neisseria gonorrhoeae, Streptococcus* and *Staphylococcus* species, *Mycobacterium tuberculosis,* genital strains of *Chlamydia,* and cytomegaloviruses. Heavy purulent discharge, postcoital and intermenstrual bleeding, pain, and tenderness to palpation, are all manifestations of cervicitis. If not treated, chronic infections can result, and extension to the uterus, through the Fallopian tubes (salpingitis) to the ovaries, is possible. Particularly life threatening is infection of the uterus (endometritis), which may result from coitus, pregnancy, or delivery and can become chronic through obstruction of intrauterine (contraceptive) devices, polyps, or fibroids. Complications are serious and can lead to thrombophlebitis and dissemination throughout the body, parametritis, and peritonitis. Before Semmelweiss took doctors to task for not washing their hands between deliveries, death due to puerperal sepsis or childbed fever, caused by *Streptococcus pyogenes,* was commonplace. Therapy using penicillin G and gentamicin may be combined with curettage and surgical removal of any obstruction.

TREATING DISORDERS: HERBOLOGY

In herbal medicine the same plants are often prescribed for treating such diverse ailments as renal and bladder stones, and infections of various kinds. Therefore the following list describes plants used to treat both metabolic and infectious disorders. Many are ancient remedies, one of the oldest being handed down from Pliny the Elder (AD 23–79), who prescribed infusions of peony (*Paeonia officinalis*), mint (*Mentha* spp.), and chick pea (*Cicer arientinum*) to dissolve stones in the bladder and kidney.[2] Other examples:

GYMNOSPERMS

Ephedra nevadensis seeds, when roasted and ground into flour, served to alleviate urogenital diseases of the southwestern American Indians. Other *Ephedra* species (Fig. 13-2b) were also employed. For example, stem decoctions of *E. antisyphilitica* of western Texas and northern Mexico and *E. aspera* of Mexico were used to cure renal diseases.

ANGIOSPERMS

ANACARDIACEAE

Rhus aromatica. Root bark was employed by eastern North American Indians to treat excessive discharges from the bladder and kidney.

ANNONACEAE

Asimina reticulata (Seminole tea). A tea from flowers reportedly relieved the Seminole Indians of Florida of kidney troubles.

APIACEAE

Eryngium campestre (snakeroot). Root extracts were used throughout Europe to treat diseases of the bladder and also uterine irritation.

ASTERACEAE

Eupatorium maculatum (snakeweed). All parts were used as an astringent in kidney ailments. Rhizomes of *E. purpureum* (gravel root) aided treatment of kidney ailments and urinary organs, as well as bladder stones. Both species were widely used in domestic medicine in eastern North America throughout the nineteenth century.

In Hindu medicine extracts of *Siegesbeckia orientalis* are recommended for diseases of the urethra.

CARYOPHYLLACEAE

Arenaria serpyllifolia. Extracts are used in Chinese medicine for the treatment of bladder ailments.

Spergularia rubra (red sandwort) of southern Europe has long been used to treat bladder catarrh and kidney stones.

CLUSIACEAE

Ascyrum hypericoides (St. Andrew's cross) of eastern North America has been considered efficacious for kidney ailments and stones.

ERICACEAE

Arctostaphylos uva-ursi (bearberry: Fig. 13-3a) was used by early settlers of

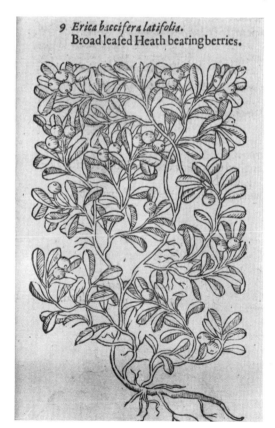

Figure 13-3a *Arctostaphylos uva-ursi* (from J Gerard, *The Herball*, 1597).

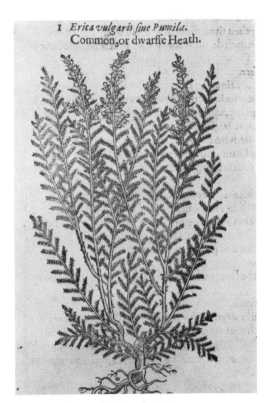

I *Erica vulgaris siue Pumila.*
Common, or dwarffe Heath.

Figure 13-3*b* *Calluna vulgaris* (from J Gerard, *The Herball,* 1597).

eastern North America as an astringent to treat nephritis, kidney stones, and other diseases of the urinary system.

Calluna vulgaris (heather: Fig. 13-3*b*). Extracts have long been used in homeopathic medicine to treat bladder ailments.

Chimaphila umbellata (spotted wintergreen). Leaves of this North Temperate plant were used for treatment of bladder stones.

EUPHORBIACEAE

Croton humilis roots are used in Brazil to treat urinary disease (as well as skin infections).

FABACEAE

Caesalpinia nuga roots are used in tropical Asia for gravel and stones in the bladder.

Copaifera coriacea (copaiba). Balsam from this plant is used in tropical South America as a urogenital disinfectant.

LAMIACEAE

Orthosiphon aristatus and *O. stamineus* leaf teas are used in Java for ailments of the bladder and kidney.

POACEAE

Arundo kakao stems have been employed in New Zealand for kidney ailments.

SOLANACEAE

Fabiana imbricata from Chile and Peru. Leaves and twigs are used to treat functional diseases of the kidney (the extracts also reportedly used as diuretic and tonic).

Solanum mammosum. Leaf decoctions are valued in Costa Rica for ailments of the bladder and kidney, and leaves of *S. paniculatum* are employed to treat bladder catarrh in Brazil.

ULMACEAE

Ulmus fulva (slippery elm). Inner bark collected in the spring contains a thick mucilage or demulcent that was long used in domestic North American medicine to treat urinary tract inflammations (also used as a poultice for abscesses).

REPRODUCTIVE SYSTEM

The genital system of the human female (Fig. 13-4) is composed of two ovaries, the Fallopian tubes (which connect the ovaries to the uterus and where fertilization takes place), the uterus (where a fertilized egg may become attached), and the external opening of the system, the vagina. The ovaries are the principal source of the female sex hormones, which are activated by the pituitary gland dis-

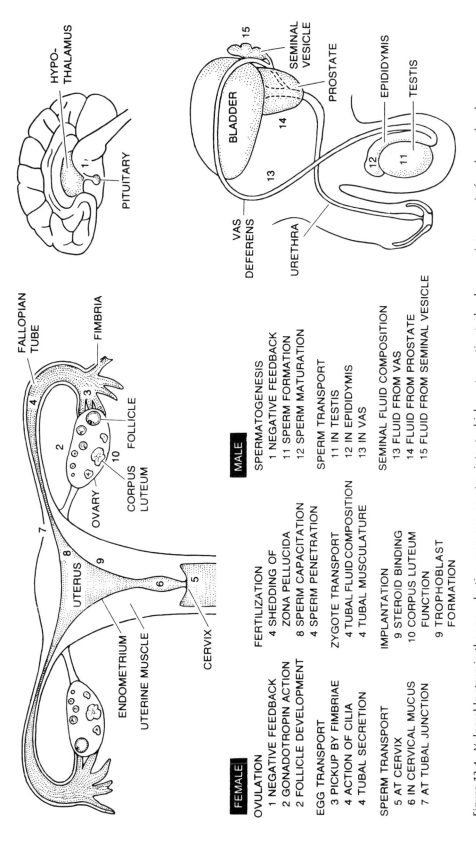

Figure 13-4 Vulnerable steps in the reproductive process suggest points at which contraceptive technology can intervene in females and males. (From SJ Segal, "The physiology of human reproduction," *Scientific American* September 1974, p 62. Copyright © by Scientific American, Inc., and reprinted with their permission.)

FEMALE

OVULATION
1 NEGATIVE FEEDBACK
2 GONADOTROPIN ACTION
2 FOLLICLE DEVELOPMENT

EGG TRANSPORT
3 PICKUP BY FIMBRIAE
4 ACTION OF CILIA
4 TUBAL SECRETION

SPERM TRANSPORT
5 AT CERVIX
6 IN CERVICAL MUCUS
7 AT TUBAL JUNCTION

FERTILIZATION
4 SHEDDING OF
  ZONA PELLUCIDA
8 SPERM CAPACITATION
4 SPERM PENETRATION

ZYGOTE TRANSPORT
4 TUBAL FLUID COMPOSITION
4 TUBAL MUSCULATURE

IMPLANTATION
9 STEROID BINDING
10 CORPUS LUTEUM
   FUNCTION
9 TROPHOBLAST
  FORMATION

MALE

SPERMATOGENESIS
1 NEGATIVE FEEDBACK
11 SPERM FORMATION
12 SPERM MATURATION

SPERM TRANSPORT
11 IN TESTIS
12 IN EPIDIDYMIS
13 IN VAS

SEMINAL FLUID COMPOSITION
13 FLUID FROM VAS
14 FLUID FROM PROSTATE
15 FLUID FROM SEMINAL VESICLE

charge of two gonad-influencing hormones (gonadotropins). One stimulates the hormone-secreting cells of the follicle, which contain the immature eggs, to produce increasing amounts of estrogens, female steroid sex hormones. This brings the egg to a state of maturation necessary for ovulation. The other gonadotropin triggers the ovulation process: the mature egg leaves the follicle, and the empty follicle is stimulated to produce large amounts of progesterone, the second female sex steroid. The endometrium lining the uterus responds to progesterone by thickening and becoming a highly vascular, spongy nest, ready to accept and nurture a fertilized and dividing egg if one arrives from the Fallopian tube. In this case (i.e., in pregnancy), the crisis of menstruation is avoided when there is an uninterrupted supply of progesterone. Eventually the placenta takes over the role of producing sufficient quantities of progesterone to maintain the pregnancy.

In the human male's reproductive system (Fig. 13-4), the center of the process is the testis, which produces sperm and sex hormones. The testis is stimulated by pituitary gonadotropins to produce male steroid hormones, mainly testosterone, which in turn must be in high concentration to maintain sperm production. Sperm pass through the vas deferens and urethra at ejaculation. When the sperm are forced rapidly into the urethra by muscular contractions, they are mixed with the fluid secretion of several accessory glands that serves primarily as a vehicle to carry the sperm into the vagina. The sperm are still immature, and only in the female reproductive tract do they reach maturity in response to estrogen domination around the time of ovulation. Few reach the upper part of the Fallopian tube, where one may penetrate and fertilize the egg. For a more detailed account of the physiology of human reproduction, the reader should refer to Segal.[3]

PRODUCTION OF HORMONES

Estrogens may be extracted from the urine of horses, but most hormones obtained in a pure state and on a large scale must be synthesized by combined chemical and microbiological processes. However partial synthesis (i.e., starting with a preformed steroidal nucleus) is far more practical than total synthesis, as the list from plant sources attests (Table 13-1).

Progesterone, for example, can be synthesized from diosgenin in only four steps. Since diosgenin is found in the rhizomes of various species of Dioscorea (Fig. 13-5) having a steroidal content of about 40% diosgenin and from 50 to 60% other sapogenins, it is available in quantity for conversion. Diosgenin is treated with acetic anhydride (Ac_2O) and yields an ester of the pseudosapogenin. This, when oxidized with chromium trioxide (CrO_3) followed by hydrolysis, yields two intermediate compounds and finally progesterone (Fig. 13-6).

In 1952 it was discovered that the fungus Rhizopus was capable of performing 11-α-hydroxylation when progesterone, which by then was readily available by partial synthesis from diosgenin of yams, was used as substrate. This

Table 13-1 Major Plant[a] Starting Materials for Hormone Synthesis[b]

Source	Compound
Glycine max (soy bean)	Stigmasterol
Physostigma venenosum (calabar bean)	Stigmasterol
Saccharomyces spp. (yeast and other microorganisms)	Ergosterol
Cereal grains	β-Sitosterol
Dioscorea spp. (yams)	Diosgenin
Agave sisalana (sisal)	Hecogenin
Solanum spp. fruit	Solasodine
Strophanthus spp. seed	Sarmentogenin
Holarrhena spp.	Conessine and holarrhimine

[a] Animal sources include cattle spinal cord for cholesterol, and bile for cholic acid and deoxycholic acid.
[b] Modified from A Burger (1960).[4]

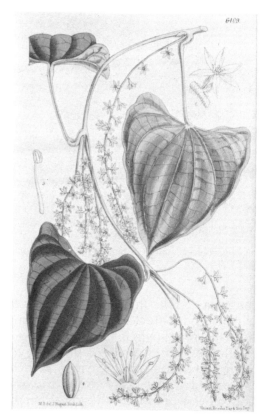

Figure 13-5 *Dioscorea vittata* (from *Curtis's Botanical Magazine* **105:** 6409, 1879).

11-α-hydroxyprogesterone can eventually be converted to cortisone (Fig. 13-7). Other transformations involving different fungi allow circumvention of some difficult and costly chemical conversions. Thus very recently sex hormones have become available at reasonable cost for a host of therapeutic uses, including the treatment of menopause, amenorrhea, dysmenorrhea, premenstrual tension, and testicular deficiency.

CONTRACEPTION

The development in the early 1950s of semisynthetic steroids opened the way for the mass use of these compounds as oral contraceptives. The standard female contraceptive pill combines an estrogen with a progestin, a progesteronelike chemical. These hormones have two major functions: to suppress the pituitary hormones through negative feedback, and to stimulate the endometrium of the uterus, initiating a menstrual cycle. The combination of hormones is taken 21

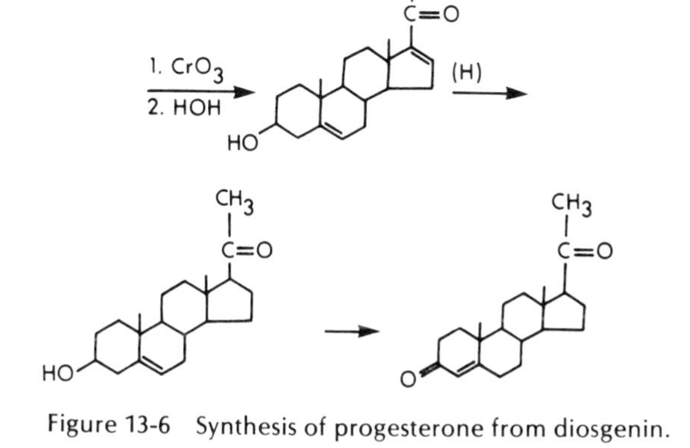

Figure 13-6   Synthesis of progesterone from diosgenin.

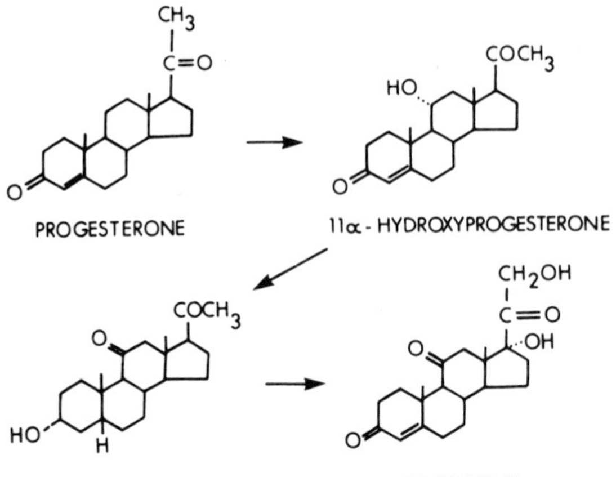

Figure 13-7 Conversion of progesterone to cortisone by combining chemical and microbiological (using *Rhizopus*) synthesis.

days each month, during which time the brain recognizes the high steroid levels in the blood. In turn, the pituitary production of ovary-influencing hormones is suppressed, signaling the cessation of further ovarian function. On completion of a pill cycle, endometrial breakdown occurs, accompanied by menstrual flow.

Even though the oral contraceptive tablet combining estrogen and progestin is the most effective and convenient form of birth control, it does generate a risk of adverse effects. Effectiveness, for example, is illustrated by the very low rate of 0.1 to 1.5 accidental pregnancies per 100 woman-years of use, compared with 15 pregnancies per 100 woman-years using contraception by the rhythm method; however, the major risk with the pill, the formation of blood clots in veins, is about seven to eight times higher in users than in nonusers.[5] Since the risk of clotting is apparently related to the dose of estrogen, the concentration of this substance must be rigidly controlled. Other negative side effects include increased blood pressure, gallbladder disease, headaches, anemia (supplements of vitamin B_2 and E may be indicated), and increased incidence of yeast vaginitis. On

the positive side, the pill can improve or eliminate menstrual disorders, acne, and noncancerous lumps in the breast.

After discontinuation of the pill, abnormal abortuses are increased, particularly a highly significant rise in triploidy and other types of chromosomal abnormalities, which are almost always lethal early in embryonic life. Depression, also, is more common among women who have stopped taking the pill.

About the time of the introduction of oral contraceptives, a second modern form of birth control was introduced, the intrauterine device (IUD). Its development was based on the empirical observation that the presence of an intrauterine foreign body prevented pregnancy. Up to 5 million American women use IUDs, but recent reports indicate a sharp increase in the number of deaths and uterine infections among users, as well as an increase in menstrual bleeding.[6]

Among folk medicines, not many contraceptives are known to us. However, as examples the Barasana Indians of Colombia ingest the unripened spadix, dried and pulverized, of *Urospatha antisylleptica* (Araceae) as their oral contraceptive, and the Shoshonis and other Nevada Indians at one time used a root decoction of *Veratrum californicum* (false hellebore, Liliaceae) taken daily for 3 weeks to ensure sterility. The latter species is known to be highly teratogenic in domestic animals (Chapter 4), but the effectiveness of either species as contraceptives in man must await experimental data.

For a long time responsibility for contraception was left to the male, and recently there has been revived interest in methods to be used by men. These largely involve interfering with sperm production, or blocking the path of the sperm by severing the vas deferens. Recent studies have shown, however, that the latter procedure may have physiological complications entailing autoimmunity, which could increase male susceptibility to disorders like rheumatoid arthritis and other side effects not hitherto associated with vasectomies.[7]

REPRODUCTIVE ORGANS

Uterine Stimulants

Oxytocic agents stimulate the motility of the uterus, hastening the rapidity of labor. Only a limited number of these potentially dangerous compounds are recommended for clinical use: oxytocin, an animal hormone, induces and stimulates labor in selected cases requiring such treatment; and two ergot alkaloids from the fungus *Claviceps purpurea* (Fig. 13-8)—ergonovine and a semisynthetic derivative, methylergonovine. The latter two are used after parturition to produce firm uterine contractions and to decrease postpartum uterine bleeding. They combine low toxicity, rapid onset, and sustained action and are preferred over oxytocin or other agents for these purposes.

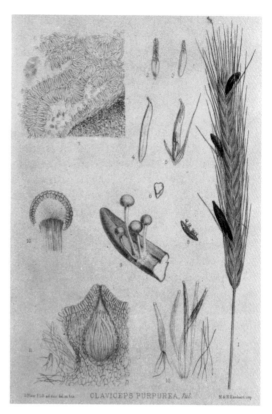

Figure 13-8 *Claviceps purpurea* (from R Bentley and H Trimen, *Medicinal Plants* **4:** 303, 1880).

Oxytocic action is known for other compounds, such as the alkaloids quinine and quinidine originally obtained from species of *Cinchona* (Rubiaceae), but the high incidence of fetal distress and intrauterine death associated with their use indicates that they should not be administered to induce labor unless the fetus has died *in utero*.

The medieval midwife aided mothers by feeding rye grains contaminated with ergot to women in labor, for they had observed that this course resulted in speedier births and recoveries with far less loss of blood. The midwives were prescribing the ergot alkaloids without knowing why the black moldy grains worked; yet this bit of European folk medicine has passed directly into modern medicine.

We know virtually nothing of the hundreds of other plants used by expectant mothers throughout the world who live outside the realm of modern medical practice. A number of these plant extracts apparently help with labor, some serve as parturition tonics, others help relieve the pain of childbirth, or by reducing hemorrhage, and still others undoubtedly are used as fertility drugs. Those listed below must have some efficacy beyond placebo, or surely they all would not be used generation after generation by women who seek relief from the suffering of parturition and its complications.

An exception to this general vacuum is the recent research with *Oldenlandia affinis* (Rubiaceae).[8] A decoction of stems and leaves of this herb is drunk during labor by Lulua women of Kasai Province, Zaire, just before the actual childbirth. Strong uterine contractions and short delivery time are normally observed (yet in some cases cervical spasms supervene, necessitating an artificial delivery). Two active, chemically distinct oxytocic principles have been isolated from this species—namely, serotonin and a uteroactive polypeptide.

CHILDBIRTH AIDS

AIZOACEAE

Trianthema portulacastrum. Root decoction causes mild contractions of the uterus, but in large doses it is abortive. It is widely used in the tropics.

ASTERACEAE

Arctium lappa (burdock). Root formed an important ingredient in the medicine used by the Meskwaki women while in labor.

Erigeron philadelphicus (Philadelphia fleabane). A volatile oil extracted from leaves and flowering tops was used by

physicians in this century for hastening uterine contractions.

Montanoa tomentosa from Mexico is used to aid women in childbirth.

Senecio aureus (squaw weed), as the vernacular name implies, was used by the Catawba women as a tea to check the pains of childbirth as well as to hasten labor.

CAPRIFOLIACEAE

Sambucus canadensis (elderberry). Tea made from the bark was taken by Meskwaki women in difficult cases of childbirth.

DIOSCOREACEAE

Dioscorea villosa. Tea made from the roots was taken by the Meskwakis to relieve the pain of childbirth.

LILIACEAE

Trillium grandiflorum (white trillium). Tea from the root of this and other species was employed by eastern North American Indians to facilitate parturition; it was also used to regularize menstruation.

MALVACEAE

Gossypium spp. (cotton). Boiled root tea was taken by the Alabamas and the Koasatis to ease labor.

MYRICACEAE

Comptonia aspleniifolia (sweet fern). Leaf extracts were used by the Menominees of Wisconsin as a potent medicine to hasten parturition.

RUBIACEAE

Mitchella repens (partridge berry). Tea made from its small fruit reportedly aids labor and acts as a parturient. At one time, the tea was widely used in female medicines by North American Indians.

POSTPARTURITION AIDS

APIACEAE

Angelica polymorpha var. *sinensis.* Extracts have long been used in Chinese medicine to stimulate uterine contraction.

Neonelsonia acuminata. Extracts are used by natives of the northern Andes after childbirth "to prevent the death of the mother."

BETULACEAE

Betula pumila (low birth). Tea made from the "cones" was taken by the Pillager women as a postparturition tonic, as well as an aid through difficult menses.

FABACEAE

Caesalpinia nuga. Powdered leaves are used in tropical Asia as a uterine tonic following childbirth.

LORANTHACEAE

Phoradendron serotinum (American mistletoe). Plant extracts were long used by North American Indians as oxytocic agents, namely, in arresting postpartum hemorrhage.

ONAGRACEAE

Fuchsia excorticata. As used in New Zealand, extracts supposedly arrest hemorrhage after childbirth.

POACEAE

Paspalum scorbiculatum (koda millet). Root and rhizome decoctions have been employed in the Philippines as an alterative during and following childbirth.

ABORTIFACIENTS

"Abortion is one of society's oldest and most effective fertility control mechanisms. Although historically it has been associated with considerable censure and medical risk, abortion nonetheless has been sought even under the most adverse conditions."[9] A few examples gleaned with relative ease from reported functions of plants, illustrate the existence of numerous abortifacients among most peoples of the world, now and in the past.

APOCYNACEAE

Kibatalia blancoi. Roots and bark extracts are used in the Philippines as abortifacients.

ASTERACEAE

Chrysanthemum parthenium (feverfew). Dried flowers have been used in home remedies in Europe to induce abortion and also to promote menstruation.

CELASTRACEAE

Celastrus paniculata. Bark extract is used from India to the Philippines to terminate pregnancy.

LILIACEAE

Urginea burkei. Bark decoction is used by the natives of South Africa to induce abortion.

RHAMNACEAE

Colubrina asiatica. Fruit decoction is an abortifacient, especially favored in Malaya.

THYMELAEACEAE

Daphne gnidium, native to the Mediterranean region. Powdered bark is considered an abortive.

VERBENACEAE

Avicennia marina, possessing an aromatic bitter juice, is abortive as used in tropical Africa and Asia.

Petrea kohautiana. Tea is used as an abortive on Dominica in the West Indies.

ANTIABORTIFACIENTS

MENISPERMACEAE

Cissampelos pareira roots are used in tropical areas to prevent a threatened miscarriage. The herb is also used to stop uterine hemorrhages.

Uterine Disorders

The skin of the mango fruit (*Mangifera indica,* Anacardiaceae) is used in some tropical areas to treat uterine hemorrhages. In India a decoction of the dried bark of *Saraca indica* (Fabaceae) is taken for various ailments of the uterus.

Menstruation

Omitted from the plants listed in Table 13-2 is nutmeg or mace (*Myristica fragrans*), a presumed emmenagogue or promoter of menstruation as well as an abortifacient. Late in the nineteenth century such uses were widely reported for this spice, even though earlier papers on the subject never mentioned efficacy in these regards. This folk belief seemed to be restricted to western Europe and North America, and it has persisted well into this century. For example, in 1959 a Virginia lady of 28 ate 18.3 g of finely ground nutmeg in an attempt to induce menstruation when only two days overdue.[10] She failed, but became violently ill and was hospitalized in a serious toxic state for a week.

The value of the plants listed in our table is unknown; they have been used for long periods of time, however, and presumably would have been abandoned if they had failed consistently to induce menstruation or if they had caused serious illness. No phylogenetic pattern appears for the plants used among the many cultures sampled, nor is there a major compound common to most (e.g., alkaloids in the Rubiaceae, volatile oils in the Lamiaceae).

Advice from a physician writing in the colony of Virginia in 1734 for "suppression of the courses" reads as follows:

Young Women must shake off Sloath, and make Use of their Legs, as well as their Hands. They should be cautious of taking *Opiats* too often, or *Jesuits-Bark* [quinine], except in Cases of great Necessity; nor must they long for *pretty Fellows,* or any other *Trash,* whatsoever.[11]

Vagina

Yoghurt has been used as a home remedy for treating vaginitis, which is possibly caused by *Candida* species. Its efficacy, however, has yet to be illustrated with clinical trials. Other remedies using extracts from flowering plants to treat various vaginal discharges, grouped under the general term leukorrhea, are listed in Table 13-3. Their effectiveness is unknown.

Male Reproductive Organs

Venereal diseases and difficulties relating to sexual drive and performance are the chief genital problems, real or imaginary, of the male. Women, of course, are not immune to these difficulties.

Infertility in some males may be corrected following treatment with clomiphene, which increases sperm concentration and motility.[12] The recent clinical study just cited is far removed from the treatment in Zaire, in which

Table 13-2 Plant Extracts Used to Promote Menstruation

Plant Group and Species	Vernacular Name	Locality and/or People	Plant Part
FERN			
(POLYPODIACEAE)			
Oleandra colubrina			Stipe (very efficient)
GYMNOSPERM			
(TAXODIACEAE)			
Taxodium mucronatum	Cypress	Mexico	Bark
ANGIOSPERMS			
ARACEAE			
Cyrtosperma merkusii		Western Oceania	Flower
ARISTOLOCHIACEAE			
Asarum canadense	Wild ginger	North American Indians	Root[a]
ASTERACEAE			
Diotis candidissima		Arabs	Plant
BERBERIDACEAE			
Caulophyllum thalictroides	Blue cohosh	North American Indians	Root[a]
BRASSICACEAE			
Cheiranthus cheiri	Wallflower	Europe	Flower
COCHLOSPERMACEAE			
Cochlospermum planchoni		Tropical Africa	Plant
DIPSACACEAE			
Dipsacus asper		China	Seed
EUPHORBIACEAE			
Euphorbia atoto		Indochina	Latex[a]
FABACEAE			
Cassia laevigata		Mexico	Plant
Dalbergia ferruginea, D. stipulacea		Western Oceania	Wood[a]
IRIDACEAE			
Crocus sativus	Saffron crocus	Mostly Europe	Flower Styles
LAMIACEAE			
Lavandula latifolia	Broad-leaved lavender	Mediterranean and domestic medicine	Leaf and flower
Leonotis leonurus	Drug lionsear	South Africa	Leaf
MENISPERMACEAE			
Cocculus filopendula		Brazil	Plant
RHAMNACEAE			
Colubrina ferruginea		West Indies	Leaf
RUBIACEAE			
Psychotria tomentosa		Colombia	Leaf
Rubia peregrina		Mediterranean	Powdered root
RUTACEAE			
Ruta graveolens	Common rue	Mediterranean	Plant[a]
SCROPHULARIACEAE			
Curanga fel-terrae		Indochina-Philippines	Leaf
ZINGIBERACEAE			
Renealmia domingensis		Brazil	Seed

[a] Also considered an abortifacient.

Table 13-3   Plant Extracts Used to Treat Vaginal Discharges (Leukorrhea)

Angiosperm Family and Species	Vernacular Name	Locality and/or People	Plant Part
ASCLEPIADACEAE			
Hemidesmus indicus		India	Plant
ASTERACEAE			
Erigeron canadensis	Fleabane	North American Indians (Houma)	Root
BETULACEAE			
Alnus incana	Speckled alder	North American Indians (Potawatomi)	Bark
CELASTRACEAE			
Celastrus scandens	American bittersweet	Eastern North America	Plant
MALVACEAE			
Sida cordifolia		Pantropic	Plant
MELIACEAE			
Cedela fissilis		Brazil	Bark
RANUNCULACEAE			
Hepatica nobilis		North American Indians (Menominee)	Root mixed with Maidenhair (*Adiantum* sp.) roots

root decoctions of *Xylopia antunesii* (Annonaceae) are taken to remedy male sterility. In South Africa similar decoctions of *Waltheria americana* (Sterculiaceae) are used.

The flow of semen from the penis without sexual stimulation (spermatorrhea) has long been treated in Europe in domestic medicine by drinking seed decoctions of *Oxalis acetosella* (wood sorrel) or *Nymphaea alba* (white waterlily). In Africa an infusion of fruit from *Pedalium murex* (Pedaliaceae) is considered effective.

Aphrodisiacs (Fig. 13-9)

Sexual drive (libido) and sexual performance (erection and orgasm) in man are governed mainly by psychic factors. Hormonal influences are important, however, especially the androgens, which affect libido in men and women.

Claims for the classical sexual stimulants (aphrodisiacs), cantharides or Spanish fly and yohimbine, have never been adequately supported. Cantharides,

consisting of the dried insect *Cantharis vesicatoria*, contains the blistering principle cantharidin, which is the lactone or anhydride of cantharidic acid. If taken internally, it is excreted by the kidney and irritates the genitourinary tract, sometimes including congestion of the erectile tissue of the clitoris or penis. This results in priapism, an abnormally persistent erection of the penis, thus the popular reputation of the drug as an aphrodisiac. However there is no evidence that congestion or erection so induced is accompanied by increased sexual desire or improved performance. Serious damage to the genitourinary tract can result, and there have been fatalities from cantharides ingestion. Yohimbine, an alkaloid derived from the bark of *Corynanthe yohimbe* (Rubiaceae) indigenous to the Cameroons, and chemically related to reserpine, has been employed for centuries as an aphrodisiac, but with little evidence that it has an effect on sexual desire or performance. It is available commercially as yohimbine hydrochloride combined with methyl-

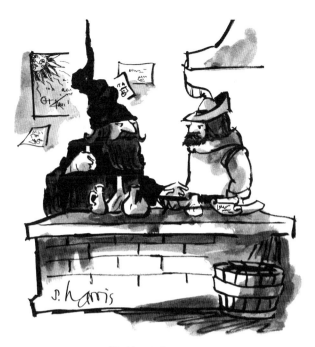

*"Gold and silver from
base metals is OK, but what
I'm trying to transmute is angelica root, mugwort and
tincture of marigold into an
effective aphrodisiac."*

Figure 13-9   The search continues. (Reproduced by special permission of PLAYBOY Magazine; copyright © 1974 by Playboy.)

testosterone and nux vomica (dried seeds of *Strychnos nux-vomica*); but the manufacturer's claim of relieving male impotence, as judged by the number of erections and orgasms per week achieved by patients apparently deserves no great credence.[13] Also available commercially as a sexual stimulant and tonic is a combination of strychnine (*Strychnos nux-vomica* and other species), caffeine (*Coffea arabica*), and theophylline. There is no evidence that these alkaloids are effective, singly or combined.

It is possible, however, that man has always used some kind of presumed sexual stimulant. The number of plants claimed for this purpose is certainly large, and some are listed in Table 13-4. The plants considered to be aphrodisiacs are generally those that have nutritive value,

contain volatile oils, or affect the neuromuscular system. A number probably do little more than calm or tranquilize; yet once agitation is eliminated, the individual is able to act normally. The volatile oils present in many plants undoubtedly stimulate respiration and cause a rise in blood pressure and a feeling of well-being. These effects are often coupled with the application of volatile oil extracts to the genitalia: the substances are irritant and slightly anesthetic and may aid in obtaining an erection while delaying ejaculation.

Alcoholic drinks have long been held to be aphrodisiac. Alcohol in moderation may help free sexual desire by lessening inhibitions, but in excess it depresses the central nervous system, hence sexual performance.

Table 13-4   Plants Used as Aphrodisiacs[a]

Angiosperm Family and Species	Vernacular Name	Plant Part	Locality	Remarks
ACANTHACEAE				
Crossandra infunduliformis	Priya-darsa	Plant	India	
Hygrophila auriculata		Seed	India	Highly esteemed
Rhinacanthus nasuta		Plant	Pakistan	Extraordinary powers
ANACARDIACEAE				
Heeria reticulata			Tropical Africa	Also galactogogue (increases flow of milk)
APIACEAE				
Eryngium coeruleum	Dudhali	Root	Kashmir and north-western India	Also nerve tonic
E. ternatum		Root	Crete	
Heracleum wallichii		Root	Nepal, Sikkim	Also tonic
Malabaila sekakul	Sekakul	Plant	Mediterranean area (Arabs)	
Pimpinella alpina		Root	Java	Great strengthening properties; also diuretic
APOCYNACEAE				
Aspidosperma quebracho-blanco	Quebracho	Bark	Central South America	Alkaloid quebrachine; occasionally sold commercially
Holarrhena antidysenterica		Seed	Arabian and Hindu medicines	Also tonic
Tabernanthe iboga	Iboga	Root	Western Africa	See Hallucinogens, Chapter 18
ARALIACEAE				
Cussonia nigerica			Sudan	Also antiblenorrhea (combats excessive vaginal secretions)
ARISTOLOCHIACEAE				
Aristolochia indica		Rhizome	India	Especially helpful for impotence
ASCLEPIADACEAE				
Schizoglossum shirense		Plant	Eastern Africa	
ASTERACEAE				
Anacyclus pyrethrum	Pellitory	Root	India	Powerful stimulating action
Chrysactinia mexicana			Mexico	Also diuretic and diaphoretic
Eupatorium purpureum	Joe-pye weed	Root	North America	Meskwakis used decoction as a love potion
E. staechadosmum		Plant	Vietnam	Also tonic
Saussurea lappa	Costus	Root	Kashmir	
Sphaeranthus indicus		Seed	India	Seed fried in sesame oil
Tricholepis glaberrimum	Brahmadandi	Plant	Hindu medicine	Also tonic

Table 13-4   (Continued)

Angiosperm Family and Species	Vernacular Name	Plant Part	Locality	Remarks
BIGNONIACEAE				
Anemopaegma mirandum	Catuabu	Root	Brazil	Also stimulant and nervine
BOMBACACEAE				
Bombax malabaricum	Roktosimul	Gum	Tropical Asia	Source of Malabar gum; also tonic
CAMPANULACEAE				
Codonopsis tangshen	Hupeh	Root	China	Important Chinese drug; also tonic
Lobelia cardinalis	Cardinal flower	Root	North America	Meskwakis considered
L. siphilitica	Blue lobelia			them love potions
CANNABACEAE				
Cannabis sativa	Bhang	Dried pistillate flowers, seeds, resinous exudate	India	Used in Old World for centuries, moderate doses were considered as exhilarants and powerful aphrodisiacs, but habituation was thought to lead to melancholia and impotence
CARYOPHYLLACEAE				
Paronychia argentea	Silver nailroot	Herb	Morocco	Also diuretic
CELASTRACEAE				
Celastrus paniculata	Kanguni	Seed	Hindu medicine	Also stimulant, emetic, cathartic
Maytenus senegalensis	Confetti tree	Root	Zambia	Chipped into beer
CONVOLVULACEAE				
Ipomoea digitata	Fingerleaf morning glory	Root	Southern Asia	Also as tonic and alterative
EUPHORBIACEAE				
Richeria grandis		Bark	West Indies	
FABACEAE				
Butea monosperma	Bastard teak	Flower and leaf	India to Malaya	
B. superba		Tuber	Thailand	Activates hormones
Prosopis africana	Guele, laddo	Macerated leaf	Especially Sudan	Also considered effective against male sterility
GERANIACEAE				
Geranium macrorrhizum	Bigroot geranium	Herb	Bulgaria	
ICACINACEAE				
Alsodeiopsis poggei	Bonsoko	Root	Congo	
A. rowlandii	Bungwingwi	Root	Congo and Southern Nigeria	
IRIDACEAE				
Crocus sativus	Saffron crocus	Dried stigmas and style tips	India	Considered a fine aphrodisiac
LAMIACEAE				
Lallemantia royleana		Seed	Iran	Also cardiac stimulant

Table 13-4 (Continued)

Angiosperm Family and Species	Vernacular Name	Plant Part	Locality	Remarks
LILIACEAE				
Hypoxis aurea		Herb	Tropical Asia	Also panacea
Liriope graminifolia		Candied tuber	Eastern Asia	Also tonic
Smilax calophylla, *S. china,* *S. myosotiflora*	Greenbriers	Rhizome	Eastern Asia	Also tonics and panaceas
MAGNOLIACEAE				
Kadsura coccinea	Re pa	Plant	China	Also tonic and for respiratory diseases
MELIACEAE				
Pterorhachis zenkeri		Fresh bark	Cameroon	
MYRISTICACEAE				
Myristica fragrans	Nutmeg and mace	Seed and aril	Yemen	Also a hallucinogen
OLACACEAE				
Liriosma ovata	Muirapuama	Balsam	Brazil	Also tonic
ORCHIDACEAE				
Eulophia campestris	Salibmisri	Rhizome	India	Also tonic
Orchis latifolia (and other spp.)	Broad-leaved orchid	Tuber	Asia	Very valuable as restorative, tonic, and aphrodisiac; taken with milk as nutritive drink
PAPAVERACEAE				
Papaver somniferum	Opium poppy	Capsule latex	Asia	Taken to delay male ejaculation; after temporary stimulus, diminishes sexual desire and causes impotence
PIPERACEAE				
Piper excelsum		Seed and fruit	New Zealand	Also diuretic
PORTULACACEAE				
Talinum cuneifolium	Ndele	Herb	Tanzania	
RUBIACEAE				
Corynanthe yohimbe	Yohimbi	Bark	Cameroons	Alkaloid yohimbine; available commercially
Rubia peregrina	Levant madder	Flower	Morocco	
RUTACEAE				
Fagara pilosiuscula	Elondo	Root	Angola and Congo	
SOLANACEAE				
Brunfelsia grandiflora		Root	Latin American Indians	Also for shamanistic purposes
Datura sp.		Flowers and root	Californian Indians	Also considered narcotic
Datura spp.	Jimson weed, stramonium, etc.	Seed	India	Powdered seed mixed with butter taken internally for impotence; mixture also applied to genitalia to obtain sexual vigor
Mandragora officinarum	Mandrake	Root	Mediterranean region	See Chapter 18

Table 13-4   (Continued)

Angiosperm Family and Species	Vernacular Name	Plant Part	Locality	Remarks
Withania somnifera		Root	India	Mixed with honey and butter, recommended for sexual debility
THEACEAE				
Laplacea semiserrata		Seed	Brazil	Also diuretic
TURNERACEAE				
Turnera diffusa	Hierba de la pastora	Dried leaves	Mayans (Mexico)	As a tea
ZINGIBERACEAE				
Alpinia galanga	Greater galangal	Tuber	India	Good for impotence; also stimulates respiration
ZYGOPHYLLACEAE				
Peganum harmala	Harmela shrub	Seed	Egypt	Also alterative
Tribulus terrestris		Fruit	Pantropics	Restore sexual potency

[a] For additional aphrodisiacs used in India, see HS Puri (1971).[14]

A well-known European natural healer uses plants having volatile oils in his creams for regular massage at the base of the spine. Included are celandine poppy (*Chelidonium majus*), cow parsnip (*Heracleum sphondylium*), and savory (*Satureja montana*), to which may be added peppermint (*Mentha piperita*) and broad-leaved plaintain (*Plantago major*). These cream massages, along with foot baths and vaginal douches, apparently work miracles for the frigid female.[15]

Two recent drug or drug combinations reportedly have aphrodisiac effects: methaqualone, a nonbarbiturate sedative-hypnotic that enhances sex drive (while resulting in loss of muscle control!), and reportedly phenelzine (monoamine oxidase-inhibitor), combined with L-tryptophan and psychotropic (tranquilizing) medication, had an aphrodisiac effect on women hospitalized with chronic schizophrenia.[16] Sexual excitement was definitely exaggerated and even provoked compulsive, pathological sexual behavior among the women.

Anaphrodisiacs

Some drugs are capable of inhibiting sexual desire and performance. Impairment of libido and erection may result from the use of barbiturates, narcotics, tranquilizers, and other depressant drugs in doses having more than a mild sedative effect, and from the use of ganglion-blocking drugs. Failure to ejaculate, without loss of libido, is occasionally encountered following treatment with thioridazone and guanethidine. The reputed anaphrodisiac effect of saltpeter (KNO_3) has never been confirmed.

Released in Great Britain in 1974, and not yet available in the United States, is a new drug that lowers the male sex drive by blocking the function of testosterone, the male sex hormone. The drug, cyproterone acetate, is being used primarily in treating rapists and others convicted of sex crimes in various European countries. However the drug may also be used for couples who are sexually incompatible as, for example, to reduce a hypersexual husband to a "once-a-week" man, if that in fact is what his wife wants. Estrogens also powerfully inhibit the libido in males, but they cause feminizing changes.

Folk medicine also has its anaphrodisiacs, but they are few. *Vitex agnus-castus* (Verbenaceae) of the Mediterranean area, and also cultivated, has been known since antiquity as the symbol of chastity; the ground fruit substituted for pepper is supposed to reduce libido. Likewise, the seeds of *Nymphaea alba* and other species of waterlily found in Eurasia have long been considered effective in deadening sexual desire.

Hormones influence sexual desire and performance. Testosterone given to women in large doses causes intensified libido and genital sensitivity, but virilism (having external genitalia with male characteristics) is often a consequence. In small doses for treatment of frigidity, the androgens may be helpful. Estrogens do not increase sexual responsiveness. There is no satisfactory demonstration of sexual benefit from administration of androgens to males who are physically normal. In fact, repeated large doses of testosterone diminish or suppress sperm formation.

VENEREAL DISEASE

Since the introduction of oral contraceptives and the near abandonment of the condom for contraception, the incidence of venereal disease has increased rapidly: in the United States it has been estimated that a new case occurs every two minutes. This is further complicated by the general public's attitude that a "shot of penicillin always does the trick." Unfortunately, penicillin-resistant mutants of *Neisseria gonorrhoeae* have been found, and treatment is not always the easy regimen it once was.

Gonorrhea may be transmitted through venereal contact to the genitals or oral cavity,

at birth to the eyes, and through fomites to the vulvovagina of prepubertal girls. Regardless of the site of infection, purulence is a common symptom. In the male, urethritis occurs through invasion of the epithelium of the anterior urethra and urethral glands. Extension of the site of infection to the posterior urethra, prostatic ducts, seminal vesicles, and epididymis may result in chronic infection or dissemination through the bloodstream to cause arthritis, tynosynovitis, endocarditis, and skin lesions. Similar complications may occur in the female, since infection can extend from the urethra and cervix to the uterus, Fallopian tubes and ovarian surfaces, thence to the bloodstream. Women may or may not have the tell-tale purulent discharge; backache, micturition, and pain in the lower abdomen are the usual symptoms. Vulvovaginitis of the prepubertal girl is characterized by vulvar pain, erythema, edema, and purulent discharge. In the infant, the conjunctivitis may be severe, possibly resulting in impairment of vision or total blindness if not treated. The prophylactic installation into newborn eyes of neomycin or silver nitrate drops has dramatically reduced the incidence of ophthalmia neonatorum.

Syphilis has a much lower incidence than gonorrhea, but the increase in the number of cases has paralleled that of other venereal diseases. Although the disease is a continuous process, there may be long intervals between the development of its three distinct stages. Of approximately 100 individuals who develop the initial lesion (a hard, black, painless chancre), only two-thirds will develop the maculopapular eruptions characteristic of the secondary stage, and only one-third of these, the autoimmune gummas and cardiovascular and nerve damage of the tertiary stage. Symptoms of primary and secondary syphilis can resolve themselves naturally, and many cures attributed to numerous medicaments can be related to developed immunity or the natural history of the infection, rather than to many of the plants listed in Table 13-5. Infection *in utero* may result in fetal death or the development of congenital malformations (Chapter 4), particularly of the teeth (Hutchinson's incisors, mulberry molars) and bones (scaphoid scapulas, perforated nasal

Table 13-5   Plant Extracts Used to Treat Venereal Diseases

Disease; Plant Group and Species	Vernacular Name	Locality	Remarks
GONORRHEA			
Fern			
Drynaria rigidula		Malaya	
Gymnosperm			
Pinus palustris	Southern pine	Southern United States	Resin oil ointment; also skin diseases
Angiosperms			
AIZOACEAE			
Mesembryanthemum crystalinum	Ice plant	South Africa, cultivated	Considered a sure cure by early cowboys of western North America
APIACEAE			
Thapsia montana		Southwestern United States and Mexico (Apaches and Pimas)	Shrub decoction; also a tonic
ASCLEPIADACEAE			
Marsdenia reichenbachii	Condorvine	Ecuador and Colombia	Cundurango bark an early Indian remedy
ASTERACEAE			
Arctium lappa	Great burdock	Europe	Seventeenth century European remedy, usually the root
Erigeron canadensis	Fleabane	North Temperate	Leaves and tops; also for other urogenital diseases
Liatris spicata	Blazing star	New England	Plant chewed
FABACEAE			
Cassia surattensis	Kembang	Indonesia	Root decoction
Copaifera lansdorffii			Balsam
C. reticulata			Copaiba balsam, an early remedy
Paradaniellia oliveri	Balsam copaiva tree	Western Africa	Root decoction; also for treating skin diseases
MYRSINACEAE			
Labisia pumila	Kelimparan tooli	Malaysia	Root decoction a popular medicine
RUBIACEAE			
Galium umbrosum		New Zealand	Plant
SOLANACEAE			
Solanum agrarium		Brazil	Leaf decoction
URTICACEAE			
Urera baccifera	Ortega de caballo	Puerto Rico	Root
SYPHILIS			
Angiosperms			
APOCYNACEAE			
Tabernaemontana corymbosa	Djelotong badak	Malaya	Bark decoction, used in tertiary stage

333

Table 13-5   (Continued)

Disease; Plant Group and Species	Vernacular Name	Locality	Remarks
BIGNONIACEAE			
Jacaranda oxyphylla		Brazil	Bark; remedy called ca-roba still in use
CAMPANULACEAE			
Lobelia siphilitica	Blue lobelia	North American Indians	Root
CUCURBITACEAE			
Cayaponia espelina		Brazil	Root
LILIACEAE			
Smilax medica, *S. ornata*	Sarsaparilla	Tropical America	Root; standby in Europe when disease first appeared
S. leucophylla		Philippines	Root
MONIMIACEAE			
Atherosperma moschatum	Southern sassafras	Australia	Bark used by aborigines, settlers followed suit; supposedly an effective remedy in the secondary stage
PAPAVERACEAE			
Corydalis gavaniana	Bhutakesi	India	Root; also for cutaneous and scrofulous ailments
URTICACEAE			
Urera caracasana		Mexico	Plant
ZYGOPHYLLACEAE			
Guaiacum officinale, *G. sanctum*	Lignum-vitae	West Indies	Guaiac wood extracts

septum, and ulnar deviations of the fingers). The typical congenital triad of malformed incisors, interstitial keratitis, and eighth nerve deafness is known as Hutchinson's triad.

Penicillin is the drug of choice in the treatment of all stages of syphilis and should be used unless the patient is allergic to it. At the initiation of treatment during the secondary stage, an exaggerated period of increased signs and symptoms, known as the Jarisch-Herxheimer reaction, occurs as a result of the sudden release of treponemal antigens, disappearing soon after 24 hours.

Surveillance through blood testing of the entire population, especially in premarital clinics, has aided in the detection and treatment of syphilis. It should always be assumed that patients with gonorrhea are also likely to have syphilis.

Other venereal diseases are chancroid, lymphogranuloma venereum, and granuloma inguinale. Chancroid, or soft chancre, is characterized by one or more painful genital ulcerations and associated with regional adenitis. This infection by *Hemophilus ducreyi* is successfully treated with erythromycin and tetracycline.

Lymphogranuloma venereum, due to infection with *Chlamydia* spp., is much more severe. Lymphadenitis and draining buboes are common, as are proctocolitis and stricture of the lower bowel. Moreover, destructive lesions of the labia and vagina and strictures of the female urethra are common. If the organisms disseminate through the blood and lymphatic glands they can cause meningo-encephalitis, pneumonitis, cystitis, and ocular-glandular syndrome. Treatment with sulfa drugs, erythromycin, and tetracycline has been successful.

Granuloma inguinale is a chronic, mildly infectious venereal disease characterized by ulcerogranulomatous lesions involving the skin and mucosa of the genital and inguinal areas. It is more common in the tropics than in temperate climates and appears to be decreasing in occurrence. The disease is most prevalent among black males. Treatment with erythromycin and tetracycline successfully eradicates the infection of *Donovania granulomatis*.

Although the etiology of nonspecific urethritis and cervicitis remains obscure, genital strains of *Chlamydia trachomatis* have been implicated. This recurrent disease is difficult to control with known antibiotics, such as tetracycline, and only new therapeutic measures will assure complete resolution.

LITERATURE CITED

1. Mathison RR. 1958. *The Eternal Search*. GP Putnam's Sons, New York. 381 p.

2. Murphy LJT. 1972. *The History of Urology*. Charles C Thomas, Springfield, Ill. 531 p.

3. Segal SJ. 1974. The physiology of human reproduction. *Sci Am* **231**(3): 53–62.

4. Burger A. 1960. *Medicinal Chemistry*, ed 2. Wiley-Interscience, New York. Table 38-VIII, p 722.

5. Topical and systemic contraceptive agents. 1974. *Med Lett* **16**(9): 37–40.

6. Sharp rise reported in IUD infections. *St Louis Post-Dispatch* 21 Aug 1974: 16D.

7. Sackler AM, Weltman AS, Pandhi V et al. 1973. Gonadal effects of vasectomy and vasoligation. *Science* **179**: 293–295; Alexander NJ, Sackler AM. 1973. Vasectomy: long-term effects. *Science* **182**: 946–947.

8. Gran L. 1973. Oxytocic principles of *Oldenlandia affinis*. *Lloydia* **36**: 174–178.

9. Sklar J, Berkov B. 1974. Abortion, illegitimacy, and the American birth rate. *Science* **185**: 909–915.

10. Green RC Jr. 1959. Nutmeg poisoning. *JAMA* **171**: 1342–1344.

11. Anonymous [J Tennent]. 1734. *Every Man His Own Doctor: or, The Poor Planter's Physician*, ed 2. William Parks, Williamsburg and Annapolis. Reprint edition, St Louis Medical Museum, St Louis. 56 p + index.

12. Palti Z. 1970. Clomiphene therapy in defective spermatogenesis. *Fertil Steril* **21**: 838–843.

13. Drugs influencing sexual desire and performance. 1963. *Med Lett* **5**(12): 45–46.

14. Puri HS. 1971. Vegetable aphrodisiacs of India. *Quart J. Crude Drug Res* **11**(2): 1742–1748.

15. Mésségué M. 1973. *Of Men and Plants*. Macmillan, New York. 327 p.

16. Doust JWL, Huszka L. 1972. Amines and aphrodisiacs in chronic schizophrenia. *J Nerv Ment Dis* **155**: 261–264.

Chapter 14
Skin

A panacea or old wives' tale is surely indicated for a plant that improves conditions of general debility, enhances sexual excitement, promotes menstruation, develops mammary glands, relieves headaches, heals skin injuries, and acts as a purgative. These powers at one time or another have been attributed to *Aloe barbadensis* (Liliaceae) and other aloes native to Africa and also widely cultivated; but only two of these claims have persisted for centuries: purgation (Chapter 11) and the healing of skin.

Modern medical reports using the fresh juice from aloe leaves (or the concentrated extract incorporated into a cream or ointment base) date from 1935, when a patient suffering from facial X-ray burns was treated. Itching and burning subsided in 24 hours, and within 5 weeks the 4 by 8 cm area had completed regeneration with no scar. After 3 months the area was pigmenting normally along with other exposed skin surfaces.[1] A similar experience of X-ray hand burns was reported a few years later.[2] More recently, Brown[3] also advocated the use of aloe gel in radiation burns for relief from pain and itching, and to keep down keratosis and ulceration, thus slowing any possible change toward malignancy.

There has been little experimental research on the effectiveness of aloe gel, although the study by Rovatti and Brennan[4] using rabbits showed that when it was used to treat deep dermal burns from heat, the skin remained pliable and soft

336

during the first week without gross or microscopic separation of an eschar (hard crust) and the lesions healed in two weeks without gross evidence of scarring. Other groups of rabbits were treated variously, as, for example, with trinitrophenol ointment, and all died within 10 days. Obviously no other procedure was as successful as that using aloe.

Antibacterial properties have also been attributed to *Aloe* species extracts[5]. The interested reader is referred to additional papers on the subject.[6]

The chemistry of aloe extracts is inadequately known. Water-soluble principles contain anthraquinones, anthranols, anthrones, and their glycosides, but perhaps most significant has been the isolation of chrysophanic acid, thought to be beneficial to healing of skin.

In domestic medicine the popularity of aloes as an aid to burning, itching, minor cuts, and first and second degree thermal burns, is spreading rapidly. No household should be without its aloe plant; it is undoubtedly among the easiest plants to grow indoors (Fig. 14–1).

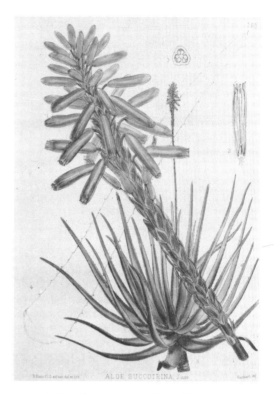

Figure 14-1 *Aloe succotrina* (from R Bentley and H Trimen, *Medicinal Plants* **4:** 283, 1880).

BODY COVERING

The external surface of the body is circumscribed by the skin, by such derivates of the skin as hair, nails, and glandular structures, and by several specialized types of receptors. The skin is the largest organ of the body. This pliable, protective covering over the body surface acts as a regulator of body temperature, a control of excessive loss of water, as well as organic and inorganic materials, an important area of storage, and a synthesizer of several important substances used in the body. In addition, it receives a variety of sensations.

Skin may be thick (hands, feet), thin (eyelids, penis), or typically intermediate, about 1 to 2 mm thick. It possesses a superficial epidermis consisting of up to five distinct layers of cells, from the internal layer, which renews the epidermis by mitosis, to the outermost corneum having 25 to 30 layers of flat, dead scalelike cells filled with keratin. The outer cells are constantly being shed. Below the epidermis is a tough, flexible, and elastic layer, the dermis; it contains many blood vessels and is much thicker than the epidermis. Not clearly demarked from the dermis is the fat-infiltrated subcutaneous layer consisting of connective tissue loose enough to accommodate significant volumes of fluid.

A downgrowth of epidermal cells into the dermis forms a hair follicle. Hair has a bulb on its lower end, a visible shaft, and an oil-producing gland that keeps the hair pliable and the surrounding skin moist. Nails are modifications of the two uppermost layers of epidermis, and each has an active growing region, the lunula or whitish half-moon-shaped area at the base. Besides the sebaceous or oil glands already mentioned, the skin possesses sweat glands, which produce a watery secretion important in temperature regulation.

Skin is normally under tension and retracts if cut, with age skin loses some elasticity and tends to sag. The application of estrogenic hormone preparations to nonresilient skin can lead to redevelopment of elastic fibers and an increase in blood supply of the dermis. At one time the skin was thought to be impermeable to all substances, but we now know that fat solubility increases the capacity of many materials to penetrate it. For example, fat-soluble hormones, vitamins A, D, and K, and organic bases are absorbed through the skin surface, as well as animal and vegetable fats through hair follicles.

Although the skin manufactures substances for its own use (e.g., keratin), its production of vitamin D from the sterol dehydrocholesterol, which is acted on by ultraviolet light when absorbed into the bloodstream, is important in the metabolism of calcium and phosphate throughout the body.

A variety of pigments are found in the skin. Skin color is largely due to the presence of melanin and carotene. Melanin is a yellow to black pigment located in the basal epidermal layer among Caucasians and found in all epidermal layers among Negroids. Exposure to ultraviolet radiation increases the amount and darkens the color of melanin, leading to tanning and protection against radiation. Carotene, a yellow-orange pigment, is found in the fatty areas of the dermis and outer epidermal layer in Orientals.

COSMETICS

The makers of cosmetics and perfumes have long experimented with different plants for their scents and beautifying properties. The beautician can produce any number of cosmetics containing some kind of herbal ingredient, including steroids, hormones, vitamins, volatile oils, and astringents. In cosmetology it has become fashionable to use "biological vegetable complexes," to produce preparations with a nurturing and curative or preventive effect. Many recom-

mended plants are used in folk medicine, but their principles must be more carefully examined, and controlled experiments must be conducted, before cosmetic values can be attributed to them. For example, an extract from deoiled wheat germ has been shown by clinical tests to have an estrogenic action, and beautifying effects have been attributed to amino acids, glucose, and rutin.[7] Little is known, however, of the absorption of these compounds through the skin and of their ability to improve skin elasticity once they have been absorbed.

Nonetheless a number of plants are major basic components of facial and toilet creams, salves, and shaving creams: *Carica papaya* (papaya) fruit pulp, the "meat" of *Cocos nucifera* (coconut) seeds, carob gum from *Ceratonia siliqua* and similar lubricants, the balsamic exudate from *Cistus ladaniferus*, and the colloidal algin from *Laminaria digitata* and *Macrocystis pyrifera* (both Algae) for thickening of pharmaceuticals, cosmetics, and dentifrices.

Any number of herbs are used for perfume and for scenting creams, salves, soaps, oils, and shampoos. Volatile oils are the more usual scents obtained from such well-known genera as *Abies, Angelica, Cedrus, Citrus, Eucalyptus, Gardenia, Hibiscus, Iris, Jasminum, Lavandula, Mentha, Narcissus, Rosa, Rosmarinus, Salvia, Sassafras, Vanilla,* and *Viola.*

Herbologists believe that many tonics will inevitably improve hair condition. Interestingly, numerous home remedies used for washing and conditioning hair do contain a foamy saponin or volatile oil. For example, to brighten, stimulate, and strengthen blonde hair, a rinse made from equal parts of chamomile (*Matricaria* or *Chamomilla*: Fig. 14-2a) and yarrow (*Achillea millefolium*) is said to be most effective; chamomile in particular has long been used in European households

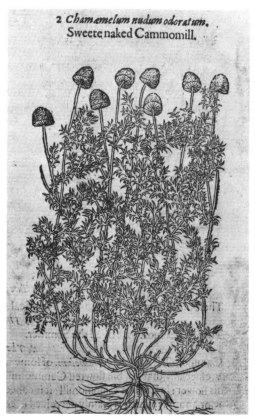

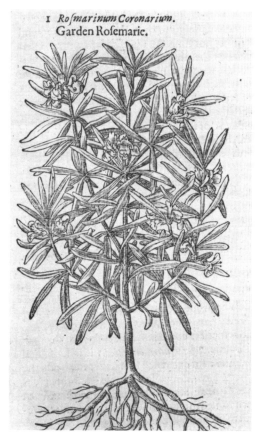

Figure 14-2a *Chamomilla suaveolens* (from J Gerard, *The Herball,* 1597).

Figure 14-2b *Rosmarinus officinalis* (from J Gerard, *The Herball,* 1597).

for keeping a golden tint. For brunettes, a mixture of rosemary (*Rosmarinus officinalis:* Fig. 14-2b) and garden sage (*Salvia officinalis*) reputedly maintains a dark sheen and also strengthens and stimulates hair growth.

The base of a homemade shampoo might be the leaves of *Saponaria officinalis* (soapwort); with which any herb extract may be mixed for suitable individual results. Thus soapwort (long used in the European countryside as a soap substitute), with powdered or extract of chamomile, should make a suitable natural shampoo.

An infusion of rosemary mixed with a little borax, used daily and massaged into the root hairs, is considered to be an efficacious home remedy for dandruff.

A sampling of plants from around the world which are used to wash and treat hair is as follows.

Asparagus africanus (Liliaceae), South Africa. Leaves are used in an ointment by women to stimulate hair growth.

Canarium oleosum (Burseraceae), Indonesia. Oil from the stem (like an olive oil), mixed with coconut oil, is used as a stimulating hair oil by women.

Caryocar glabrum (Caryocaraceae), Guyana. Inner bark is used to wash hair as well as clothes.

Claytonia sibirica (Portulacaceae), Pacific

Northwest. Indians used stem juice as a hair tonic and stimulator, and to prevent dandruff.

Coleus aromaticus (Lamiaceae), tropics. Herb decoction is used for washing hair and clothes.

Eclipta erecta (Asteraceae), tropics. Elderly women use an herb decoction to rinse hair; the plant possesses a bluish-black dye, and they say there is no need for white hair as long as *Eclipta* is available.

Euphorbia thomsoniana (Euphorbiaceae), Kashmir. Crushed roots are recommended for washing hair.

Eurotia lanata (Chenopodiaceae), western North America. Indians used plant decoctions as a hair and scalp tonic; hot decoctions were also used to remove lice from hair.

Fallugia paradoxa (Rosaceae), Southwestern United States. Hopi Indians used leaf infusions as a hair rinse; supposed to promote growth.

Nardostachys jatamansi (Valerianaceae), Alpine Himalayas. Volatile oil from the plant is supposed to improve hair growth.

Pithecellobium bigeminum (Fabaceae), India. Leaf decoction is prepared for promoting hair growth.

Urtica dioica (Urticaceae), North Temperate zone. The herb extract containing volatile oils has long been used in Europe as a nettle hair rinse. The root is an ingredient in commercial hair growth preparations, and the seeds are used as a home remedy for hair troubles generally.

Vanilla griffithii (Orchidaceae), tropical Asia. The irritating juice from the crushed leaves is rubbed into the hair to produce a healthy, thick growth.

Vernonia missurica (Asteraceae), central North America. A flower decoction is considered efficacious for dandruff.

Yucca glauca (Liliaceae), Western United States and Mexico. The root, which contains a foamy saponin, is used as a soap to wash hair as well as clothing.

WOUNDS AND BLEEDING

A wound is a breach in the continuity of any body tissue. Wounds may be open or they may show no external opening in skin covering. In the case of a bruise, the wound is obvious because of the rupture of blood vessels.

Wounds should be washed with sterile water and soap, and wrapped in sterile gauze. Then the body takes over, and healing should result, provided nature's defenses are able to overcome the initial bacterial infections present in all wounds. If secondary infections occur, penicillin or other appropriate antibiotics and the sulfa drugs may be indicated. The ancient Egyptians were very familiar with this procedure, for they stuffed moldy bread in wounds, and, when the mold contained members of the genus *Penicillium,* a form of penicillin would be produced.

Widely used in domestic medicine, especially in tropical areas, are various balsams and resins to arrest bleeding and possibly to aid in wound healing. They are considered efficacious by many native peoples on several continents. Other plants found useful have astringent properties, probably due to the presence of tannins and similar compounds.

FERN ALLIES

Cyathea mexicana (treefern). Fronds are used to arrest hemorrhages in tropical parts of Mexico.

Equisetum heleocharis (horsetail). Plant decoctions are used in the Ukraine to stop hemorrhage.

GYMNOSPERMS

Pinus montezumae (Montezuma pine). Resin is used in Mexico to heal open wounds.

Tsuga canadensis. Ojibwa Indians found that bark from this and other species of hemlock healed wounds and cuts and stopped bleeding.

ANGIOSPERMS

ANACARDIACEAE

Pistacia lentiscus (Pistachio), Fig. 14-3a). Gum has long been used in Europe and the Middle East to arrest bleeding.

Rhus glabra root bark tea was used by the Ojibwas and Potawatomis as a hemostatic.

APIACEAE

Ferula galbaniflua, source of a gum-resin stem exudate called Galbanum, is widely used in Asia to treat wounds. In Kashmir, *F. jaeschkeana* gum is also applied to wounds and bruises.

ARECACEAE

Caryota mitis leaf base fibers are used in Cambodia to cauterize wounds.

ASCLEPIADACEAE

Asclepias tuberosa roots were pulverized and used by the Menominees for cuts, wounds, and bruises. The Omahas chewed the root and placed the macerated material on wounds and sores.

ASTERACEAE

Cnicus japonicus stems and leaves are considered to have hemostatic properties in China.

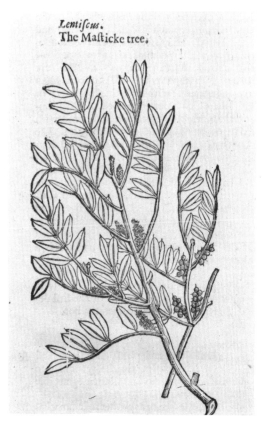

Figure 14-3a   *Pistacia lentiscus* (from J Gerard, *The Herball,* 1597).

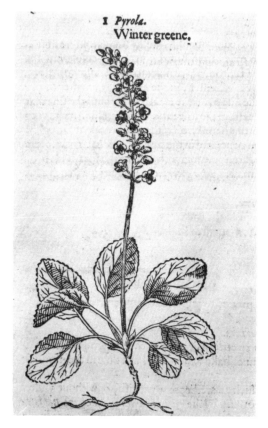

Figure 14-3b   *Pyrola* sp. (from J Gerard, *The Herball,* 1597).

Gynura pinnatifida roots are astringent and are employed in China for wounds and hemorrhages.

BOMBACACEAE

Bombax malabaricum resin, the source of gum of Malabar, is used in Asia for its hemostatic properties.

BORAGINACEAE

Cordia globosa leaves and shoots are used in Cuba for their hemostatic action.

BURSERACEAE

Commiphora opobalsam (Mecca myrrh). Balsam from the stem is used in Arabia for cleaning and healing wounds, as is the gum from *C. stocksiana* in India.

CLUSIACEAE

Caraipa fasciculata of Guyana and Brazil produces a stem balsam useful in healing wounds.

Clusia flava (monkey apple). Stem is the source of hog gummi, which is a resin employed in the West Indies to heal wounds. Similar uses are found for *C. insignis* resin in Brazil and *C. plukenetii* resin also in the West Indies.

COMBRETACEAE

Combretum glutinosum leaf decoctions are used for washing wounds in tropical Africa.

ERICACEAE

Pyrola spp. (Fig. 14-3b). Decoctions of the whole plant are excellent wound healers according to North American Indians.

ERYTHROXYLACEAE

Erythroxylum citrifolium bark is employed in Brazil to heal wounds.

FABACEAE

Cassia sericea leaves are made into a poultice in tropical America for treating wounds.

Myroxylon balsamum (balsam of Tolu), *M. pereirae* (balsam of Peru), and other balsams were long used by the Incas, and currently are employed by the Colombian Indians, to treat wounds and to arrest bleeding. Healing is supposed to take place with little or no scarring. In orthodox medicine these balsams are also used, especially when bleeding is profuse.

LAMIACEAE

Amaracus dictamnus. Whole plants were used in Crete by the ancient Greeks for treating wounds.

LILIACEAE

Bulbine narcissifolia. Fresh juice from plants is used to hasten healing of wounds in South Africa.

Dracaena cinnabari and other species found in Arabia, east Africa, and on Socotra are sources of dragon's blood resin, used to stop hemorrhages.

LOGANIACEAE

Buddleja americana. Roots, bark, and leaves are used as healing agents for wounds in Mexico to South America. The plant is also a diuretic.

MORACEAE

Ficus cotinifolia. The Indians of Mexico have long used the milky juice mixed with its powdered bark, for treating wounds and bruises. *F. trichopoda*, having latex that readily coagulates on exposure, is similarly employed in Madagascar.

NYCTAGINACEAE

Boerhaavia plumbaginea. A leaf decoction reportedly heals wounds, as used in tropical Africa.

ORCHIDACEAE

Bletia purpurea. Bulbs are split and placed on open wounds for treatment in the West Indies and Central America.

RANUNCULACEAE

Hydrastis canadensis (golden seal). Dried rhizomes have been used in eastern North America as a hemostatic because of their astringent properties.

SAPOTACEAE

Lucuma glycyphloea bark is astringent and is used in Brazil as a hemostatic (also as a tonic).

VERBENACEAE

Lippia scaberrima. Dried plants are considered hemostatic in South Africa.

VITACEAE

Vitis compressa. Juice from plants, as used in tropical Asia, is reported to heal wounds quickly.

ZINGIBERACEAE

Curcuma longa. Fresh juice from roots is used in tropical Asia for treatment of wounds, bruises, and leech bites.

ZYGOPHYLLACEAE

Larrea mexicana (greasewood). A decoction of leaves or twigs has been used in the southwestern United States and Mexico for healing wounds and sores.

BURNS

Skin is very susceptible to damage by flame, scalding, or contact with hot objects. A reddening or first degree burn of the skin is due either to direct damage to capillaries, causing their dilation, or to the release of chemicals such as histamine, which dilate vessels. A sunburn is a common example. A second degree burn results in blistering and usually only involves the epidermis or occasionally the uppermost dermal layer. Third degree burns destroy the deep tissues of the skin.

A word of caution for those inclined to sunbathe. A suntan may be cosmetic, but it comes at a price to Caucasians; melanin is manufactured on exposure to sunlight, and each time this happens, skin degeneration takes place. Young skin can be made old by this accumulation of sun damage, which includes premature wrinkling. Because of the protective effect of natural melanin among blacks, their facial skin remains undamaged and free of wrinkles until old age.

If whites must sunbathe, they should shield the skin with a sun-screening agent that will help prevent sunburn. Paraaminobenzoic acid (PABA), or one of its derivates in alcohol, is widely used.[8]

Treatment of burns is related to reducing pain and excluding infection. It is important to apply large, sterile, firm dressings to the area. Wet dressings incorporating silver nitrate solutions are used for antisepsis and to promote protein coagulation in the treatment of second degree burns and deeper ulcerations. Antibiotics are also important in the treatment of some of the complications of large and deep wounds. If, however, the width of the area burned extends more than an inch, skin grafting is indicated.

Home remedies for treating minor burns are numerous (Table 14-1) and probably relate to decreasing pain (e.g., cold water bath). Yet actual aid in the healing process with certain extracts can-not be excluded, as has been illustrated for *Aloe barbadensis* preparations.[4] Chinese medicine advocates other plant preparations for burns: first degree—*Zizyphus vulgaris* (Rhamnaceae) stem

Table 14-1 Plants Used as Remedies for Burns

Plant Group and Species	Vernacular Name	Locality and/or People	Remarks
Fungus			
Xylaria obovata		Malaya	Powdered fruiting bodies mixed with coconut oil
Angiosperms			
ASTERACEAE			
Parthenium integrifolium	Wild quinine	Eastern North America (Catawba Indians)	Leaves
BETULACEAE			
Alnus spp.	Alders	North American Indians	Bark decoction used to reduce pain from burn or scald
Betula spp.	Birches	North American Indians	Boiled bark used to relieve pain of burns and scalds; also used for wound treatment
CRASSULACEAE			
Sempervivum tectorum	Hen-and-chickens	Europe	Infusion of leaves; ointments and salves made from leaves or volatile oils of this species mixed with *Glechoma hederacea* (Lamiaceae)
IRIDACEAE			
Iris versicolor	Blue flag	North American Indians	Lightly boiled root, crushed, and made into poultice for burns, bruises, and sores
LILIACEAE			
Aloe barbadensis	Aloe	Africa and cultivated	Leaf sap for burns and sunburn (including radiation)
MELIACEAE			
Carapa procera		Tropics	Seeds source of touloucouna oil for curing burns, yaws, and mosquito bites
PIPERACEAE			
Peperomia leptostachya		Oceania	Juice from leaves used for burns (and skin and eye infections)
RANUNCULACEAE			
Anemone cylindrica	Thimbleweed	North America (Meskwaki Indians)	Leaf poultice for severe burns
RHAMNACEAE			
Trevoa trinervia		Chile	Bark is important home remedy for burns
VERBENACEAE			
Clerodendron buchananii		Malaya and Indonesia	Leaf paste for burns
VIOLACEAE			
Melicytus camiflorus		New Zealand	Bark used for burns

powdered in 80% alcohol; second degree—*Ulmus campestris* (Ulmaceae) endodermal powder (5 parts) and powdered *Phellodendron chinensis* (Rutaceae) (2 parts); third degree—4 parts *Z. vulgaris*, 3 parts *P. chinensis*, 3 parts *Sanguisorba officinalis* (Rosaceae), and 1 part *Glycyrrhiza uralens* (Fabaceae). This basic therapy is supplemented by skin grafting, antishock treatment, and appropriate replacement of fluid. It was recently reported that all 500 cases of burns treated mainly with these traditional herb drugs were cured.[9]

ANIMAL BITES

INSECT AND CHIGGER BITES

Over much of their near cosmopolitan distributions, leaves of *Anthemis cotula* (mayweed) and *Plantago major* (plantain) are rubbed on the skin to relieve bee stings. The Dakota and Winnebago Indians bruised wild onions for both bee and wasp stings, and reportedly these gave almost instant relief from pain. Other Indians used *Hedeoma pulegioides* (American pennyroyal) to repel chiggers and remedy their bites. Balsam from *Liquidambar orientalis* in China and *L. styraciflua* in North America have also been used to treat chigger bites and other skin afflictions. Mosquitoes are a worldwide plague. The extensive use of touloucouna oil from seeds of *Carapa procera* (Meliaceae) in tropical areas, however, suggests that man has located a remedy there to relieve the pain and irritation of mosquito bites.

In eastern North America the juice from *Eupatorium capillifolium* (dog fennell) has long been used in domestic medicine to treat insect bites, much as *Carapa guineensis* (andiroba oil) ointment has been found efficacious in tropical America and west Africa. In Mexico leaves of *Cassia emarginata* are applied to most insect stings and bites for relief (see Chapter 15, Insecticides).

SCORPION AND CENTIPEDE STINGS

Coleus aromaticus (Lamiaceae) is of tropical Asian origin but widely cultivated throughout the world. Poultices made of the leaves are used to relieve both scorpion bites and centipede stings. Relief from the pain of scorpion bites is also obtained from macerated roots of *Achyranthes aspera* (Amaranthaceae) in India, plant juices of *Elettariopsis sumatrana* (Zingiberaceae) in southeastern Asia, roots of *Lobelia nicotinaefolia* (Campanulaceae) in India, from roots and fruit of *Luvunga scandens* (Rutaceae) in Malaya, and from most parts of *Oberonia longibracteata* (Orchidaceae) in Cambodia.

SNAKEBITES

Venom of snakes contains a number of enzymes or proteinaceous substances that attack the blood, the nervous system, or other tissues. Certain venoms produce direct toxic effects, some are systemically lethal (e.g., rattlesnake venom), whereas others are destructive primarily to the tissues in the vicinity of the bite. Not all are lethal.

Most types of snake venom poisoning can be treated with the use of antivenins prepared by the immunization of animals, especially horses, against the venoms. The effectiveness of the antivenin varies considerably and largely depends on the antibody titer and purity of antivenins.

Plants reputedly efficacious against poisonous snakebites can be obtained from all parts of the world inhabited by poisonous snakes. Very probably the

Table 14-2   Plants Used as Snake Bite Antidotes

Angiosperm Family and Species	Vernacular Name	Locality; Snake, if Known	Remarks
ACANTHACEAE			
Blepharis capensis		South Africa	Herb used by natives
ANNONACEAE			
Annona nana		Angola	Root bark
APOCYNACEAE			
Tabernaemontana sralensis		Indochina	Root
Urechites suberecta		Tropical America	Plant
Wrightia tomentosa		India and Pakistan	Bark
ARACEAE			
Arisaema speciosum		Himalayas	Root
Rhaphidophora pertusa		India to Indonesia	Black pepper
ARALIACEAE			
Aralia spinosa	Angelica tree	Southern United States (rattlesnake)	Root bark decoction widely used internally by blacks, as well as powdered root for wounds
ARISTOLOCHIACEAE			
Aristolochia barbata		Brazil	Rhizome
A. longa		Mediterranean to Iran	Root
A. maxima		Yucatan to Venezuela	Root
A. taliscana		Sinaloa, Mexico	Root
A. theriaca		Brazil	Root
Bragantia corymbosa		Java	Stems and leaves
ASCLEPIADACEAE			
Blepharodon mucronatum		Mexico and Central America	Crushed leaves
ASTERACEAE			
Antennaria plantaginifolia	Everlasting pussy toes	Eastern North America (rattlesnake)	
Echinacea angustifolia	Purple coneflower	North American Plains Indians (rattlesnake)	Plant; also used for other venomous bites, stings, etc.
Prenanthes serpentaria	Lion's foot	Eastern North America (rattlesnake)	Plant used in homeopathic medicine
BIGNONIACEAE			
Bignonia unguis-cati		Mexico	Plant
CARYOPHYLLACEAE			
Polycarpaea corymbosa		India	Leaves and flowers
CONVOLVULACEAE			
Ipomoea arborescens		Sinaloa, Mexico (rattlesnake)	Bark
EUPHORBIACEAE			
Cluytia similis		South Africa	Root
FABACEAE			
Alysicarpus zeyheri		Tropical Africa	Root
Cassia alata	Ringworm senna	Pantropic	Juice from leaf; also employed for skin diseases
Machaerium angustifolium		Brazil	Gum resin
Uraria picta		Eastern India (phursa)	Leaves

Table 14-2   Continued

Angiosperm Family and Species	Vernacular Name	Locality; Snake, if Known	Remarks
GENTIANACEAE			
Gentiana andrewsii	Closed gentian	Moskwakis, Eastern North America	Root
Sebaca crassulaefolia		South Africa (puff adder)	Plant
LAMIACEAE			
Leonotis leonurus	Drug lionsear	South Africa	Plant
Leucas aspera		Tropical Asia	Leaves
L. zeylanica		Cambodia	Boiled leaves
MELIACEAE			
Trichilia capitata		Mozambique	Root
MELIANTHACEAE			
Melianthus comosum		South Africa	Leaves or root bark
MENISPERMACEAE			
Cissampelos capensis		Cape, South Africa	Leaves
Cocculus filipendula		Brazil	Fruit?
PIPERACEAE			
Piper medium		Costa Rica	Plant
POLYGALACEAE			
Polygala senega	Seneca snakeroot	Eastern North America, Senecas	Root
RUBIACEAE			
Chiococca alba		Tropical America	Plant
Psychotria jackii		Malaysia	Leaf, also used against insect bites
SIMAROUBACEAE			
Simarouba versicolor		Brazil	Bark
TACCACEAE			
Tacca fatsiifolia, T. palmata		Philippines and Indonesia	Plant or root
VERBENACEAE			
Clerodendron buchananii		Indonesia and Malaya	Root

length of the list of such plants (Table 14-2) reflects the great number of poisonous reptiles rather than the value of the plant extracts; but this is speculation.

RASHES, DERMATITIS, AND ITCHES

Rashes and dermatitis due to allergic or other causes are commonly treated with antihistamines, which suppress histamine release. Many antihistamines also relieve pruritus (itching). Often wet dressings of water or ethanol are used, or lotions having anti-inflammatory and cooling effects (zinc oxide, talc, glycerin, water, and often calamine).

For relief from pain and itching, home remedies include applying the juice of dock or sorrel (Rumex spp.), or the leaves of houseleek, onion or plantain. The stinging rash obtained from brushing against stinging nettles (Urtica spp.) is best treated by Rumex spp. juice, which often is found growing nearby.

The Indians of North America employed a number of remedies against poison ivy, poison oak, and poison sumac: *Grindelia robusta* was used by tribes in California, *Lactuca canadensis* latex by the Menominees, and *Impatiens capensis* (jewel weed) juice by the Potawatomis. The last is widely used today by Indians living in the Appalachian area, both as a prophylactic and after poison ivy sores have erupted. Extracts from jewel weed are also found in a number of commercially available preparations.

In the American tropics extracts of *Bignonia unguis-cati* are used to treat contact dermatitis caused by manchineel (*Hippomane mancinella*); in Ceylon oil from *Calophyllum calaba* (Clusiaceae) is specific for itch. Other itch preparations include those from *Coprosma australis* (Rubiaceae) bark in New Zealand, *Canarium oleosum* (Burseraceae) stem oil in Indonesia, and *Knema corticosa* (Myristicaceae) seed oil in Vietnam. Other contact dermatitis treatments are: *Copaifera lansdorffii* (Fabaceae), from which copaiba balsam is obtained and used for eczema in Brazil; ground leaves of the fern *Drymoglossum heterophyllum* a remedy for eczema in tropical Asia; *Ervatamia cylindrocarpa* leaves, pounded with rice and turmeric, used for eczema and itch in Malaya; and in Brazil leaf juices from *Philodendron cordatum* mixed with soap for treating eczema, as well as other skin difficulties.

Additional treatments for itching include the use of *Mollugo hirta* and *M. oppositifolia* (Aizoaceae) plant juices in India and *Leucas zeylanica* (Lamiaceae) decoctions in Malaya; at one time the Mayans crushed the leaves of *Croton eluteria* (Euphorbiaceae) to use for erysipelas and itching, and the Indians of Canada and the United States employed a decoction of *Achillea* spp. (yarrow), or juice scraped from the inner bark of *Alnus incana* (Betulaceae) for similar disorders.

RUBEFACIENTS AND COUNTERIRRITANTS

Dried seeds of black mustard (*Brassica nigra*, Fig. 14-4), leaves of *Capparis horrida*, dried ripe fruit of green pepper (*Capsicum frutescens*), whole plants of *Cneorum tricoccum*, and in Hindu medicine *Drosera burmannii*, are all considered powerful rubefacients. These skin irritants, often in the form of plasters or poultices, increase blood supply to the skin and create a warm, tingling sensation. They are also widely used in the home for respiratory ailments.

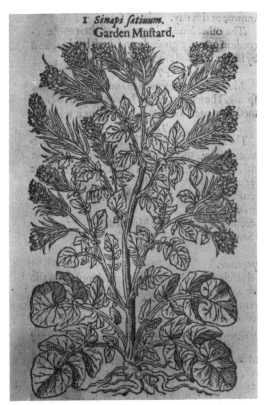

Figure 14-4 *Brassica nigra* (from J Gerard, *The Herball*, 1597).

SKIN INFECTIONS

WOUND INFECTIONS

Cutaneous anthrax, the most common anthrax in the United States, results through contact with animal hair that has been infected with *Bacillus anthracis*. Spores enter the epidermis and germinate, and the bacilli multiply and manifest a toxin that produces the characteristic black eschar of the "malignant pustule." High doses of penicillin have been used to avert the development of septicemia and death. The rare pulmonary (woolsorters' disease) and gastrointestinal types are almost always fatal.

The entry into deep tissue wounds after trauma or surgery of spores of the anaerobic species of *Clostridium perfringens, C. septicum, C. oedematiens,* and *C. histolyticum* can result in gas gangrene. These organisms can elicit such necrotizing infections as anaerobic cellulitis, anaerobic myositis, and anaerobic puerperal sepsia (uterine gangrene) by producing a wide range of potent tissue-dissolving enzymes. Such infections are sometimes fatal.

Another skin infection, due to *Erysipelothrix insidiosa,* is much more slowly evolving and self-limiting. Erysipeloid is generally restricted to persons handling edible (meat and poultry) and inedible (bones and shells) animal products contaminated with this saprophyte. Only rarely does arthritis or endocarditis also develop. Penicillin, erythromycin, and tetracycline are used in therapy.

PRIMARY SKIN INFECTIONS

Boils, pimples, and large carbuncles extending to the subcutaneous tissue result from infection with strains of *Staphylococcus aureus,* producing the enzyme coagulase. Over the years, antibiotic-resistant strains have developed and are especially prevalent in hospital-related wound infections. Therefore when the organism produces penicillinase, and penicillin G is not applicable, the semisynthetic penicillins, such as methicillin, oxacillin, nafcillin, cloxacillin, and decloxacillin, are used; also employed are the cephalosporin antimicrobics cephalothin, cephaloridine, and cephalexin.

Pemphigus neonatorum, impetigo resulting from staphylococcal infection in the newborn, is bullous, superficial, and crusting. Rarely seen in school children nowadays, especially in temperate climates, impetigo may also be due to *Streptococcus pyogenes* alone or in combination with *Staphylococcus aureus.* In this form of the disease, the lesions found on exposed parts of the body are vesiculopustular or ulcerated. Furthermore, following oral streptococcal infections, a spreading inflammation of the dermis of the face and neck known as erysipelas may develop. To avoid sequelae from any of these streptococcal infections, prompt antibiotic therapy with penicillin G should be instituted.

Superficial infections may also be due to *Corynebacterium* species common to the skin. Erythrasma, due to infection with *C. minitissimum,* appears in body folds and clefts as scaly, wrinkled skin that at times is also inflamed and weeping. In another condition called trichomycosis axillaris, *C. tenuis* and other *Corynebacterium* species invade the keratin and cuticles of pubic or axillary hairs to form yellow, black, or red nodules. Moreover acne can result from infection with a related anaerobe, *Proprionibacterium acnes,* when hypersecretion of sebum occurs. Treatment involves cleaning with antibacterial soap and systemic use of erythromycin. Tetracycline is preferred for acne because it can penetrate sebaceous secretions.

Leprosy, a chronic skin disease endemic to tropical and subtropical areas, is caused by *Mycobacterium leprae.* Although it has the potential to produce mutilation of the extremities and disfigurement of the face (Fig. 14-5), it is rarely fatal. Seen in two forms or as an intermediate between the two, the tuberculoid type may be limited to a few nerves and skin areas, whereas the lepromatous type is disseminated throughout the body. The drug of choice is dapsone (DDS, 4,4'diamindopdiphenyl sulfone); when drug resistance occurs, B653 (Lampren, clofazimine) or rifampin may be used. Plant extracts, mostly oils, have long been used to treat leprosy, probably with only limited success (Table 14-3). As a prophy-

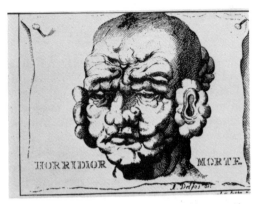

HORRIDIOR   MORTE.

Figure 14-5   Typical disfigurement of leprosy (from G. Schilling, 1778).

laxis, contacts can be immunized with the tuberculosis vaccine BCG for protection. Other *Mycobacterium* species, that are clearly saprophytic (*M. ulcerans*) or associated with aquatic environments (*M. marinum*) or aquatic animals (*M. fortuitum*) can also produce skin abscesses, ulcers, and chronic granulomas.

These conditions are treated with antituberculous drugs or by surgical excision.

A large number of fungi can elicit superficial skin infections. Some may only affect the skin (*Malassezia furfur, Cladosporium werneckii*), whereas others go to the hair (*Piedraia hortai, Trichosporon beigelii*). Cutaneous mycoses involving the hair, skin, and nails are produced by species of the genera *Microsporum* and *Trichophyton*. Various types of ringworm are in this group (Table 14-4). Subcutaneous invasion by such genera as *Sporotrichum, Phialophora, Streptomyces, Nocardia, Madurella, Allescheria, Basidiobolus,* and *Candida* may produce more severe, chronic, and even disseminating infections. Furthermore, as part of the systemic disease, mucocutaneous lesions may also be a manifestation of coccidiomycosis, blastomycosis, and histoplasmosis. Treatment of these diseases involves use of both topical and systemic antimycotic agents such as fungizone (amphotericin B) and griseofulvin. The latter antibiotic is unique in that it has the ability to

Table 14-3   Plant Extracts Used to Treat Leprosy

Angiosperm Family and Species	Locality	Remarks
ASCLEPIADACEAE		
Calotropis procera	India	Root bark
ASTERACEAE		
Siegesbeckia orientalis	Old World tropics, especially India	Tincture of whole plant; also for ringworm and other such diseases
CISTACEAE		
Cistus villosus	Brazil	Labdanum balsam
CLUSIACEAE		
Calophyllum inphyllum	Old World tropics	Relieves pain of lepers by intramuscular injection of refined oil
DIPTEROCARPACEAE		
Dipterocarpus lamellantus	China	Gurjim oil from seeds
FLACOURTIACEAE		
Casearia sylvestris	Brazil	Oil from seeds; also for wounds
Hydnocarpus alcalae	Philippines	Oil from seeds
H. anthelmintica	China	Oil from seeds
H. wightiana	India	Oil from seeds
Oncoba echinata	Cultivated in tropics	Gorli oil
Taraktogenos kurzii	Eastern India	Chaulmoogra oil
LOGANIACEAE		
Strychnos gaulthieriana	Indochina	Bark
OCHNACEAE		
Gomphia parviflora	Brazil	Oil from seeds

Table 14-4   Plant Extracts Used to Treat Ringworm

Angiosperm Family and Species	Locality	Remarks
ACANTHACEAE		
Rhinacanthus nasuta	India	Fresh roots, leaves, or seeds mixed with lime juice; also used for other skin diseases
ANACARDIACEAE		
Microstemon velutina	Southeast Asia	Bark latex
Pentaspadon motleyi	Malayan archipelago	Acrid balsam from stem; also other skin diseases
FABACEAE		
Cassia occidentalis	Tropics	Seeds; also for eczema
C. sophera	Tropics	Leaf juice
C. tora	India	Leaves; also for other skin diseases
LILIACEAE		
Bulbine asphodeloides, *B. narcissifolia*	South Africa	Juice from leaves and stalks; also used like iodine for treating wounds
PASSIFLORIACEAE		
Adenia singaporeana	Malaya	Root decoction
VITACEAE		
Leea macrophylla	India	Root

concentrate in the keratinized areas of the skin after being administered orally.

HERBOLOGY

Antibiotics for treatment of primary skin infections may not be available to the majority of those living in equatorial areas; thus their suffering must be alleviated by using extracts readily available from local vegetation, such as the following.

FUNGUS

Daldinia concentrica powdered stromata are used by Indonesians to treat ulcers (yaws?) and other skin diseases.

ANGIOSPERMS

AMARANTHACEAE

Celosia trigyna leaves are used for pustular skin eruptions in Africa.

ASTERACEAE

Ambrosia psilostachya tea (from whole plant) has been used by the Kiowas of western North America to heal sores.

BURSERACEAE

Commiphora stocksiana gums are used in India to clean sores.

CAPPARIDACEAE

Capparis horrida leaves are used to make poultices for treating boils, swellings, and piles; also employed as a counterirritant.

LILIACEAE

Allium spp. (onions) bulbs and stems were applied as a poultice to carbuncles by the Cheyennes. When the sores were opened, the pus was washed out with a similar decoction.

MELIACEAE

Azadirachta indica (neem tree), having seeds as a source of margosa oil, is widely used in

India as an anti-inflammatory for treating skin diseases.

OLEACEAE

Fraxinus americana (white ash) bark infusion was used by the Meskwakis for sores and to cure itch.

ORCHIDACEAE

Bletia hyacinthina (whole plant) is used to treat abscesses in China.

Oberonia anceps (whole plant) is crushed to make poultices for treating boils in Indonesia (Malacca).

RHAMNACEAE

Poultice of *Gouania javanica* root is applied to sores in southeastern Asia.

RUBIACEAE

Coprosma australis leaf infusion is used in New Zealand to treat sores as well as cuts and bruises.

SAXIFRAGACEAE

Heuchera americana (alum root). Powdered root, when applied to ulcers, wounds, and other skin conditions, was considered very beneficial by eastern North American Indians, whereas leaves, as an astringent for healing sores, were valued greatly by the Meskwakis.

SCROPHULARIACEAE

Scrophularia auriculata (water betony, Fig. 14-6) and *S. nodosa* (figwort) were used in Europe for various cutaneous eruptions including abscesses and ulcers. A decoction of the whole plant was used.

ULMACEAE

Ulmus fulva (slippery elm). Meskwakis made poultices of the bark for cold sores, Potawatomis poultices for boils; elm bark was widely used by North American Indians for cutaneous diseases and sometimes wounds.

VERBENACEAE

Avicennia officinalis. A green fruit poultice is used in India for treating boils.

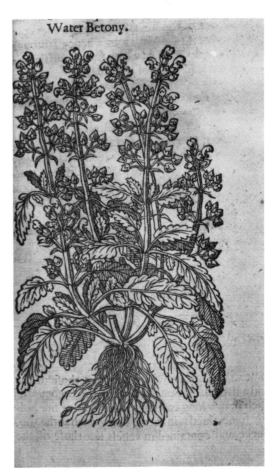

Figure 14-6 *Scrophularia auriculata* (from J Gerard, *The Herball,* 1597).

EXANTHEMS RELATED TO SYSTEMIC DISEASE

Systemic infection may also produce various exanthems. For example, the nonvenereal treponematoses of yaws, pinta, and bejel are found almost exclusively among the young of primitive peoples. With better personal hygiene and increased use of penicillin, however, these diseases are rapidly disappearing. A home remedy for curing yaws throughout the tropics is the application of touloucouna oil obtained from *Carapa procera* (Meliaceae).

Tetracyclines and chloramphenicol have been used for treatment of rickettsial infections, which are characterized by rashes, severe headache, and fever, and the fatality rate has been reduced dramatically. Control of these diseases may also involve eradication of either the vector (louse, tick, flea) or reservoir (mouse, rodent); in typhus and Rocky Mountain spotted fever, vaccines have been used as well. Vaccines are also available for such viral exanthems as measles, rubella, and smallpox, but none exist for the more exotic, though severe, infections of the epidemic hemorrhagic group such as dengue.

WARTS

Transmitted from man to man, warts or verrucae can be found among all human populations. Infections with this papovavirus is more common in children, among whom the incidence appears to be rising. The typical skin wart is a solid growth, but the appearance may vary if the soles and palms, eyelids, or genitalia are affected; pigmented warts have occurred on the face, forehead, and dorsal surfaces of the hands. Normally after a prolonged indolent course, spontaneous remissions occur. Immunity is not long lasting and reinfections are possible.

Available therapies are destructive and include excision, cryotherapy, electrodesiccation, curettage, and application of chemicals such as trichloroacetic acid or 40% salicylic acid. A number of home remedies are used in different parts of the world.

In Mexico warts are removed by applying the caustic milky juice from *Cecropia peltata* (Moraceae); elsewhere in tropical America the similar appearing milky latex of *Tabernaemontana citrifolia* (Apocynaceae) is used. The juice from leaves of *Sempervivum tectorum* (hens-and-chickens) or the white latex from *Taraxacum officinale* (dandelion) are popular home remedies for wart removal. In Asia, too, warts and similar growths are removed using a milky latex, this one from *Euphorbia neriifolia* (Euphorbiaceae).

Finally, there are plant extracts commonly

Table 14-5 Plants Used to Treat Generalized Skin Diseases and Complaints

Angiosperm Family and Species	Locality	Remarks
APIACEAE		
Chaerefolium sylvestre	Europe	Leaf juices common home remedy
Laserpitium prutenicum	Europe	Root a home remedy
APOCYNACEAE		
Rauvolfia vomitoria	Western Africa	Latex from leaves
BORAGINACEAE		
Cordia alliodora	West Indies	Ointment using pulverized seeds
CAPPARIDACEAE		
Capparis flexuosa	West Indies	Leaf decoction
CLUSIACEAE		
Calophyllum inophyllum	Old World tropics to Polynesia	Source of dilo oil applied
C. wallichianum	Indonesia	Stem resin boiled with coconut milk
EUPHORBIACEAE		
Croton cortesianus	Mexico	Caustic juice from plant
FABACEAE		
Cassia alata	Pantropic	Leaf juices (due to chrysophanic acid)
Copaifera reticulata (and others)	Brazil	Balsam (also for healing wounds)
FLACOURTIACEAE		
Caloncoba echinata	Western and central Africa	Gorli oil from seeds
JUGLANDACEAE		
Juglans insularis	Cuba	Herb decoction used in baths, especially for treating children's skin diseases

Table 14-5   (Continued)

Angiosperm Family and Species	Locality	Remarks
LILIACEAE		
Curculigo orchioides	Philippines	Plant
PAPAVERACEAE		
Chelidonium majus	Europe	Fresh yellow latex
RANUNCULACEAE		
Clematis dioica	Tropical America	Ointment from leaves
C. thunbergii	Senegal	Leaves
RHAMNACEAE		
Gouania leptostachys	Java	Pulped stems, roots, and leaves
SCROPHULARIACEAE		
Veronica officinalis	North Temperate	Herb for chronic skin diseases
SOLANACEAE		
Cestrum dumetorum	Mexico	Plant decoction
URTICACEAE		
Urtica dioica	North Temperate	Used in homeopathic medicine
XYRIDACEAE		
Xyris caroliniana	Eastern North America	Leaves and roots

used to treat generalized conditions involving skin diseases and complaints (Table 14-5). A number appear repeatedly in the literature, and these may possess efficacious properties worthy of note.

LITERATURE CITED

1. Collins CE, Collins C. 1935. Roentgen dermatitis treated with fresh whole leaf of *Aloe vera. Am J Roentgen* **33**: 396–397.

2. Loveman AB. 1937. Leaf of *Aloe vera* in treatment of roentgen ray ulcers. *Arch Dermatol Syphilol* **36**: 838–843.

3. Brown JB. 1964. Prevention and treatment of radiation-induced cancer, including pure atomic and cathode-ray lesions. *Ca—Cancer J Clin* **14**: 14–15; Brown JB, Fryer MP, Killiopoulos P. 1963. Long-term control of cancer of head and neck with planned use of natural survival and healing tendencies. *Arch Surg* **86**: 945–954; Brown JB. 1967. Management of cancer of the skin of the face and neck, 91–98. In J Conley (ed), *Cancer of the Head and Neck*. Butterworths, Washington, DC. 1967.

4. Rovatti B, Brennan RJ. 1959. Experimental thermal burns. *Industr Med Surg* **28**: 364–368.

5. Lorenzetti LJ, Salisbury R, Beal JL et al. 1964. Bacteriostatic property of *Aloe vera. J Pharm Sci* **53**: 1287.

6. Bouchey GD, Gjerstad G. 1969. Chemical studies of *Aloe vera* juice II. *Quart J Crude Drug Res* **9**(4): 1445–1453; Bovik EG. 1966. Panacea or old wives' tales? [healing after gingivectomy] *Tex Dent J* **84**: 13–16; Cheney RH. 1970. Aloe drug in human therapy. *Quart J Crude Drug Res* **10**(1): 1523–1530.

7. Janistyn H. 1961. The active principles of plants in cosmetology. *Am Perfum* **76**(1): 19–21.

8. Topical sun screening agents. 1972. *Med Lett* **6**: 27–28.

9. Burns treated principally with traditional herb medicine. 1973. *Chinese Med J* (**8**): 111–112.

GENERAL REFERENCES

Pusey WA. 1912. *The Care of the Skin and Hair*. Appleton, New York and London. 182 p.

Wells FV, Lubowe II. 1964. *Cosmetics and the Skin*. Reinhold, New York. 690 p.

Marples MJ. 1965. *The Ecology of the Human Skin*. Charles C Thomas, Springfield, Ill. 970 p.

Beedel S. 1972. *Herbs for Health and Beauty*. Sphere Books, London. 174 p.

Montagna W, Parakkal PF. 1974. *The Structure and Function of Skin*, ed 3. Academic Press, New York. 433 p.

Chase D. 1975. *The Medically Based No-nonsense Beauty Book*. Knopf, New York. 285 p.

Chapter **15**

Deterrents: Antibiotics, Antiseptics, and Pesticides

Control of particular organisms is extremely relevant to man's health, his well-being, and often his life. The astonishing changes that antibiotics and pest inhibitors have fashioned in medicine and agriculture during the twentieth century are testimonials to this, as well as to the ingenuity of man.

THE MAGIC MOLD AND OTHER ANTIBIOTICS

Folk medicines from countless countries allude to the use of infusions of moldy bread for the treatment of wound infections. Therefore the discovery by early bacteriologists that molds contaminating bacterial plate cultures possessed antibacterial activity was not surprising.

Fortunately for mankind, however, Fleming in 1929 reported the bactericidal action of *Penicillium notatum* contaminating a culture of *Staphylococcus aureus,* and the work came to the attention of Florey and his team at Oxford, who were investigating antibacterial substances for therapeutic value.[1] Unlike pyocanin from *Pseudomonas pyocyanea,* which was briefly used therapeutically by Freudenreich (1888),[2] penicillin lacked

355

toxicity and could be successfully used to combat many human infections.

When the initial human trials were carried out in 1941, the yield of penicillin from known strains was as low as 2 units per milliliter. Bombing during World War II forced an exodus of the British group to the United States, and research was resumed with the collaboration of American scientists and pharmaceutical companies. Breakthroughs occurred rapidly, and a phenomenal increase in yield resulted (3000 U/ml) from the use of cultural additives such as corn extract and genetically manipulated strains. Within 2 years enough penicillin was available for Allied consumption. This drug was very crude, however, and actually contained a mixture of many penicillins. During early clinical trials it was found that massive, repetitive oral doses had to be administered to maintain optimum therapeutic blood levels, and an alternative regimen was devised whereby penicillin was mixed with adjuvant and administered intramuscularly. After the war, when the various penicillins were separated by purification, penicillin G was isolated; it has subsequently proved to have a broad spectrum of activity and to maintain high blood levels when administered orally.[3]

The success with penicillin prompted the search for other antibiotic substances in nature. Tenacity was the byword of these massive screening programs, for it became apparent that finding a good antibiotic was a rare event indeed. Of perhaps the 1000 mold species examined by Waksman in his search for streptomycin, 100 possessed antibiotic activity, but only 5% of these were sufficiently nontoxic to be clinically applicable.

Unlike penicillin, which is derived from a few imperfect fungi having ascomycetous correlates, more than half of the therapeutic antibiotics are now produced by the bacterial Actinomycetales and especially from

Streptomyces. Examples are streptomycin, the tetracyclines, chloromycetin, the macrolide family of compounds including erythromycin, and the polyene compounds such as nystatin (Fig. 15-1). Other antibiotics have been produced by additional bacteria (Fig. 15-2), fungi (Fig. 15-3), algae, higher plants and some animals.

The majority of antibiotics are active against Gram positive microorganisms, and a smaller proportion effective against those which are Gram negative or acid-fast. In general, antibiotics exert their bactericidal or bacteriostatic effects by either inhibiting synthesis of cell walls, protein, or nucleic acid, or by affecting the permeability of the cytoplasmic membranes. By preventing further multiplication of bacteria, bacteriostatic agents enable the defense mechanisms of the host to eliminate the offending organism. Other antibiotics may be used against protozoa, spirochetes, and plant and animal viruses; a few also possess anthelmintic or insecticidal properties. Germination of seeds may be inhibited by some unpurified antibiotics, or enhanced by others, in purified form.[6] By changing the balance of intestinal bacterial flora, the drugs may also act as growth factors for animals.

Many criteria must be satisfied for every new candidate antibiotic before it is accepted for general therapeutic use. Obviously its yield from biological material must be high, its stability and shelf life prolonged, and its toxicity to humans relatively low. Once its antimicrobial spectrum has been determined, a practical therapeutic regimen for treating various infections is established to ensure that the proportions excreted or detoxified by the body are balanced to maintain optimal levels in infected tissue. There should be a minimum of side effects, particularly nerve damage, immune suppression, or allergy. Finally, selection of the new antibiotic as a primary or

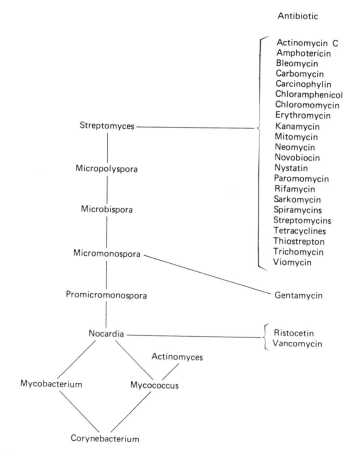

Figure 15-1 Phylogeny of the Actinomycetales and related groups illustrating the numerous antibiotics produced by the genus *Streptomyces*. (From A Zähner and WA Mass, Heidelberg Science Library, Volume 4, 1972. Copyrighted © Springer-Verlag, New York, Heidelberg and Berlin, and reprinted with permission.)

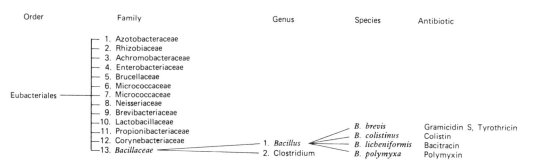

Figure 15-2 Antibiotic producers among the Eubacteriales. (From A Zähner and WA Mass, Heidelberg Science Library, Volume 4, 1972. Copyrighted © by Springer-Verlag, New York, Heidelberg and Berlin, and reprinted with permission.)

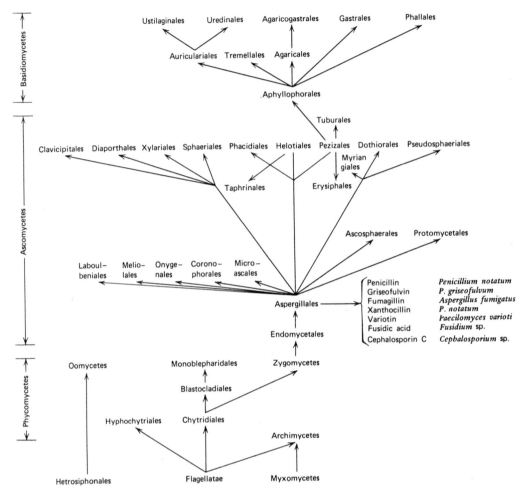

Figure 15-3 Phylogeny of the fungi (excluding Fungi Imperfecti and Lichens), including the antibiotics produced by the Aspergillales. (From E Gäumann, *Die Pilze*, 1964. Copyrighted © by Birkhauser-Verlag, Basel, and reprinted with their permission.)

secondary drug of choice may be influenced by the degree of drug resistance arising from its use with susceptible bacterial populations that cause disease.

Generally, antibiotics are low molecular weight compounds with a wide range of chemical structure, elemental composition, and physicochemical properties. Classification on a chemical basis is difficult because all have not been characterized or purified. For these reasons antibiotics are classified either taxonomically by the organism producing them or according to their biological activity spectrum. It is usually far more practical to utilize the biological machinery of the organism producing the drug than to attempt chemical synthesis. With the delineation of the penicillin nucleus, however, semisynthetic molecules have been derived that are refractory to the penicillinases produced by resistant strains. In other cases, once the antibiotic's chemically active nucleus has been defined, biological activity has been enhanced by chemical manipulation of prosthetic groups.

As already noted, the majority of isolated antibiotics are produced by species of *Streptomyces* (about 58%), and an additional 9% come from other bacteria. Other lower plants, which include the fungi, algae, the symbiotic lichens, and mosses, account for 19%; and the higher plants produce about 14% of known antibiotics.

We suspect that the total of 909 antibiotics known in 1967 represents only a fraction of those to be found in nature. Moreover, not a single one used therapeutically is from the higher plants, even though these possess the largest single group of antibiotics for which there is no known use. This represents an extraordinary reservoir among, for example, the many trees resistant to attack by fungi, and other organisms that have recently been shown to produce antibiotics in their wood and bark as well as leaves and presumably other plant parts. In fact, many intact leaves produce water-soluble fungistatic substances that are probably responsible for the plant's natural resistance to fungal action.[8] The adaptive value of these Gymnosperm and Angiosperm antibiotics is probably very great. They are certainly widespread and variable chemically, having in many instances a long history of use against bacterial and fungal infection by those practicing folk medicines throughout the world (Table 15-1). It is of particular note that many plants producing antibiotics also produce mitogens (Chapter 4), an association which needs exploration.

ANTISEPTICS AND DISINFECTANTS

In 1865 Joseph Lister began sterilizing surgical wounds with dilute carbolic acid, a postoperative practice that was to save countless lives. Mortality from amputations in Lister's wards, for example, had been reduced from 43 to 15%, and the areas were freed of the stench from pus in patients' wounds. Surgeons refused to accept asepsis for nearly another generation, but Lister remained steadfast in the face of scathing criticism for having disturbed the old order of surgical technique.

Antiseptics are chemical agents applied to living tissues, either to destroy microorganisms or to inhibit their reproductive activity. Care must be exercised, however, for they may retard the healing of clean wounds. The ideal antiseptic should destroy all types of bacteria, fungi, viruses, and other infective agents without harming living tissues; but no agent is known to possess these properties. Disinfectants are similar to antiseptics. They are used on inanimate objects to destroy microorganisms (but not spores); sterilization is the complete destruction of all microbial and viral life. Sterilization is often accomplished by physical means or agents (e.g., heat, radiation).

The most widely used antiseptics and disinfectants are alcohols, chlorine-containing compounds, iodine preparations, phenol compounds, inorganic and organic mercurial and silver preparations, quaternary ammonium compounds, boric acid, oxidizing agents, and aldehyde derivatives. They kill by coagulating or denaturing protoplasmic protein, by causing cell lysis, or by denaturing enzymes.

Most soaps used for personal hygiene are efficient cleansers and are nonirritating, although excessive use by older persons may irritate the skin. Many antiseptic and disinfectant agents used today are of botanical origin, and still others were important for the hygiene of our forefathers.

Table 15-1 Antibiotics from Higher Plants

Plant Group and Species	Vernacular Name	Antibiotic	Active Against	Plant Part Used; Use in Folk Medicines; Other Remedies
GYMNOSPERMS				
Chamaecyparis nootkatensis	Yellow or sitka cypress	Nootkatin	Fungi	Wood[a]
Gingko biloba	Gingko or maidenhair tree	Gingkolic acid	Tubercle bacilli	"Fruit"
Juniperus sabina and other spp.	Junipers	Podophyllotoxin	Tumor	Leaves; also found in *Podophyllum* (Berberidaceae)
Pinus sylvestris	Scotch pine	Pinosylvine	Bacteria and fungi	Heartwood[a]
Thuja plicata	Western red cedar	Tetrahydroxystilbene, thujaplicins	Cellulose-decomposing fungi	Wood[a]
ANGIOSPERMS				
Phylogenetic Group 1				
ARISTOLOCHIACEAE				
Aristolochia clematitis, A. fimbriata, A. foetida		Substances A and B	Broad-spectrum bacteria and fungi	Several species used for colds, chills, fevers, asthma
Asarum canadense, A. europaeum, A. maximum	Wild ginger	Substances A and B	Broad-spectrum bacteria and fungi	Root; treating coughs
RANUNCULACEAE				
Anemone spp., *Ranunculus* spp.		Anemonin, protoanemonin	Broad-spectrum bacteria	Plant; used to treat abrasions, toothache, rheumatism
Hydrastis canadensis	Golden seal	Berberine	Broad-spectrum bacteria and protozoa	Root; inflammations
BERBERIDACEAE				
Berberis vulgaris	European barberry	Berberine	Broad-spectrum bacteria and protozoa	
Phylogenetic Group 3				
POLYGONACEAE				
Rheum officinale	Medicinal rhubarb	Rhein (cassic acid)	Gram + and acid-fast bacteria	Some species used as vermifuge

Phylogenetic Group 4

CLUSIACEAE				
Garcinia morella	Gamboge	Morellin, guttiferins	Gram + and − bacteria	Seeds; extract for ointments
ERICACEAE				
Arbutus unedo	Strawberry tree	Ethyl gallate	*Mycobacterium*	
PLUMBAGINACEAE				
Plumbago europaea	Common plumbago	Plumbagin	Bacteria and fungi	Root; used for toothache, swellings, and as substitute for highly irritating Catharidens (insects)

Phylogenetic Group 5

FLACOURTIACEAE				
Hydnocarpus anthelmintica, H. wightiana	Chaulmoogra trees	Hydnocarpic acid	Leprosy	Seed oil; against leprosy
Taraktogenos kurzii		Chaulmoogric acid	Leprosy	Seed oil; against leprosy
SALICACEAE				
Populus candidans, P. trichocarpa	Poplars	Trichocarpin	Fungi	Bark[a]
P. tacamahaca		Bisabolol	Tubercle bacilli	Young shoots
BRASSICACEAE				
Brassica oleracea	Cabbage	Rapine	Fungi	Plant
B. rapa	Turnip	Rapine	Fungi	
Cheiranthus cheiri	Wallflower	Cheirolin	Bacteria and many pathogenic fungi	Seeds; remedy for oral ulcers
Armoracia rusticana	Horseradish	Undefined	Bacteria	Root
Raphanus sativus	Radish	Raphanin	Gram + and − bacteria	Seeds and stems
MORINGACEAE				
Moringa oleifera	Horseradish tree	Pterigospermin	Gram + and − bacteria	Roots

Phylogenetic Group 6

MORACEAE				
Chlorophora excelsa	African oak	Chlorophorin	Fungi	Wood[a]; tree not attacked by termites
Maclura pomifera	Osage orange	Tetraphydroxystilbene	Cellulose-decomposing fungi	Wood[a]
CANNABACEAE				
Humulus lupulus	Hops	Lupulon, humulon	Gram + and acid-fast bacteria	Hops (inflorescence); prevent bacteria from growing in beer or wort

361

Table 15-1 (Continued)

Plant Group and Species	Vernacular Name	Antibiotic	Active Against	Plant Part Used; Use in Folk Medicines; Other Remedies
EUPHORBIACEAE				
Cnidoscolus urens		Uresin	Gram + and acid-fast bacteria	Roots
Croton sellowii		Selovicin	Acid-fast bacteria	Roots; different species used for toothache, skin diseases, rheumatism, worms, fever, eye disease, as insecticide
Phylogenetic Group 7				
ROSACEAE				
Malus spp., *Prunus* spp., *Pyrus* spp.	Apples, pears, plums	Phloretin	Gram + and − bacteria	Bark and root
Sorbus aucuparia	European mountain ash	Parasorbic acid	Gram +bacteria and protozoa	Fruit; used for coughs and catarrh
Spiraea aruncus		Undefined	Bacteria	Leaves and flowers
FABACEAE				
Acacia adonsonii, *A. seyal*		Ethyl gallate		
Canavalia ensiformis	Jack bean	Canavanine	Bacteria and fungi	Seeds
Cassia reticulata		Rhein (cassic acid)	Gram + and acid-fast bacteria	Leaves; to treat gonorrhea, ringworm, skin diseases
Dalbergia nigra		Dalbergions	Broad-spectrum bacteria and yeasts	Sawdust[a]; used as anthelmintic and to remove pimples
Haematoxylum campechianum	Logwood	Ethyl gallate	Mycobacterium	Leaves
Melilotus spp.	Sweet clover	Dicumarol	Broad-spectrum bacteria	Plant; seeds used against colds and moths
Phaseolus vulgaris	Common bean	Phaseollin	Fungi	Seed
Prosopis ruscifolia		Vinaline	Broad-spectrum bacteria	Used to make alcoholic beverages
Vicia faba	Broad bean	Undefined	Fungi	Stem and root; plant is very immune to fungal attack

362

Phylogenetic Group 9				
ZYGOPHYLLACEAE				
Larrea divaricata	Creosote bush	Nordihydroguaiaretic acid	Skin bacteria	Plant; against venereal diseases and rheumatism
BALSAMINACEAE				
Impatiens balsamina	Jewel balsam weed	2-Methoxy-naphthoquinone	Fungi	Plant
RUTACEAE				
Zanthoxylum clava-herculis	Toothache tree	Berberine	Broad-spectrum bacteria	Used for toothache and rheumatism
ANACARDIACEAE				
Anacardium occidentale	Cashew	Anacardic acid	Gram + bacteria, Nemathelminthes	Oil from fruit; against leprosy and as anthelmintic; gum from stem used in varnishes to protect books and woodwork against ants and other insects
JUGLANDACEAE				
Juglans nigra	Black walnut	Juglone	Dermatomycosis	Bark and fruit; used in Greek and Roman medicine for cutaneous mycoses
Phylogenetic Group 10				
CELASTRACEAE				
Pristimera grahamii, *P. indica*		Pristimerin	Gram + bacteria	
APIACEAE				
Centella asiatica		Asiaticoside	Tubercle bacilli	Plant; treat leprosy
Phylogenetic Group 11				
APOCYNACEAE				
Allamanda violacea		Allamandin	Protozoa	
Plumeria multiflora		Plumericin	Fungi especially	
Tabernaemontana sp.		Undefined	Fungi	
BIGNONIACEAE				
Tabebuia avellanedae and other spp., *Tecoma* spp.		Lapachol	Gram + and acid-fast bacteria, fungi	Root; against rheumatism (leaves), for cough (bark), syphilis (bark) and warts (juice)
				Sawdust[a]; resistant to termites (deoxylapachol)
		Xyloidone	*Brucella* and *Candida*	Wood[a]

Table 15-1 Continued

Plant Group and Species	Vernacular Name	Antibiotic	Active Against	Plant Part Used; Use in Folk Medicines; Other Remedies
SCROPHULARIACEAE				
Capraria biflora		Biflorin	Fungi	Root
ACANTHACEAE				
Adhatoda vasica	Malabar nut tree	Undefined	Tubercle bacilli	Plant; long used in India to treat colds, coughs, bronchitis, and asthma
SOLANACEAE				
Lycopersicon pimpinellifolium		Tomatine	Gram + bacteria	
Solanum tuberosum	Potato	Tuberosines	Protozoa	Plant; used for alcoholic beverages; many species of genus used to treat sores and for coughs
Withania somnifera		Withaferin	Broad-spectrum bacteria and viruses	Leaves
ASTERACEAE				
Crepis taraxacifolia		Crepin	Gram + bacteria	Buds, flowers, and roots
Phylogenetic Group 14 POACEAE (many members of family have antibiotic principles)				
Zea mays	Corn	Undefined	Fungi	Young stalks
ZINGIBERACEAE				
Curcuma longa, C. rotunda, C. tinctoria, C. viridiflora		Curcumin	Broad-spectrum bacteria and fungi	Root juice used in India as anthelmintic
Phylogenetic Group 15 LILIACEAE				
Allium sativum	Garlic	Allcin, allistatin	Broad-spectrum bacteria and fungi	Bulk; widely used to treat tuberculosis, coughs, colds, toothache and earache
Aloe barbadensis		Barbaloin	Tubercle bacilli	Plant; used against ringworm

GYMNOSPERM

Pinus mugo (mountain pine: (Fig. 15-4*a*) is the source of pine needle oil, widely used as a mild antiseptic.

ANGIOSPERMS

ASCLEPIADACEAE

Blepharodon mucronatum. Leaf juice is used as an antiseptic in Mexico.

ASTERACEAE

Arnica cordifolia, A. fulgens, A. montana, and others. Dried flowering heads are

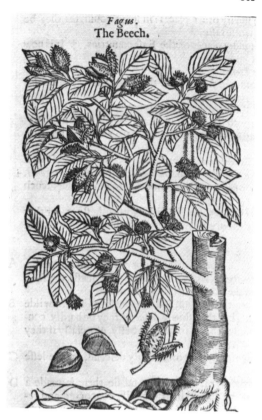

Figure 15-4*b* *Fagus sylvatica* (from J Gerard, *The Herball*, ed 2, 1636).

bactericidal and at one time were widely esteemed in Europe and North America for their value in treating slight wounds and abrasions.

FABACEAE

Myroxylon pereirae (balsam of Peru) is mildly antiseptic as well as being hemostatic.

FAGACEAE

Fagus ferruginea (American beech) and *F. sylvatica* (European beech: Fig. 15-4*b*) are sources of creosote, which is antiseptic and is also used in the manufacture of certain soaps.

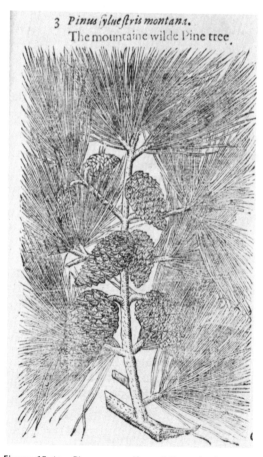

Figure 15-4*a* *Pinus mugo* (from J Gerard, *The Herball*, 1597).

MELIACEAE

Azadirachta indica (neem tree). Very bitter leaves are used as an antiseptic in Asia.

MENISPERMACEAE

Arcangelisia flava, a source of berberine, is used as a germicide in tropical Asia.

MYRTACEAE

Melaleuca alternifolia and *M. linariifolia* of Australia are sources of a volatile oil having a highly germicidal activity. The oil is used in surgery and dentistry and as an ingredient of antiseptic soaps.

ZYGOPHYLLACEAE

Larrea mexicana (greasewood) of the southwestern United States and Mexico. Twigs and leaves, when steeped in boiling water, release principles that are used in commercial antiseptic lotions.

PESTICIDES

All pesticides block some metabolic process. They differ, however, in their composition, potency, mode of action, speed of effect, and dose requirements. These agents can be classified according to the organism they are intended to control—insecticide, fungicide, herbicide, and so forth.

INSECTICIDES

Stomach poisons were once widely used against insects with biting mouth parts and are toxic when ingested; examples are arsenic (paris green, lead arsenate) and fluoride compounds (cryolite). These agents are now largely replaced by contact insecticides.

The contact poisons penetrate the integument of the pest and are particularly effective against insects with sucking mouth parts. The naturally occurring contact insecticides are nicotine from leaves of *Nicotiana rustica* (Solanaceae: Fig. 15-5a), pyrethrum from flowers of *Chrysanthemum cinerariifolium* and other species (Asteraceae: Fig. 15-5b), and rotenone from roots of *Derris* and *Lonchocarpus* (Fabaceae). These insecticides, whose effects are short-lived, are listed in Table 15-2 together with many other natural insecticides and parasiticides used by native populations. Most are probably contact poisons.

Synthetic contact insecticides are now the primary agents of chemical control. Some, like the pyrethrins, have been synthetically modeled on plant extracts;

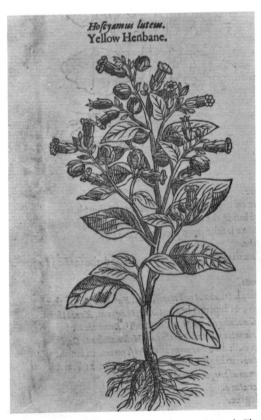

Figure 15-5a *Nicotiana rustica* (from J Gerard, *The Herball*, 1597).

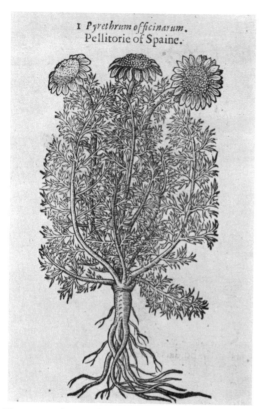

I *Pyrethrum officinarum.*
Pellitorie of Spaine.

Figure 15-5b   *Chrysanthemum cinerariifolium*
(from J Gerard, *The Herball*, ed 2, 1636).

but many stem from the development of a series of chlorinated hydrocarbons in the 1940s following the discovery of DDT as an insecticide. These include chlordane, lindane, toxaphene, aldrin, and dieldrin; most are long lasting, and their toxic effects are cumulative. Toxic action is not fully understood; the substances probably affect neurochemical transmitters, leading to a disorganization of the nervous system.

When DDT first appeared it seemed almost as miraculous as the first antibiotic—it was cheap, it efficiently destroyed pests, it brought bumper harvests, and it reduced such diseases as malaria. Yet data accumulated over several decades indicate that the chemical is a threat to a wide variety of animals, including man.[9] When long-lasting pesticides become linked with food chains, for example, the consequences are significant. The chemicals are concentrated as they pass along the food chain, which means that predators at the top are usually severely affected. For example, earthworms are resistant to DDT and accumulate it without difficulty. If robins eat about 100 DDT-ingesting worms, however, they will die. If the birds happen to live, DDT affects their calcium metabolism, and their egg shells are too fragile for proper incubation. Extinction is the ultimate end of this chain for a number of predatory birds, including the peregrine falcon and the bald eagle. DDT also poisons a wide spectrum of insects, and thus breaks the food chain by destroying many aquatic insects that serve as food for fish or birds. DDT is now recognized as an uncontrollable, durable chemical that persists in aquatic and terrestrial environments, and because it lasts so long and accumulates in fish and other animals, it may have serious effects on human beings. With this realization, the federal government banned DDT in 1972, except for use under special circumstances such as a malarial epidemic, and in 1974 the manufacture of aldrin and dieldrin, which cause cancerous tumors in mice, was also prohibited.

Members of a second series of insecticides known as organophosphates (e.g., parathion, malathion) are also very toxic, but many of them break down shortly after use. Some can be used systemically, for they are absorbed into the plant if the leaves are sprayed or if solutions are applied to the soil, since sucking insects that feed on the plants later are killed. These insecticides are widely used today, but a word of caution is needed. Whereas DDT and some of the earlier insecticides are not very toxic to man, a lethal dose of the more common organophosphates is less than 1 g. The toxic

Table 15-2   Plants Used as Insecticides and Parasiticides

Angiosperm Family and Species	Locality	Remarks
ANNONACEAE		
Annona cherimola	Tropical America	Resins of seed used against lice
A. squamosa		
APOCYNACEAE		
Trachelospermum stans	Mexico	Used to poison cockroaches
ASCLEPIADACEAE		
Cynanchium arnottianum	India	
Funastrum clausum	Tropical America	Latex a powerful insecticide
ASTERACEAE		
Chrysanthemum cinerariifolium	Yugoslavia	Widely cultivated, source of Pyrethrum insect powder of dried, unexpanded flowerheads containing the toxic principle pyrethron
C. coccineum	Southern Russia to Iran	Source of Persian insect powder
C. marschallii	Iran	Insect powder from dried flowerheads
C. parthenium	Mediterranean	Insect powder from dried flowerheads
Eupatorium capillifolium,	Eastern North America	Herb used on floor to ward off insects
E. compositifolium		
BIGNONIACEAE		
Jacaranda filicifolia	Panama	Possibly contains lapachol as deterrent
CELASTRACEAE		
Tripterygium wilfordii	China	Powdered root as insecticide
CHENOPODIACEAE		
Anabasis aphylla	Near East	Plant source of insecticide
CISTACEAE		
Cistus ladaniferus	Mediterranean region	Gum labdanum as insecticide and deodorant
CLUSIACEAE		
Mammea americana	Tropical America	Flowers, leaves, and roots are insecticides
CONVOLVULACEAE		
Ipomoea quamoclit	Tropical America	Seeds as insecticide
Jacquemontia tamnifolia	Tropical America	Seeds as insecticide
CUCURBITACEAE		
Momordica schimperiana	Tropical Africa	
EUPHORBIACEAE		
Croton texensis	New Mexican Indians	Plant as insecticide
FABACEAE		
Derris elliptica, D. uligonosa	Old World tropics	Powdered root widely used as insecticide, source of rotenone
Dolichos pseudopachyrrhizus	Tropical Africa	
Lonchocarpus nicou, L. urucu,	South America	Roots source of rotenone
L. utilis		
Mucuna spp.	Tropical America	Seeds contain L-dopa, repel insects
FLACOURTIACEAE		
Patrisia pyrifera	Tropical South America	Source of insecticide Ryanex
HAMAMELIDACEAE		
Liquidambar orientalis,	China and Eastern North America	Balsam used in fumigating powders
L. styraciflua		
LILIACEAE		
Schoenocaulon officinale	Central America	Seeds an insecticide; also an extract strongly toxic to house flies

368

Table 15-2   (Continued)

Angiosperm Family and Species	Locality	Remarks
MELIACEAE		
Melia azedarach	Western Asia	Fruit powder an insecticide against flies
POACEAE		
Cymbopogon nardus	Tropical Asia and cultivated	Source of Citronella, used as insecticide and disinfectant
RANUNCULACEAE		
Delphinium consolida,	Southern Europe and	Seed tincture active insecticide and
D. staphisagria	Near East	parasiticide (against lice and nits in hair)
ROXBURGHIACEAE		
Stemona burkelii, S. collinsae,	Tropical Asia	Roots contain stemorin
S. sessilifolia, S. tuberosa		
RUBIACEAE		
Adina cordifolia	India	Sap an insecticide
Gardenia lucida	Burma	Source of combee resin, used to ward off flies
RUTACEAE		
Clausena anisata	Tropical Africa	Anise-scented leaves used to combat mosquitoes
SIMAROUBACEAE		
Simarouba versicolor	Brazil	Powdered bark as insecticide
SOLANACEAE		
Nicotiana rustica, N. tabacum	North America	Leaf dust containing nicotine widely used in former times by Indians against insects and now commercially available

action of these chemicals is related to inhibiting cholinesterase. Free acetylcholine increases, with the result that organs responding to acetylcholine undergo prolonged and intense stimulation. After a lethal dose has been ingested or inhaled, convulsions occur and the individual dies from respiratory failure. A striking increase in the number of cases of poisoning by these pesticides has already been recorded,[10] for example, from fumes of malathion.[11]

Fumigants (hydrogen cyanide, naphthalene, methyl bromide, nicotine) are toxic when they enter the respiratory system of the pest; repellents ward off rather than kill (e.g., L-dopa, creosote, lime, certain oils); sterilants inhibit reproduction of pests (e.g., alkylating agents, antimetabolites); pheromones affect insect behavior (e.g., sex attractant secretion); viruses infect insects; and hormones regulate insect growth and maturation.[12] All such weapons may be important for our pest control programs.

FUNGICIDES

Compounds that either prevent or stop the development of fungal diseases on crop plants are known as fungicides. They are based on such chemicals as sulfur, mercury, and copper, and usually have a broad spectrum of action. Their use must be carefully controlled, for they can be highly toxic if ingested by man. A tragic example was an outbreak of mercury poisoning in Iraq during 1971–1972: misuse of seed grain treated with methylmercury led to the loss of 459 lives because many farmers baked bread with the treated wheat, despite warnings printed on the sacks of grain.[13]

HERBICIDES

Herbicides may kill most vegetation on contact or they may be selective. Nonselective chemicals include sodium chlorate, sulfuric acid, and the bipyridyls, but selective agents have important applications in agriculture. Thus 2,4-D, dalapon, and MCPA possess individual properties that enable agriculturists to use them selectively, some to control broad-leaved weeds in cereal plantings, others to control weedy grasses in broad-leaved crops. Still other herbicides, such as the carbamates, triazines, and ureas, selectively destroy germinating weeds over prolonged periods without harming established plants in the same region. This is due partly to insolubility of the compounds, which do not affect crop seeds or their developing roots when plantings are deeper than the more shallow zone of herbicidal action.

Insecticide activity is greatly enhanced by a number of herbicides (atrazine, simazine, monuron, 2,4-D) which otherwise are nontoxic to insects.[14] This synergism could have important applications in controlling insects. A number of herbicides are teratogenic in experimental animals. At present, however, these compounds are not considered hazardous to human health.

As the study of pesticide effects becomes more sophisticated, embracing the total exposed environment, the use of these agents will certainly change. The naturally occurring pyrethroids, for example, are becoming increasingly important in insect control, for they combine a number of desirable properties: exceptional insecticidal activity, low mammalian toxicity, rapid biodegradation, and little or no persisting residues.[15] These characteristics should be universal for all pesticides, and it is to be hoped that this goal will be achieved in the near future.

But what if you wish to eliminate pests in your yard? Besides using pyrethroids, you might purchase ladybugs and praying mantises, which thrive on other insects, as another way to rid pests. Still another is to intersperse among your plants a number of herbs that have proved to be particularly obnoxious to insects. These include the many culinary herbs containing volatile oils (basil, peppermint, rosemary, sage, and tansy), as well as strong-smelling marigolds, onions, garlic, radishes, and nasturtiums. In addition, many insects, including mosquitoes, are repelled by the lemony or citronella herbs (lemon verbena, lemon balm, pelargonium), which are pleasant to smell or to have as herb teas; a garden well stocked with these plants is not only attractive and utilitarian, it also deters pests without danger to people, their pets, or the wild creatures of the area.

LITERATURE CITED

1. Fleming A. 1929. On the antibacterial action of cultures of a *Penicillium,* with special reference to their use in the isolation of *B. influenzae. Brit J Exp Pathol* 10: 226–236; Florey WH, Chain E, Heatly NG et al. 1949. *Antibiotics.* 2 vols. Oxford University Press, New York; Böttcher HM. 1963. *Miracle Drugs.* Heinemann, London. 285 p.

2. Freudenreich E. 1888. Sur une variété particulièrement chromogène du Bacille *Pyocyaneus. Ann Microgr.* 5: 183.

3. Galdston I. (ed). 1958. *The Impact of the Antibiotics on Medicine and Society.* International University Press, New York. 222 p.

4. Zahner A, Maas WK. 1972. *Biology of Antibiotics.* Heidelberg Science Library, Vol 4. Springer-Verlag, New York. 125 p.

5. Gäumann E. 1964. *Die Pilze.* Birkhauser-Verlag, Basel.

6. Lewis WH, Elvin-Lewis M. 1961. Medium for growing small rubiaceous seeds from herbarium material. *Castanea* 26: 146–155.

7. Korzybski T, Kowszyk-Gindifer Z, Kurylowicz W. 1967. *Antibiotics.* 2 vols. Pergamon Press, Oxford; Gjerstad G. A quarter of a century of

antibiotic therapy. *Quart J Crude Drug Res*—I. **6**(2): 841–852, 1966; II. **7**(4): 1093–1096, 1967; III. **9**(1): 1317–1322, 1969; IV. **9**(2): 1360–1365, 1969; V. **12**(3): 1909–1922, 1972.

8. Topps JH, Wain RL. 1957. Fungistatic properties of leaf exudates. *Nature* **179:** 652–653.

9. Carson R. 1962. *Silent Spring.* Houghton Mifflin, Boston. 368 p; Graham F. 1970. *Since Silent Spring.* Houghton Mifflin.

10. DDT substitutes pose more medical hazards. 1971. *Mod Med* **39**(25): 46, 50.

11. Sare WM. 1972. Chronic poisoning by a phosphate ester insecticide, malathion. *New Zealand Med J* **75:** 93–94.

12. Marz JL. 1973. Insect control (I): use of pheromones. *Science* **181:** 736–737; Insect control (II): hormones and viruses. **181:** 833–835.

13. Bakir F, Damluji SF, Amin-Zaki L et al. 1973. Methylmercury poisoning in Iraq. *Science* **181:** 230–241.

14. Lichtenstein EP, Liang TT, Anderegg BN. 1973. Synergism of insecticides by herbicides. *Science* **181:** 847–849.

15. Abernathy CO, Casida JE. 1973. Pyrethroid insecticides: esterase cleavage in relation to selective toxicity. *Science* **179:** 1235–1236.

Chapter 16
Panaceas

Universal remedies or panaceas could not form a chapter of this book if it were not for the acclaim of one genus, *Panax*, better known as ginseng. The worth of all other plants pales in comparison with the value proclaimed for ginseng by millions. Ginseng is the only plant used routinely by so great a number of more or less healthy individuals for stimulation, added energy, and a sense of well-being—a panacea for the healthy who want to remain well for a long time and if possible become healthier.

Root extracts are also taken by less healthy as an alterative, to modify favorably the course of a disease or difficulty, specifically tuberculosis, coughs, nausea, diabetes, indigestion, diarrhea, kidney degeneration, gout, rheumatism, and suppurating sores.[1] Many believe that ginseng also has aphrodisiac properties, maintaining sexual potency in the male. These beliefs have been held by Oriental peoples since ancient times: ginseng is "a tonic to the five viscera, quieting animal spirits, establishing the soul, allaying fear, expelling evil effluvia, brightening the eye, opening up the heart, benefiting the understanding, and if taken for some time it will invigorate the body and prolong life."[2]

This cure-all reputation of the eastern Asian *Panax ginseng* is shared by the eastern North American species *P. quinquefolium* (Fig. 16-1). Roots of this species have been shipped to the Orient

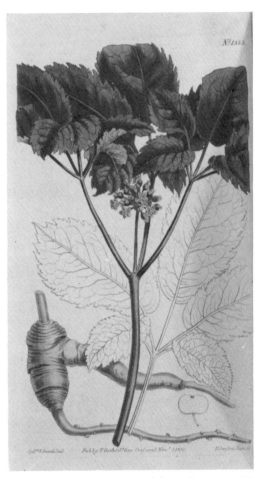

Figure 16-1 *Panax quinquefolium* (from *Curtis's Botanical Magazine* **33:** 1333, 1811).

for several centuries at huge profits and at the expense of this species, which is nearly eradicated in much of the eastern woodland where it once thrived. The Indians, it appears, used the roots only sparingly and then only after being hired to gather them for export,[3] although the Ojibwas (Chippewas) may have had a tradition of ginseng use for prolonging life and relieving pain.[1] A third member of the family Araliaceae, *Eleutherococcus senticosus*, native to Siberia, reportedly shares the panacean properties of *Panax*.

What modern evidence exists of the efficacy of these species? In recent research undertaken largely by Chinese, Japanese, and Russian scientists, physiologically active glycosides have been isolated, but none has been fully characterized. Among the compounds isolated from roots and leaves are (1) panaxin, acting as a stimulant for the midbrain, heart, and vessels; (2) panax acid, as a stimulant for the heart and general metabolism; (3) panaquilin, as a stimulant for internal secretions; (4) panacen and sapogenin, volatile oils that stimulate the central nervous system; and (5) ginsenin that lowers blood sugar.[4]

Several pharmacological trials illustrate the effectiveness of these extracts. Ginseng as a regulator has received considerable attention in experiments with rats and mice. Under conditions of extreme cold or heat, the animals treated with ginseng extracts were better able to withstand variations in their environment, for they appeared normal during the stress and none convulsed, whereas the controlled animals were unable to move after stress, showed clonic convulsions, and did not regain normal activity until up to one hour after the stress. Levels of ascorbic acid and cholesterol in the adrenal glands, and of eosinophil cells in the peripheral blood were recorded during these times, and the conclusions suggested that ginseng has a stimulating effect on the adrenal cortex. Corticosteroid content in the urine increased by more than 60%, and eosinophil cell counts decreased. All research demonstrated a reduced mortality and morbidity of animals exposed to temperature stress. Ginseng also promoted defenses against other kinds of stress such as acute hemorrhagic shock, asphyxia, and histamine shock, and it demonstrated specific effects on carbohydrate metabolism, such as partial control of hyperglycemia and increasing the force of cardiac contraction, especially during acute circulatory failure. Antimicrobial and antineoplastic activity has also been reported.

In double-blind clinical studies male radio operators were tested for speed and accuracy in transmitting messages. In this experiment there was no noticeable increase in the number of characters transmitted by either group, but the operators who had taken ginseng had mistakes in only 17% of their messages, and the others had an error rate of 31%. Based on these and similar experiments, researchers concluded that ginseng increases mental and physical efficiency, improves the accuracy of work, contributes to concentration, and prevents overfatigue. Its action is distinct from that of synthetic stimulants, such as the amphetamines, for ginseng neither provokes subjective excitation nor disturbs normal sleep. Administration may be prolonged and repeated without side effects, and a generalized tonic effect is usually demonstrated after about two weeks and is consolidated after a month of treatment.[4]

There is no question among those in the Orient, continental Europe, and a growing number of users in North America that ginseng is the best tonic by far, but over the years many other plants have been utilized to give a lift. Of the sample given in Table 16-1 (see also

Table 16-1 Plants Considered Significant Tonics

Plant Group and Species	Vernacular Name	Locality	Remarks
FUNGUS			
Cordyceps sinensis		China	Tonic and stimulant for convalescents
ANGIOSPERMS			
APIACEAE			
Angelica archangelica	Angelica	Eurasia	This and following species
Peucedanum ostruthium	Masterwort	Eurasia	rich in coumarin derivates; herbs considered as tonic to
Pimpinella saxifraga	Black caraway	Mediterranean region	improve well-being and mental harmony
ARALIACEAE			
Eleutherococcus senticosus	Siberian ginseng	Eastern Asia	Leaves and roots make miracle tonic similar to *Panax*
Panax ginseng	Oriental ginseng	Eastern Asia	See text
P. quinquefolium	American ginseng	Eastern North American Indians	See text
P. repens		China, Indochina	Tonic for convalescents
ARISTOLOCHIACEAE			
Asarum caudatum	Wild ginger	Western Washington State (Skagits)	Boiled leaves as tonic tea
ASTERACEAE			
Centaurea cyanus	Cornflower	Mediterranean region	Tea of flowerheads tonic and stimulant
C. nigra	Knapweed	Europe, North America	
Doronicum falconeri		Himalayas and Kashmir	Root tonic helps nervous depression
D. pardalianches		Europe	Cardiac tonic, also used for nervous depression and melancholia
Eupatorium perfoliatum	Boneset	North America	Leaves and flowering tops virtual panacea among Indians and whites
Matricaria chamomilla	Chamomile	Eurasia	Widely cultivated for bitter tonic tea
Senecio jacobaea	Tansy ragwort	Eurasia	Leaves home remedy as stimulant and tonic
Xanthium canadense	Burweed	Eastern North America	Herb alterative
X. strumarium	Sea burweed	Cosmopolitan	Herb alterative
BERBERIDACEAE			
Jeffersonia diphylla	Twinleaf	New York to Iowa	Roots used as stimulant and tonic
Mahonia aquifolium	Oregon grape	Western North America	Rhizomes and roots bitter tonic and alterative
COCHLOSPERMACEAE			
Cochlospermum niloticum		Sudan (Nuba Mountains)	Swollen below-ground parts chewed as tonic
CONVOLVULACEAE			
Cressa cretica		Sudan	Plant as tonic
Ipomoea digitata	Fingerleaf Morning glory	India to Malaya	Root as tonic, alterative, and aphrodisiac
CYPERACEAE			
Cyperus iria		India	Herb as stimulant and tonic
ERICACEAE			
Calluna vulgaris	Heather	Europe	Health tea from plant

Table 16-1 (Continued)

Plant Group and Species	Vernacular Name	Locality	Remarks
EUPHORBIACEAE			
Croton eluteria		West Indies (Bahamas)	Dried cascarilla bark is aromatic bitter and tonic
C. reflexifolius		Central America	Tonic
FABACEAE			
Caesalpinia bonduscella	Molucca bean	India	Seeds mixed with black pepper as a tonic
C. nuga		India	Roots used as tonic
Cassia occidentalis	Coffee senna	Tropics	Seeds used as tonic and diuretic
GENTIANACEAE			
Canscora diffusa		Philippines	Herb as tonic tea
Gentiana spp.		North America	Roots as bitter tonics for Indians and whites
Swertia carolinensis	Columbo	Eastern North America	Roots as tonic and stimulant
LAMIACEAE			
Leonurus cardiaca	Common motherwort	Eurasia	Herb tonic for heart ailments, female weakness, and hysteria
LILIACEAE			
Hypoxis aurea		Tropical Asia	Herb considered rejuvenating, reconstructive, tonic, and aphrodisiac; a panacea similar to ginseng
Smilax calophylla		Malaysia	Rhizomes tonic and aphrodisiac
S. china	China root	China, Japan	Root decoction as stimulant, alterative, and aphrodisiac; source of sarsaparilla
S. ornata		Central America	Dried roots source of commercial Jamaica sarsaparilla, tonic, and alterative
S. regelii (and other spp.)		Central America	Root source of brown sarsaparilla
MENISPERMACEAE			
Cyclea peltata		China	Tubers tonic
PAPAVERACEAE			
Corydalis gavaniana		India	Roots tonic, alterative, diuretic
Dicentra canadensis, D. cucullaria	Squirrel corn, Dutchman's breeches	Eastern North America	Dried tubers tonic and alterative
Fumaria officinalis		Temperate Eurasia and Northern Africa	Herb as home remedy for tonic and blood purifiers
F. parviflora		Iran and Afghanistan	Herb and fruit as blood purifiers
PIPERACEAE			
Piper methysticum	Kava	Oceania	Cold water extract of roots tonic and stimulant
RANUNCULACEAE			
Clematis hexasepala		New Zealand	Bark and stem infusion a mild alterative
Coptis teeta		Assam	Root containing berberine as bitter tonic

Table 16-1   (Continued)

Plant Group and Species	Vernacular Name	Locality	Remarks
C. trifolia	Goldenthread	North America	Dried plant as tonic
RUBIACEAE			
Cinchona calisaya	Yellowbark cinchona	Bolivia	Bark as tonic
C. ledgeriana	Ledgerbark cinchona	Bolivia	Bark as tonic
RUTACEAE			
Euodia lepta		Southeast Asia	Whole plant as bitter tonic
E. lunuankenda	Vanashempaga	Malaya	Leaf or flower infusion as tonic
Ptelea trifoliata	Common hop tree	North America	Menominees and Meskwakis considered bark a sacred medicine and panacea; also used to render other medicines potent
VERBENACEAE			
Lantana camara		Tropical America	Leaves as stimulant and tonic
L. microphylla		Tropical America	Fruit as stimulant and tonic

stimulating teas, Table 17-2), *Hypoxis aurea* and several species of *Smilax* of the Liliaceae have at one time approached ginseng in local popularity. Many tonics contain volatile oils, steroidal sapogenins, and bitter glycosides.

LITERATURE CITED

1. Harriman S. 1973. *The Book of Ginseng.* Pyramid Books, New York. 157 p.
2. Stuart GA. 1928. *Chinese Materia Medica: Vegetable Kingdom.* Presbyterian Mission Press, Shanghai.
3. Vogel VJ. 1970. *American Indian Medicine.* University of Oklahoma Press, Norman. 583 p.
4. Brekhman II, Dardymov IV. 1969. Pharmacological investigation of glycosides from ginseng and *Eleutherococcus. Lloydia* 32: 46–51; Kim C, Kim CC, Kim MS et al. 1970. Influence of ginseng on the stress mechanism. *Lloydia* 33: 43–48; Li CP, Li RC. 1973. An introductory note to ginseng. *Am J Chin Med* 1: 249–261; Nabata H, Saito H, Takagi K. 1973. Pharmacological studies of neutral saponins (GNS) of *Panax ginseng* root. *Japan J Pharm* 23: 29–41; Popov IM, Goldwag WH. 1973. A review of the properties of clinical effects of ginseng. *Am J Chin Med* 1: 263–270; Saito H, Morita M, Takagi K. 1973. Pharmacological studies of *Panax ginseng* leaves. *Japan J Pharm* 23: 43–56.

Section Three
"PSYCHOACTIVE" PLANTS

Psychoactive drugs act on the central nervous system. They are here divided into three broad categories: *stimulants,* which excite and enhance psychomotor activity, *hallucinogens,* which are capable of inducing a dreamlike state as well as hallucinations, and *depressants,* which reduce mental and physical performance. A wide range of plant derivates are involved in these mind-altering drugs. Cocaine, coffee, and tea are well-known stimulants; peyote, certain mushrooms, morning glory seeds, and marihuana are frequently used hallucinogens; and alcohol and tranquilizers are the best known examples of depressants. Nicotine obtained from smoking, chewing, and sniffing tobacco may act as a depressant, but it serves usually as a stimulant, where it is here grouped. Plants having psychoactive potential are discussed in Chapters 17 to 19, together with a number of synthetically derived drugs such as the barbiturates and amphetamines.

Chapter 17

Stimulants

Stimulants have long been enjoyed by man. They give him a sense of well-being and exhilaration, self-confidence and power, and they alleviate fatigue and drowsiness. Why should man not seek drugs with these attributes that help him so much? To some, there is the inevitable price to be paid: increased agitation, apprehension and anxiety, mild mania (flight of ideas), as well as increased tolerance and often dependency, are direct results of using stimulants.

Two of the most powerful natural stimulants, however, have never been generally available to man. One, coca, is native to the Andes area of South America; the other is chat, which is commonly used in eastern Ethiopia and neighboring states. An extract of coca, well-known as cocaine, has been available since the nineteenth century, but then only for medicinal purposes and, to the very few who could afford it, for pleasure. In contrast to these powerful stimulants are the many mildly stimulating beverages, like tea and coffee, as well as numerous tonics and panaceas purportedly giving the same effect.

In 1932 Benzedrine® was introduced commercially, and this and other amphetamines were widely used beginning with World War II. The Germans first employed amphetamines to enhance and extend performance of their paratroopers and other forces in 1938 and, as the war progressed, both sides were dispensing "pep pills" to their personnel to increase fighting effective-ness. In Japan the use of amphetamines was even more general, particularly by the war's end; they were taken almost compulsively by the air force, and by construction and factory workers in-volved in the war effort to maintain production at a high level of efficiency for many hours. At the end of the war the Japanese drug companies dumped their surplus stock on the open market with the slogan "elimination of drowsiness and repletion of the spirit." After a de-vastating war, amphetamines were exactly what the people wanted to counter feelings of frustration and loss of confidence. Within a few years Japan was in the midst of the first central nervous system stimulant epidemic known to man. Chronic amphetamine abusers were everywhere. By 1951 arrests for illegal use totaled 17,528, by 1955, 55,664; but by 1958 the epidemic was brought to an abrupt end following stern governmental measures against the illegal manufacture and sale of the drugs. That year only 271 persons were arrested.[1] The discussions of the natural stimulants coca (cocaine) and chat are followed by treatments of the synthetic amphetamines and the mild beverage stimulants containing caffeine, theobromine, theophylline, and other al-kaloids. Nicotine from tobacco also has stimulating effects and a section on smok-ing concludes this chapter.

COCA AND COCAINE[2]

Native and widely cultivated in the Andean highlands of South America is a plant long used as a stimulant and as a hunger depressant—the divine coca (*Erythroxylum coca*, Fig. 17-1, Eryth-roxylaceae) from which cocaine is derived. This shrub was considered the property of the Incan royal family, to be dispensed as desired and so revered by

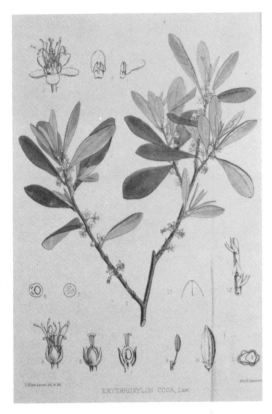

Figure 17-1 *Erythroxylum coca* (From R Bentley and H Trimen, *Medicinal Plants* 1: 40, 1880).

the Incas that leaves of the plant were in-cluded in the graves of noblemen to give a sense of exalted well-being and freedom from fatigue and hunger in the hereafter.

The Spanish soon learned of coca's powers from the Incas, and for economic reasons the distribution of leaves became widespread among the Indian workers of Ecuador, Peru, and Bolivia. Today millions chew quids mixed with a little alkali for intensified effects. A handful of leaves chewed daily, with fresh ones added to the quid every hour or so, gives sustained energy and the will to work hard even under the most deplorable conditions. This dosage represents about 2 ounces of dried leaves containing approximately 0.7 grain of cocaine, a tropane alkaloid isolated from coca in the 1840s. Cocaine was popularized in Europe during the latter half of the nineteenth century by such advocates as Sigmund Freud (to counteract the effects of morphine and for his depression), and Sir Arthur Conan Doyle, whose fictional detective Sherlock Holmes took the drug to stimulate and clarify the mind, and for mental exaltation. In addition, thousands routinely purchased Mariani's Coca Wine from France and Coca-Cola in North America. (Coca-Cola contained cocaine until 1904, when use of this ingredient was prohibited.) Various tonics and other patent medicines also included cocaine for treating catarrh. The drug has the effect of reducing mucous membrane swelling, thus enlarging the nasal and bronchial passages, an action similar to that of the amphetamines. Many cases of cocaine habit originated from the popular catarrh medicines, which contained from 2 to 4% cocaine.

Not long after its extraction, cocaine was found to possess local anesthetic properties and was widely used in eye surgery and in dentistry. The potential for misuse was clear, however, and a search for synthetic drugs not having stimulatory effects on the central nervous system was rewarded with the discovery of procaine (Novocaine®) and Xylocaine®. Consequently there is little medical use of cocaine today.

Cocaine arousal of the central nervous system and enhancement of all adrenergic neurons, resulting in a stimulation of the sympathetic nervous system, produces effects very similar to those of the amphetamines, but the duration of action is very different. To maintain exhilaration, cocaine must be injected intravenously every 5 to 15 minutes, whereas the misuser of amphetamines, for example, injects methamphetamine every 2 to 4 hours to maintain a high.

Cocaine addiction differs from addiction to the depressant drugs in at least two respects. A cocaine user (cocaine sold illegally in New York in 1970 reportedly was about 6% pure) does not suffer dramatic physical effects on withdrawal, and this has led many to classify cocaine as a nonaddictive drug. Cocaine withdrawal, however, is characterized by a profound manifestation, depression, for which cocaine is considered by the user to be the only remedial drug. Consequently the compulsion to return to cocaine is very strong.

In South America the use of coca among the Indian labor force is associated with poverty and malnutrition. No fewer than 15 million use coca regularly in the Andes region of South America, and there are many users in Java, India, and Ceylon, where the shrub was introduced years ago. Studies on long-range effects of such use are wanting. Use is spreading in South America as coca is planted and incorporated into rituals among the Cubeo of Colombia, for example, thus closing the gap left when other tribal rites were lost.[3]

CHAT

The leaves of *Catha edulis* (Celastraceae), native from Arabia through eastern Africa to the Cape of South Africa, and the source of chat, have been used for centuries as a central nervous system stimulant by Moslem peoples and by the Copts of Ethiopia. The use of chat is now spreading, as east Africans and others learn of the exhilarating properties of this "flower of paradise."[4]

In the mountainous Harar Province of eastern Ethiopia the history of chat as a social stimulant is lost in antiquity. The species grows well in these highland regions and today is widely cultivated on terraced hills (Fig. 17-2). The fresh leafy upper branches are shipped by air, wrapped in banana leaves, to neighboring

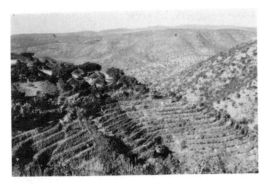

Figure 17-2 Terracing chat above Dire Dawa, Ethiopia, altitude about 5000 feet (courtesy W Burger, Field Museum Natural History, Chicago).

countries throughout the year. These harvests are very profitable to the Ethiopian farmer and account for much of the foreign currency earned by Ethiopia. According to some habitués, however, chat loses much of its effect if not chewed within three days of picking, and this factor, whether real or imagined, has limited the spread of chat to far-flung parts of the world.

To obtain the desired effect, leaves and/or branchlets of chat are chewed for about 10 minutes as a quid until all juices are extracted. The residue is then swallowed, along with copious amounts of water, or preferably sweet soda, to counter the bitter taste of the plant. The amount ingested during any day varies greatly among men and women, schoolboys and the aged, and farmers and businessmen; but where found, use is usually quite high.

What are the desired effects? Euphoria, increased alertness, general excitement, and hyperactivity, accompanied by relief from hunger and fatigue, are common experiences. Like coca, the drug gives a constant mild high to those who chew throughout the day. Its use is now common in eastern Ethiopia and in urban areas elsewhere, no longer just by the ·farmers but among all walks of life. Traditionally farmers ingested chat in the early

morning followed by a major working spurt; and still more chat later in the day produced more stimulation and work. For some, excessive use, or lack of it, leads to disputes and serious fights that often result in grave injuries.[4]

Undesirable effects, besides irritability, include dry mouth and thirst, and decrease in appetite, thus potentiating poor dietary habits (although chat contains vitamin C, niacin, calcium, and iron principally);[4] also reported are inflammation of the mouth and gastric disturbances from the abundant tannins present, constipation, and initially a heightened sexual interest followed by depressed libido and even sexual impotence in chronic users.[5] Some complain of a typical hangover the morning after use. Physical dependence apparently does not occur; and tolerance is reputedly at a very low level.

There is general agreement that central nervous system stimulation involves the alkaloid D-norpseudoephedrine, but there has been too little critical research with this and other compounds to permit a categorical statement. Other alkaloids are present, and probably a holistic approach involving total content and activity in relation to saliva is needed before pharmacological action can be explained satisfactorily.[6]

AMPHETAMINES

Amphetamines stimulate the central nervous system and induce a transient sense of well-being, self-confidence, and alertness. Although synthesized in the 1930s as cheap substitutes for ephedrine and adrenaline in inhalers as nasal decongestants, they are now used to combat fatigue, curb appetite, and reduce mild depression. Benzedrine® was the first outstanding compound for constricted blood vessels to relieve nasal congestion.

Generally the action of amphetamines is opposite that of the barbiturates—namely, fatigue is reduced and general activity, speech, and concentration are increased. The amphetamines are adrenergic drugs and as such mimic the action of neural transmitters like noradrenaline and produce a stimulating action on the sympathetic nervous system. Moreover, they stimulate nervous impulses across the synapses in parts of the central nervous system by substituting for the brain's transmitter substances, 5-hydroxytryptamine (serotonin). After taking these drugs, the body is in a general state of stress as if threatened or expecting a violent fight, and this state of tension is maintained for prolonged periods.

Among the more common synthetic stimulants are Benzedrine® (bennies, purple hearts), Dexedrine® (brownies, orange hearts), biphetamine (black beauties), Preludin®, Ritalin®, and Methedrine® (speed). About 8 billion capsules are manufactured annually in the United States; the majority are dispensed to relieve depression, but nearly 40% are unaccounted for by the Department of Justice. This suggests the extent of their abuse, especially considering that an unknown, and likely enormous, number of amphetamines manufactured in black-market laboratories are not included in this percentage. Among those who use amphetamines are people who work irregular hours (members of the medical profession, truck drivers, students); and athletes and others who must put forth almost superhuman physical effort during particular periods. Much more debilitating than pill taking, perhaps the most disastrous form of drug abuse, is the intravenous use of amphetamines, as practiced by the speed freak who mainlines methedrine alone or in combination with heroin (speedball). Such heavy use almost inevitably leads to a paranoid psychosis with feelings of persecution, delusions of reference, feelings of omnipotence, and formication hallucinations (imaginary snakes or insects crawling on or under the skin). Amphetamines are dispensed also in combination with barbiturates (Dexamyl®), but the value of such compounds for alleviating depression and chronic fatigue has never been clinically established.

Continued use of amphetamines beyond several weeks establishes psychological dependency. Tolerance increases rapidly. The sense of power, self-confidence, and exhilaration artificially created by these stimulants is so pleasant, and the depression and fatigue that follow discontinuance so severe, that the user is strongly tempted to continue taking amphetamines. But prolonged use or large doses is nearly always followed by mental depression and fatigue, and many individuals experience headache, palpitation, vasomotor disturbances, agitation, apprehension, delirium, and hallucinations. Even more serious cases of malnutrition, progressive inflammatory disorders of the arteries, generalized organ damage (kidney, liver, pancreas), and abnormal pregnancies, as well as the amphetamine psychosis just described, may be the outcome of continued abuse.[1]

STIMULATING BEVERAGES

For fifteenth-century Europeans, there were few mind-altering substances. The population had no coffee, no tea, little opium, no cocaine, no tobacco, and no hallucinatory drugs in general use. To be sure they had a few spices and mildly stimulating teas made from mint, lavender, rosemary, and so forth; but by and large there were no major stimulants, sedatives, or intoxicants, except for alcohol. Because of this, alcohol was widely used in a variety of ways, permeating every aspect of European culture from the richest to the poorest.

Following the explorations of Columbus and other Europeans, however, many foreign mind-affecting drugs were brought home. Tobacco was discovered on Columbus' first voyage; coffee arrived from the Moslem world and became available in coffeehouses, which first appeared in England in the mid-seventeenth century, and soon afterward tea from China and cocoa from tropical America completed the trilogy of caffeine-containing drinks. In a short time, there evolved a multidrug culture in western Europe, which for centuries had had little more than a single psychoactive drug.

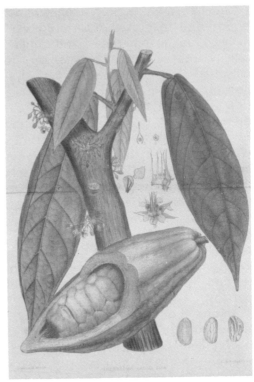

Figure 17-3b *Theobroma cacao* (from R Bentley and H Trimen, *Medicinal Plants* 1: 38, 1880).

Caffeine is a xanthine alkaloid common to the stimulatory beverages coffee, tea, cocoa or chocolate, and soft (cola) drinks. Coffee is made from the ground, roasted seeds of *Coffea arabica* (Fig. 17-3a), native to Ethiopia and long cultivated in parts of the Arab world as a beverage and as a medicine; it contains on the average 1% caffeine and is the widely cultivated species. Many other plants from Africa also contain caffeine, however, and a few are cultivated (Table 17-1).

In the United States 68% of those over 10 years of age drink coffee; in 1969 2.8 billion pounds were consumed—150 billion cups of coffee. Most coffee drinkers enjoy two cups in the morning (= about 300 mg of caffeine) to get a quick lift. Without it, users become irritable, nervous, and restless, they are un-

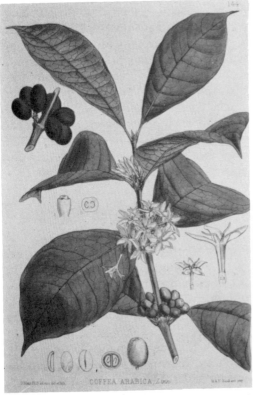

Figure 17-3a *Coffea arabica* (from R Bentley and H Trimen, *Medicinal Plants* 2: 144, 1880).

able to work, and they often develop headaches. Those who ordinarily do not drink coffee find the reverse effects when asked to drink the equivalent of 300 mg of caffeine: they report unpleasant stimulating effects such as nervousness, as well as gastrointestinal complaints.[7] Tolerance to caffeine is of a low grade, but dependence is more significant; lethargy and headache are typical withdrawal symptoms among habitual users.

Recent reports suggest that heavy coffee drinkers have a higher incidence of myocardial infarctions than those who do not use coffee (Chapter 7). Since there is apparently no link between heavy tea drinking and heart disease, presumably the correlation is not a function of the presence of caffeine. This relationship is under debate, however, for the higher incidence of death from cardiovascular disease among men who drink seven or more cups of coffee per day can be directly linked to their smoking habits. A study reports that this group smokes 21.8 cigarettes daily, compared to an average of only 8.7 cigarettes for the non-coffee-drinker.[8] It appears certain, however, that heavy coffee drinking is harmful for those with heart problems for whom increased heart rate and respiration are disadvantageous.

Similar stimulating effects are obtained from other beverages containing caffeine. Tea from *Camellia sinensis* (Theaceae), of Oriental origin, spread into Europe on the heels of coffee during the seventeenth century. Public houses dispensing these stimulants as social drinks were considered rowdy places, and contemporary prophets of doom foresaw speedy death for those who indulged in tea and coffee. This gave the beverages much notoriety and so increased popularity that by 1700 most Europeans were drinking one or both of these stimulants, as well as cocoa.

The most popular form of tea in the West is black tea prepared by drying, rolling, and crushing fresh young leaves, which are then kept in a damp area to promote the absorption of oxygen. Oxidation turns the leaves a copper color. Green teas (without oxidation) are also available and are especially enjoyed in the Orient. Black tea is particularly popular among English-speaking peoples and former colonials, as a hot drink (British) or cold (iced tea was invented during the St. Louis World's Fair of 1904). Caffeine content per cup is a little less than that of coffee, but tea possesses small amounts of a second active stimulant, theophylline (Table 17-1).

The active ingredient of cocoa or chocolate from the seeds of *Theobroma cacao* (Sterculiaceae: Fig. 17-3b), a small tree of American origin but widely cultivated especially in western Africa, is theobromine, another xanthine alkaloid. Up to 3% of this alkaloid is present, along with minute quantities of caffeine and large amounts of cocoa butter in the kernel of the seed, which is ground after fermentation. This product accounts for the main ingredients and flavor of powdered chocolate, liqueurs (creme de cacao), milk chocolates, and other confectionaries. Theobromine is the least stimulating of the xanthine alkaloids, caffeine the most active.

The cola soft drinks contain caffeine (30–45 mg per 12 oz bottle) obtained from seeds of western African species of *Cola* (Sterculiaceae). It is interesting that North Americans unhesitatingly allow children to drink these caffeine-containing beverages as well as hot chocolate, while at the same time discouraging the use of tea and, particularly, of coffee.

Other plants which contain xanthine alkaloids that are used as beverages in various parts of the world are also noted in Table 17-1.

But many individuals do not drink

Table 17-1   Mildly Stimulating Beverages Containing Xanthine Alkaloids

Angiosperm Family and Species	Vernacular Name	Alkaloid	Remarks
AQUIFOLIACEAE *Ilex paraguensis*	Yerba maté	to 2% Caffeine	Leaves for Paraguay tea or maté in Central America, much cultivated in northern Argentina to southern Mato Grosso (Brazil)
I. amara, I. conocarpa, I. pseudobuxus, I. theezans		Caffeine	Species widely substituted in Maté
I. cassine	Dahoon holly, cassina	Caffeine	Leaves sold for tea in southern North America; especially popular during Civil War when the South was blockaded; long used by Creek and other Indians as beverage and for ceremonials
I. vomitoria	Yaupon		
I. opaca *I. verticillata*	American Holly Winterberry	?	Dried leaves substituted for tea in eastern North America during Civil War; probably little or no caffeine
MELASTOMATACEAE *Miconia willdenowii*		0.2% Caffeine	Leaves for tea in Brazil
RUBIACEAE *Coffea arabica*	Arabian coffee	1–2% Caffeine[a]	Seed roasted, the widely cultivated coffee in South and Central America, eastern Africa; native to the highlands of eastern Africa
C. excelsa, C. liberica, C. maclaudii, C. robusta, C. stenophylla, and others		Caffeine	Western Africa and cultivated, often grown in lower, more tropical elevations than *C. arabica*

xanthine-possessing beverages: they find such drinks detrimental to their health, their religion forbids the practice, or they wish to avoid minor nervousness or irritability associated with use. It has long been traditional, particularly in continental Europe and parts of the tropics, to drink various and sundry herb teas or coffee substitutes probably lacking stimulants (although the chemical compositions of most are not well known). In times of deprivation man characteristically turns to other sources; but recently, these nonxanthine drinks have become popular throughout North America and Great Britain, even though coffee, tea, and chocolate are all readily available (Table 17-2).

Coffee substitutes and adulterants, all presumably lacking xanthine alkaloids, but perhaps containing compounds such as volatile oils that may impart pleasant flavors and possibly a stimulating effect, are common in temperate and tropical regions. In the southern United States, *Cichorium intybus* (chicory) roots are added to impart a desired strong (more bitter) taste to coffee; in tropical America

Table 17-1 (Continued)

Angiosperm Family and Species	Vernacular Name	Alkaloid	Remarks
SAPINDACEAE			
Paullinia cupana	Guarana	2.5–5% Caffeine	In Brazil a paste from pulverized seeds mixed with cassava is dried into bars and used as needed in beverage, also contains 5% tannin; alcoholic drink prepared from seeds and cassava
P. yoco		2.8% Caffeine	Beverage in Colombia chiefly from bark
STERCULIACEAE			
Cola acuminata, C. nitida	Cola	±2.5% Caffeine	Cola nuts (seeds) infusion for stimulating tea in western Africa and cultivated throughout tropics; seeds also chewed; popular chewing stick; ingredient of cola soft drink beverages (Coca-Cola, Pepsi-Cola)
Theobroma cacao	Cacao tree	(Minute) caffeine; to 3% theobromine	Seeds long a beverage among Mexican Indians, native to tropical America, widely cultivated esp. western Africa, source of powdered chocolate, cocoa
THEACEAE			
Camellia sinensis	Tea	1–4% Caffeine (small) theophylline	Of Asian origin and widely cultivated since ancient times for dry tea leaf
C. kissi		Caffeine and theophylline	Leaves for tea in the Himalayan region
Eurya theoides			Leaves for tea in Cuba

[a] Decaffeinized coffee is prepared by extracting most of the caffeine (normally up to 0.8% remains), yet retaining the pleasant aroma of coffee.

seeds of *Cassia laevigata, C. occidentalis,* or *C. sericea* form the base of coffee senna, whereas around the Mediterranean fruits of *Castanea sativa* (Spanish chestnut) are boiled and roasted like coffee, as are the seeds and roots of *Cicer arietinum* (chick pea). Other substitutes include roasted parts of such well-known plants as *Asparagus* (seeds), *Canavalia* (jack bean seeds), *Ceratonia* (carob coffee from seeds), *Crataegus* (hawthorn seeds: Fig. 17-4a), *Daucus* (carrot root), *Dioscorea* (yam tuber), *Galium* (bedstraw fruit), *Glycine* (soybean seed), *Gym-* *nocladus* (Kentucky coffee tree seeds), *Iris* (seeds), *Ligustrum* (privet seeds), *Sorbus* (mountain ash fruit, Fig. 17-4b), and *Taraxacum* (dandelion root).

Whereas coffee and its substitutes often begin as roasted roots or seeds, which are then boiled, teas are usually made by adding the plant part, commonly leaves, to boiling water and allowing them to steep. Tea substitutes presumably contain no caffeine or xanthines, but they nevertheless are intended to relax or stimulate in addition to quenching thirst. Many teas act simultaneously as alteratives. In most cases their contents are imperfectly known, but volatile oils are commonly found, and the beverages may act as gastric stimulants (e.g., mint tea); vitamins may be present and beneficial (e.g., vitamin C in rose hip tea), and aromatic bitters to stimulate the appetite may be found in chamomile and other teas.[9] (Indiscriminate drinking of teas may be harmful: e.g., chamomile tea should be avoided by those allergic to ragweed; see Chapter 3.) The number of teas seems enormous because each culture and · ethnic group has made selections for various reasons from the vast supply afforded by the local vegetation. Many plants noted in Table 17-2 are available in health food stores, including some listed as tonics and panaceas in Table 16-1.

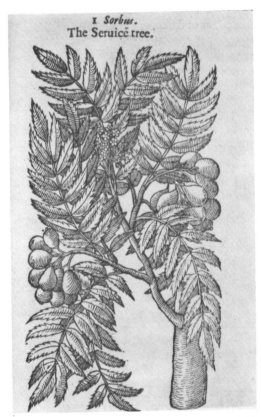

Figure 17-4b *Sorbus aucuparia* (from J Gerard, *The Herball*, ed 2, 1636).

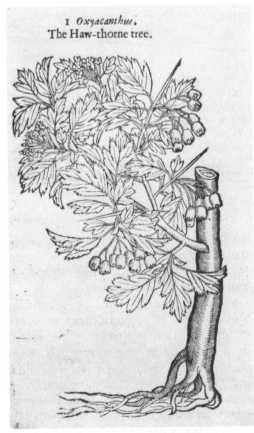

Figure 17-4a *Crataegus monogyna* (from J Gerard, *The Herball*, ed 2, 1636).

Volatile oils and aromatic compounds are commonly used for flavoring oral preparations and beverages, of which the majority possess a stimulating effect as additives.[10]

TOBACCO AND NICOTINE

Nicotine no longer has medicinal uses. Taken in tobacco—cigarette, cigar, pipe, chewing, and snuff—its effects are variable; it can act as a stimulant, depressant, or tranquilizer. Tobacco is one of the most physiologically damaging substances used by man. When smoked in cigarettes it is the chief cause of lung cancer. Tobacco is also a factor in other cancers, in coronary artery disease, in emphysema of the lungs, and in other

Table 17-2   Teas Used Throughout the World (not Known to Contain Xanthine Alkaloids)

Plant Group and Species	Vernacular Name	Locality	Remarks
GYMNOSPERM			
EPHEDRACEAE			
Ephedra trifurca	Desert, teamster, or Mormon tea	Southwestern United States, Mexico	Tea from branches, very popular among early settlers in the west, Indians, and Mexicans
ANGIOSPERMS			
ANACARDIACEAE			
Rhus aromatica	Fragrant sumac	Eastern North America	Ripe fruit for refreshing drink
R. integrifolia	Lemonade berry	California and Baja California	Ripe fruit for refreshing drink
R. trilobata, R. typhina	Indian lemonade	Eastern and central North America	Acidic fruit for drink
ANNONACEAE			
Artabotrys uncinatus		India, Ceylon	Flowers for tea
APIACEAE			
Anethum graveolens	Dill	Cultivated	Dried ripe seeds for tea
Angelica archangelica	Angelica	Eurasia and cultivated	Ripe fruit for tea
Carum carvi	Caraway	Cultivated	Dried fruit a stimulating tea
C. roxburghianum		Southern Asia	Seeds for stimulating tea
Foeniculum vulgare	Fennel	Eurasia and cultivated	Fruit for tea
ASTERACEAE			
Artemisia abrotanum	Southern wood	Southern Europe, temperate Asia	Leaves a stimulating tea
Solidago virgaurea	European goldenrod	Europe	Leaves for a tea and tonic
BORAGINACEAE			
Borago officinalis	Borage	Europe and all Mediterranean	Refreshing tea from flowers and dried stems (well known since Middle Ages)
Ehretia buxifolia		Philippines	Leaves for tea
Lithospermum officinale	Gromwell	Europe	Leaves for Bohemian or Croatian tea
CAPRIFOLIACEAE			
Viburnum cassinoides	Sweet viburnum	Eastern North America	Leaves as a tea
V. theiferum		China	Leaves as a tea
CELASTRACEAE			
Catha edulis	Chat	Ethiopia, Arabia	Leaves a stimulating tea
Celastrus paniculata	Kanguni	India to Philippines	In Hindu medicine leaves as stimulating tea; seed oil powerful stimulant
CHLORANTHACEAE			
Chloranthus officinalis		Malaya, Java	Leaf decoction for tea
CISTACEAE			
Cistus albidus		Algeria	Leaves for tea
ERICACEAE			
Chamaedaphne calyculata		North American Ojibwas	Fresh or dried leaves for tea
Gaultheria procumbens	Wintergreen	North America	Tea from plant is "mountain tea"
EUPHORBIACEAE			
Croton argyratus		Indochina	Leaves for tea
C. crymbulosus	Chaparral tea	Southwestern United States	Infusion of flowering tops

389

Table 17-2   (Continued)

Plant Group and Species	Vernacular Name	Locality	Remarks
C. linearis		West Indies	Leaves for tea
Mallotus anamiticus, M. furetianus		Indochina	Leaves for tea
FABACEAE			
Cyclopia genistoides		South Africa	Leaves for tea
C. subterenata		South Africa	Leaves as a source for commercially available caspa tea
Trigonella coerulea	Sweet trefoil	Mediterranean and cultivated	Herb decoction for tea
FRANKENIACEAE			
Frankenia portulacaefolia		St. Helen	Leaves for tea
LAMIACEAE			
Cedronella triphylla		Canary Islands	Leaves for Canary tea
Clinopodium laevigatum		Western Mexico	Leaves with sugar a popular tea
Glechoma hederacea	Ground ivy	North Temperate	Leaves as tea (also diuretic and tonic)
Rosmarinus officinalis	Rosemary	Europe, cultivated	Plant for mildly stimulating tea and relief of nervous headaches
Satureja douglasii	Yerba buena	West coast North America	Leaves and stems for tea
Sideritis thuzans		Greece	Leaves and flowering tops as aromatic tea
Stachys officinalis	Common betony	Europe, cultivated	Plant for tea
Teucrium thea		China	Leaves for tea
LAURACEAE			
Aniba canelilla		Peru	Stimulating tea from cinnamon-flavored bark
Cinnamomum tetrageonum		Indochina	Leaves and wood as stimulating beverage
Litsea novoleontes		Mexico	Leaves for tea

diseases. Since nicotine is one of the most perniciously addicting drugs in common use, most tobacco users are "hooked" and, in effect, *locked* to the damaging effects of the tobacco.[7]

HISTORY

Wherever Columbus went in the Caribbean during the last decade of the fifteenth century, native Americans were smoking rolled dried leaves of a plant new to the Europeans. The Indians inhaled the smoke, "drinking" smoke, and were never without their leaves. Sailors were taught how to use them, and they soon learned to enjoy the unique combinations of effects—tranquilizing when they felt anxious, stimulating when stimulation was needed. They also learned that after smoking a while they had to continue day after day, or an insatiable craving developed that only tobacco, whether smoked, chewed, or sniffed, could satisfy. This created a need for a guaranteed ready supply of the leaves, and the sailors of the sixteenth century and later took the plant with them. Small farms of tobacco were

Table 17-2   (Continued)

Plant Group and Species	Vernacular Name	Locality	Remarks
MALVACEAE			
Malva sylvestris	High mallow	Cosmopolitan	Leaves for tea (flowers for gargle)
ONAGRACEAE			
Epilobium angustifolium		Russia	Leaves for kapporie or kapor tea
PROTEACEAE			
Roupala montana		Trinidad	Bark infusion as nerve stimulant
RHAMNACEAE			
Ceanothus americanus	New Jersey tea	Eastern North America	Leaves used as tea during revolutionary times
ROSACEAE			
Rosa canina (dog rose), R. pomifera and other spp.		North Temperate	Leaves for tea, but especially rose hips (fruit) containing vitamin C
Rubus caesius	European dewberry	Europe	Leaves for tea
R. idaeus	European red raspberry	Europe	Leaves for tea
RUTACEAE			
Citrus limon and other spp.	Lemon	Cultivated	Fruit juices or peel for drink
C. sinensis	Seville orange	Cultivated	Dried peel as stimulating tonic
TILIACEAE			
Tilia cordata	Linden	Europe	Flowers for tea
VERBENACEAE			
Lippia citriodora	Lemon verbena	South America	Leaves for tea
L. multiflora	Gambia tea bush	Western Africa	Leaves for tea
L. pseudothea		Cultivated	
Stachytarpheta jamaicensis	Bastard vervain	Tropics	Dried leaves for Brazilian tea
Verbena officinalis	Vervain	Europe	Leaves for tea

planted in settlements along all major trade routes beyond the New World—in Europe, Africa, Asia, and even Australia—where the sailors and their charges tended tobacco plants with zeal.

Before long all native populations who had even the remotest connection with European sailors and their way of life were taking up smoking. Likewise there was great demand for this mind-altering plant, which was said to cure scores of illnesses, in disease and plague-ridden Europe during the Middle Ages. None should be deprived access to a plant considered by Gerard[11] in 1597 to be therapeutic for several dozen infirmities from headaches ("The drie leaves are used to be taken in a pipe set on fire and suckt into the stomacke, and thrust forth againe at the nostrils against the pains of the head . . ."), toothaches, skin problems, burns, to wounds, dropsy, piles, colic, and deafness, besides acting as a purgative, emetic, and anthelmintic. Gerard was astute enough to observe, however, that "Some use to drink it (as it is termed [for inhaling smoke]) for wantonnesse or rather custome, *and cannot forbeare it, no not in the midst of their dinner* [italics added], which kind of taking is unwholesome and very dangerous. . . ." This clear statement of the craving engendered by tobacco, written in 1597, is no less applicable today to the condition of millions who must have a continuous supply of cigarettes. It is probably correct to generalize that man is more addicted to the pyridine alkaloid nicotine than he is to any other naturally occurring plant product.

NICOTINE

Tobacco leaves contain 0.6 to 9% nicotine as well as lesser amounts of nornicotine and an aromatic principle known as tobacco camphor. Roots of *Nicotiana tabacum* (Solanaceae: Fig. 17-5) contain the additional pyridine alkaloids anabasine and anatabine. Only one other species is widely cultivated today, *N. rustica*, the source of the aromatic Turkish tobacco. Many other species, however, have been used in the Western Hemisphere, where many species of tobacco are native (Table 17-3).

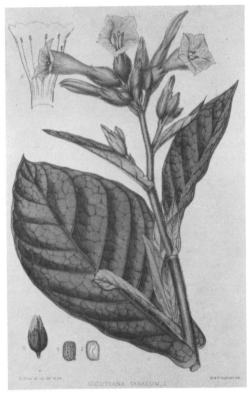

Figure 17-5 *Nicotiana tabacum* (from R Bentley and H Trimen, *Medicinal Plants* **3**: 191, 1880).

A typical filter cigarette contains 20 to 30 mg of nicotine, of which 10% is absorbed by inhalation. Nicotine appears to act in the central nervous system at the level of the cortex by increasing arousal. Much better understood are its effects on the autonomic nervous system, where it mimics acetylcholine, thereby stimulating neurotransmission at the cholinergic receptors. Since nicotine is not rapidly deactivated, however, its continued action prevents incoming impulses from being effective, thus partially blocking the transmission of new information. It also activates adrenergic response by causing the release of adrenaline from the adrenal glands and the sympathetic nervous system. Other actions involve a stimulation, then a blockage, of certain sensory receptors such as those in the skin and tongue responsible for heat and pain. In acute nicotine poisoning, tremors and convulsions develop, and frequently the individual dies of respiratory paralysis. Nicotine when inhaled inhibits hunger contractions of the stomach and slightly increases blood sugar levels; these actions, along with the deadening of sensebuds, probably account for a decrease in hunger after smoking.

It is far easier to become dependent on cigarettes than on alcohol or barbiturates, for most users of alcohol or sleeping pills can limit themselves to intermittent use and are able to tolerate periods free of the chemical effect; not so with cigarettes. Occasional use is rare and is found in only about 2% of smokers. Usually a continuous supply is necessary, and most smokers are not aware of the addicting nature of nicotine until the supply is cut off. Limited tolerance is quickly acquired to nicotine, although it may take several years before the smoker becomes tolerant of high nicotine intake.

HAZARDS OF TOBACCO AND SMOKING

The meteoric rise in the popularity of cigarette smoking in the twentieth century was stimulated by several factors: improved flax wrapping paper (made from the fiber of *Linum usitatissimum*), automatic manufacturing machinery (which lowered the price), and intense advertising campaigns. Ultimately concern developed for those inhaling hourly doses of this drug. Data indicating deleterious effects began to accumulate in the 1950s, but it took the well-publicized *Report of the Surgeon General's Advisory Committee on Smoking and Health* of 1964 to convince most people that cigarettes are injurious to health. It was stated that cigarette smoking shortens life, causes lung and other kinds of cancer, exacerbates heart disease, emphysema, bronchitis, and other illnesses, and greatly increases the risk of dying of these causes. For example, the coronary death rate among smokers is 1.5 to 2 times as great as among nonsmokers, and for a man aged 45 to 54, who smokes a pack or more of cigarettes a day, the rate is 3 times as high. Hazards to the unborn were also revealed; not only were babies born to women who smoked during pregnancy lighter on the average than those of nonsmokers, but more were premature, and they were twice as likely as babies of nonsmoking mothers to be aborted, stillborn or to die soon after birth.[12] The increased level of carbon monoxide in closed areas where smokers are is often

sufficiently great to impair skills required for driving, flying, or other activities. Tars also increase in such areas to a level considered unsafe. The smoker is harming not only himself but also the nonsmokers in his immediate environment.

By 1970 the consumption of cigarettes in the United States had fallen from an all-time high of 4345 (annual per capita consumption over 18 years old) in 1963 to 3985. During this time an estimated 10 million smokers had given up cigarettes, and by 1970 the population's smokers 17 years old and over totaled 36.7%. In addition, there was a decided reduction in the tar content of cigarettes, with 90% of all cigarettes falling between 14 and 29 mg in 1972, compared to a 1954 tar content of 95% of cigarettes between 35 and 53 mg. Lower tar and nicotine levels are important, and this trend should continue as "improved" or less hazardous cigarettes are manufactured for those unable to kick the habit.[13] Equally important is a serious effort to prevent young people from beginning to smoke, a trend that is apparently increasing in momentum, particularly among girls.

TO CURE THE SMOKING HABIT

The only known cure for smoking is abrupt stopping and suffering the distress of withdrawal. Some relief may be found in chewing gum or sucking candy or in resorting to commercial preparations containing lobeline, the alkaloid allied to nicotine, from *Lobelia inflata* (Table 17-3). All these approaches are of marginal value. A search among "ancient" medicines practiced today might reveal something worthwhile as, for example, the recent report of using tincture of oats (*Avena sativa*) to reduce the craving for cigarettes suggests.[14] However there is no reason to assume that addiction to nic-

Table 17-3 Smoking: Tobacco, Its Substitutes and Flavorings, and Other Plants[a]

Angiosperm Family and Species	Vernacular Name	Remarks
ANACARDIACEAE *Rhus glabra, R. triloba,* *R. sempervirens, R. virens*	Sumac	Dried leaves mixed with tobacco or alone smoked by eastern and central North American Indians and occasionally by early settlers
APIACEAE *Angelica archangelica*	Angelica	Root used to flavor cigarette tobacco (source of volatile oil of angelica)
A. atropurpurea	Purple angelica	Root mixed with tobacco for smoking by Arkansas Indians
Coriandrum sativum	Coriander	Fruit for flavoring cigarette tobacco (source of aromatic volatile oil of coriander)
ASTERACEAE *Matricaria chamomilla*	Chamomile	Dried flowering heads contain a volatile oil for flavoring cigarette tobacco
Trilisa odoratissima	Deer's tongue	Leaves containing coumarin added to cigarette tobacco to give a sweet taste (southeastern United States)
BETULACEAE *Corylus avellana*	European hazel	Leaves smoked in Eurasia
BORAGINACEAE *Tournefortia argentea*		Leaves smoked in the Seychelles
CAMPANULACEAE *Lobelia excelsa*		Leaves smoked in India
L. inflata	Indian tobacco	Contains an alkaloid lobeline allied to nicotine and leaves often smoked by North American Indians with or without tobacco; lobeline is substituted for nicotine in commercial products to help stop smoking (Bantron®, Lobidan®, Nikoban®)
L. tupa	Tobaco del diablo	Contains lobeline and other piperidine alkaloids, smoked by Mapuches of Chile
CORNACEAE *Cornus stolonifera*	Red-osier dogwood	Inner bark smoked by eastern North American Indians with or without tobacco
DAPHNIPHYLLACEAE *Daphniphyllum humile*		In Japan the Ainu smoke its leaves in place of tobacco
ERICACEAE *Arctostaphylos uva-ursi*	Bearberry	Eastern North American Indians and colonists mixed leaves with tobacco for smoking
EUPHORBIACEAE *Sauropus quadrangularis*		Leaves smoked for tonsilitis in Hindu medicine
FABACEAE *Dipteryx odorata*	Tonka tree	Fermented tonka beans produce coumarin and are used for flavoring cigarette tobacco; also supposed to be narcotic and stimulant

Table 17-3 (Continued)

Angiosperm Family and Species	Vernacular Name	Remarks
LAMIACEAE		
Mentha arvensis	Mint	Mint oil containing 90% menthol for flavoring mentholated cigarettes
MORACEAE		
Dorstenia contrajerva		Dried rhizomes for flavoring cigarettes (from tropical America)
MYRISTICACEAE		
Myristica fragrans	Nutmeg and mace	Mace containing volatile aromatic oil used for flavoring cigarettes
POACEAE		
Zea mays	Corn	Dried silks are a traditional tobacco substitute in the New World
ROSACEAE		
Crataegus oxyacantha	Hawthorn	Young leaves substituted for tobacco
Prunus spp.		Essences of prune or peach added to flavor cigarettes
SOLANACEAE		
Datura fastuosa		Leaves smoked in Africa to relieve asthma
D. metel	Hindu datura	Leaves smoked in India and elsewhere to relieve asthma
D. stramonium	Jimson weed	Leaves at one time widely smoked to relieve respiratory complaints (Chapter 12)
Nicotiana tabacum	Common tobacco	See text
N. alata		Leaves smoked in South America and also chewed
N. attenuata		Dried leaves smoked in pipes and as cigarettes by New Mexican Indians
N. glauca	Tree tobacco	Contains an alkaloid anabasin[b]
N. quadrivalvis		Indians in western United States used leaves for smoking
N. rustica	Aztec tobacco, yellow henbane	Leaves for smoking in Mexico and North American Indians, also cultivated in Old World[b]
N. trigonophylla		Smoked by Indians of southwestern United States and Mexico
Solanum inaequilaterale		Leaves smoked in the Philippines
TILIACEAE		
Tilia cordata	Linden	Leaves used to adulterate tobacco

[a] Cigarettes are often smoked in India and southeastern Asia as "beedi" or "bidi" which is sundried, uncured tobacco wrapped in a dried leaf of temburni (*Diospyros melanoxylon*) or banana (*Musa sapientum*) and secured at one end by a thin string. Other domestic wrappings for cigarettes include young leaves of the palms of *Licuala pumila* and *Nypa fruticans*.

[b] Nicotine content may be as high as 9%, and these species are the source of the widely used natural contact insecticide obtained from tobacco leaves (Chapter 15).

otine is any less difficult to overcome than addiction to any other drug.

Perhaps the most effective control is provided by the full awareness that smoking is harmful and by firm resolution, perhaps enforced by a group therapy, to overcome this undesirable habit.

LITERATURE CITED

1. Amphetamines. Fourth report by the Select Committee on Crime, 91st Congress, 2d Session, House Report No. 91-1807, pp 1–44, Government Printing Office, Washington, DC. 1971.

2. Mortimer WG. 1901. *Peru History of Coca.* JH Vail, New York. 576 p.

3. Salser JK Jr. 1970. Cubeo acculturation to coca and its social implications. *Econ Bot* **24:** 182–186.

4. Getahun A, Krikorian AD. 1973. Chat: coffee's rival from Harar, Ethiopia. I. Botany, cultivation and use. *Econ Bot* **27:** 353–377.

5. Margetts EL. 1967. Miraa and myrrh in east Africa—clinical notes about *Catha edulis. Econ Bot* **21:** 358–362.

6. Krikorian AD, Getahun A. 1973. Chat: coffee's rival from Harar, Ethiopia. II. Chemical composition. *Econ Bot* **27:** 378–389.

7. Brecher EM, Editors of *Consumer Reports.* 1972. *Licit and Illicit Drugs.* Little, Brown, Boston. 623 p.

8. Dawber TR, Kannel WB, Gordon T. 1974. Coffee and cardiovascular disease. *New Eng J Med* **291:** 871–874.

9. Nagy M. 1972. Do herb drinks have less effect on the nervous system than coffee or tea? *JAMA* **219:** 626; Farnsworth NR, Morgan BM. 1972. Herb drinks: camomile tea. *JAMA* **221:** 410.

10. Hocking GM. 1969. Plant flavor and aromatic values in medicine and pharmacy, 273–288. In JE Gunckel (ed), *Current Topics in Plant Science.* Academic Press, New York.

11. Gerard J. 1597. *The Herball or General Historie of Plantes . . .* John Norton, London.

12. Fletcher CM, Horn D. 1970. *World Health Organization Chronicle* Vol 24, 345–370.

13. Tiggelbeck D. 1972. Improved cigarettes-comments on the state-of-the-art, 1971. *J Nat Cancer Inst* **48:** 1825–1832.

14. Anand CL. 1971. Effect of *Avena sativa* on cigarette smoking. *Nature* **233:** 496.

Chapter **18**

Hallucinogens

Hallucinogens are unique compounds. In nontoxic doses they produce changes in perception, thought, and mood, without causing major disturbances of the autonomic nervous system. A variety of hallucinations may be characteristic. Addiction and withdrawal symptoms are unknown.[1]

Psychic changes and abnormal states of consciousness induced by hallucinogens differ utterly from ordinary experiences. The user of hallucinogens forsakes the familiar world and, in full consciousness, embraces a quasi-dream world operating under other standards, strange dimensions, and in a different time. These drugs are a means of escaping from reality as it is commonly understood.

Most hallucinogens are of plant origin.* They do not, however, occur at random throughout the plant kingdom, but rather are dispersed among two groups only—the fungi and, more commonly, the flowering plants. As the arrangement of Table 18-1 indicates, 11 phylogenetic groups of angiosperms possess hallucinogens, again not at random, because more than half the total occurs in phylogenetic group 11 among such well-known and allied families as the Loganiaceae, Rubiaceae, Apocynaceae, Acanthaceae, Solanaceae, and Convolvulaceae. There are remarkably few of these compounds in the monocotyledons. Table 18-1 also reveals that these plants

---

* A few are found among animals; for example, taraxein, a substance producing schizophrenia, is the only hallucinogen extracted from humans.[2]

Table 18-1   Plants of Hallucinogenic Use

Plant Group and Species	Vernacular Name	Active or Presumed Active Hallucinogenic Principle	Comments
FUNGI: ASCOMYCETES			
Clavicepitales			
Claviceps purpurea	Ergot	D-Lysergic acid amide	Visual hallucinations; St. Anthony's fire from other ergot alkaloids (see text)
FUNGI: BASIDIOMYCETES			
Lycoperdales			
Lycoperdon marginatum, L. mixtecorum	Puffballs	Unknown	Auditory hallucinations characterize intoxication as experienced by the Mixtecs (Oaxaca, Mexico)
Agaricales (Mushrooms)			
Amanita muscaria	Fly agaric	Ibotenic acid, muscimol	Major hallucinogen of Eurasia in times gone by (see text)
Conocybe cyanopus, *C. siliginoides;* *Gymnopilus spectabalis;* *Panaeolus sphinctrinus,* *P. subbaltatus;* *Psilocybe acutissima,* *P. aztecorum, P. baesystis,* *P. caerulescens,* *P. cordispora,* *P. fagicola,* *P. hoogshagenii,* *P. isauri,* *P. mexicana,* *P. mixaeensis,* *P. semperviva,* *P. wassonii,* *P. yungensis,* *P. zapotecorum;* *Stropharia cubensis*		Psilocybin, psilocin	Sacred mushrooms (Teonanactl) of Mexico (see text)
ANGIOSPERMS			
Phylogenetic Group 1			
Annonales			
HIMANTANDRACEAE			
Galbulimima belgraviana[a]		Piperidine derivates: himbacine, himbosine, etc.	In Papua, leaves and bark are taken with leaves of *Homalomena* sp. (Araceae) to induce violent intoxication that progresses into sleep and hallucinations
MYRISTICACEAE			
Myristica fragrans	Nutmeg and mace	Nonnitrogenous phenylpropenes: in aromatic fraction; possibly a synergism between elemicin, myristicin, and safrole[b]	See text

Table 18-1 (Continued)

Plant Group and Species	Vernacular Name	Active or Presumed Active Hallucinogenic Principle	Comments
Virola calophylla, *V. calophylloidea,* *V. cuspidata,* *V. elongata,* *V. peruviana,* *V. punctata, V. rufula,* *V. sebifera, V. theidora*	Yakee and yato (Colombia), paricá, epená, and nyak- wana (Brazil)	Tryptamine: *N,N*-di- methyltryptamine (DMT), *N*-methyltryp- tamine (MMT), and others; derivatives (β- carbolines)	Snuff powder hallucinogens of South America (see text)
GOMORTEGACEAE			
Gomortega keule[a]	Keule or hualhual (Chile)	Volatile oils?	Mapuche Indians (Chile) value fruit for intoxicating ef- fects, possibly hallucino- genic
LAURACEAE			
Sassafras albidum[a,b]	Sassafras	Safrole (chemically like myristicin and asarone)	Suspected of being hallucin- ogenic in large doses; source of sassafras oil, the principal component being safrole (carcinogenic and he- patotoxic)
PIPERACEAE			
Piper methysticum[a]	Kava		A depressant, see Chapter 19
P. nigrum[a]	Pepper	Volatile oils?	
Berberidales			
PAPAVERACEAE			
Corydalis cava[a]		Bulbocapnine?	Temperate Europe
Phylogenetic Group 3			
Chenopodiales			
AIZOACEAE			
Sceletium *(Mesembryanthemum)* *expansum,* *S. tortuosum*		Tropanelike alkaloid: mesebrine	In South Africa natives make a preparation of leaves, stems, or roots, called kou- goed—produces visions and "moral degeneration" re- garding veracity and sex
CACTACEAE			
Ariocarpus retusus[a]		Unknown	Used as peyote substitute by Indians of northern Mexico; said to drive ingestants mad
Epithelantha *micromeris[a]*		Unknown	Valued in northern Mexico for its narcotic properties (also native to southwestern United States)
Lophophora williamsii (+ *L.* *diffusa*)	Peyote	β-Phenylethylamines: mescaline and deri- vates	South Texas and Mexico (see text)
Pachycereus *pectenaboriginum[a]*	Cawe	Carnegine	Used in Mexico as a narcotic
Trichocereus pachanoi	San Pedro	Mescaline, hordenine, and other compounds	Basis of hallucinogenic bev- erage called cimora in Peru and other Andean areas
T. terschekii[a]		*N,N*-Dimethyl mesca- line	Andean region

Table 18-1 (Continued)

Plant Group and Species	Vernacular Name	Active or Presumed Active Hallucinogenic Principle	Comments
Phylogenetic Group 4			
Ericales			
ERICACEAE			
Pernettya furens[a]	Hush-hued or hierba loca (Chile)	Unknown	Fruit in Chile known to be toxic, producing mental confusion and madness; in excess said to be an intoxicant similar to *Datura* (Solanaceae)
P. parvifolia[a]	Taglli (Ecuador)	Andromedotoxin	Fruit said to induce hallucinations and other psychic and motor alterations
Phylogenetic Group 6			
Urticales			
MORACEAE			
Maquira (Olmedioperebea) sclerophylla[a]	Rape dos Indios (Portuguese)	Unknown	At one time utilized in hallucinogenic snuff by Brazilian Indians (Pariana region)
CANNABACEAE			
Cannabis sativa (+ C. indica, C. ruderalis)	Hemp, marihuana, hashish, bhang	Nonnitrogenous dibenzopyrans: Δ'-tetrahydrocannabinol	See text
Euphorbiales			
EUPHORBIACEAE			
Alchornea floribunda[a]		Unknown	Additive to *Tabernanthe* (Apocynaceae) or employed in the same way as that hallucinogen in Gabon
Phylogenetic Group 7			
Rosales			
FABACEAE			
Anadenanthera (Piptadenia) peregrina	Cohoba, yopo	Tryptamines and derivates (β-carbolines)	Hallucinogenic snuff of northern South America and the West Indies (see text)
A. colubrina[a]			Perhaps hallucinogenic snuff of central South America
Cytisus (Genista) canariensis		Cytisine	Originating in the Canary Islands, but widely cultivated; used by Yaqui (Mexico) as hallucinogen
Erythrina spp.[a]	Coral bean	Unknown	Reddish seeds valued as hallucinogens in Mexico
Mimosa hostilis	Ajuca or vinho de Jurema (eastern Brazil)	N,N-Dimethyltryptamine (nigerine)	Roots source of potent hallucinogenic drink used by Indians of eastern Brazil
Rhynchosia longeracemosa,[a] R. pyramidalis[a]		Unknown	Toxic seeds thought to be narcotic and hallucinogenic (pictured together with mushrooms in Aztec paintings), Oaxaca, Mexico

Table 18-1 (Continued)

Plant Group and Species	Vernacular Name	Active or Presumed Active Hallucinogenic Principle	Comments
Sophora secundiflora	Mescal bean, red bean	Cytisine	Red seeds used by south-western United States and Mexican Indians in visionary rites
Phylogenetic Group 8 **Myrtales** LYTHRACEAE			
Heimia salicifolia	Sinicuichi	Quinolizidines: cry-ogenine, lythrine, heimine, etc.	Fermented leaves provide a mildly intoxicating drink called sinicuichi (Mexico) that produces euphoria and hallucinations (common from Texas to northern South America)
Phylogenetic Group 9 **Geraniales** ZYGOPHYLLACEAE			
Peganum harmala	Syrian rue	β-carbolines: har-mine, harmaline, etc.	Seeds possess undoubted hallucinogenic components (from Mediterranean to Manchuria)
Polygalales MALPIGHIACEAE			
Banisteriopsis caapi, *B. inebrians*	Ayahuasca (uascá), caapi, yajé, or cipó (Brazil)	β-carbolines: har-mine, harmaline, D-te-trahydroharmine	In northern South America one or both species used as basis of narcotic drink (see text)
B. rusbyana, Tetrapteris methystica		N,N-Dimethyltryptam-ine, β-carbolines?	Leaves added to ayahuasca bark cold water infusion, narcotic drink in northwest-ern Brazil
Phylogenetic Group 11 **Gentianales** LOGANIACEAE			
Desfontainia spinosa var. *hookeri*[a]	Taique	Unknown	Leaves employed in south-ern Chile as a narcotic, but hallucinogenicity not estab-lished
RUBIACEAE			
Corynanthe yohimbe[a]		Yohimbine, a harmine analog	Considered an aphrodisiac in western Africa and avail-able commercially; hallucin-ogenic in large doses
Mitragyna speciosa[a]		Mitragynine, a har-mine analog	Intoxicant in southeast Asia; hallucinogenic in large doses
Psychotria catharginensis, *P. viridis*		N,N-Dimethyltryptam-ine	Added to ayahuasca to en-hance hallucinogenic bever-age
APOCYNACEAE			
Aspidosperma quebracho-blanco[a]		Quebrachine, proba-bly yohimbine, a har-mine analog	Aphrodisiac (Argentina); hal-lucinogenic in large doses

Table 18-1 (Continued)

Plant Group and Species	Vernacular Name	Active or Presumed Active Hallucinogenic Principle	Comments
Prestonia amazonica[a]		N,N-Dimethyltryptamine	Hallucinogenic in large doses
Tabernanthe iboga	Iboga	Ibogaine and other alkaloids	Visual and other hallucinations associated with severe anxiety (in whites); stimulant and aphrodisiac (see text)

Bignoniales
ACANTHACEAE

Justicia pectoralis var. *stenophylla*		N,N-Dimethyltryptamine?	Pulverized leaves added to *Virola*, hallucinogenic snuff in Colombia and adjacent Brazil

Solanales
SOLANACEAE

Atropa belladonna	Belladonna	Hyoscyamine, scopolamine and other alkaloids	Hallucinations sometimes occur largely because of scopolamine; ingredient of magic brews of Middle Ages
Brunfelsia spp.		Alkaloid components not well characterized	Hallucinogenic drink from leaves and bark in tropical South America, may be added to ayahuasca (*Banisteriopsis*)
Cestrum laevigatum,[a] *C. parqui*[a]	Dama da noite	Unknown (contain saponins, gitogenin, and digitogenin, *C. parqui* the steroidal alkaloid solasonine)	Reputedly sold in ports of southern Brazil as a substitute for marihuana
Datura spp.		Scopolamine and other tropane alkaloids	Pulverized seeds in fermented drinks, or infusion of leaves and twigs lead to intoxication and hallucination (see text)
Hyoscyamus niger, *H. muticus*	Henbane	Hyoscyamine, scopolamine, and other alkaloids	Ingredient of magic and witches brews of earlier days producing visual hallucinations and flights of fancy
Iochroma fuchsioides[a]		Unknown	Reports of hallucinogenic properties as used by Indians of Colombian Andes, added to ayahuasca
Latua pubiflora	Arbol de los brujos	Hyoscyamine, scopolamine	Leaves used by medicine men to produce delirium and hallucination (central Chile)
Mandragora officinarum	Mandrake	Hyoscyamine, scopolamine, and other alkaloids	Like *Atropa*, an undoubted ingredient of magic brews of earlier times in Europe

Table 18-1 (Continued)

Plant Group and Species	Vernacular Name	Active or Presumed Active Hallucinogenic Principle	Comments
Methysticodendron amesianum	Cuebra borrachera	Scopolamine chiefly	Leaf infusion highly psycho-tropic and used carefully by Indians of Colombian Andes
CONVOLVULACEAE			
Argyreia nervosa	Wood rose	Ergoline alkaloids	Seeds contain 3 mg of alka-loidal material per gram
Ipomoea violacea	Morning glory	D-Lysergic acid amide (ergine); other "er-got" alkaloids may be active	Seeds—tlitliltzen—have long use in Mexico as hallucino-gen (see text)
Rivea corymbosa	Morning glory	As for *Ipomoea*	Seeds—ololiuqui—as hallu-cinogen in Mexico
Lamiales			
LAMIACEAE			
Coleus blumei,[a] *C. pumilus*[a]		Unknown	Leaves reputedly hallucino-genic (Oaxaca Indians, Mex-ico)
Lagochilus inebrians[a]		Lagochiline (perhaps)	Tea from roasted leaves is made into a narcotic, intoxi-cating drink in Turkestan—it may be hallucinogenic
Nepeta cataria	Catnip	Unknown (contains volatile oils and bitter principle)	Smoked like marihuana, pro-ducing euphoria and visual hallucinations, but sample is small
Salvia divinorum	Yerba de Maria	Unknown	Crushed leaves used in di-vine rites for their hallucino-genic properties (whenever mushrooms or morning glory seeds not available, Oaxaca, Mexico)
Campanulales			
CAMPANULACEAE			
Isotoma longiflora[a]		Unknown	Added to hallucinogenic drink prepared from *Tricho-cereus* (Peruvian Andes) and may be psychotropic
Lobelia tupa[a]	Tupa	Unknown (contains piperidine alkaloids lobeline, lobelanidine, norlobelanidine)	Herb smoked by Mapuches of Chile but not certain that narcotic effects are hallucin-ogenic
Asterales			
ASTERACEAE			
Calea zacatechichi	"Leaf of God"	Unknown	Leaf infusion of dried crushed leaves used as hallu-cinogen in Oaxaca, Mexico, by Chontal Indians (leaves also smoked)

Table 18-1   (Continued)

Plant Group and Species	Vernacular Name	Active or Presumed Active Hallucinogenic Principle	Comments
Phylogenetic Group 13 **Arales** ARACEAE			
Acorus calamus[a]	Sweet flag	Asarone (chemically like mescaline), β-asarone (chemically like myristicin and kava alkaloids)	Cree Indians of northern Canada chewed roots as a strong stimulant, perhaps hallucinogenic
Homalomena sp.	Ereriba	Unknown	Leaves eaten with leaves and bark of *Galbulimima* (Himantandraceae) as narcotic and hallucinogen (Papua)
Phylogenetic Group 14 **Zingiberales** ZINGIBERACEAE			
Kaempferia galanga[a]	Galanga	Unknown	Rhizome perhaps used as hallucinogen in New Guinea
Zingiber officinale[a]	Ginger	Unknown	Widely used aromatic stimulant, possibly hallucinogenic in large doses
Phylogenetic Group 15 **Liliales** LILIACEAE			
Pancratium trianthum		Unknown	The Botswana Bushmen reportedly rub the bulb on an incision made in the head, thereby inducing visual hallucinations

[a] Plants of possible or suspected hallucinogenic use and effect, especially in large doses.
[b] Other sources of safrole from oils of *Illicium parviflorum* (Illiciaceae), the yellow star anise of southeastern United States, and *Mespilodaphne sassafras* (Lauraceae), the Brazilian sassafras, and also as a minor component of *Cinnamomum camphora* (camphor), *C.* spp. (cinnamon leaf), *Umbellularia californica* (Californian laurel), all in the Lauraceae, and *Chenopodium ambrosioides* var. *anthelminticum* (American wormseed, Chenopodiaceae).

are not scattered evenly throughout the world; rather, there are centers of concentration, especially in the New World, in Mexico, and in northern South America, where the use of hallucinogens has deep traditional roots among the indigenous populations.

Just as plants having hallucinogens are not found at random and the number of taxa involved is limited, the compounds responsible for hallucinations are composed of very few chemical types. Most are nitrogen-containing compounds, thus alkaloids. Marihuana is nonnitrogenous, however. The alkaloids include the protoalkaloids or amino alkaloids, which lack nitrogen in their central structure though usually not in the side chains, and the more complex alkaloids, having nitrogen in their heterocyclic ring structure. The majority of the latter are indoles derived from tryptamines.

Figure 18-1 illustrates the basic chemical structures of the hallucinogens, which consist first of the primitive protoalkaloid compounds mescaline (peyote cactus) and myristicin (nutmeg and mace), as well as synthetic amphetamine (not illustrated). The second and largest group of compounds are indole alkaloids, all derivatives of tryptamine, which, following our sequence, includes psilocybin and psilocin (sacred mushrooms), various methyltryptamines and β-carbolines (South American snuffs and drinks), lysergic acid derivates (LSD, morning glories, and ergot), and ibogaine (iboga). Being tryptamine derivates, these indolic hallucinogens are structurally akin to the neurohumoral factor serotonin (5-hydroxytryptamine), common to warm-blooded animals. This substance accumulates in the brain, where it is involved in the biochemistry of central nervous regulations. It appears that certain tryptamines that occur frequently as hallucinogens, as well as in the neurohormone serotonin, are in fact centrally important in the metabolism of psychic functions.[1] Another distinct group of complex alkaloids found in the Solanaceae are the tropane derivatives, and finally a second group of alkaloids, well removed structurally from the indoles, are the isoxazoles of *Amanita* (fly agaric mushroom).

The active nonnitrogenous compound found in the resin of marihuana, Δ'-3,4-*trans*-tetrahydrocannabinol (Δ'-THC), differs markedly from the hallucinogenic alkaloids in respect to both its chemistry and the symptoms of intoxication in which the euphoric state predominates.

In this all too brief introduction to the hallucinogens, we urge the reader to augment his appreciation for these interesting compounds by reading further

about some of the major hallucinogens we have chosen for discussion. This review is of necessity superficial when compared to the detailed and extraordinary accounts published in recent years by Prof. Richard E. Schultes[1,3] and his students at Harvard University, and by his collaborator R. Gordon Wasson,[4] whose achievements in unveiling the mysteries of mushroom-induced hallucinations are truly remarkable. Their writings together with those of Norman R. Farnsworth,[5] Peter T. Furst,[6] Albert Hofmann,[1] Weston La Barre,[7] and numerous others,[8] will lead the reader interested in hallucinogens into one of the most enlightening adventures involving man and the plants around him.

PEYOTE[7,9,10]

A number of cactus species possess psychoactive properties (Table 18-1), but none is more significant or more spectacular as a vision-inducing plant than peyote, *Lophophora williamsii* (Cactaceae: Fig. 18-2). Known as peyotl in the Aztec Empire, this cactus, native from southern Texas to central Mexico, was one of the earliest North American hallucinogens to be firmly established in religious rites before the Spanish conquest. The peyote cult withstood centuries of civil and ecclesiastical opposition, and today in the United States, Mexico, and Canada use of the plant as part of the Indian religious experience continues unabated. It is legally incorporated into the communion service of the Native American Church, whose adherents number about a quarter million.

Peyote is usually eaten as mescal buttons, the dried, brown pieces of the above-ground part of the cactus. Occasionally fresh green pieces are used. This bitter cud is swallowed after a brief mix-

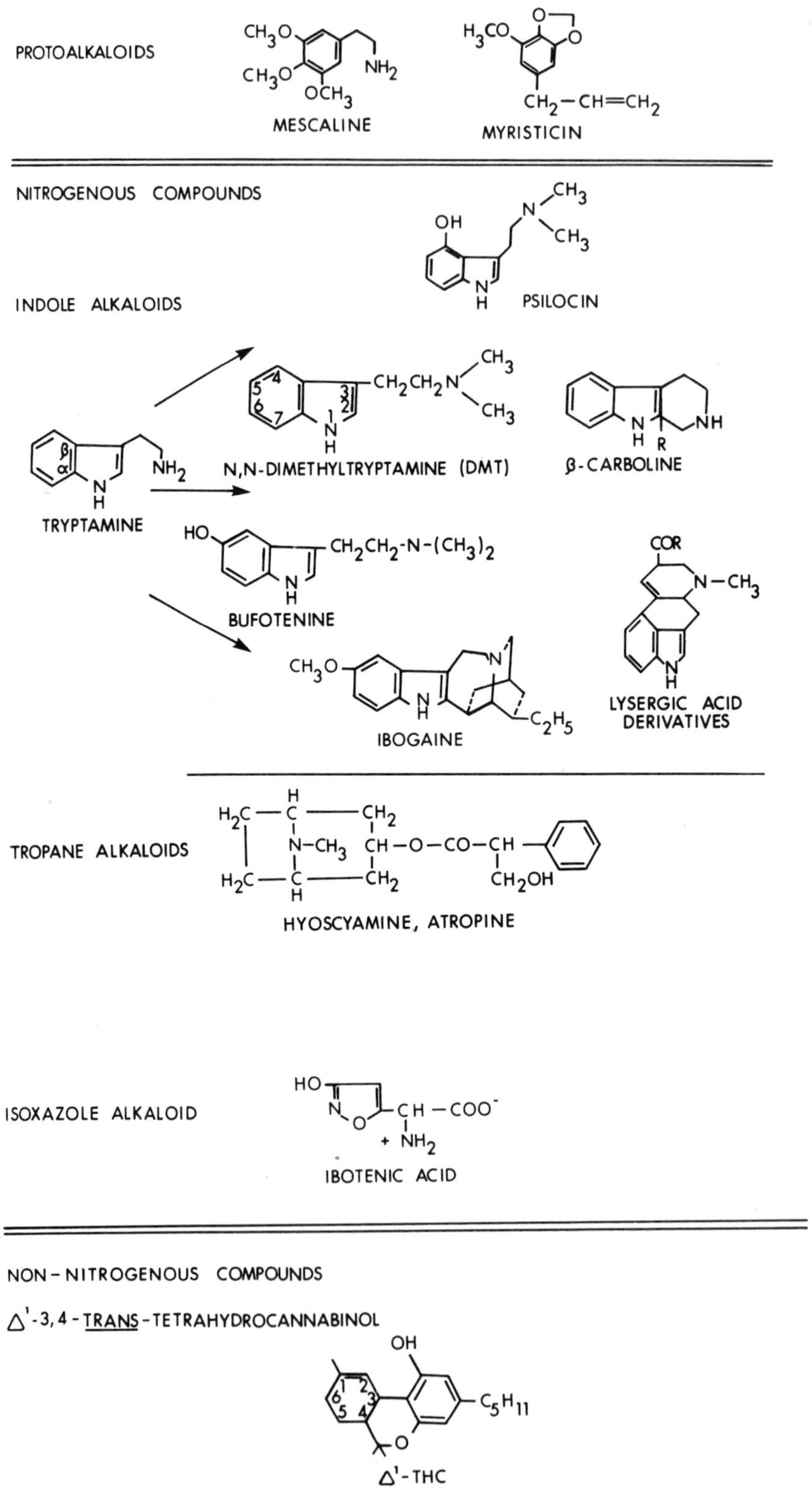

PROTOALKALOIDS

MESCALINE

MYRISTICIN

NITROGENOUS COMPOUNDS

INDOLE ALKALOIDS

PSILOCIN

TRYPTAMINE

N,N-DIMETHYLTRYPTAMINE (DMT)

β-CARBOLINE

BUFOTENINE

IBOGAINE

LYSERGIC ACID DERIVATIVES

TROPANE ALKALOIDS

HYOSCYAMINE, ATROPINE

ISOXAZOLE ALKALOID

IBOTENIC ACID

NON-NITROGENOUS COMPOUNDS

Δ^1-3,4-TRANS-TETRAHYDROCANNABINOL

Δ^1-THC

Figure 18-1 Structural types of principal hallucinogens.

406

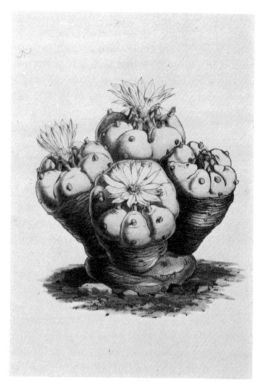

Figure 18-2 *Lophophora williamsii* (from *Curtis's Botanical Magazine* 73: 4296, 1847).

ual hallucinations for the first time. He was sitting on the floor of a room filled with music, and notes flowing from the stereo took on the form of long orange, red, and purple ribbons that permeated the room just as the music filled the air. Before long the ribbons drifted beyond the room as the walls disappeared, floating off in continuous streams from the machine to encompass the visible horizon. The whole world became a moving panorama of brightly colored, textured ribbons, drifting aloft, filling the sky: a breath-taking picture. Then Orlando slept. Some days later as he penned the first letter of his name, Orlando had a flashback, a sudden loss of reality. He was in the letter "O"; he was caught by high walls. The "O" was shrinking, the walls were getting higher; he clambered to get out, and as his fingers tore at the walls, blood dripped from his torn fingernails. There was no escape, and the walls kept contracting until Orlando felt that his life was being squeezed away. Orlando was found screaming and was hospitalized. When the fear of spontaneous hallucinations passed, he was released, but he never took peyote tea again.

No one will know for certain why Orlando had this particular experience because the action of mescaline, peyotline, anhaline, anhalamine, lophophorine, and other alkaloids found in peyote depends on the concentration of each compound, their potential synergism, the size of the dose, the physiology and mental state of the ingestor, and undoubtedly other factors. The full range of effects of peyote taken habitually is not well understood, but individually the alkaloids can be characterized. For example, lophophorine is the most toxic, having strychninelike effects: shortly after ingestion of lophophorine the user has a sickening sensation in the back of the head, a hot and flushed face, and a slight decrease in pulse. The drug also augments

ing with saliva. Peyote is also brewed and the tea drunk (with more powerful effects?). Not long after ingestion, peyote produces nausea, chills, and vomiting often accompanied by terror, anxiety, and a dislocation of visual perspective, in the majority of users. After these unpleasant symptoms subside, mental stimulation begins. There is a clarity and intensity of thought, but most characteristic of all is the motion of indescribably brilliant colored visions, as well as exaggerated sensitivity to sounds and other sense impressions.

These effects are well represented by our subject Orlando, who drank peyote tea made from sections of the stem, and containing mescaline and many other alkaloids. He suppressed an initial feeling of nausea, the tea remained down, and in a half-hour or so Orlando perceived vis-

the irritability of the spinal cord. On the other hand, mescaline acts by paralyzing the central nervous system and produces an awareness of heaviness in the limbs and eventually color visions. These alkaloids represent two extremes of action in a broad spectrum of individual and interactive effects typified by the many compounds present in the cactus.

Other cacti containing mescaline are also known for their hallucinogenic properties, though none is more interesting than *Trichocereus pachanoi* (San Pedro) of Peru and adjacent areas. The cactus is used in folk healing to diagnose illness and to effect cures, an ancient practice to help those facing the fears and uncertainties of disease.[11]

NUTMEG[12]

Those who do not live in southern Texas or Mexico cannot step out the back door to find a natural peyote patch, but they can stay in the kitchen, almost any kitchen in the world, and locate on the spice shelf a potent drug. We know this exotic drug from the Old World tropics as nutmeg and it is a powerful hallucinogen, capable of removing one completely from the world of reality in a hypnotic trance accompanied by golden dreams and euphoric bliss.

In Ayurvedic medicine nutmeg is called madashaunda, a term for "narcotic fruit," and today it is often added by betel chewers to their quid for its intoxicating effects. Nutmeg is also added to tobacco and chewed or snuffed in Asia, but it is in Europe and North America that nutmeg has been used by more sophisticated societies, such as the jazz set after World War I in New Orleans, or more commonly by those deprived of their preferred drugs. This is especially true of prisoners who have difficulty obtaining psychoactive drugs.

Powdered nutmeg or mace is taken orally or sniffed; dose requirements vary greatly. For some a single tablespoon mixed in water as a hot toddy is sufficient to induce hallucinations, for others as many as six tablespoons are necessary. Results vary from no hallucinogenic effect to experiences roughly equivalent to those of hashish. Almost always, however, there are unpleasant initial side effects—headache, dizziness, nausea—and sickening hangovers, which indicate that nutmeg is generally toxic when used in large amounts.[1] It is, for example, mildly inhibiting to monoamine oxidase, thus disturbs neural transmission.

Nutmeg or mace intoxication is characterized by a feeling of detachment from reality. Visual hallucinations may occur, but auditory and other hallucinations are more common. There are also sensations of floating or flying, a separation of limbs from the body, which typify a number of the more toxic hallucinogens (e.g., the solanaceous genera, *Atropa, Hyoscyamus, Mandragora*). Perhaps these recollections by a prisoner most vividly portray the effects of nutmeg:

For some strange reason nutmeg is a drug that seems to be used only in prison, and then only by the rare individual. I believe the reason for this is that in the first place it is a revolting concoction to take. One has to have between six and eight tablespoonfuls. This is mixed into a mug of hot water. It is stirred frantically until the water turns a milky brown. Drinking this mixture is only the beginning. The nutmeg does not dissolve and the user then has to spoon the horrible bitterness into his rebellious stomach as quickly as possible. For the next half hour his stomach tries to get rid of it but heroically the user fights the nausea and doesn't vomit it back up.

After approximately 45 minutes the user finds himself giggling in a silly manner at everything. Regardless what is said; what is done; what is thought; it all seems so ridiculously humorous. Anyone who has smoked marijuana has experienced this complete inability to control laughter at sometime. Some even have had this experience with LSD.

After 30 to 60 minutes of this gut-tearing silliness the mouth and throat begin to dry up as though one has taken atropine. I believe the whole system becomes dehydrated because one may go 36 hours without a bowel movement or a desire to urinate. When the dehydration sets in then the laughter stops and a great lethargy creeps over one. Although one might think they'll lie down and read this is impossible because the eyes become dry, red, contracted to pinpoints and it's impossible to keep them open. The natural thing to do is lie down.

A strange thing happens when one begins to "coast" on nutmeg. I've taken it in solitary confinement where the bed was only the hard cement floor; and I've taken it where I had a comfortable bed and mattress to lie on. It didn't matter. Once the lethargy took over both felt like I was resting on a cloud. It seems that one has a tendency to lie flat on the back and the lethargy is so great not even a finger or a muscle will be moved unless forced to.

It's when the drug really takes over that beautiful visions replace reality. These are usually very exotic visions. Mine, possibly because I lived in the Far East and still love it, immediately take me back to some tropical isle. But now is when the nutmeg begins to have many of the characteristics of an LSD session. The visions and dreams one experiences begin to lose their continuity and come in chunks of unrelated experiences. One may find his childhood becomes his reality except that it is invariably a happy childhood. Then his visions will jump into a whole vortex of revolving, unexplainable colors. Suddenly, as though it is coming from thousands of miles, music will take on such sweetness and lucidity and color that one becomes lost in it. You find yourself hung up on a bar and then hurry like hell to catch up with the rhythm and notes again. Usually the music you've been listening to is from the prison radio. Sometimes, just as in marijuana, one can hear a whole symphony played in the most exquisite manner when there's no music being played at all. Voices, speaking to you, are also part of the experience.

Unlike the LSD and marijuana—I'm speaking only of my own experiences now—when someone speaks to me while in a nutmeg coma I can wrench myself back to reality and know what they're saying. The only problem is that it seems like ten minutes between their question and my answer and my speech is very slow and thick.

Time loses all meaning just as in LSD. One also likes themselves when under nutmeg and you almost become childlike in the ability to understand yourself and forgive yourself. The user becomes very sensual under its influence and although the effects are with him from 24 to 36 hours he usually has an erection most of the time.

Whether the drug of nutmeg stays with one 24 or 36 hours one really doesn't sleep. But he is in a sleep stupor and capable of shutting out all noises that are obnoxious. There seems to be no sensation of cold when high. Although many nights in the "hole" were horror to me because of the cold and I had no covers, on the days or nights that a buddy was able to smuggle in nutmeg I felt no discomfort at all. Neither does it matter whether one is in a lighted place or in pitch darkness. The eyes are closed and one sees most of the visions in erotic colors anyway. I think possibly the greatest similarity nutmeg has to LSD is the sensation of going back in time to ages one has only read about. Another is the complete loss and the lack of need for time as we know it.

When the drug finally wears off one sinks into a deep slumber. But the awakening is torture. The after-effects of nutmeg are actually painful. Every bone and muscle in the body aches as though one had malaria. The eyeballs set up a throbbing pain all their own. The nose runs frantically and a great deep depression sets in. . . .[2]

Thus like other spices (cinnamon, ginger, see Table 18-1), a spice of southern Asia obtained from the seeds and surrounding aril of the tree *Myristica fragrans* (Myristicaceae) may cause hallucination in overdose as well as other intoxicating symptoms. Probably the volatile oils of these spices are responsible; in nutmeg it is undoubtedly the aromatic ether fraction of which myristicin, elemicin, and safrole are the primary constituents. Action may be the result of synergism between these and other aromatic fractions that leads to a full psychoactive experience.

Nutmeg is reputed to possess aphrodisiac powers, and is used for this purpose in Yemen today (Table 13-4). It is also claimed to induce abortions, but its use results more often in serious toxic effects than in the effect desired.

AMPHETAMINES

Although the stimulant drugs called amphetamines as such are not hallucinogenic, certain derivates containing methoxy substitutes on the benzene ring have hallucinogenic properties similar to mescaline. Thus 3,4,5-trimethoxyamphetamine (TMA) is twice as psychoactive as mescaline. Among the more chemically interesting of the substituted amphetamines are the methylenedioxyamphetamines (MDA), which resemble myristicin of nutmeg. The most powerful, however, is dimethoxymethylamphetamine (DOM or specifically 2,5-dimethoxy-4-methylamphetamine); known as STP, this is the amphetamine of abuse, responsible for a large number of "bad trips." STP is 80 times more potent than mescaline, and the usual illegal dose of about 10 mg produces a reaction that may last 2 or 3 days. The abuser probably believes the reactions will last forever—a state of normality is lost—thereby producing a panic effect. Illicit use of these powerfully acting hallucinogens with their terrifying side effects is decreasing.

SACRED MUSHROOMS[13]

Many hallucinogenic alkaloids are tryptamine derivates; of these, psilocybin (4-phosphoryloxy-N,N-dimethyltryptamine) and psilocin (4-hydroxy-N,N-dimethyltryptamine) are the active principles of Teonanacatl or "flesh of the gods," the sacred mushrooms of Mexico. These mushrooms are found in the genera *Conocybe*, *Panaeolus*, *Psilocybe*, and *Stropharia* (Table 18-1 gives species), and a number are common throughout tropical and subtropical regions, reaching well into the United States. Except for their recent adoption by the youth of western North America, they do not appear to be used now to induce hallucinations outside Mexico and northern Central America. There, however, the Indians had "openly" used them to commune with the spirit world until European persecution drove the practice underground—to the isolated highlands of Oaxaca and like regions. The sacramental eating of these mushrooms has continued, however, and today the shaman relies on the natural power of the mushroom coupled with Christian rites in order to evolve a supernatural experience (see below).

The powerful vision-inducing powers of these hallucinogens are typified by a number of symptoms: muscular relaxation, flaccidity, and pupil dilation in the early stages; then emotional disturbances, visual and auditory hallucinations; and eventually lassitude and mental and physical depression. The subject feels isolated from the world around him, for without loss of consciousness he is indifferent to his environment, which becomes unreal as his dreamlike condition becomes apparently real.[1]

A former student of ours went to Oaxaca with several acquaintances and reported the following adventure in the house of a shaman, one night atop a rainy, wind-swept mountain.

We arrived from our hotel up the long trail above the village drenched from the torrential rain, in the dark night, tired and physically miserable. We sat on the floor in candle light in the one-room house while prayers were offered at the homemade altar, a rite reflecting both Catholic and native influences. Our names were asked and included in the blessing. Then the shaman turned from the altar and, using the sign of the cross, anointed both elbows of each of us with earth moistened by saliva while continuing her chant.

Before long we were each handed a small swatch of newspaper holding several mushrooms. They included newly budded specimens about 2 cm in diameter to mature and gangly ones with caps up to 4 cm. The total weighed about an ounce. We ate the mushrooms promptly, the candles were blown out, and we sat in silence.

Amid the haunting chants of our shaman, the first sign I had that something was happening was a hint of geometric patterns, very confused and very rapidly changing. I could barely perceive a design before it would change; the images were as faint as they were fleeting, but becoming more vivid with time. Effects heightened: they were clear and normal looking as an array of brilliant fibers of light passed overhead in a horizontal plane, only to break up and reattach to a central point forming a starlike pattern that began to swirl slowly one way, then another. The swirling slowed and stopped, and my fantasy acquired a third dimension in the form of a hemisphere in bluish hue, and from the center of its radiating lines came a stem colored green.

The most dramatic incident of the night was one that has since caused me to reconsider scoffing at references to the "spirit of the mushroom." At some point soon after the hallucination had begun, I had gotten off on a distressing tangent. Various emotional problems which had been concerning me began to command more and more of my attention, and before long my entire being was focused on them. Their proportions became so ominous that no amount of intellectual rationalization could control them. Feeding on this state and perhaps catalyzed by my

physical discomfort, I rapidly approached an almost unbelievable state of despair. Suddenly, completely out of context, came a vision which immediately and miraculously removed me from this condition: my first impression was that someone was checking on things by shining a flashlight in my face, but on second glance, this light, though as bright and taking up most of my field of vision as would a flashlight beam, had no glare and had an incredibly rich golden hue. As I stared agape at the brilliance, its dark periphery turned green and then coalesced into a jungle vegetation—of giant herbs, trees, and lianas. Before this had finished forming, the central glow began to coalesce into a golden scene, a clearing on which were constructed stepped pyramids and other buildings. In the foreground was a giant column with an abstract carved face at the top like the god seen on Aztec and Mayan displays. When I tried to form a conscious series of thoughts about this scene, the whole faded from view.

As I returned to my former state and again confronted the emotional gargoyles that had so bothered me, I saw how truly insignificant they were compared to the visions I had just witnessed. How apparently coincidental that this spectacular display came to me at the most incredible point of despair, and then, with unimaginable ease, placed everything in its proper perspective.

At this point someone lighted the candles, we huddled together, now more fully in reality, and we talked quietly sharing blankets and warmth. We talked for perhaps two hours and finally, exhausted yet euphoric, we settled into a warm heap and into a total sleep unwarranted by the hard dirt floor. We arose next morning and went our separate ways, a little dazed by the night's experience and the power of the sacred mushroom.

SOUTH AMERICAN SNUFFS

These snuffs are prepared by scraping the inner bark stripped from certain trees, boiling until all water has evaporated, toasting the sediment over a slight fire, and finely powdering. Alternately, the bark is stripped from the trees early in the cool of morning, and the blood-red resin is scraped from the soft inner bark. The scrapings are kneaded in water, strained, and boiled to a thick syrup. When sun-dried, the material is pulverized, sifted, and mixed with the ashes of the bark of *Theobroma subincanum* (Sterculiaceae), a source of inferior cocoa. These ash snuffs are sniffed through reeds or bird bone tubes (Fig. 18-3).

Only as recently as 1954[14] has snuffing been described in detail and the plants identified as *Virola* (Myristicaceae, Table 18-1), often mixed with other genera probably to enhance the intoxicating effects. The most prominent additive is *Justicia pectoralis* (Acanthaceae), whose pulverized aromatic leaves are said to make the snuff smell better. To mixture of approximately equal amounts of *Virola* and *J. pectoralis* is added a similar amount of the ashed bark of *Elizabetha princeps* (Fabaceae). The whole powder, ready for use as snuff, is greyish and extremely fine.[1]

The effect of *Virola* or yakee intoxication usually includes initial excitability shortly after the first sniffing, followed by numbness of limbs, facial muscle twitching, lack of muscular coordination, nausea, visual hallucinations, and ultimately a deep disturbed sleep. According to Schultes and Hofmann,[1] objects often

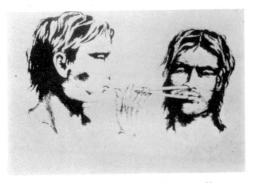

Figure 18-3   Tubes for sniffing snuff.

appear unnaturally large (macropsia), and this experience undoubtedly enters into the belief by some Indians that a spirit dwells in the plant.

In some parts of the Amazon, pellets of the resin are ingested for similar intoxicating effects, with three to six said to last up to two hours. Others drink the resin of *Virola,* and the inner bark may be dried and smoked for curing fevers or driving away evil spirits. Regardless of how *Virola* is taken, its highly active components and possibly its additives have long been used by Indians of northern parts of South America, often only by witch doctors, for the diagnosis and treatment of disease, for prophecy and divination, and for purposes of magic.

The biodynamic properties of *Virola* resin are due to several tryptamines: N,N-dimethyltryptamine (DMT, which was synthesized before being found in nature), N-methyltryptamine (NMT), 5-methyoxy-N,N-dimethyltryptamine (5-MeO-DMT), and other derivates, as well as β-carboline alkaloids, which are apparently present in sufficient concentrations to exert their effect as monoamine oxidase inhibitors, thus serving to activate the hallucinogenic properties of the tryptamines when the plant product is taken orally.[15] For example, DMT taken by itself, orally, is inactive, but it may be smoked with marihuana or tobacco, sniffed, or injected, with essentially instantaneous effects beginning in 2 minutes and lasting less than an hour (60–150 μg). At one time it was called the "businessman's high," a peak during the quick lunch instead of a martini.

These tryptamines, commonly DMT, are also found among the Fabaceae. They occur, for example, in the seeds of *Anadenanthera (Piptadenia) peregrina* along with β-carbolines; in fact the snuff called cohoba or yopo is chemically closely allied to that of *Virola*. At least one other species, *A. colubrina*, is implicated in these snuffs, and a number of legumes and other plants containing tryptamines are known or suspected of being hallucinogenic. One new derivative 5-hydroxy-*N,N*-dimethyltryptamine (5-OH-DMT or bufotenine),which was originally isolated from the skin glands of toads and is known in numerous *Bufo* spp., may also possess synergistic effects with other hallucinogens, even though it is not certain that it has such properties alone.

SOUTH AMERICAN DRINKS[16]

No more interesting or complex narcotic drink can be found than ayahuasca, caapi, or yaje, prepared basically from the bark of the liana *Banisteriopsis caapi* or *B. inebrians* (Malpighiaceae) with additives of a number of other species. Most critical for maximum hallucinogenic effect appear to be *Psychotria catharginensis*, *P. viridis* (Rubiaceae), or *Banisteriopsis rusbyana*, all of which contain DMT. This combined with the β-carbolines (harmine, harmoline, tetrahydroharmine) of the basic *Banisteriopsis* component suggests the same enhanced effect noted for the hallucinogenic snuffs, which also contain the tryptamines and β-carbolines. Other occasional additives include *Malouetia tamaquarina* and *Tabernaemontana* sp. (Apocynaceae) leaves, powdered tobacco (*Nicotiana tabacum*), and other Solanaceae (*Brunfelsia* sp., *Iochroma fuchsioides*, *Juanulloa ochracea*), *Teliostachya lanceolata* var. *crispa* (Acanthaceae), *Calathea veitchiana* (Marantaceae), and many others such as cacti, mints, sedges, and ferns.[3] In most instances the biodynamic compounds remain unknown.

From Amazonian Brazil, Prance[17] vividly reports how the drink is prepared not only by the Indians but also by the Brazilian townsmen who belong to a growing spirit worship cult centered around ayahuasca (called cipó in Brazil). The vine of *Banisteriopsis* is cut into sections and allowed to almost boil in a saucepan of water; the leaves of *Psychotria* are added at this point and the two are simmered together for about half an hour. The rust-brown liquid is cooled, then bottled and corked. It is acrid tasting and may be stored for up to 4 weeks.

Families use the beverage apparently without harm or addiction, and individuals frequently gather in groups for large drinking bouts. Always there is one person who does not drink (to bring anyone out of a bad hallucinating experience). The participants shut their eyes and wait for the hallucinations while background music is played. A few vomit, but soon the visions begin: bright colors and large objects and animals, particularly snakes and jaguars. Some report seeing cities they have never visited, and others are able to describe ocean liners and large stores in considerable detail. Prance tells the story of an air force captain who showed the Indians in an isolated area of Amazonia a film on cowboys and a documentary film about Brazil. The Indians were distinctly disappointed by the movies, for as they told him, they had seen all that before and even more while under the influence of cipó. In the future they were going to stick with their drink.

The hallucinogenic experiences of this group are not unlike those known to the Indians deep in the upper Amazon, as described by a Peruvian youth who had been captured by the Amahuacas. The ayahuasca, prepared ritualistically by the medicine man, was passed among a group of 12, gathered in a secluded jungle glade to bid farewell to the dying chief (Fig. 18-4).

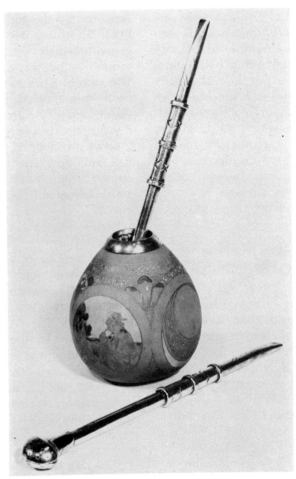

Figure 18-4 Ceremonial gourd for drinking maté and other drinks prepared from several South American species (courtesy May W Elvin).

We drank in unison amid a quiet chant. Color visions began to evolve into immense vistas of enchanting beauty with the chief chanting and taking control of the progression of our visions. Soon the animals appeared, first the jungle cats, many of which I had not seen before, including a giant rosetta-spotted jaguar (all murmured in recognition), then snakes and birds passed in review, each holding some significance to the tribe in their domination over the forest.

These Indians were experiencing inter-individual communication and perception, their collective unconsciousness was an immediate reality. Characteristically, the drug had intensified their ability to telepathize and to enhance extrasensory perception beyond usual conscious levels.[18] Such simultaneous vision perception by many as a part of their hallucinogenic experience needs critical study for potential application in psychiatry and other fields.

LYSERGIC ACID DERIVATIVES

Other tryptamine residues are lysergic acid and its derivatives. The best known hallucinogenic derivative is D-lysergic acid diethylamide (LSD-25), which was synthesized from ergometrine (ergonovine), one of the ergot alkaloids of the fungus *Claviceps purpurea*. A less powerful hallucinogenic derivative is D-lysergic acid amide (LAA), or ergine, found in the seeds of morning glories as well as in ergot.

LSD-25 (LSD)

Four stereoisomers can by synthesized from lysergic acid, but only D-lysergic acid diethylamide (LSD) has unique psychoactive properties. It is the most powerful psychic drug known to man, being 4000 times more powerful than mescaline. The substance was synthesized by Hofmann in 1938, but it was not until 1943 that he accidentally discovered LSD's hallucinogenic properties, as described in this famous passage:

In the afternoon of 16 April, 1943, when I was working on this problem, I was seized by a peculiar sensation of vertigo and restlessness. Objects, as well as the shapes of my associates in the laboratory, appeared to undergo optical changes. I was unable to concentrate on my work. In a dreamlike state I left for home where an irresistible urge to lie down overcame me. I drew the curtains and immediately fell into a peculiar state similar to a drunkenness, characterized by an exaggerated imagination. With my eyes closed, fantastic pictures of extraordinary plasticity and intensive color seemed to surge toward me. After two hours this state gradually wore off.

Later LSD was "discovered" and popularized in the 1960s by such advocates as Timothy Leary.[19] The subculture included the curious, those out for kicks, and others in quest of religious or philosophical insights. Its use illegally for nonmedical purposes has been on the wane since the early 1970s.

Ingesting or injecting only 100 μg of

LSD has a striking impact on the senses. Perception is greatly modified: colors become bright, even brilliant; sounds become louder and more important. Sense impressions overflow into one another (synthesia—thus the user hears music and watches sounds) and become confused and distorted, as picture frames waver, walls appear to move, colors of paintings run together, and ordinary objects suddenly become luminous, a glow, for instance, appearing around someone's head. These effects represent a loss of the normal boundaries of perception. Under the effects of LSD, emotions become heightened, defenses and reserves are lessened, and mood changes may become extreme. Time may appear to stand still, and this effect may reduce the user's anticipation of future events, even dimming, for example, the desire to continue working, going to school, or pursuing a goal. Normally those taking LSD remain fully conscious and aware.

Another characteristic of the LSD trip is that memories and experiences from the past flood the user with all the reality of the day they occurred. If these experiences are unpleasant, the user may become extremely frightened, and once begun, such a bad trip may last for many hours. If, however, the experience is pleasant, the subject maintains a pleasant, satisfied feeling for 6 or more hours in a state of comfortable detachment. Many months later flashbacks may occur spontaneously, or they may be triggered by other drugs such as marihuana or by medication like antihistamines. These experiences can be terrifying (see discussion under Peyote).

Although certain effects of LSD may be disturbing to the psyche for a time, perhaps even a long time, what are the physical consequences of using the drug? Many studies have shown that it can cause chromosomal damage in cultured human cells, that it can cause birth defects in laboratory animals and humans, and that it is carcinogenic. Yet an equally large number of studies have demonstrated that there is insufficient evidence for such effects, particularly at concentrations encountered in drug abuse. Perhaps these conflicting results have in recent years generated a complacency about the potential hazards of LSD, but two recent reports suggest that indifference to the problem may be premature.[20]

The first investigation implies that there is a greatly increased rate of spontaneous abortions and birth defects among LSD users,[21] and the second suggests that LSD may disrupt the body's immune system by interfering with the production of antibodies. These data correlate with an increased incidence of infectious diseases among typical drug abusers.[22] In both instances, there is cause to reflect on the potential hazards of LSD to human reproduction, but fortunately the drug is not physically addictive and tolerance develops and disappears rapidly.

OLOLIUQUI: THE MORNING GLORIES

Seeds of *Rivea corymbosa* and *Ipomoea violacea* (Convolvulaceae) were associated by the Aztecs and other Mexican Indians with divination. As noted by early Spanish writers: "when the Aztec priests want to commune with their gods and to receive a message from them, they eat this plant to induce delirium during which time a thousand visions and satanic hallucinations appear to them."[1] For several centuries no one outside Mexico was certain of the identity of "this plant"—it remained for Schultes[23] in 1941 to connect these early writings with *Rivea corymbosa*, and it was not until 1960 that an ergot alkaloid D-lysergic acid amide was found in its seed. Hofmann proved

this substance, like LSD-25, to be hallucinogenic.[24].

As morning glory is used today by the Indians of Oaxaca, the seeds are finely ground to flour and soaked in cold water. After a short time the liquid is passed through a strainer and drunk. A dose includes sufficient seeds to fill a beer cap or the cup of a hand: those of *Rivea* are considered less potent and women use them; the more potent black seeds of *Ipomoea* are taken by men. The hallucinations are similar to those of peyote and psilocybin. The seeds are commercially available as the varieties Heavenly Blue and Pearly Gates (*I. violacea*).[25]

ERGOT

Ergot is the sclerotium of *Claviceps purpurea*, the fungus that parasitizes the growing kernels of rye and wheat principally, but also other less known members of the grass family. Ergot destroys the ovaries of the grain, and the kernel is replaced by a brownish violet, horn-shaped mass that protrudes from the head of the grain.

The ergot alkaloids are derivatives of lysergic acid and the hallucinogenic D-lysergic acid amide. The chief effects of these alkaloids are gangrenous and convulsive. In gangrenous ergotism the fingers start to tingle, vomiting and diarrhea follow, and within a few days gangrene appears in the toes and fingers. Entire limbs are affected, and amid excruciating pain as circulation is decreased, they separate from the body (Fig. 18-5). The convulsive form starts the same way but is followed by painful spasms of the limb muscles, culminating in epileptic-like convulsions. Known as St. Anthony's fire, it was a dreaded disease wherever infected rye bread was eaten.[26] Dark

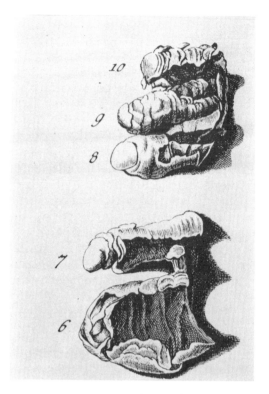

Figure 18-5a Gangrenous fingers of ergotism (from J Toube, 1782).

must have appeared absolute. Under the circumstances, it was easy to be among the faithful, and the many visions undoubtedly seen as a result of ingesting the hallucinogenic D-lysergic acid amide surely added to this conviction. Because the church embraced all aspects of life, the hallucinations would manifest themselves in one direction—to the Holy Family, their supporting disciples and angels, and the church hierarchy. Through the Dark and Middle Ages, visions and ergot intoxication went hand in hand; in Europe today there are few reports of visions, and there is very little ergot.

Hallucinating may not have been restricted to Europe, for ergotism during the Salem, Massachusetts crises of 1692 could explain the convulsions, mental

bread—dark from the rye and darker when the brownish violet ergot contaminates it—was a staple of the poor of Europe, and with continued ingestion of the alkaloids thousands perished from this unknown malady. An epidemic in France in 994 killed about 40,000; thousands died of it during the Middle Ages, and even in the present small outbreaks are reported. In earlier days seeking God's protection against this terrifying affliction, the affected poor would flock to the churches. They were fed the bread eaten by the clergy (lighter-colored loaves, often made from uncontaminated rye or even wheat), and before long their symptoms disappeared, as daily consumption of ergot alkaloids was reduced or eliminated. For those who survived, the power of the church and God to heal

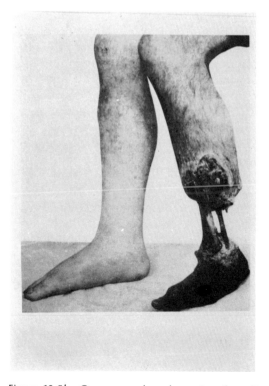

Figure 18-5b Gangrenous leg of ergotism (from P Haushalter, 1892).

disturbances, and perceptual distortions of the girls whom the New England Puritans considered possessed by witchcraft. During that year 20 witches were executed and at least two died in prison. Were they victims of ergot-induced hallucinations?[26]

IBOGA[27]

Among a dozen or so of the complex indole alkaloids derived from tryptamine and found in *Tabernanthe iboga* (Apocynaceae), ibogaine is the most important hallucinogen, not only in iboga, but perhaps of all those species indigenous to the African continent.

Found in Gabon, the Republic of the Congo, a large area of Zaire, and also cultivated in west Africa beyond this natural range, iboga is an important element of life, not only for its hallucinogenic powers but also as an aphrodisiac prized more by the natives for this purpose than the famous African yohimbine (*Corynanthe yohimbe*). The use may be justified, for the stimulating properties of this drug may well increase confidence and stave off fatigue. Iboga is also taken during religious festivals and rites, especially by shamans to enhance their psychic powers, increase inspiration, and assist in contemplation. The drug is also consumed by those who believe it can reveal objects (ogbanje) reputedly buried by individuals subjected to the intoxicant during their former lives. Mostly young women and children are "led" under the influence of iboga to reveal where they hid their treasures in their fore-lives during these strange ogbanje rituals. Failure to expose the possessions, they believe, may result in sudden and mysterious deaths among the villagers.

One of the most interesting uses of iboga, however, is as a hallucinogen. It is prepared from dried root bark and masti-

cated into a fine powder, often with other plants; or the root raspings are chewed until the desired effect is obtained. There are visual hallucinations (i.e., seeing the Bwiti, god, among a Gabon cult), accompanied by anxiety and apprehension among the few whites having taken the drug, but for the African natives the drug represents an unmatched power with strong spiritual, animistic overtones. Today the use of iboga is spreading, and the societies associated with it are immensely popular. Here is a condensed report of an all-night party:

Priests and assistants prepared the Iboga, shared their concoction, and the men began dancing around each of the poles in the temple—they jumped, stamped, leaped in a compulsive sort of way. The torsos of the men streamed with sweat and from time to time they rushed over to a pail of water, drank great draughts, and then resumed their intoxicating motions. Some women shook their rattles, others sang, and the rhythm accelerated. The group became as a single creature, tensed for an impossible victory.[28]

So wrote a European observer, who added that he felt "foreign, separate, trapped by his human dignity, encumbered by a body that had lost even the memory of its potentialities. . . . like a cripple to whom no one need pay the slightest attention."

How little we understand of this fascinating hallucinogen and supposed aphrodisiac. We know that concoctions are often made up of numerous species besides *Tabernanthe iboga,* among them *Alchornea floribunda* (Euphorbiaceae), which apparently acts as a hallucinogen and aphrodisiac in its own right (Byeri secret society). But the shamans and herbalists of west Africa have long been guarding their secrets from prying queries of Western physicians and scientists, and they will undoubtedly continue to do so in the future.

TROPANE ALKALOIDS: SOLANACEAE

Except for the stimulant cocaine, all the significant tropane alkaloids are found in the potato family, the Solanaceae. They include scopolamine (hyoscine), and atropine ((+)-hyoscyamine), present in varying concentrations in different parts of the plants, during various stages of development, and even under different environmental conditions (e.g., fewer alkaloids are found in *Datura stramonium* following a rainy period than after clear weather, and decreases occur during the day and increases at night).

The pharmacological action of the tropane alkaloids is well known (Chapter 6): they are autonomic nervous system blocking agents that inhibit effector organs innervated by postganglionic cholinergic neurons. Because of this effect they commonly stimulate, then depress, the medulla and higher cerebral centers; they inhibit glandular secretions of the nose through bronchi and relax smooth muscles there; they alter cardiac rate; they allow vasodilation of blood vessels; they reduce gastric secretion and motility; they increase body temperature and alveolar ventilation; and they may block the sphincter muscle of the iris. There is no report of hallucinogenic effects induced by the pure chemicals hyoscyamine or atropine below toxic doses, but scopolamine is known to produce intoxication followed by unconsciousness, and hallucinations sometimes occur in the transition between consciousness and sleep. Species of *Datura* contain mainly scopolamine, and they enjoy side use as hallucinogens. However without data on potential synergistic effects between scopolamine, hyoscyamine, and atropine, as well as with the minor alkaloids tropine, scopine, and others as a part of the whole biodynamic component of these plants, valid conclusions cannot be reached. Minute amounts of the right combinations well below toxic levels may be important in triggering unusual states of consciousness.

Of the hallucinogens discussed thus far, use has been generally by ingestion, and more occasionally by sniffing and smoking. We also noted that in Europe particularly there was no native plant in common use having hallucinogenic or even psychoactive effects. An exception is the ergot alkaloid ingested with "bad" bread, but this hallucinogen was not taken to achieve voluntary removal from reality. Ingestion of plant concoctions related to the deadly nightshades was not normally attempted except by those contemplating suicide, or in controlled doses carefully administered, by those desiring medication. It is now clear, however, that some Europeans did stumble on a way to use their native hallucinogens which eliminated the (immediate) risk of poisoning: they boiled plants and incorporated the extracts into fats or oils, which were rubbed on the skin or orifice areas (rectum, vagina). In this manner flights from reality as intense as any we have described were obtained.

At one time the skin was thought to be impermeable to all substances; fat solubility, however, increases penetration of many materials. For example, fat-soluble hormones, vitamins, and organic bases are absorbed through the skin surface, as are animal and vegetable fats through the hair follicles (p. 601). The tropane alkaloids are fat soluble and are readily absorbed through the skin. Thus the witches' brews of the Middle Ages and back at least to Roman times were not necessarily for ingestion but were used externally by those who knew the power of the solanaceous alkaloids for propelling midnight flights through the air to rendezvous with the devil (Fig. 18-6).

Realizing the power of the church in

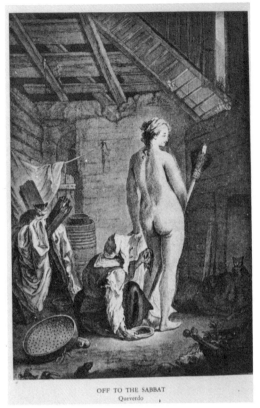

OFF TO THE SABBAT
Queverdo

Figure 18-6 Preparation for the Sabbat (By Queverdo, artist eighteenth century).

anoint a staff and ride on it to the appointed place or anoint themselves under the arms and in other hairy places and sometimes carry charms under the hair.

As Harner[29] notes, the use of a broom or staff was undoubtedly more than a symbolic Freudian act, for it served to apply the salves to the sensitive vaginal membranes as well as providing a means of conveyance, a ride on a broom being a typical illusion of how a witch arrived at the Sabbat (Fig. 18-7). Still another account (1523) supplies unusual detail.

But there is also a story commonly told among us, that at the time when the Inquisition in the diocese of Como was being carried on by our people, in the walled city called Lugano, it happened that the wife of a notary of the Inquisition was accused by due process of law of

medieval Europe, it is not surprising that only those who had cast aside Christianity would dare indulge in such heretical practices. Grave risks were also involved during the Inquisition, when even a hint of witchery meant burning. Biological understanding has now caught up with the empirical knowledge of the psychoactive experimentalists among our forefathers; the execution and torture of perhaps thousands might have been avoided if their persecutors had realized the power inherent in the specially prepared salves and ointments. Records from the Inquisition files attest to the reality of their "trips":

But the vulgar believe, and the witches confess, that on certain days or nights they

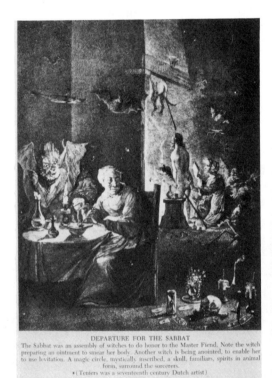

DEPARTURE FOR THE SABBAT
The Sabbat was an assembly of witches to do honor to the Master Fiend. Note the witch preparing an ointment to smear her body. Another witch is being anointed, to enable her to use levitation. A magic circle, mystically inscribed, a skull, familiars, spirits in animal form, surround the sorcerers.
*(Teniers was a seventeenth century Dutch artist.)

Figure 18-7 Departing for the Sabbat, including depiction of hallucination as a lycanthrope (from D Teniers).

being a witch and a sorceress. Her husband was exceedingly troubled at this, since he had thought her a holy woman. Then, through the will of the Lord, early on Good Friday, since he could not find his wife, he went to the pigsty. There he found her naked, displaying her genitals, completely unconscious and smeared with the excrement of the pigs. Now then, made more certain of that which he had not been able to believe, he drew his sword in sudden wrath, wishing to kill her. Returning to himself, however, he stood waiting for a little while that he might see the outcome of all this. And lo, after a little while she returned to her senses. When she saw that her husband was threatening to kill her, she prostrated herself before him and, seeking pardon, promised that she would reveal the whole truth to him. So she confessed that she had gone that night on the journey, etc. Hearing these things, her husband left at once and made an accusation of her in the house of the Inquisitor, so that she might be given to the fire. She, however, though sought at once, was nowhere to be found. They think that she drowned herself in the lake above whose shore that area is situated.[29]

Another example is that of Porta (1562), a colleague of Galileo, who suggested a physiological explanation of the witches' salve:

They [witches] take boys' fat and boil it in a copper vessel, then strain it; they knead the residue. With it they mix eleoselinum, aconite, poplar branches, and soot . . . or sometimes sium, common acorum, cinquefoil, the blood of a bat, sleep-inducing nightshade, and oil. . . . As soon as it is finished, they anoint the parts of the body, having rubbed them very thoroughly before, so that they grow rosy, and heat returns, and that which was stiff with cold becomes penetrable. So that the flesh may be loose and the pores open, they add, moreover, fat or, alternately, flowing oil that the force of the juices may descend inward, and be more powerful and lively.

Thus, on some moonlit night they think that they are carried off to banquets, music,

dances, and coupling with young men, which they desire most of all. So great is the force of the imagination and the appearance of the images, that the part of the brain called memory is almost full of this sort of thing; and since they themselves, by inclination of nature, are extremely prone to belief, that take hold of the images in such a way that the mind itself is changed and thinks of nothing else day or night.

While I was working on this matter—for I was still in a state of ambivalent judgment—an old woman came to my notice . . . who promised of her own accord to bring me answers in a short while. She ordered all of us who were gathered there with me as witnesses to go outside. Then she stripped off all her rags and rubbed herself very thoroughly and heartily with some ointment (she was visible to us through the cracks of the door). Then she sank down from the force of the soporific juices and fell into a deep sleep. We then opened the doors and gave her quite a flogging; the force of her stupor was so great that it had taken away her senses. We returned to our place outside. Then the powers of the drug grew weak and feeble and she, called from her sleep, began to babble that she had crossed seas and mountains to fetch these false answers. We denied; she insisted; we showed her the black-and-blue marks; she insisted more tenaciously than before.[29]

Inspired by the accounts of Porta and others, and after employing a seventeenth-century formula of *Atropa belladonna, Hyoscyamus,* and *Datura* ointment, twentieth-century investigators gave the following account: they rubbed the ointment on their foreheads and armpits and fell into a 24 hour sleep in which they dreamed of wild rides, frenzied dancing, and other weird adventures of the type connected with medieval orgies.[30] There is no better example of the modern use of solanaceous alkaloids to induce hallucinations of this type than the experience described by Castaneda. During his apprenticeship with don Juan, a Yaqui Indian of northwestern Mexico,

Castaneda rubbed himself with a lard ointment made from *Datura inoxia*. After he had drunk a root extract, the unguent was thoroughly smeared on his feet and legs, and the largest amount on his genitalia. The paste was cold and had an odor so strong that Castaneda could hardly breathe. He tried to breathe through his mouth and tried to talk to don Juan, but he couldn't.

Don Juan kept staring at me. I took a step toward him. My legs were rubbery and long, extremely long. I took another step. My knee joints felt springy, like a vault pole; they shook and vibrated and contracted elastically. I moved forward. The motion of my body was slow and shaky; it was more like a tremor forward and up. I looked down and saw don Juan sitting below me, way below me. The momentum carried me forward one more step, which was even more elastic and longer than the preceding one. And from there I soared. I remember coming down once; then I pushed up with both feet, sprang backward, and glided on my back. I saw the dark sky above me, and the clouds going by me. I jerked my body so I could look down. I saw the dark mass of the mountains. My speed was extraordinary. My arms were fixed, folded against my sides. My head was the directional unit. If I kept it bent backward I made vertical circles. I changed directions by turning my head to the side. I enjoyed such freedom and swiftness as I had never known before. The marvelous darkness gave me a feeling of sadness, of longing, perhaps. It was as if I had found a place where I belonged—the darkness of the night. I tried to look around, but all I sensed was that the night was so serene, and yet it held so much power.

Suddenly I knew it was time to come down; it was as if I had been given an order I had to obey. And I began descending like a feather with lateral motions. That type of movement made me very ill. It was slow and jerky, as though I were being lowered by pulleys. I got sick. My head was bursting with the most excruciating pain. A kind of blackness enveloped me. I was very aware of the feeling of being suspended in it.

The next thing I remember is the feeling of waking up. I was in my bed in my own room. I sat up. And the image of my room dissolved. I stood up. I was naked! The motion of standing made me sick again.

I recognized some of the landmarks. I was about half a mile from don Juan's house, near the place of his *Datura* plants. . . .[31]

The solanaceous alkaloids also lead the user into believing he is a lycanthrope (changed into a wolf or similar predatory animal). How common are the accounts of witches partially transformed into animals, or men as werewolves stalking the medieval European forest. And how essential the ointment was, according to an account by Boguet (1602):

I have seen those named go on all-fours in a room just as they did when they were in the fields. But they said that it was impossible for them to turn themselves into wolves since they had no more ointment by being imprisoned. Thus, for some the solanaceous ointment was a means of metamorphosizing to werewolves while for others of experiencing the witches' flight.[29]

These hallucinogens did not come into general use in Europe because their anti-Christian aspects were avoided at a time when the church was an intimate part of most people's lives. Furthermore, there surely are health risks associated with the use of any tropane alkaloids, and this must have been recognized by the same persons who knew of their extraordinary powers.

BELLADONNA, HENBANE, MANDRAKE

Native throughout Europe, the non-European Mediterranean, and with henbane extending into western Asia, the species *Atropa belladonna, Hyoscyamus niger,* and *Mandragora officinarum* have a centuries-long association with magical

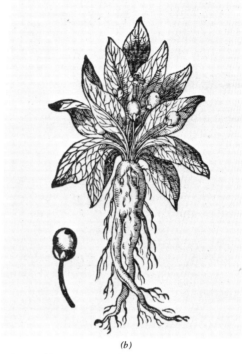

Figure 18-8 *Mandragora officinarum* containing scopolamine and long associated with mysticism and magic. According to folklore the male-appearing plant (a) was more robust, the female (b) more delicate.

practices and mysticism. All contain scopolamine, which is known to be hallucinogenic, as well as hyoscyamine and atropine. Belladonna is well known as a highly toxic species, and it has been employed as a poison since early classic times. *Hyoscyamus* species (henbanes) are also extremely toxic, but in limited doses they have a long history of use in domestic medicine for inducing sleep, for nerves, and for toothaches.

Of these genera *Mandragora* (mandrake) is surrounded by the greatest folklore. Like henbane it is recommended as a sedative and for nervous conditions; it once served as a pain killer during surgery, and in some parts of Europe as an aphrodisiac as well. Notwithstanding these virtues, it was greatly feared in the Middle Ages, not just because of toxicity but because its folklore was bound up

with the doctrine of signatures, according to which the stouter, more robust, male-looking roots would be appropriate for certain masculine diseases and difficulties, and the more delicate parts were useful for treating more female-oriented problems (Fig. 18-8). Mandrake plants also had orgiastic and magical applications involving the sexes.

DATURA AND ALLIED GENERA

Datura, a genus of about 20 species, distributed worldwide, and *Methysticodendron,* a monotypic genus of Andean Colombia, are rich in scopolamine. Their epicenter of diversity is in the New World, with two areas of concentrated use as hallucinogens: Andean South America (*Datura* subg. *Brugmansia* and *Methysticodendron*), and southwestern

United States and Mexico (*Datura inoxia*, the most used, and *D. discolor, D. ceratocaula, D. stramonium, D. wrightii*).

Methysticodendron is usually used as an infusion of the leaves by the Indians. It is today known only from cultivation and is propagated by the natives specifically for medicinal and narcotic purposes. Its reputation as potent and dangerous to use correlates well with the high proportion of scopolamine—up to 80% of total alkaloids that consist of 0.3% of leaves and stems. Very often the trees are the exclusive property of the medicine men, who employ the hallucinogen in difficult cases of diagnosis of disease, divination, prophecy, or witchcraft.

Among the Mexican and adjacent American Indians today, the local *Datura* species are widely used ceremonially. The roots often belong only to the priests, sorcerers, and diviners, and no one else is allowed to collect them. The rain priests, for example, chew the roots and ask the spirits of the dead to intercede with the gods for rain. Extracts as a concoction or as a salve are basic to adolescent initiation rites of many tribes, while others believe it possible to obtain supernatural allies through the drug and gain much power by the induced visions. Still its use was always considered dangerous, and much care is necessary in preparation and use, as don Juan so clearly outlined to Castaneda in relation to the devil's weed, *Datura inoxia*.[31]

Any part of these plants causes hallucinations. The oldest known record is of jimson weed (*Datura stramonium*), as reported in 1705 from Virginia:

The *James-Town* Weed (which resembles Thorny Apple of *Peru*, and I take to be the Plant so call'd) is supposed to be one of the greatest Coolers in the World. This being an early Plant, was gather'd very young for a boil'd Salad, by some of the Soldiers sent thither, to pacifie the Troubles of *Bacon*; and some of them eat plentifully of it, the Effect of which was a very pleasant Comedy; for they turn'd natural Fools upon it for several Days: One would blow up a Feather in the Air; another wou'd dart Straws at it with much Fury; and another stark naked was sitting up in a Corner, like a Monkey, grinning and making Mows at them; a Fourth would fondly kiss, and paw his Companions, and snear in their Faces, with a Countenance more antick, than any in a *Dutch* Droll. In this frantick Condition they were confined, lest they should in their Folly destroy themselves; though it was observed, that all their Actions were full of Innocence and good Nature. Indeed, they were not very cleanly; for they would have wallow'd in their own Excrements, if they had not been prevented. A Thousand such simple Tricks they play'd, and after Eleven Days, return'd to themselves again, not remembring any thing that had pass'd.[32]

Intentional use varies from smoking *Datura* leaves for respiratory diseases (Chapter 12) to using *D. fastuosa* for ensuring fertility during female puberty initiations in southern Africa.[33] There is a growing use of *D. stramonium* to induce hallucinations (e.g., homemade tea extract of boiled seeds). In one sample, as many as one-half hallucinated and one-quarter exhibited delirium and serious toxic symptoms.[34] The severely intoxicated user is usually acutely ill with fever, flushed, with dilated pupils, and in an incapacitating state of confused delirium. The usual hallucinations appear as a parade of material objects: flowers, sport cars, girls. One sees these objects usually in their simple colors, certainly not in the brilliant and shifting interplay of light and color seen during LSD or mescaline intoxication. Some users show marked tendencies to aggressive and violent behavior, similar to that observed during amphetamine abuse. Few deaths result from poisonings with these alkaloids, despite these alarming clinical signs, but the user must be controlled or he may harm himself or others. On analyzing five deaths brought on by the mental state of those using stramonium, Gowdy[34] observed that two wandered into the desert and died of exposure, one walked into a lake and drowned, and two drowned in a pond while searching for red-eyed dolphins. If the five could have been restrained, all would probably have recovered from the acute phase in 24 hours, although pupil dilation may continue for a week. Experimenting with these anticholinergic agents is dangerous, especially when no one is around to attend the user.

FLY AGARIC, THE PLANT GOD

The second group of compounds, removed structurally from the typical tryptamine derivates, are the isoxazoles found in *Amanita muscaria*. This mushroom, known as fly agaric, is widely distributed in the North Temperate zone, although the Eurasian race appears to have important morphological and chemical differences from the North American forms (Fig. 18-9). The active hallucinogenic compounds are ibotenic acid and pantherine (muscimol).

From this sober introduction of fly agaric, we begin to discuss one of the most exciting deductive books ever written on plant-man interrelations. We refer to R. Gordon Wasson's incredible *SOMA*,[4] a document that evolved around the identification of probably the only plant man has ever deified. In his introduction Wasson describes how a people calling themselves Aryans some 2000 years before the birth of Christ swept into Afghanistan and India from the northwest. Their language was Indo-European, the Vedic tongue, and they possessed a hereditary priesthood with elaborate and sometimes bizarre rituals and sacrifices. They had many gods, but unique among them was Soma: a god, a

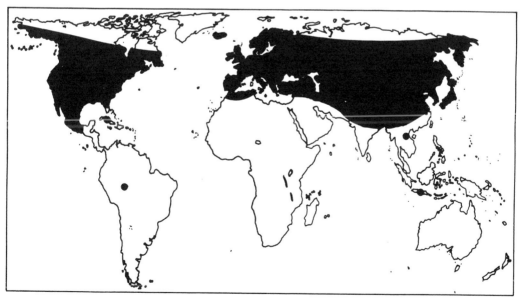

Figure 18-9 Generalized world distribution of *Amanita muscaria* (Adapted from R Singer, "Hongos alucinogenos," *Bol Acad Nac Cienc* **41**(1): 36, 1959, and reprinted with permission of the author.)

plant, and the juice of that plant. It was a very real god, something quite tangible, not just a symbol of a spiritual truth, like bread and wine in the Christian communion, but a miraculous drink that spoke for itself.

Fortunately for civilization the hymns of this religion were written, as they are today the only source of information about the period. This material, the Rig Veda, tells of an amazing hallucinogen used in the Aryan religion; but our inability to translate the Vedic descriptive words prevented us from identifying the kind of plant involved until Wasson delved into the past and presented us with a logical answer to this historic mystery. Soma, he concluded, is the mushroom fly agaric.

What is the evidence, circumstantial and direct, for this decision? According to the Rig Veda, Soma is without leaves, seeds, or branches. Its dazzling red skin is like the hide of the bull, its dress like that of a sheep, with woolly fragments remaining when the envelop bursts. Soma has a head (mushroom cap) and a stem or stalk (mainstay of the sky or pillar of the world). Does this description not fit the fly agaric (Fig. 2-3b)?

There is much more. Wasson was able to relate a reference in one of the Vedic hymns describing ceremonial urine drinking to a similar ritual practiced by scattered tribes in Siberia. Muscimol from this mushroom is the only known hallucinogen excreted by our kidneys unaltered, or at least with active metabolites, and many tribesmen practiced ritualistic drinking of the urine of intoxicated individuals until very recent times.

But with time and the absence of the mushroom in their new home, succeeding generations of Aryans lost the identity of their god Soma and with it hallucinogenic power. It was clear that the priesthood controlled the people's accessibility

to the plant, undoubtedly the seeing of gods was not open to all:

We have drunk the Soma, we are become immortals
We are arrived at the light, we have found the gods
What now can hostility do to us, what the malice of mortals,
O immortal Soma!

There is even a symbiotic relationship between the fungus and a higher plant. Wasson notes that in the forests of Siberia, the Siberian birch was much revered by custom, for it was always the tree the shaman chose, building his shelter around its base and climbing when in his trances. Why? Because this birch is the preferred symbiont for the fly agaric. Such an apparently inexplicable association of the two plants would not be missed by a primitive people surviving by observations of natural events such as this, even if clouded with magic and mystery. Are these the legendary Tree of Life and the Marvelous Herb? It would seem so. Furthermore, as the tribes of Siberia thousands of years before Christ spread their way to the subcontinent of Asia and elsewhere, perhaps even to the shores of the Mediterranean, it is not difficult to imagine the words of the parables eventually written and passed to us in Genesis. There is a haunting similarity in Genesis 3:1-5:

The serpent was more crafty than any wild creature that the Lord God had made. He said to the woman, "Is it true that God has forbidden you to eat from any tree in the garden?" The woman answered the serpent, "We may eat the fruit of any tree in the garden, except for the tree in the middle of the garden; God has forbidden us either to eat or to touch the fruit of that; if we do, we shall die." The serpent said, "Of course you will not die. God knows that as soon as you eat it, *your eyes will be opened and you will be like gods knowing both good and evil.*"[35] (italics added)

Others propose that even Christ was the personification of a fertility cult based on the use of the hallucinogenic *Amanita muscaria*.[36]

It happens that one of the most widespread of all the hallucinogens, with a long history in Asia and perhaps Europe, is only rarely used today. A notable exception is among the young people of the west coast of North America, where use of several hallucinogenic indole mushrooms has in some places reached epidemic proportions. This legacy from the "hippie generation" has been known from California to British Columbia for some years. For hallucinogenic purposes experienced pickers have been eating *Conocybe cyanopus, Gymnopilus spectabilis, Panaeolus subbalteatus, Psilocybe baecystis, P. cyanescens, P. pelliculosa, P. semilanceata,* and *P. silvatica,* in addition to *Amanita muscaria*. Inability to differentiate these from the more harmful species has caused serious cases of mushroom poisoning.[37]

MARIHUANA

Plants having hallucinogenic properties usually possess active compounds containing nitrogen, but one important compound is nonnitrogenous. This is Δ'-3,4-*trans*-tetrahydrocannabinol (Δ'-THC), largely responsible for the psychoactivity of marihuana or *Cannabis sativa* (Cannabaceae), although other tetrahydrocannabinols are present and may help induce a euphoric state. These compounds are found in varying amounts in the resin of a species botanically so notorious for variation that it may represent three closely allied species.[38] The fresh plant contains almost exclusively cannabidiolic acids, the precursor of the active THCs, which are transformed during the drying and storage of the material, during extraction. Transformation may also occur

during smoking; indeed, the effective dose on smoking is 200–250 μg/kg; on ingestion it is 300–480 μg/kg.

The more fibrous type of plant, which became widely disseminated throughout Europe and North America as escapes from the eighteenth-century hemp plantations is very low in biologically active material. In the flowering tops of the plants, Δ'-THC content is often less than 0.2% and rarely reaches 1%. This type is commonly sold for smoking in western Europe, Canada, and the United States, and is used in India (bhang) as a weak drink or in candy. The plants having more druglike properties have been selected over the centuries, especially in Asia where greatest diversity would logically exist among the indigenous species, not for their fibrous quality but rather for their high Δ'-THC concentrations, which range between 3.4 and 4.8% and may reach 6%. This is the popular marihuana of India (e.g., ganja when smoked and often mixed with tobacco), southeastern Asia, the Arab world (as hashish, the resin from pistillate flowers being eaten), parts of Africa, and much of tropical America. Millions of Arabs, for example, ingest hashish in significant amounts; consumption unexpectedly rose in the United States in 1973 to a level sufficient to provide the equivalent of 20 joints for every man, woman, and child. 420,700 were arrested that year on marihuana charges, a 43% increase over the previous year.

Early use and domestication of *Cannabis sativa* (Fig. 18-10) is lost in the antiquity of Asia. It was valued as long ago as 6000 BC in China; the Assyrians used it as incense, and in India and Africa the drug played major roles in religion and magic, as an aphrodisiac, and in activities requiring endurance or physical effort. An early mention of its intoxicating resin dates from 600 BC when Herodotus wrote that the Scythians burned its seeds to produce

428

a narcotic smoke. Galen recorded the use of hemp in cakes (the first magic brownies) which, if eaten in sufficient quantity, would induce intoxication. In the thirteenth century the notorious hashishans committed political murders throughout Asia Minor in return for *Cannabis* resin.[1] Yet its most universal value is as an euphoric narcotic: the user finds himself in a dreamy state of altered consciousness, often with a feeling of well-being, exaltation, and inner joy. But this extremely good feeling may alternate with states of depression where panic and fear of death are experienced. Commonly ideas are disrupted, uncontrollable, and sometimes plentiful. Vivid hallucinations may be experienced—they sometimes are pleasant and have sexual overtones.

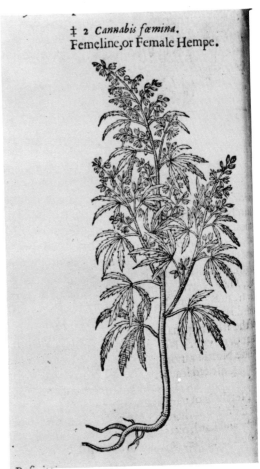

Figure 18-10b *Cannabis sativa,* male (from J Gerard, *The Herball,* ed 2, 1636). (Gerard often had male and female plants identified incorrectly—if a plant produced fruit, i.e., gave rise to the next generation, it had to be male in 16th century eyes.)

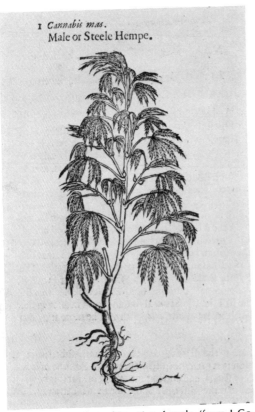

Figure 18-10a *Cannabis sativa,* female (from J Gerard, *The Herball,* ed 2, 1636).

Marihuana has been used to treat glaucoma, and it shows antibiotic activity against Gram + bacteria; but by and large cosmopolitan medicine maintains that it does not present a pharmacological property that could justify its use as a therapeutic agent more effective than any presently in use.[39]

What are the physical, pharmacological, and physiological effects of using marihuana? A dose-related increase in heart rate is the most consistent physical symptom observed. Daily users develop physiological and psychological tolerance to the drug leading to increased dosage. Δ'-THC is highly fat soluble and binds to plasma and cellular proteins; its metabolites accumulate in the brain and other tissues, and it affects the central nervous system by altering the turnover rate of the major neurotransmitters norepinephrine, serotonin, and acetylcholine.

Do these characteristics affect man to any important degree? Until very recently, the notion that marihuana is harmless has enjoyed a high degree of acceptability. Since 1969, however, evidence suggesting potential hazards has accumulated at a rapid pace and, if corroborated, we may find that marihuana is far more dangerous than originally believed.

We are not saying that smoking only a few cigarettes will cause permanent harm, for the chances are that such moderate use will not prove injurious to most people, but the new evidence does suggest that the effects are cumulative and dose related and that prolonged heavy use of marihuana, or less frequent use of hashish, is associated with a number of potential hazards. In summary the most current research indicates that *Cannabis* use:

1. May cause chromosomal damage that could affect the user's health.
2. May cause the disruption of cellular metabolism (e.g., synthesis of DNA) and may interfere with the functioning of the immune system.
3. May mimic hormones or act on hormonal regulators and so produce impotence, temporary sterility, and femalelike breasts in men.
4. May cause potentially irreversible brain damage.
5. *Is severely debilitating to the bronchial tract and lungs with heavy smoking.*
6. *Causes personality changes that lead*

to a marked deterioration in what is normally considered good mental health.[40]

Our italics serve to emphasize the relatively noncontroversial dangers to our health of *Cannabis* spp.; more research is required before the questionable status of the others is changed.

Cannabis intoxication prevails almost throughout the world and should be considered on a worldwide basis. Medically and botanically our knowledge of this plant and its action on man is little known, but we must not lose sight of its prevalent use under two completely different sets of social circumstances:

Endemically in poor agrarian societies (Middle East, India, Jamaica) or amidst an impoverished proletariat to escape from the daily dreariness of a marginal existence. *Cannabis* is the most available drug and is preferentially used; it is the opium of the poor. These societies are stagnant.

Epidemically amidst the educated affluent young who are disenchanted by the offerings of a technological society and who seek instant pleasure. . . . Marihuana intoxication . . . is part of the pandemic toxicomania which has developed in the second half of this century in the Western world dominated by Anglo-Saxon technology.[39]

The reader is referred to the reports on marihuana use[41] presented to the governments of the United States and Canada, and to a few of many books on the subject.[42]

LITERATURE CITED

1. Schultes RE, Hofmann A. 1973. *The Botany and Chemistry of Hallucinogens.* Charles C Thomas, Springfield, Ill. 267 p.
2. Hoffer A, Osmond H. 1967. *The Hallucinogens.* Academic Press, New York and London. 626 p. Copyright © by Academic Press, Inc., and reprinted with their permission and that of the second author, p. 53–55.

3. Schultes, RE. 1972. The ethnotoxicological significance of additives to New World hallucinogens. *Plant Sci Bull* 18(4): 34–40; Hallucinogens of plant origin. 1969. *Science* 163: 245–254.

4. Wasson RG. 1969. *SOMA Divine Mushroom of Immortality.* Harcourt Brace Jovanovich, New York. 381 p; Wasson RG. 1972. *SOMA and the Fly-agaric.* Botanical Museum of Harvard University, Cambridge, Mass. 58 p.

5. Farnsworth NR. 1968. Hallucinogenic plants. *Science* 162: 1086–1092; Farnsworth NR. 1969. Some hallucinogenic and related plants, 367–399. In JE Gunckel (ed), *Current Topics in Plant Science.* Academic Press, New York, London; Farnsworth NR. 1972. Psychotomimetic and related higher plants. *J. Psychedelic Drugs* 5: 67–74.

6. Furst PT (ed). 1972. *Flesh of the Gods.* Praeger, New York and Washington. 304 p.

7. La Barre W. 1969. *The Peyote Cult,* enlarged edition. Schocken Books, New York. 260 p.

8. Aaronson B, Osmond H. 1970. *Psychedelics: The Use and Implications of Hallucinogenic Drugs.* Doubleday-Anchor, Garden City, NY. 512 p; Brown FC. 1972. *Hallucinogenic Drugs.* Charles C Thomas, Springfield, Ill. 154 p; Efron DH (ed-in-chief). 1967. *Ethnopharmacologic Search for Psychoactive Drugs.* US Public Health Service Publ No 1645, Government Printing Office, Washington, DC. 468 p; Emboden WA Jr. 1972. *Narcotic Plants.* Macmillan, New York. 168 p; Gjerstad G. Naturally occurring hallucinogens I. *Quart J Crude Drug Res* 11(3): 1774–1784, 1971; II. 11(4): 1797–1805, 1971; III. 12(1): 1849–1864, 1972; Taylor N. 1949. *Flight from Reality.* Duell, Sloan and Pearce, New York. 237 p; Weil GM, Metzner R, Leary T (eds). 1965. *The Psychedelic Reader.* University Books, New York. 260 p.

9. Huxley A. 1968. *The Doors of Perception* and *Heaven and Hell.* Chatto & Windus, London. 152 p. (Originally published in 1954 and 1956, respectively.)

10. Der Marderosian A. 1966. Current status of hallucinogens in the Cactaceae. *Am J Pharm* 138: 204–212; Marriott A, Rachlin CK. 1971. *Peyote.* New American Library, New York. 128 p; Bergman RL. 1971. Navajo peyote use: its apparent safety. *Am J Psychiatr* 128: 695–699.

11. Dobkin M. 1968. Folk curing with a psychedelic cactus in the north coast of Peru. *Int J Soc Psychiatr* 15: 23–32; Dobkin M. 1968. *Trichocereus pachanoi*—a mescaline cactus used in folk healing in Peru. *Econ Bot* 22: 191–194.

12. Weil AT. 1969. Nutmeg and other psychoactive groceries, 356–366. In JE Gunckel (ed), *Current Topics in Plant Science.* Academic Press, New York.

13. Wasson RG. 1962. The hallucinogenic mushrooms of Mexico and psilocybin: a bibliography. *Bot Mus Leafl, Harvard Univ* 20: 25–73.

14. Schultes RE. 1954. A new narcotic snuff from the northwest Amazon. *Bot Mus Leafl, Harvard Univ* 16: 241–260.

15. Agurell SB, Holmstedt B, Lingren JE et al. 1968. Identification of two new β-carboline alkaloids in South American hallucinogenic plants. *Biochem Pharmacol* 17: 2487–2488.

16. de Rios MD. 1972. *Visionary Vine.* Chandler, San Francisco. 161 p; Rivier L, Lindgren J-E. 1972. "Ayahuasca," the South American hallucinogenic drink: an ethnobotanical and chemical investigation. *Econ Bot* 26: 101–129; Schultes RE. 1957. The identity of the malpighiaceous narcotics of South America. *Bot Mus Leafl, Harvard Univ* 18: 1–56.

17. Prance GT. 1970. Notes on the use of plant hallucinogens in Amazonian Brazil. *Econ Bot* 24: 62–68.

18. Weil A. 1972. *The Natural Mind.* Houghton Mifflin, Boston. 229 p.

19. Leary T. 1968. *High Priest.* World, New York and Cleveland. 353 p.

20. Maugh TH II. 1973. LSD and the drug culture: new evidence of hazard. *Science* 179: 1221–1222.

21. Jacobson CB, Berlin CM. 1972. Possible reproductive detriment in LSD users. *JAMA* 222: 1367–1373.

22. Voss EW Jr, Babb JE, Metzel P et al. 1973. In vitro effect of D-lysergic acid diethylamide on immunoglobulin synthesis. *Biochem Biophys Res Commun* 50: 950–956.

23. Schultes RE. 1941. A contribution to our knowledge of *Rivea corymbosa,* the narcotic ololiuqui of the Aztecs. Harvard Botanical Museum, Cambridge, Mass.

24. Hofmann A, Tscherter H. 1960. Isolierung von Lysergsäure-Alkaloiden aus der mexikanischen Zauberdroge Ololiuqui (*Rivea corymbosa* [L.] Hall.f.). *Experientia* 16: 414.

25. Der Marderosian A. 1967. Psychotomimetic indoles in the Convolvulaceae. *Am J Pharm* 139: 19–26.

26. Bove FJ. 1970. *The Story of Ergot.* S. Karger, Basel and New York. 97 p; Fuller JG. 1969. *The Day of St. Anthony's Fire.* Hutchinson Publ

Group, London. 310 p; Taylor N. 1965. *Plant Drugs That Changed the World.* Dodd, Mead, New York. Doctor Hosack and St. Anthony's Fire, Chapter 5, pp 58–71; Caporael LR. 1976. Ergotism: the satan loosed in Salem? *Science* **192:** 21–26.

27. Pope HG Jr. 1969. *Tabernanthe iboga:* an African narcotic plant of social importance. *Econ Bot* **23:** 174–184.

28. Balandrier G. 1957. *Ambiguous Africa: Cultures in Collision.* Pantheon, Paris. (Translated by H. Weaver, 1966).

29. Harner MJ. 1974. The role of hallucinogenic plants in European witchcraft, 125–150. In MJ Harner (ed), *Hallucinogens and Shamanism.* Oxford University Press, New York. Copyright ©1973 by Oxford University Press and reprinted by permission, p 130–1, 133–4, 138–9.

30. Kreig MB. 1966. *Green Medicine.* Bantam Books, New York (p 53). 336 p.

31. Castaneda C. 1968. *The Teachings of Don Juan: A Yaqui Way of Knowledge.* University of California Press, Berkeley and Los Angeles. 196 p. Copyright © by *The Regents of the University of California*; reprinted by permission of the University of California Press, p 127–129. Also *A Separate Reality: Further Conversations with Don Juan.* 1971. Simon & Schuster, New York. 317 p; *Journey to Ixtlan: The Lessons of Don Juan.* 1972. Simon & Schuster, New York. 315 p; *Tales of Power.* 1974. Simon & Schuster, New York. 287 p; Don Juan and the sorcerer's apprentice. *Time* (cover story) 5 Mar 1973: 36–38, 43–45.

32. Beverley R. 1705. *The History and Present State of Virginia,* Book 2. London.

33. Johnston TF. 1972. *Datura fastuosa:* Its use in Tsonga girls' initiation. *Econ Bot* **26:** 340–351.

34. Gowdy JM. 1972. Stramonium intoxication. *JAMA* **221:** 585–587.

35. *The New English Bible, The Old Testament.* Oxford and Cambridge Univ Presses, 1970.

36. Allegro JM. 1970. *The Sacred Mushroom and the Cross.* Doubleday, Garden City, NY.

37. Wieland T. 1968. Poisonous principles of mushrooms of the genus *Amanita. Science* **159:** 946–152; *Mushroom Poisoning in the Pacific Northwest.* Puget Sound Mycological Society, Seattle. 1972.

38. Schultes RE, Klein WM, Plowman T et al. 1974. *Cannabis:* an example of taxonomic neglect. *Bot Mus Leafl, Harvard Univ* **23:** 337–367; Anderson LC. 1974. A study of systematic wood anatomy in *Cannabis. Bot Mus Leafl Harvard Univ* **24:** 29–36.

39. Nahas GG. 1973. *Marihuana—Deceptive Weed.* Raven Press, New York. 334 p; Nahas GG. 1974. Marihuana: toxicity, tolerance, and therapeutic efficacy. *Drug Ther* **4**(1): 33–35, 38–39, 43, 46–47.

40. Maugh TH II. 1974. Marihuana: the grass may no longer be greener. *Science* **185:** 683–685; Maugh TH II. 1974. Marihuana (II): does it damage the brain? *Science* **185:** 775–776; Maugh TH II. 1975. Marihuana: new support for immune and reproductive hazards. *Science* **190:** 868–867; Tinklenberg JR (ed). 1975. *Marijuana and Health Hazards.* Academic Press, New York. 188 p.

41. *Marihuana: A Signal of Misunderstanding.* 1972 First Report of the National Commission on Marihuana and Drug Abuse. Government Printing Office, Washington, DC. 184 p, appendix 1252 p; *Cannabis.* 1972. A Report of the Commission of Inquiry into the Non-Medical Use of Drugs. Information Canada, Ottawa. 426 p.

42. Andrews G, Vinkenoog S (eds). 1967. *The Book of Grass.* Grove Press, New York. 242 p; Grinspoon L. 1971. *Marihuana Reconsidered.* Harvard University Press, Cambridge, Mass. 443 p; Lewis B. 1970. *The Sexual Power of Marijuana.* PH Wyden, New York. 177 p; Mikuriya TH (ed). 1973. *Marijuana: Medical Papers 1839-1972.* Medi-Comp Press, Oakland, Calif. 465 p; Paton WDM, Crown J (eds). 1972. *Cannabis and its Derivatives.* Oxford University Press, London. 198 p; Saltman J. 1969. *Marijuana and Your Child.* Grosset & Dunlap, New York. 123 p.

Chapter 19
Depressants

A number of drugs that act to depress the central nervous system produce effects of euphoria and well-being beginning with sedation (calming, tranquilizing), followed by hypnosis (sleep), general anesthesia, and coma, and ending with death from respiratory failure as the dose increases to higher levels. When controlled, all are enormously useful drugs in medicine and society, but all are subject to abuse. With depressant drugs abuse may lead to addiction, a compulsion characterized by three features: a tendency to increase dose because tolerance develops, appearance of physiological changes when drug use is discontinued (i.e., withdrawal symptoms occur), and a strong desire to continue taking the drug.[1] This addictive property of many depressants, which include alcohol, barbiturates, tranquilizers, and opium and its derivatives morphine, heroin, and methadone, is their great danger to mankind.

We know little of the composition of native and domestic depressants used in treating convulsions and insomnia, and as sedatives (Chapter 6).

ALCOHOL

Alcohol in several forms—beer from cereals, wine from fruits and berries, and mead from honey—was well known by the beginning of recorded history. Some authorities suggest that mead, possibly the oldest of alcoholic beverages, appeared during the Paleolithic Age (ca. 8000 BC), and unquestionably man has indulged in alcohol for religious, social, and medicinal purposes ever since.

Medicinal use by the Egyptians is recorded among the papyri, which attest to the use of beer and wine as vehicles for other medicines, and as tranquilizers and soporifics. Once distillation had been developed by the Moslems, many of the distillates, such as brandy from wine and whisky from beer, were mixed with sweeteners and herbs for use by physicians to counter a variety of illnesses. Ethanol was the potent constituent in many such concoctions, causing recognizable physiological effects of relaxation and tranquility, and its effective role in these and numerous patent medicines of today must not be discounted. Alcohol has numerous other uses: as a solvent to remove oils such as those from poison ivy, as an evaporator to cool the skin during fevers, as a disinfectant, as a pain reliever, as an appetite stimulator, and as a treatment for the common cold (to make the patient sleepy enough to rest).

Most alcohol is consumed not for medicinal purposes, however, but for pleasure and solace in this hectic world, where hundreds of millions drink liquor, beer, or wine; however an estimated 9 million persons or about 10% of the drinkers in the United States, have become enslaved by alcohol.

ALCOHOLIC BEVERAGES

The basis for all alcoholic beverages is fermentation, the chemical action of yeast (commonly *Saccharomyces cerevisiae*) acting on sugar in the presence of water. Yeast recombines the carbon, hydrogen, and oxygen of sugar and water into ethyl alcohol (ethanol, C_2H_5OH) and carbon dioxide. The source of sugar is most fruit, frequently grapes, or malted barley (sprouted grain that when killed retains the enzymes necessary to convert the starch of grains and mashes to sugar). The appropriate yeasts, often widespread wherever the grapes or other plants grow, are selected for their tolerance to the alcohol they metabolize, which normally has an upper limit of about 15%.

To obtain alcohol at concentrations higher than that produced by fermentation, alcohol is heated and vapors are collected and condensed into liquid again, in a process known as distillation. This increases the percentage of alcohol, because the distillate has a lower boiling point than water, and thus becomes more concentrated in the condensed liquid than in the original solution.

When man mastered the process of distillation he increased to five the basic forms of alcoholic beverages available: table wines, fortified or dessert wines, beers, liqueurs, and distilled beverages (spirits).[2] Wines, containing about 12% alcohol, are widely produced throughout temperate regions, using grapes as the chief source of sugar. Dessert wines (e.g., port, sherry) are ordinary wines that have been fortified with additional alcohol to reach concentrations of about 20%. Beers are all made by fermenting carbohydrate extracted from malted barley and boiling with hops (dried flowers of *Humulus lupulus*), the latter giving beer its characteristic pungent flavor. The types of beer vary in alcoholic content (e.g., lager 3–6%, stout 4–8%) as well as in hop and malt content.

Liqueurs have a high sugar content (up to 50%), an alcoholic concentration between 20 and 50%, and they contain various herbs, spices, and extracts, often in complex and secret mixtures that impart distinctiveness to the final beverage. Brandy, distilled from grape wine, is probably the oldest of the commercial liqueurs. Probably the first whiskey was made commercially in Ireland during the twelfth century, and there are now several major types: bourbon from corn with rye and malted barley, scotch from malted barley, Irish whiskey from malted and unmalted barley, and rye from rye or malt barley and unmalted rye. These grains are brewed with water to form a strong beer (5-10% alcohol) minus the hops, then distilled and aged in oak barrels for 2 to 8 years before blending. Generally the final product contains 40% to 50% alcohol. Other distilled beverages include rum (distillate of fermented molasses containing 40-70% alcohol), gin (distillate of any fermentable carbohydrate, flavored during a second distillation with juniper berries and containing 35-50% alcohol), and vodka (distillate of potatoes or most other carbohydrates, but free of other flavors, and with 35-50% alcohol). There are many other distilled spirits, including tequila and mescal, and a wide variety of undistilled beverages made locally throughout the world by indigenous peoples (Table 19-1). There are dangers associated with home brewing, however, for during fermentation various yeasts and bacterial contaminants may metabolize fusel oil components, and n-butyl and n-amyl alcohols that render the final product undesirable and even dangerous to health.[3] Headaches are a common consequence.

The origin of bourbon whiskey in the United States is an example of ingenuity typical of man anywhere in the world who wants an intoxicating beverage. Faced with mounting costs for transportation and little income from their grain

Table 19-1 Examples of Plants Used as Carbohydrates Sources in Making Alcoholic Beverages for Domestic Use

Plant Group and Species	Locality	Remarks
RED ALGA		
Rhodymenia palmata	Kamchatka, Siberia	Natives use this seaweed as a base
FUNGUS		
Fomes auberianus	Tropics	Intoxicant, also causes fits and frenzy
ANGIOSPERMS		
ANACARDIACEAE		
Sclerocarya caffra	South Africa	Fruit
S. schweinfurthii	Tropical Africa	Fruit to prepare a beerlike beverage
APIACEAE		
Heracleum sphondylium	Eastern Europe	In Slavic countries boiled leaves and fruit used to prepare bartsch
ARECACEAE		
Hyphaene crinata	South Africa	Stem sap (this and other species of palm widely used)
ELAEAGNACEAE		
Elaeagnus multiflora	Japan	Fruit
FABACEAE		
Hymenaea courbaril	Brazil	Seed pulp
Prosopis nigra	Argentina	Fruit
P. pubescens	Southwestern United States and Mexico	Fruit used by Indians
RHAMNACEAE		
Zizyphus abyssinica	Malawi	Fruit for potent alcoholic beverages
SAPINDACEAE		
Paullinia cupana	Guarana, Brazil	Seeds mixed with cassava and water

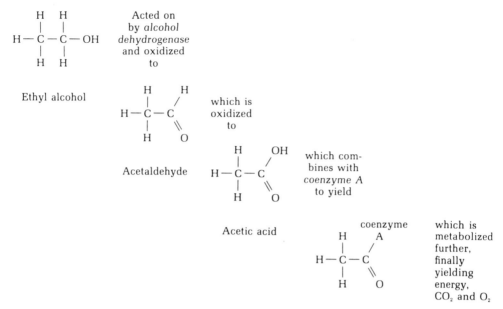

Figure 19-1   Metabolism of ethyl alcohol. (From OS Ray, *Drugs, Society, and Human Behavior*, p 85, fig 6-1, 1974 updated, The CV Mosby Co, St. Louis, reprinted with permission.)

crops west of the Appalachian Mountains, the eighteenth-century farmers of western Pennsylvania, western Virginia, and eastern Kentucky, decided to take matters into their own hands. Six barrels of flour made one barrel of whiskey. This could profitably be shipped east over the mountains, and distillation began on a grand scale. One of the first to realize the potential here was Elijah Craig, a Baptist minister in Bourbon County, Kentucky, who about 1789 began storing his whiskey in charred new oak barrels, thereby originating a technique that gives bourbon its characteristic flavor.[1]

EFFECTS OF ALCOHOL

Alcohol requires no digestion and is absorbed rapidly and unchanged from the stomach and small intestine through the bloodstream. There it passes to the liver, is acted on by the enzyme alcohol dehydrogenase, and is eventually oxidized to carbon dioxide and oxygen (Fig. 19-1). The ability of alcohol dehydrogenase to metabolize alcohol varies greatly from individual to individual, but generally among moderate drinkers between 0.25 and 0.33 ounce of alcohol is oxidized per hour. If intake is faster than oxidation, blood concentration increases, and with that increase behavioral effects as described in Fig. 19-2 become apparent. In the United States the legal level of alcohol concentration in the blood is 0.15%, which for modest drinkers is gross intoxication; but levels beyond this are well known, individuals with 0.35% being described as dead drunk, those having 0.60% probably dead.

Besides passing to the liver, alcohol reaches the central nervous system, where it slows or anesthetizes brain activity. Though alcohol is a depressant, the initial feeling created is just the opposite as the barriers of self-control are

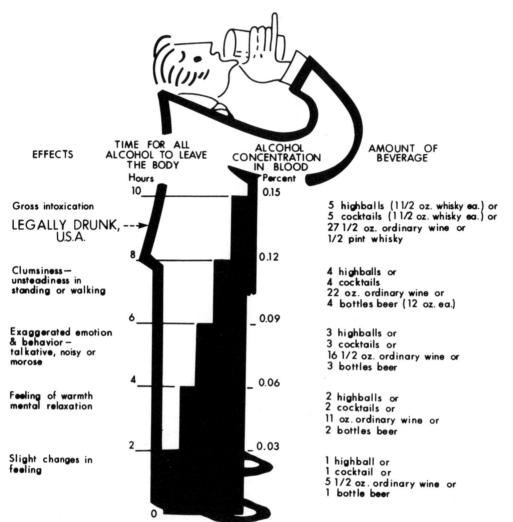

EFFECTS

Gross intoxication

LEGALLY DRUNK, ---
U.S.A.

Clumsiness—
unsteadiness in
standing or walking

Exaggerated emotion
& behavior —
talkative, noisy or
morose

Feeling of warmth
mental relaxation

Slight changes in
feeling

**TIME FOR ALL
ALCOHOL TO LEAVE
THE BODY**

Hours
10
8
6
4
2
0

**ALCOHOL
CONCENTRATION
IN BLOOD**

Percent
0.15
0.12
0.09
0.06
0.03

**AMOUNT OF
BEVERAGE**

5 highballs (1 1/2 oz. whisky ea.) or
5 cocktails (1 1/2 oz. whisky ea.) or
27 1/2 oz. ordinary wine or
1/2 pint whisky

4 highballs or
4 cocktails
22 oz. ordinary wine or
4 bottles beer (12 oz. ea.)

3 highballs or
3 cocktails or
16 1/2 oz. ordinary wine or
3 bottles beer

2 highballs or
2 cocktails or
11 oz. ordinary wine or
2 bottles beer

1 highball or
1 cocktail or
5 1/2 oz. ordinary wine or
1 bottle beer

Figure 19-2   Alcohol levels in the blood (after drinks taken on an empty stomach by a 150 lb individual). (Adapted from Time magazine, 22 April 1974, p. 77. Reprinted by permission from TIME, The Weekly Newsmagazine; Copyright Time Inc.) [4]

lifted and the drinker acts or speaks in ways his well-trained, sober self normally forbids. After a number of drinks, the motor centers of the brain are affected, causing clumsiness and unsteadiness in movements.

Nausea and Hangover

The nausea and upset stomach typically experienced by those who overindulge can probably be attributed to gastric irritation by alcohol. These reactions, and also headaches, may be partly an allergic response to congeners; also some natural products of fermentation found in aged, distilled spirits are quite toxic. The complete basis for the symptoms of the hangover is not known. Consequently a cure is elusive, although aspirin may alleviate the headache, and for some, fruit and vegetable juices help reduce fatigue, thirst, and other symptoms. We know of two native remedies, a leaf tea of *Dorstenia drakena* (Moraceae) used in Mexico to relieve hangovers, and an herbal tea of *Elsholtzia cristata* (Lamiaceae) consumed by the Ainu of Japan for treatment of alcoholic aftereffects. The value of these infusions, however, has not been ascertained.

Withdrawal

The nervous system usually becomes rapidly adapted to high levels of alcohol, although the upper limit of this tolerance is unclear. Few chronic alcoholics, however, are able to consume more than 28 to 32 ounces of 100 proof (50% alcohol) liquor per day and still function.

Withdrawal from alcohol may involve tremors, seizures, visual or auditory hallucinations or both, delirium tremens (frenzied excitement with tremors), and blackouts. Sobering a highly intoxicated alcoholic may take up to 48 hours. An intravenous infusion of fructose in which the sugar apparently speeds the metabolism of alcohol may rapidly relieve the sufferer from delirium tremens, the very drunk individual, or intoxicated persons who are unconscious and may be suffering from acute conditions such as head injury or other drug overdose.[5] Fructose treatment speeds the elimination of blood ethanol by approximately 25%.

Effect on Specific Organs

Heavy drinking provides abundant calories and energy that must be used immediately, for unlike most other foods, alcohol has no nutritional value. Since the calories in alcohol are not stored, they do not alone make one fat. The alcoholic usually has a weak appetite, however, and often suffers from malnutrition and vitamin deficiency.

Excessive intake of alcohol also affects the production and activity of white blood cells, which may lower one's disease-resisting capabilities. Characteristically, the alcoholic develops a fatty liver, and his chances of developing cirrhosis (liver cells replaced by fibrous scar tissue) are greatly increased. A damaged liver cannot adequately manufacture bile, which is necessary for the digestion of fats; thus the alcoholic often feels weak and suffers from chronic indigestion.

Recent research links heavy drinking to heart-muscle damage, deterioration of the brain, and damage to fetuses. Damage to the central nervous system and hormonal imbalance may result in impotence.

Who are the 10% of our population who become alcoholics? Recent metabolic and clinical studies suggest that genetic factors are active in the predisposition toward alcoholism. It is quite possible that complex polygenic inheritance may account at least in part for a tendency toward alcohol abuse, whether from inherited metabolic differences or inherited personality differences.[1,6] Whatever the basis for misuse of alcohol heavy drinkers were largely responsible for 25,000 auto deaths and 800,000 auto accidents in the United States during 1971.

BARBITURATES

The next most widely used depressant drugs of the central nervous system after alcohol are the barbiturates. About 10 billion sedative doses are manufactured each year in the United States.

Barbiturates are all synthetic compounds derived from barbituric acid, which is a combination of urea and malonic acid. The term is thought to have been derived from the name of the patron saint of artillery officers, St. Barbara.

At any rate, the saint's day was supposedly being celebrated, at a tavern frequented by Bayer, on the day he synthesized from urea the compound barbituric acid.[7] Depending on their use, dosage, and administration, barbiturates—commonly known as sleeping pills—produce all degrees of depression ranging from mild sedation to coma. They act on the cerebral centers and interfere with the passage of impulses in the brain. They depress brain function, and in large doses depress the brain centers responsible for maintaining the rhythm of respiration.

As noted, the barbiturates exert a powerful sedating action on the central nervous system; and properly prescribed and taken in small doses, they relieve tension and anxiety. Tranquilizers, however, are normally used today for sedation. In large doses (100–200 mg) they produce drowsiness and sleep for 6 hours or so.

Increasing use of barbiturates quickly produces tolerance and may create physical and psychic dependency considered by some to be as serious as that caused by heroin addiction. Indeed addiction to barbiturates may occur, and these depressant drugs represent an underrated current drug problem: the fatality rate is higher than that of any other type of addiction (more than 3000 barbiturate suicides per year, or 20% of all suicides in the United States, and more than 1500 deaths from accidental poisonings). Alcohol potentiates the barbiturates—the two depressants are synergistic—and the practice of using both undoubtedly accounts for the unusually high number of accidental self-poisonings and deaths from respiratory depression.

Since all barbiturates are considered dangerous addictive drugs, they should never be used except under a physician's supervision. Some depressants are barbital, phenobarbital, pentobarbital, secobarbital, amobarbital, butabarbital, cyclobarbital, heptabarbital, probarbital, talbutal, vinbarbital, and methaqualone (see under Aphrodisiacs, p. 331) and other nonbarbiturate drugs used as sleeping pills (chloral hydrate, Doriden). According to the Bureau of Narcotics and Dangerous Drugs, barbiturates are the principal drugs of abuse in the United States, outranking even heroin.

TRANQUILIZERS

Like alcohol and the barbiturates, tranquilizers depress the central nervous system, relieve tension and anxiety, and sometimes relax the skeletal muscles.

The minor tranquilizers, meprobamate (Miltown®, Equanil®), chlordiazepoxide (Librium®), and diazepam (Valium®) have effects so similar to the barbiturates that distinction is difficult. The major difference is that minor tranquilizers produce a little less sleepiness and interfere less with motor activities than do the barbiturates. As such, they are not normally chosen by those contemplating suicide; but in other respects, including the withdrawal and tolerance syndrome, they are similar.

The major tranquilizers belong to a group of derivates of phenothiazine, a drug synthesized in the last century but not developed until the 1950s. They are used for treating patients in acute or chronic psychoses, especially schizophrenia, which includes about 50% of the mental patients in North America. Since even massive doses will not make a patient unconscious, the drugs can be administered to calm the violent, the hyperexcited, and the fearful sufficiently to render them receptive to therapy. For example, the wide use of chlorpromazine for treating the schizophrenics, replacing insulin and electroconvulsive therapies, had reduced the population of mental hospitals in the United States from a peak of more than 550,000 patients in 1955 to 338,000 in 1970. There is no more dramatic evidence of the effectiveness of tranquilizers on the acutely disturbed.

The first tranquilizer was found in *Rauvolfia serpentina* (Apocynaceae), which proved to be an indole alkaloid reserpine.

Whenever Mahatma Gandhi felt the need to induce a state of philosophic detachment, he sipped tea brewed from the leaves of the plant that grows wild in India and in most of the world's tropical lands. For centuries, the plant was widely used for its calming effect. Holy men chewed it while meditating. Native medicine men employed it to treat highly agitated mental patients. It was even used to soothe fretful babies.

For a long time the plant was ignored by Western scientists. It was considered just mumbo-jumbo stuff that couldn't possibly live up to all the extravagant claims made for it. But in 1952, the plant made its debut in American medicine. . . .[8]

Today the drug is not much used in mental health therapy, but it remains the most important drug employed in the relief of a major killer, high blood pressure (Chapter 7).

KAVA

For a very long time, the natives of the South Pacific islands used the rhizomes and roots of *Piper methysticum* (Piperaceae) or kava to make a beverage that relaxed body and mind, induced refreshing sleep, and eased pain.

The rootstocks are initially handled in two ways: (a) they are reduced to fragments and chewed to a soft mass with saliva, the quid is mixed with cold water or coconut milk, and the foamy liquid is strained and consumed a few hours later; (b) they are grated and macerated in cold water or coconut milk, and the liquid is filtered before drinking. The kava prepared by chewing has a narcotic effect. It paralyzes muscles, particularly the lower limbs; it increases the force, but decreases the rapidity of the heart's action; and it at first stimulates, then depresses, respiration. Unlike alcohol, the drug does not impair mental alertness. A small quantity gives rise to a euphoric state of short duration characterized by tranquility and friendliness. In larger doses, the kava prepared by chewing disturbs vision (pupils become enlarged and respond slowly to light) and muscle coordination (staggering), and acts as a powerful hypnotic.[9] When the drink is prepared by grating, it is tonic and stimulant only and is often given to the sick and convalescent as well as to young mothers as a galactagogue.

Chewed kava is a cerebral depressant; the drug apparently steadies the pulse, does not raise body temperature, is diaphoretic, and counteracts obesity. The deep, dreamless sleep from kava is not followed by a hangover. The substance is addicting, however, and with continued use many natives, as well as patients using the extract dihydromethysticin, develop exfoliative dermatitis.[10]

From the root of kava have been isolated methysticin, yangonin, dihydromethysticin, and dihyrokawain, mostly lactones and resins variously estimated at between 3 and 4% of the root. Several compounds have been synthesized, but the principle (or principles) responsible for narcotic action is still unknown. Since physiological activity is significantly enhanced after the roots are chewed, it seems logical to suppose that the active components are acted on by digestive enzymes to produce their full effect.

Other species of *Piper* (e.g., *P. plantagineum* of the West Indies) are considered narcotic, but none has been studied.

OPIATES

Opium is a powerful drug derived from the poppy *Papaver somniferum* (Fig. 19-3), native to the Middle East. If its capsule is cut between the time the petals drop and before the capsule is mature—a period of about 10 days during the year-long growth of this annual—a milky sap emerges. When left in the open, the sap dries into the brown, gummy substance known as opium.

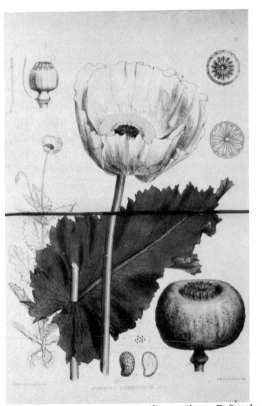

Figure 19-3 *Papaver somniferum* (from R Bentley and H Trimen, *Medicinal Plants* **1:** 18, 1880).

HISTORY

Throughout history opium has been a servant to man, but many men have also been dependent and addicted servants to it. Opium is possibly the oldest narcotic known, for as early as 4000 BC the Sumerians referred to it as the joy plant. The drug was used medicinally in ancient Greece and Rome, and Arabian traders introduced it into China. During the Middle Ages a variety of opium preparations appeared in the form of a laudanum or tincture (opium in about 10% ethanol), to ease pain and to create general euphoria. Thus the stage was set for the popularity of patent medicines containing opium in the nineteenth century.

In Europe, opium had by this time become widespread and popular. Notable writers, such as Thomas De Quincey, who was addicted by the age of 20 after initially using a laudanum to dull the pain of a toothache, wrote: "Opium gives and takes away. It defeats the steady habit of exertion; but it creates spasms of irregular exertion. It ruins the natural power of life; but it develops preternatural paroxysms of intermitting power" (*Confessions of an English Opium-Eater,* 1821). Similarly addicted were Elizabeth Browning and Samuel Coleridge (his *Kubla Khan* was said to have been composed in an opium reverie); in fact, little social or other stigma was associated with the frequent use of opium by the wealthy or for medicinal purposes. Godfrey's Cordial, for example, consisting of a mixture of opium, molasses, and sassafras, was very popular in England as a teething syrup for young children, a cough remedy, a cure for diarrhea and dysentery, and as an overall soothing syrup for neuralgic or rheumatic maladies among the old, miserable, and impoverished. Without opium, according to the nineteenth-century saying, the healing art would cease to exist.

There was little difference in North America. Some ladies took opium medicinals for the "vapors," others to counter pain and diarrhea; use was so general that a survey of Boston drugstores in 1888 revealed that of 10,000 prescriptions filled, 1481 contained opiates, and among those refilled three or more times, 78% had opiates.[11] By the turn of the century one out of every 400 Americans was caught in some kind of opiate habit, and there was little popular outcry to outlaw these substances. They were not viewed as a menace to society and perhaps, used as they were, they were not.

At other times opium use has assumed major international proportions. Probably introduced into China in about AD 1000, it was essentially monopolized by the elite, but was used only modestly. In the view of the last Ming emperor (1628–1644), it was not opium that was evil but the American plant called tobacco, being smoked by so many of his people. He forbid the use of tobacco, and gradually more and more opium was mixed with the New World plant; eventually only pure opium was smoked, from specially made pipes. Thus the Chinese introduced the world to opium smoking.

The use of opium in Asia was not limited to the Chinese. In India the drug had been cultivated and widely used for several centuries, and when the powerful East India Company and British suzerainty extended their influence over the subcontinent, opium became a major commercial crop, a virtual world monopoly by 1831. The huge market was China, where millions were addicted, even though smoking had been banned by the emperor a century before. Although the East India Company could not sell or transport opium directly to China, massive public auctions were held in India, and tons of opium were sold to British and American merchants (e.g., the opium clipper fleets from Boston and New York), who smuggled it into China through Canton. Everyone made vast sums of money—the East India Company, the merchants who bought and transported the goods, the Chinese middlemen, and the Hong merchants (a guild that enjoyed the foreign trade monopoly at Canton) who dispensed the opium throughout China. Only the Chinese people suffered from this addicting drug and from the staggering loss of currency and of goods (tea) used as payment.

The volume of the illicit opium trade continued to rise until in 1838 the emperor changed viceroys in Canton and installed an official whose integrity astonished the world. He took the imperial edicts literally and confiscated and destroyed all opium found on British and American ships in the river leading to Canton, as well as that found in the Hong warehouses. In one swoop this amounted to 2,640,000 pounds of opium. Few were happy about such a turn of events, and a year later, following a racial incident, the ignoble Opium Wars began. Within two years 10,000 British troops backed by the largest fleet in the world were victorious over 350 million Chinese. The emperor conceded Hong Kong island, but the victors got much more: reimbursement for the destroyed opium at Canton, broad trading rights within China including commerce in opium, and the opening of concession ports along the China coast for Western countries, which virtually owned and governed these areas as colonial states.

A decade later the Second Opium War weakened China further, and by this time all European powers and the United States got their pieces of China. Finally, in the Boxer Rebellion, bands of Chinese, dedicated to throwing foreigners out of their country, illustrated to the world the frustration of the Chinese people with both opium and foreigners. It was too much in a single package. In 1913, with about 25% of the Chinese addicted, great pressures within China and cries in Parliament and from the British people forced the British-Indian trade in opium to an end. By this time, however, much poppy was grown in China, and it was not until after World War II and the establishment of the People's Republic of China that illicit use of opium was virtually eliminated.

PHARMACOLOGY

Of the more than twenty-five alkaloids obtained from opium and its extracts, the most important are morphine (4–21%), codeine (0.8–2.5%), noscapine or narcotine (4–8%), papaverine (0.5–2.5%), and thebaine (0.5–2%). By far the most significant are morphine and its salts, which are strongly analgesic, hypnotic, and narcotic. Heroin, formed by the acetylation of morphine, has similar but more pronounced action.

Isolated in 1803, morphine came into general use as a painkiller in the 1830s, but only after the perfection of the hypodermic needle in 1853 could the drug be used to obtain rapid relief. It was so widely dispensed thereafter that during the American Civil War and the Franco-Prussian war addiction to morphine became known as the soldier's disease. Substitutes were sought, and in 1898, with major acclaim, heroin was placed on the market as a harmless, nonaddicting substitute for morphine and codeine. Heroin, they said in 1900, "is the perfect drug, more potent yet less harmful, and as a sufficiently long period has elapsed since its introduction during which time it has been used very extensively, we are able to pass judgment on its real value.

Habituation has been noted in a small percentage of cases, but all observers agree, however, that none of the patients suffer from this habituation, and that none of the symptoms which are so characteristic of chronic morphinism have ever been observed even after prolonged use."[12]

By 1905, however, a leading text asserted that "although heroin is stated not to give rise to habituation, a more extended knowledge of the drug would seem to indicate that this is not entirely correct."[13] In a few more years everyone knew that of the opiates, heroin was the *most addicting*. Furthermore, because the two acetyl groups added to morphine increased lipid solubility, allowing the molecule to enter the brain more rapidly, heroin was about three times as potent. This historic introduction of heroin is clearly worth repeating.

Morphine and its substitutes produce their major effects on the central nervous system and the intestine. Action in the central nervous system includes a general decrease in brain arousal to painful stimulation, that is, a diminished awareness of the pain that occurs following morphine-induced analgesia. This is probably the basis of morphine's therapeutic effect relating to pain, but an understanding of more specific action must await further research. Morphine also depresses respiration, and this is a dangerous side effect, for respiratory arrest can readily follow overdose. Actions of opiates in the gastrointestinal tract are well known, but again, the mechanisms are poorly understood. Morphine impairs digestion by decreasing secretion of digestive juices, and it slows the passage of food by decreasing peristaltic contractions. Also, water is absorbed faster than usual from the intestinal material. All these effects result in constipation, and opium-containing compounds have been used successfully against diarrhea (e.g., paregoric, a tincture of opium with camphor).

Other effects are known, such as suppression of tension, anxiety, hunger, sexual desires, feelings of depression, and panic. The opiates produce a feeling of total satisfaction. At addictive levels, morphine, the semisynthetic heroin, and the synthetic methadone may exert mild aphrodisiac action for a time, but after heavy prolonged drug use, libido is less strong and potency is commonly reduced in both men and women. Female addicts often have delayed and irregular menstruation, and likelihood of pregnancy is reduced; if pregnancy results, there is a much greater risk of a handicapped birth, such as low birth weight typical of premature babies.

WITHDRAWAL AND REHABILITATION

Heroin is not manufactured in the United States and it is not dispensed for medical purposes. Therefore, the illegal alkaloid is synthesized surreptitiously, normally in the Mediterranean area, from opium obtained from especially Turkey and the Golden Triangle (border highlands of Burma, Laos, and Thailand). Accurate measurement of dosage and of real content is rarely known, although the level of heroin reaching the streets is probably between 3 and 5%. Overdoses that fatally depressed respiration accounted for 1154 deaths during 1970 in New York City alone; most were not directly suicidal, and many undoubtedly were accidental. Other risks are certainly involved with the use of heroin; for example, infection with hepatitis virus (leading to permanent liver damage) and bacterial and protozoan diseases such as syphilis and malaria can result from use of unsterilized hypodermic needles. Despite these dangers, however, heroin addiction has reached epidemic levels in certain areas.[14]

The average person who injects heroin daily develops the habit within 2 weeks (based on normal dose of $\frac{1}{6}$–$\frac{1}{4}$ grains of morphine 4 times daily for 2 weeks). Tolerance develops swiftly, and when the addict wants to repeat the intensity of the first euphoric experiences, he must increase the heroin doses. The addict feels normal for only a short period, whereupon withdrawal symptoms appear until another dose is administered. Larger doses are soon taken, to enable the addict to break through his tolerance threshold, but now the high feeling lasts very briefly. High tolerance develops, and the addict begins to inject heroin not to feel good but to prevent feeling sick (Fig. 19-4).

Abstinence by the addict induces the withdrawal symptoms tabulated in Table 19-2. Generally, the longer it takes for the initial symptoms to develop, the less intense the withdrawal effects. Muscle twitching of the feet and legs, which appears in most users, about 12 hours after the last dose of heroin, increases in intensity for several days (thus the term "kicking the habit"). Perhaps even more vivid is a description by a former addict of abrupt withdrawal from a moderate habit without medication ("cold turkey" because of extensive gross bumps resembling a plucked turkey).

Remember when you had a bad case of the 24-hour virus. You're coming out both ends—vomiting and diarrhea—and every joint in your body hurts. You wish you could die but feel too badly to do anything about it. Take that, double it, and spread it over 4 or 5 days. That's cold turkey.[1]

Many addicts, especially those with a severe habit, will not, or perhaps cannot, withdraw from addiction this way. Psychosocial methods exist to help the addict, but these have been replaced or

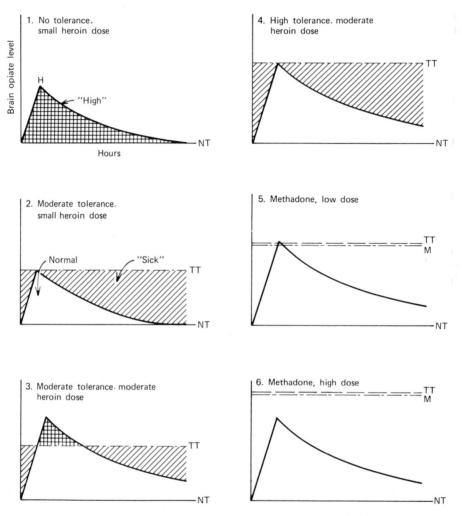

Figure 19-4 Pharmacodynamics of various aspects of opioid addiction. (From A Goldstein, "Pharmacologic basis of methadone treatment," p 27, *Proceedings, Fourth National Conference on Methadone Treatment,* National Association for the Prevention of Addiction to Narcotics (NAPAN), 1972, and reprinted with permission.) **1.** *First dose:* Normal threshold (NT); no tolerance. **2.** *Repeated dose* at frequency less than critical interval: tolerant threshold (TT) is moderate and represents cumulative increments of neuronal adaption. Small heroin dose does not "break through" TT and no "high" is obtained. Addict feels "normal" for short time but experiences "withdrawal sickness" until next dose is administered. **3.** *Greater dose* of heroin is administered in an attempt to break through the TT. Addict feels "high" for short time, but experiences "withdrawal sickness" as brain opioid level falls below TT. **4.** *High tolerance* develops as a result of increased heroin dose and TT exceeds the brain opioid level once again. Addict now injects heroin "not to feel good" but to "prevent from feeling sick." Breakthrough requires amounts of heroin not readily obtained. **5.** *Methadone, low dose* (40–50 mg): daily administration of methadone (by mouth) results in a persistently elevated TT, accompanied by suppression of opioid craving. Addict perceives little or no effect from up to 200 mg of heroin. **6.** *Methadone, high dose* (50–300 mg): same as 5 except that cross tolerance to heroin is increased proportionately.

are supplemented by pharmacological methods of treatment which in the United States have centered around methadone maintenance programs. Methadone is a synthetic addictive opiate developed in Germany during World War II; its molecular structure is similar to morphine and heroin and some of its effects are similar, but there are important differences. These differences make methadone useful: it depresses respiration less acutely than do morphine and heroin, it is equally powerful taken orally and by injection, it does not produce as much euphoria or drowsiness as the nonsynthetic narcotics, and withdrawal symptoms from it are less severe because they occur over a longer period. In treatment programs methadone is given orally once a day, with the daily dose of 10 mg increased to 40 or 50 mg during the first stage. At this level craving for opiates disappears. At still higher doses (80–140 mg) methadone prevents withdrawal symptoms, stops the desire for opiates, and blocks the pleasurable effects of opiates.

Methadone maintenance has been used to treat thousands of heroin addicts, and it is working for many patients who continue with the programs. They no longer depend on the use of opiates other than methadone, they may return to society and a constructive life, and they reduce the massive criminal element associated with illegal sale and distribution of opiates. As might be expected, the side effects accompanying methadone use resemble those of other opiates (weight gain 80%, constipation 70%, delayed ejaculation 60%, increased use of alcohol 40%, increased frequency of urination 37%, numbness in extremities 32%, and hallucinations 17%); in addition, critics cite the return of numerous patients to heroin. Still others raise the moral question of whether society should substitute one addiction for another, locking the addict into a behavioral pattern and a form of treatment, with some addicts existing as experimental animals for new opiate substitutes as they are developed. The interested student should explore the pros and cons.[16]

Table 19-2   Sequence of Appearance of Some Abstinence or Withdrawal Symptoms from Opiate Addiction[a]

Signs	Approximate Hours after Last Dose		
	Heroin	Morphine	Methadone
Craving for drugs, anxiety	4	6	12
Yawning, perspiration, running nose, teary eyes	8	14	34–48
Increase in above signs plus pupil dilation, goose bumps (piloerection), tremors (muscle twitches), hot and cold flashes, aching bones and muscles, loss of appetite	12	18	48–72
Increased intensity of above, plus insomnia, raised blood pressure, increased temperature, pulse rate, respiratory rate and depth; restlessness; nausea	18–24	24–36	
Increased intensity of above, plus curled-up position, vomiting, diarrhea, weight loss, spontaneous ejaculation or orgasm; hemoconcentration, increased blood sugar	26–36	36–48	

[a] Adapted from OS Ray (1972, p 203).[1]

Elsewhere (e.g., in Britain), addicts are registered and are administered minimum heroin dosages by the government. This makes heroin a medical problem and, like methadone use, removes the criminal element from drugs providing the treatment is adhered to.

For other medicinal uses and general utilization of the opium poppy, see Duke.[17]

OPIUM SUBSTITUTES

A number of plants are used as substitutes for opium. *Lactuca quercina* and *L. virosa* (Asteraceae) are cultivated in France; the extracted lactucarium, reputed to be a mild sedative, is used in cough mixtures to replace opium. In Thailand leaves of *Mitragyna speciosa* (Rubiaceae) are chewed and smoked as a substitute for opium, as are the seeds of *Pterygota alata* (Sterculiaceae) in Pakistan. A tincture of oats (*Avena sativa*) has been employed successfully for centuries by Ayurvedic Indian practitioners to cure the opium habit.[18] Presumably these plants have been selected for their sedative properties, and they probably act by depressing the central nervous system.

SOLVENTS

Organic solvents (ingested orally or, more recently, sniffed) have from time to time been popular substitutes for achieving the euphoria and occasional hallucinations associated with alcoholic indulgence. Ether, in particular, was drunk in place of alcohol whenever the latter was prohibited by law or simply too expensive; other substitutes include a broad range of solvents such as chloroform, paint thinners, lacquers, enamels, cigarette lighter fluid, polish and spot removers, gasoline, and glues. Glue-sniffing has received much publicity, some of it inaccurate and exaggerated, but the results are probably similar to those of inhaling gasoline fumes, which in turn is like drinking alcoholic beverages: uncoordination, restlessness, excitement, confusion, delirium, coma that may last from a few hours to several days, and even death. Repeated inhalation induces dizziness, giddiness, hallucinations, and unconsciousness, along with neurological effects such as confusion, ataxia, tremor, itching, neuritis, and paralysis of peripheral and cranial nerves.[2]

Why would anyone wish to sniff gasoline or glue? Perhaps one account of a boy nicknamed Bullet, found alone by A. E. (Tajar) Hamilton one day while the other children were on a trip, answers this question at least in part.

TAJAR: Bullet, you said you would come up the attic and tell me about the gasoline and the bicycles. Will you talk your story into the mike, just as you remember it?

BULLET: Well, I was awful mad when they said I couldn't go on the trip. Sure I picked up the axe when Martha told me not to, but I put it back again. Then she said I couldn't go . . . and Donnie was going, and when they all went I didn't have anything to do to have fun and I began to get madder and madder all the time. It made me feel kind of sick to be so mad, so I went where they keep the gasoline can and I started to smell it.

TAJAR: What made you want to smell gas, Bullet?

BULLET: Well, when you feel bad, you smell it and it makes you feel kind of hot and kind of drowsy, like you was floating through the air. It makes you feel sort of hot inside and different from the way you were before.

TAJAR: And after you smelled the gas and felt better, what did you do?

BULLET: Then I began to feel mad again and had to do something, so I found a nail. It was an old rusty one, and I got a piece of board to push it with so it wouldn't hurt my hand, and I made holes in all the tires except Donnie's.

TAJAR: Why not in Donnie's?

BULLET: Because they're solid and you can't. . . .

TAJAR: And after you had punched all those holes what did you do?

BULLET: Mary hollered to come to dinner, so I went and we had hot dogs at the Council ring and then we had some games and then I didn't feel so good, so I went and smelled the gas again.

TAJAR: How long have you liked to smell gas, Bullet?

BULLET: Well, here at camp, ever since about two weeks after I came to the farm. I showed Donnie how to smell it. It makes you feel like you was in fairyland or somewhere else than where you are. . . .

TAJAR: Bullet, how come so much gas was spilled on the cellar floor?

BULLET: Oh, I just wanted to get more on my rag. If you have a lot it makes you sort of dream. It gets all dark and you see shooting stars in it, and this time I saw big flies flying in it. They were big and green and had white wings.

TAJAR: And you feel better about yourself and about people after you have one of those dreams?

BULLET: Yep, until I begin to feel bad again, or get mad.

TAJAR: Okay, Bullet, that's all for now. Thank you for being truthful with me.[19]

There was a tragic sequel to Bullet's gasoline narcosis. Months later he was found lying on a couch with a bottle of cleaning fluid (ether) beside him. He never awakened.

LITERATURE CITED

1. Ray OS. 1972. *Drugs, Society and Human Behavior.* C V Mosby, St Louis. Chapter 6, 78–94.

2. Becker CE, Roe RL, Scott RA. 1974. *Alcohol as a Drug.* Medcom Press, New York. 99 p.

3. Amerine MA. 1966. The search for good wine. *Science* **154:** 1621–1628; Amerine MA, Kunkee RE. 1968. Microbiology of winemaking. *Ann*

Rev Microbiol **22:** 323–358; Kleyn J, Hough J. 1971. The microbiology of brewing. *Ann Rev Microbiol* **25:** 583–608.

4. The effects of alcohol [chart by W Hortens], *Time* 22 Apr 1974: 77.

5. Dalton MS, Duncan DW. 1970. The effects of fructose in the management of delirium tremens. *Med J Aust* **1:** 659–661; Brown SS, Forrest JAH, Roscoe P. 1972. A controlled trial of fructose in the treatment of acute alcoholic intoxication. *Lancet* **2:** 898–899.

6. Winokur G, Reich T, Rimmer J et al. 1970. Alcoholism: III. Diagnosis and familial psychiatric illness in 259 alcoholic probands. *Arch Gen Psychiatr* **23:** 104–111.

7. Sharpless SK. 1970. Hypnotics and sedatives, 98, 100, 103. In L Goodman, A Gilman (eds), *The Pharmacological Basis of Therapeutics.* Macmillan, New York.

8. Lentz J. 1968. 5. *Rauwolfia* plant. *Today's Health* **46**(3): 83.

9. Steinmetz EF. 1960. *Piper methysticum.* Published by the author, Amsterdam. 46 p.

10. Keller F, Klohs MW. 1963. A review of the chemistry and pharmacology of the constituents of *Piper methysticum. Lloydia* **26:** 1–15.

11. Brecher EM. 1942. *Licit and Illicit Drugs.* Little, Brown, Boston. 623 p (with the editors of *Consumer Reports*).

12. Manges M. 1900. A second report on the therapeutics of heroine. *NY Med J* **71:** 51–55; Floeckinger FC. 1900. Clinical observations on heroin and heroin hydrochloride as compared with codeine and morphine. *NY Med J* **71**:970.

13. Wilcox RW. 1905. *Pharmacology and Therapeutics.* P Blakiston's , Philadelphia. 860 p.

14. DuPont RL, Greene MH. 1973. The dynamics of a heroin addiction epidemic. *Science* **181**:716–722.

15. Goldstein A. 1972. Pharmacologic basis of methadone treatment. *Proceedings of the Fourth National Conference on Methadone Treatment,* San Francisco. National Association for the Prevention of Addiction to Narcotics, New York, p 27.

16. Bazell, RJ. 1973. Drug abuse: methadone becomes the solution and the problem. *Science* **179:** 772–775; Chambers CD, Brill L. 1973. *Methadone: Experiences and Issues.* Behavioral Publications, New York: Koran LM. 1973. Heroin maintenance for heroin addicts: issues and evidence. *New Eng J Med* **288:** 654–660; Page IH, Alvarez WC. 1970. Methadone—

we should wait no longer. *Mod Med* **38**(15): 67–69; Weppner RS, Stephen RC, Conrad HT. 1972. Methadone; some aspects of its legal and illegal use. *J. Psychiatr* **129:** 451–455; Dole VP, Nyswander ME. 1976. Methadone maintenance treatment, a ten-year perspective. *JAMA* **235:** 2117–2119.

17. Duke JA. 1973. Utilization of *Papaver*. *Econ Bot* **27:** 390–400.

18. Anand CL. 1971. Effect of *Avena sativa* on cigarette smoking. *Nature* **233:** 496.

19. Hamilton AE. 1955. *Psychology and "the Great God Fun."* Julian Press, New York. 189 p. Copyright © by Julian Press and reproduced by permission, p. 106–109.

Outline Classification of the Plant Kingdom

The plant kingdom consists of "lower" plants and "higher" plants. The former generally do not possess complex vascularization for transport of water, mineral salts, and manufactured food. Many are aquatic or at least rely on water to complete their alternation of generations (e.g., motile exposed sperm requiring moisture to locate the egg). Included in this grouping are the Bacteria, Algae, Fungi, and Bryophytes, although some phylogenists find the Bacteria and Fungi sufficiently distinct from plants to exclude them from the kingdom. The higher plants include those having sufficient vascular tissue to transport materials over considerable distances; they generally are terrestrial (although a number have evolved an aquatic habit), and most do not require a wet condition to complete their cycle of generations (some lower forms still possess naked sperm). The higher forms include the Ferns and allied groups, the Gymnosperms, and the diverse, numerous, and highest evolved Angiosperms or flowering plants.

Below are listed the classes; the vernacular names of the lower plants are grouped by major units (Bacteria, Algae, Fungi, Bryophytes) as used throughout the text. For elaboration of this classification, see a general text in botany[1] or morphology.[2]

The higher plants are also listed by simple groupings of Ferns and Fern Allies, Gymnosperms, Angiosperms—dicotyledons, and Angiosperms—monocotyledons. Each includes the family (ending -aceae) and, for Angiosperms, the order (ending -ales). Among the Angiosperms 15 phylogenetic or supraordinal groupings are recognized, a useful convenience in associating the large number of families found among flowering plants. The phylogeny is in large part taken from Thorne,[3] supplemented by others.[4] The student interested in the phylogeny of higher plants should consult these excellent works.

The angiospermous families most important as medical plants are indicated in boldface. The first listing, which is phylogenetic, is followed by an alphabetical compilation, permitting the reader to find readily the phylogenetic grouping of any family of higher plants used in this text and also the classes of lower organisms (no fossil taxa). For the Angiosperms this phylogeny may be visualized by reference to Fig. 2-2.

PHYLOGENETIC CLASSIFICATION OF PLANTS

LOWER PLANTS (NONVASCULAR)

BACTERIA. Schizomycetes.

ALGAE. Cyanophyceae (blue-greens), Chlorophyceae (greens), Euglenophyceae (euglenoids), Phaeophyceae (browns), Xanthophyceae (yellow-greens), Chrysophyceae (golden-browns), Bacillariophyceae (diatoms), Cryptophyceae (cryptomonads), Dinophyceae (dinoflagellates), Rhodophyceae (reds), Charophyceae (stoneworts).

FUNGI. Myxomycetes (slime molds), Acrasiomycetes (cellular slime molds), Phycomycetes (algalike fungi), Ascomycetes (sac fungi), Basidiomycetes (club fungi), Deuteromycetes (fungi imperfecti), Lichens.

BRYOPHYTES. Hepaticae (thallose and leafy liverworts), Anthocerotae (horned liverworts), Musci (mosses).

HIGHER PLANTS (VASCULAR)

FERNS (AND FERN ALLIES). Psilotaceae (whisk ferns), Lycopodiaceae and Selaginellaceae (club mosses), Isoetaceae (quillworts), Equisetaceae (horsetails), and the extant ferns Ophioglossaceae (adder's tongue and grape ferns), Marattiaceae, Polypodiaceae (majority of temperate ferns), Osmundaceae (royal, cinnamon and interrupted ferns), Schizaeaceae, Hymenophyllaceae (filmy ferns), Cyatheaceae (tree ferns).

GYMNOSPERMS (Cone-bearing Plants). Cycadaceae (cycads), Ginkgoaceae (*Ginkgo*), Ephedraceae (*Ephedra*), Gnetaceae (*Gnetum*), Welwitschiaceae (*Welwitschia*); Coniferales including Pinaceae (pine, fir, cedar, spruce, larch, Douglas fir, hemlock), Taxodiaceae (cypress, redwood), Cupressaceae (juniper, red cedar, Monterey cypress, white cedar, arborvitae), Araucariaceae (monkey-puzzle tree, Norfolk Island pine), Podocarpaceae; Taxales including Taxaceae (yew).

ANGIOSPERMS (FLOWERING PLANTS): DICOTYLEDONS

PHYLOGENETIC GROUP 1

Order Annonales. Winteraceae, Illiciaceae, Schisandraceae, **Magnoliaceae,** Degeneriaceae, Eupomatiaceae, Himantandraceae, Annonaceae, **Myristicaceae**, Canellaceae, **Aristolochiaceae**, Austrobaileyaceae, Chloranthaceae, Amborellaceae, Trimeniaceae, Monimiaceae, Calycanthaceae, Lactoridaceae, Gomortegaceae, **Lauraceae**, Hernandiaceae, Gyrocarpaceae, **Piperaceae**, Saururaceae.

Order Berberidales. Lardizabalaceae, Sargentodoxaceae, **Menispermaceae, Ranunculaceae, Berberidaceae, Papaveraceae** (including Fumariaceae).

Order Nymphaeales. Nymphaeaceae, Ceratophyllaceae.

PHYLOGENETIC GROUP 2

Order Hamamelidales. Trochodendraceae, Tetracentraceae, Eupteleaceae, Cercidiphyllaceae, Eucommiaceae, **Hamamelidaceae, Platanaceae**.

Order Casuarinales. **Casuarinaceae**.

Order Fagales. **Fagaceae, Betulaceae**.

Order Balanopales. Balanopaceae.

PHYLOGENETIC GROUP 3

Order Chenopodiales. **Phytolaccaceae,** Gyrostemonaceae, **Nyctaginaceae, Aizoaceae, Cactaceae**, Didiereaceae, **Portulacaceae**, Basellaceae, **Chenopodiaceae**, Halophytaceae, **Amaranthaceae, Caryophyllaceae.**

Order Polygonales. **Polygonaceae.**

Order Batidales. Batidaceae.

PHYLOGENETIC GROUP 4

Order Theales. Dilleniaceae, Paeoniaceae, Actinidiaceae, Stachyuraceae, **Theaceae, Aquifoliaceae**, Marcgraviaceae,

Caryocaraceae, Clethraceae, Cyrillaceae, Pentaphylacaceae, Ochnaceae, Quiinaceae, Scytopetalaceae, Sarcolaenaceae, Strasburgeriaceae, **Dipterocarpaceae**, Dioncophyllaceae, **Clusiaceae**, Elatinaceae, Lecythidaceae.

Order Nepenthales. Nepenthaceae.

Order Ericales. **Ericaceae**, Epacridaceae, Empetraceae.

Order Ebenales. **Ebenaceae, Sapotaceae**, Symplocaceae, Lissocarpaceae, **Styracaceae**.

Order Primulales. **Myrsinaceae, Theophrastaceae, Primulaceae.**

Order Plumbaginales. Plumbaginaceae.

PHYLOGENETIC GROUP 5

Order Cistales. **Flacourtiaceae**, Dipentodontaceae, Peridiscaceae, Scyphostegiaceae, **Violaceae**, Bixaceae, Cistaceae, Turneraceae, Malesherbiaceae, **Passifloraceae**, Achariaceae, **Caricaceae, Cucurbitaceae, Begoniaceae**, Datiscaceae, Loasaceae.

Order Salicales. **Salicaceae**.

Order Tamaricales. Tamaricaceae, Frankeniaceae.

Order Capparidales. **Capparidaceae, Brassicaceae**, Resedaceae, Moringaceae.

PHYLOGENETIC GROUP 6

Order Malvales. **Sterculiaceae**, Sphaerosepalaceae, Elaeocarpaceae, Tiliaceae, **Bombacaceae, Malvaceae.**

Order Urticales. **Ulmaceae, Moraceae, Cannabaceae, Urticaceae.**

Order Euphorbiales. **Euphorbiaceae**, Pandaceae, Aextoxicaceae, Didymelaceae, Dichapetalaceae, **Thymelaeaceae, Buxaceae.**

Order Rhamnales. **Rhamnaceae, Elaeagnaceae.**

PHYLOGENETIC GROUP 7

Order Rosales. **Rosaceae,** Chrysobalanaceae, Crossosomataceae, **Connaraceae, Fabaceae** (including Caesalpinoideae, Faboideae, Mimosoideae), Crassulaceae, Cephalotaceae, **Saxifragaceae,** Stylidiaceae, Droseraceae, Greyiaceae, Podostemaceae, Diapensiaceae, Cunoniaceae, Brunelliaceae, Davidsoniaceae, Eucryphiaceae, Medusagynaceae, Staphyleaceae, Corynocarpaceae, Coriariaceae.

Order Pittosporales. Daphniphyllaceae, Pittosporaceae, Byblidaceae, Tremandraceae, Roridulaceae, Bruniaceae, Geissolomataceae, Grubbiaceae, Myrothamnaceae, Hydrostachyaceae.

PHYLOGENETIC GROUP 8

Order Proteales. Proteaceae.

Order Myrtales. **Lythraceae,** Punicaceae, Crypteroniaceae, Trapaceae, Combretaceae, Oliniaceae, Penaeaceae, **Myrtaceae,** Melastomataceae, **Onagraceae.**

PHYLOGENETIC GROUP 9

Order Geraniales. **Linaceae,** Ancistrocladaceae, **Erythroxylaceae,** Zygophyllaceae, **Oxalidaceae, Geraniaceae, Balsaminaceae,** Tropaeolaceae, Limnanthaceae.

Order Polygalales. **Malpighiaceae, Polygalaceae, Krameriaceae,** Trigoniaceae, Vochysiaceae.

Order Rutales. **Rutaceae, Simaroubaceae,** Surianaceae, Cneoraceae, **Meliaceae,**

Burseraceae, Anacardiaceae, Sapindaceae, Sabiaceae, Melianthaceae, Akaniaceae, **Aceraceae, Hippocastanaceae,** Bretschneideraceae, Rhoipteleaceae.

Order Juglandales. **Juglandaceae.**

Order Myricales. **Myricaceae.**

Order Leitneriales. Leitneriaceae.

PHYLOGENETIC GROUP 10

Order Santalales. **Celastraceae,** Stackhousiaceae, Icacinaceae, Cardiopteridaceae, Medusandraceae, **Olacaceae,** Opiliaceae, Santalaceae, Misodendraceae, **Loranthaceae,** Balanophoraceae, Cynomoriaceae.

Order Oleales. Salvadoraceae, **Oleaceae.**

Order Rafflesiales. Rafflesiaceae, Hydnoraceae.

Order Cornales. Rhizophoraceae, **Vitaceae,** Nyssaceae, **Cornaceae,** Alangiaceae, Garryaceae, Haloragidaceae, Hippuridaceae, **Araliaceae, Apiaceae.**

Order Dipsacales. **Caprifoliaceae,** Adoxaceae, **Valerianaceae,** Dipsacaceae, Calyceraceae.

PHYLOGENETIC GROUP 11

Order Gentianales. **Loganiàceae, Rubiaceae, Apocynaceae, Asclepiadaceae, Gentianaceae,** Menyanthaceae.

Order Bignoniales. **Bignoniaceae,** Pedaliaceae, Martyniaceae, Myoporaceae, **Scrophulariaceae, Plantaginaceae,** Orobranchaceae, Lentibulariaceae, **Acanthaceae,** Gesneriaceae.

Order Solanales. **Solanaceae, Convolvulaceae,** Polemoniaceae, Fouquieriaceae.

Order Lamiales. Hydrophyllaceae, **Boraginaceae,** Lennoaceae, Hoplestigmataceae, **Verbenaceae**, Callitrichaceae, **Lamiaceae**.

Order Campanulales. Pentaphragmataceae, **Campanulaceae,** Goodeniaceae.

Order Asterales. **Asteraceae.**

ANGIOSPERMS: MONOCOTYLEDONS

PHYLOGENETIC GROUP 12

Order Alismales. Butomaceae, **Alismaceae**, Hydrocharitaceae.

Order Zosterales. Aponogetonaceae, Scheuchzeriaceae, Juncaginaceae, Potamogetonaceae, Posidoniaceae, Zannichelliaceae, Zosteraceae.

Order Najadales. Najadaceae.

Order Triuridales. Triuridaceae.

PHYLOGENETIC GROUP 13

Order Arales. **Araceae**, Lemnaceae, Sparganiaceae, **Typhaceae**.

Order Arecales. Arecaceae.

Order Cyclanthales. Cyclanthaceae.

Order Pandanales. Pandanaceae.

PHYLOGENETIC GROUP 14

Order Bromeliales. Bromeliaceae.

Order Commelinales. Rapateaceae, Xyridaceae, Pontederiaceae, Philydraceae, Juncaceae, Cyperaceae Commelinaceae, Mayacaceae, Eriocaulaceae, Flagellariaceae, Restionaceae, Centrolepidaceae, **Poaceae**.

Order Zingiberales. **Musaceae**, Lowi-

aceae, **Zingiberaceae**, Cannaceae, Marantaceae.

PHYLOGENETIC GROUP 15

Order Liliales. **Liliaceae** (including Amaryllidaceae), Roxburghiaceae, **Dioscoreaceae**, Taccaceae, Velloziaceae, **Iridaceae**, Burmanniaceae.

Order Orchidales. Orchidaceae.

ALPHABETICAL LISTING OF PLANTS

This list contains major groups Bacteria to Gymnosperms and phylogenetic group number for Angiosperms (see foregoing list and Fig. 2-2).

Acanthaceae (11), Aceraceae (9), Achariaceae (5), Acrasiomycetes (Fungus), Actinidiaceae (4), Adoxaceae (10), Aextoxicaceae (6), Aizoaceae (3), Akaniaceae (9), Alangiaceae (10), Alismaceae (12), Amaranthaceae (3), Anacardiaceae (9), Ancistrocladaceae (9), Annonaceae (1), Anthocerotae (Bryophyte), Apiaceae (10), Apocynaceae (11), Aponogetonaceae (12), Aquifoliaceae (4), Araceae (13), Araliaceae (10), Araucariaceae (Gymnosperm), Arecaceae (13), Aristolochiaceae (1), Asclepiadaceae (11), Ascomycetes (Fungus), Asteraceae (11), Austrobaileyaceae (1).

Bacillariophyceae (Alga), Balanopaceae (2), Balanophoraceae (10), Balsaminaceae (9), Basellaceae (3), Basidiomycetes (Fungus), Batidaceae (3), Begoniaceae (5), Berberidaceae (1), Betulaceae (2), Bignoniaceae (11), Bixaceae (5), Bombacaceae (6), Boraginaceae (11), Brassicaceae (5), Bretschneideraceae (9), Bromeliaceae (14), Bruniaceae (7), Brunelliaceae (7), Burmanniaceae (15), Burseraceae (9), Butomaceae (12), Buxaceae (6), Byblidaceae (7).

Cactaceae (3), Callitrichaceae (11), Calycanthaceae (1), Calyceraceae (10), Campanulaceae (11), Canellaceae (1), Cannabaceae (6), Cannaceae (14), Capparidaceae (5), Caprifoliaceae (10), Cardiopteridaceae (10), Caricaceae (5), Caryocaraceae (4), Caryophyllaceae (3), Casuarinaceae (2), Celastraceae (10), Centrolepidaceae (14), Cephalotaceae (7), Ceratophyllaceae (1), Cercidiphyllaceae (2), Charophyceae (Alga), Chenopodiaceae (3), Chloranthaceae (1), Chlorophyceae (Alga), Chrysophyceae (Alga), Chrysobalanaceae (7), Cistaceae (5), Clethraceae (4), Clusiaceae (4), Cneoraceae (9), Combretaceae (8), Commelinaceae (14), Connaraceae (7), Convolvulaceae (11), Coriariaceae (7), Cornaceae (10), Corynocarpaceae (7), Crassulaceae (7), Crossosomataceae (7), Crypteroniaceae (8), Cryptophyceae (Alga), Cucurbitaceae (5), Cunoniaceae (7), Cupressaceae (Gymnosperm), Cyanophyceae (Alga), Cyatheaceae (Fern), Cycadaceae (Gymnosperm), Cyclanthaceae (13), Cynomoriaceae (10), Cyperaceae (14), Cyrillaceae (4).

Datiscaceae (5), Daphniphyllaceae (7), Davidsoniaceae (7), Degeneriaceae (1), Deuteromycetes (Fungus), Diapensiaceae (7), Dichapetalaceae (6), Didiereaceae (3), Didymelaceae (6), Dilleniaceae (4), Dinophyceae (Alga), Dioncophyllaceae (4), Dioscoreaceae (15), Dipentodontaceae (5), Dipsacaceae (10), Dipterocarpaceae (4), Droseraceae (7).

Ebenaceae (4), Elaeagnaceae (6), Elaeocarpaceae (6), Elatinaceae (4), Empetraceae (4), Epacridaceae (4), Ephedraceae (Gymnosperm), Equisetaceae (Fern), Ericaceae (4), Eriocaulaceae (14), Erythroxylaceae (9), Eucommiaceae (2), Eucryphiaceae (7), Euglenophyceae (Alga), Euphorbiaceae (6), Eupomatiaceae (1), Eupteleaceae (2).

Fabaceae (7), Fagaceae (2), Flacourtiaceae (5), Flagellariaceae (14), Fouquieriaceae (11), Frankeniaceae (5).

Garryaceae (10), Geissolomataceae (7), Gentianaceae (11), Geraniaceae (9), Gesneriaceae (11), Ginkgoaceae (Gymnosperm), Gnetaceae (Gymnosperm), Gomortegaceae (1) Goodeniaceae (11), Greyiaceae (7), Grubbiaceae (7), Gyrostemonaceae (3), Gyrocarpaceae (1).

Halophytaceae (3), Haloragidaceae (10), Hamamelidaceae (2), Hepaticae (Bryophyte), Hernandiaceae (1), Himantandraceae (1), Hippocastanaceae (9), Hippuridaceae (10), Hoplestigmataceae (11), Hydnoraceae (10), Hydrocharitaceae (12), Hydrophyllaceae (11), Hydrostachyaceae (7), Hymenophyllaceae (Fern).

Icacinaceae (10), Illiciaceae (1), Iridaceae (15),·Isoetaceae (Fern).

Juglandaceae (9), Juncaceae (14), Juncaginaceae (12).

Krameriaceae (9).

Lamiaceae (11), Lardizabalaceae (1), Lauraceae (1), Lactoridaceae (1), Lecythidaceae (4), Leitneriaceae (9), Lemnaceae (13), Lennoaceae (11), Lentibulariaceae (11), Lichens (Fungus), Liliaceae (15), Limnanthaceae (9), Linaceae (9), Lissocarpaceae (4), Loasaceae (5), Loganiaceae (11), Loranthaceae (10), Lowiaceae (14), Lycopodiaceae (Fern), Lythraceae (8).

Magnoliaceae (1), Malesherbiaceae (5), Malpighiaceae (9), Malvaceae (6), Marantaceae (14), Marattiaceae (Fern), Marcgraviaceae (4), Martyniaceae (11), Mayacaceae (14), Medusagynaceae (7), Medusandraceae (10), Meliaceae (9), Melianthaceae (9), Melastomataceae (8), Menispermaceae (1), Menyanthaceae (11), Misodendraceae (10), Monimiaceae (1), Moraceae (6), Moringaceae (5), Musaceae (14), Musci (Bryophyte), Myoporaceae (11), Myricaceae (9), Myristicaceae (1), Myrothamnaceae (7), Myrsinaceae (4), Myrtaceae (8), Myxomycetes (Fungus).

Najadaceae (12), Nepenthaceae (4), Nyctaginaceae (3), Nymphaeaceae (1), Nyssaceae (10).

Ochnaceae (4), Olacaceae (10), Oleaceae (10), Oliniaceae (8), Onagraceae (8), Ophioglossaceae (Fern), Opiliaceae (10), Orchidaceae (15), Orobanchaceae (11), Osmundaceae (Fern), Oxalidaceae (9).

Paeoniaceae (4), Pandanaceae (13), Pandaceae (6), Papaveraceae (1), Passifloraceae (5), Pedaliaceae (11), Penaeaceae (8), Pentaphragamataceae (11), Pentaphylacaceae (4), Peridiscaceae (5), Phaeophyceae (Alga), Philydraceae (14), Phycomycetes (Fungus), Phytolaccaceae (3), Pinaceae (Gymnosperm), Piperaceae (1), Pittosporaceae (7), Plantaginaceae (11), Platanaceae (2), Plumbaginaceae (4), Poaceae (14), Podocarpaceae (Gymnosperm), Podostemaceae (7), Polemoniaceae (11), Polygalaceae (9), Polygonaceae (3), Polypodiaceae (Fern), Pontederiaceae (14), Portulacaceae (3), Posidoniaceae (12), Potamogetonaceae (12), Primulaceae (4), Proteaceae (8), Psilotaceae (Fern), Punicaceae (8).

Quiinaceae (4).

Rafflesiaceae (10), Ranunculaceae (1), Rapateaceae (14), Resedaceae (5), Restionaceae (14), Rhamnaceae (6), Rhizophoraceae (10), Rhodophyceae (Alga), Rhoipteleaceae (9), Roridulaceae (7), Rosaceae (7), Roxburghiaceae (15), Rubiaceae (11), Rutaceae (9).

Sabiaceae (9), Salicaceae (5), Salvadoraceae (10), Santalaceae (10), Sapindaceae (9), Sapotaceae (4), Sarcolaenaceae (4), Sargentodoxaceae (1), Saururaceae (1), Saxifragaceae (7), Scheuchzeriaceae (12), Schisandraceae (1), Schizaeaceae (Fern), Schizomycetes (Bacteria), Scrophulariaceae (11), Scyphostegiaceae (5), Scytopetalaceae (4), Selaginellaceae (Fern), Simaroubaceae (9), Solanaceae (11),

Sparganiaceae (13), Sphaerosepalaceae (6), Stachyuraceae (4), Stackhousiaceae (10), Staphyleaceae (7), Sterculiaceae (6), Symplocaceae (4), Strasburgeriaceae (4), Stylidiaceae (7), Styracaceae (4), Surianaceae (9).

Taccaceae (15), Tamaricaceae (5), Taxaceae (Gymnosperm), Taxodiaceae (Gymnosperm), Tetracentraceae (2), Theaceae (4), Theophrastaceae (4), Thymelaeaceae (6), Tiliaceae (6), Trapaceae (8), Tremandraceae (7), Trigoniaceae (9), Trimeniaceae (1), Triuridaceae (12), Trochodendraceae (2), Tropaeolaceae (9), Turneraceae (5), Typhaceae (13).

Ulmaceae (6), Urticaceae (6).

Valerianaceae (10), Velloziaceae (15), Verbenaceae (11), Violaceae (5), Vitaceae (10), Vochysiaceae (9).

Welwitschiaceae (Gymnosperm), Winteraceae (1).

Xanthophyceae (Alga), Xyridaceae (14).

Zannichelliaceae (12), Zingiberaceae (14), Zosteraceae (12), Zygophyllaceae (9).

LITERATURE CITED

1. Hill JB, Overholts LE, Popp HW et al. 1960. *Botany,* ed 3. McGraw-Hill, New York. 571 p.
2. Bold HC. 1967. *Morphology of Plants,* ed 2. Harper & Row, New York. 541 p.
3. Thorne RF. 1968. Synopsis of a putatively phylogenetic classification of the flowering plants. *Aliso* 6(4): 57–66.
4. Cronquist A. 1968. *The Evolution and Classification of Flowering Plants.* Houghton Mifflin, Boston. 396 p; Hutchinson J. 1959. *Families of Flowering Plants,* ed 2. 2 vols. Clarendon Press, Oxford; Hutchinson J. 1969. *Evolution and Phylogeny of Flowering Plants, Dicotyledons: Facts and Theory.* Academic Press, London and New York. 717 p; Soo R. 1967. Die modernen systeme der Angiospermen. *Acta Bot Acad Sci Hung* **13:** 201–233; Takhtajan A. 1969. *Flowering Plants.* (Translated from Russian by C Jeffrey.) Smithsonian Institution Press, Washington, DC. 310 p.

Appendix II

Bibliography of Herbal Medicine

Below are listed selected references primarily in English on herbal medicine. They are presented either under a general category or by a geographic arrangement whenever restricted to an area (North America, Latin America, Europe, Middle East and North Africa, Sub-Saharan Africa, Southern Asia, Eastern Asia, and Australia and Oceania).

GENERAL: PLANTS FROM MORE THAN ONE AREA

Aikman L. 1974. Nature' gifts to medicine. *Nat Geog* **146:** 420–444.

Amber RB, Babey-Brooke AM. 1966. *The Pulse in Occident and Orient: Its Philosophy and Practice in India, China, Iran, and the West.* Santa Barbara Press, New York. 203 p.

Arber A. 1970. *Herbals, Their Origin and Evolution,* ed 2, fascimile of 1938 ed. Hafner, New York. 326 p.

Ballard E, Garrod AB. 1846 *Elements of Materia Medica and Therapeutics.* Hogan & Thompson, Philadelphia. 516 p.

Bentley R, Trimen H. 1880. *Medicinal Plants.* Vols 1–4. J Churchill, London.

Best MR, Brightman FH (eds). 1973. *The Book of Secrets of Albertus Magnus of the Virtues of Herbs, Stones and Certain Beasts.* Clarendon Press, Oxford. 128 p.

Blackwell E. 1739. *A Curious Herbal.* 2 vols. London.

Boerhaave H. 1719. *A Method of Studying Physick.* (Translated by Mr Samber). London. 331 p.

Boyle R. 1718. *Medicinal Experiments: or, a Collection of Choice and Safe Remedies,* ed 6. W & J Innys, London. 168 + 61 p.

Brock AJ. 1929. *Greek Medicine, Being Extracts Illustrative of Medical Writers from Hippocrates to Galen.* EP Dutton, New York, JM Dent & Sons, London and Toronto. 256 p.

Buchan W. 1820. *The New Domestic Medicine,* new ed. Rider & Weed, London. 608 + 107 p.

Budge EAW. 1928. *The Divine Origin of the Craft of the Herbalist.* Culpeper House, London. 96 p. Reprinted 1971. Gryphon Books, Ann Arbor, Mich.

Celsus AC (first century AD) 1935–1938. *De Medicina.* Vols 1–3. (Translated by WG Spencer). Harvard University Press, Cambridge and Heinemann, London. Vol 1, 499 p, Vol 2 and 3, 649 p.

Chapman N. 1825. *Elements of Therapeutics and Materia Medica,* ed 4 rev. Vols 1–2. Carey & Lea, Philadelphia. 526 + 533 p.

Coffin AI. 1851. *Medical Botany: A Course of Lectures Delivered at Sussex Hall, During 1850.* WB Ford, London. 223 p.

Coles W. 1657. *Adam in Eden, or Nature's Paradise.* J Streater, London. 629 p.

Coon N. 1963. *Using Plants for Healing.* Hearthside Press, Great Neck, N.Y. 272 p.

Cruso J. 1771. *A Treasure of Easy Medicines.* London. 266 p.

Culbreth DMR. 1927. *A Manual of Materia Medica and Pharmacology,* ed 7. Lea & Febiger, Philadelphia. 627 p.

Cullen W. 1789. *A Treatise of the Materia Medica.* Vols 1–2. Charles Elliot, Edinburgh. 432 + 610 p.

Culpeper N. 1835. *The Complete Herbal.* Thomas Kelly, London. 398 p.

Dawson WR. 1934. *A Leechbook or Collection of Medical Recipes of the Fifteenth Century.* Macmillan, London. 344 p.

Dimbleby GW. 1967. *Plants and Archaeology.* J Baker, London. 187 p.

Dodge BS. 1959. *Plants that Changed the World.* Little, Brown, Boston and Toronto. 183 p.

Eberle J. 1834. *A Treatise of the Materia Medica and Therapeutics,* Vols 1–2, ed 4. Grigg & Elliot, Philadelphia. 450 + 479 p.

Ellingwood F. 1903. *A Systematic Treatise on Materia Medica and Therapeutics.* Chicago Medical Times, Chicago.

Fernie WT. 1914. *Herbal Simples,* ed 3 rev. J Wright & Sons, Bristol. 596 p.

Freeman MG. 1943. *Herbs for the Mediaeval Household (for cooking, healing, and diverse uses).* Metropolitan Museum of Art, New York. 48 p.

Gerard J. 1597. *The Herball or Generall Historie of Plantes.* John Norton, London. 1392 p. Second edition enlarged and amended by Thomas Johnson, 1633, 1631 p, and reprinted, 1636. (Translation of R Dodoens' *Stirpium Historiae Pemptades Sex,* Antwerp, 1583).

Gesner C. 1599. *The Practise of the New and Old Physicke.* (Transl by G Baker). Peter Short, London. 257 p.

Gibbons E. 1966. *Stalking the Healthful Herbs.* David McKay, New York. 303 p.

Green RM. 1951. *A Translation of Galen's Hygiene.* Charles C Thomas, Springfield, Ill. 277 p.

Grieve M. 1931. *A Modern Herbal.* Vols 1–2. Cape, London. 888 p.

Gunther RT. 1934. *The Greek Herbal of Dioscorides.* Oxford University Press, Oxford. 701 p. (Reprinted by Hafner, New York, 1959).

Hamilton E. 1852–1853. *Flora Homeopathica.* Vols 1–2. H Baillier, London. 300 + 223 p.

Harding AR. 1972. *Ginseng and Other Medicinal Plants,* rev ed. AR Harding, Columbus, Ohio. 385 p.

Harris BC. 1972. *The Compleat Herbal.* Barre Publ, Barre, Mass. 243 p.

Hill J. 1775. *The Useful Family Herbal,* ed 2. W Johnston & W Owen, London.

Hool RL. 1924. *Health from British Wild Herbs,* ed 3. "Visiter" Printing Works, Southport, England. 43 p + 31 plates.

James R. 1746. *The Modern Practice of Physic.* 2 vols. London.

Jarvis DC. 1960. *Folk Medicine.* WH Allen & Co, London.

Kariyone T. 1971. *Atlas of Medicinal Plants.* Takeda Chemical Industries, Osaka, Japan. 151 p.

Kloss J. 1971. *Back to Eden.* Lancer Books, New York. 671 p.

Kreig MB. 1964. *Green Medicine.* Rand McNally, Skokie, Ill.

Lewis W. 1791. *An Experimental History of the Materia Medica,* ed 4. 2 vols. London. Vol 1, 507 p; Vol 2, 495 p.

Leyel CF. 1926. *The Magic of Herbs.* Cape, London. 320 p.

Leyel CF. 1946. *Compassionate Herbs.* Faber & Faber, London. 224 p.

Leyel CF. 1948. *Elixirs of Life.* Faber & Faber, London. 221 p.

Leyel CF. 1952. *Green Medicine*. Faber & Faber, London. 324 p.

Lindley J. 1838. *Flora Medica*. Longman et al, London. 656 p.

Lindley J. 1856. *Medical and Oeconomical Botany*, ed 2. Bradbury & Evans, London. 274 p.

Lloyd JU. 1921. *Origin and History of all the Pharmacopeial Vegetable Drugs, Chemicals and Preparations with Bibliography*. Vol 1, *Vegetable Drugs*. Caxton Press, Cincinnati. 449 p.

Lust B. 1961. *About Herbs*. Thorsons Publ, Wellingborough, Northamptonshire. 64 p.

Lucas R. 1966. *Nature's Medicines*. Universal-Award House, New York. 251 p.

Lyte H. 1578. *A Niewe Herball or Historie of Plantes*. G Dewes, London.

Marks G, Beatty WK. 1971. *The Medical Garden*. Charles Scribner's Sons, New York. 178 p.

Mathison RR. 1958. *The Eternal Search*. GP Putnam's Sons, New York. 381 p.

Medicinal Plants of the Arid Zones. 1960. UNESCO, Paris. 96 p.

Mességué M. 1973. *Of Men and Plants*. Macmillan, New York (adapted from English translation published by Weiderfeld & Nicolson, 1972). 327 p.

Meyer JE. 1972. *The Herbalist*, 9th printing (first ed published 1918). [no publisher given.] 304 p.

Meyrick W. 1790. *New Family Herbal*. T Pearson, Birmingham, England. 498 p.

More Secret Remedies, series 2. 1912. British Medical Association, London, 282 p.

Murray J. 1824. *System of Materia Medica and Pharmacy*. E Duyckinck et al, New York. 560 p.

Nelson A. 1951. *Medical Botany*. E & S Livingstone, Edinburgh. 544 p.

Nissen C. 1958. *Herbals of Five Centuries*. (Translated by W Bodenheimer and A Rosenthal). L'Art Ancien, Zurich. 86 p.

Orbell A. 1967. *A Compendium of Botanical Remedies Physio-medical Practice*. Ilford, Exeter.

Parkinson J. 1640. *Theatrum Botanicum: The Theater of Plants*. T Cotes, London.

Perrot E, Paris R. 1971. *Les Plantes Médicinales*. 2 vols. Presses de l'Université de France, Paris.

Powell EF. 1965. *The Modern Botanic Prescriber*. LN Fowler, London. 136 p.

Potter SOL, Scott RJE. 1931. *Therapeutics, Materia Medica and Pharmacy*. Blakiston, Philadelphia. 997 p.

Reis Altschul S von. 1973. *Drugs and Foods from Little-Known Plants*. Harvard University Press, Cambridge, Mass. 366 p.

Rose J. 1972. *Herbs and Things*. Workman Publ, New York. 323 p.

Schroder J. 1669. *The Compleat Chymical Dispensatory*. (Translated by W Rowland). London. 545 p.

Singer C. 1927. The herbal in antiquity. *J Hell Stud* **47**: 1–52.

Spinelli WB. 1971. *The Primitive Therapeutic Use of Natural Products: a Bibliography*. Duquesne University Library, Pittsburgh. 106 p.

Steinmetz EF. 1954. *Materia Medica Vegetabilis*. Vols 1–3. Amsterdam.

Stephensen J, Churchill JM. 1834–1836. *Medical Botany*, new ed, Vols 1–3. J Churchill, London.

Swain T (ed). 1972. *Plants in the Development of Modern Medicine*. Harvard University Press, Cambridge, Mass. 367 p.

Taylor N. 1965. *Plant Drugs That Changed the World*. Apollo ed. Dodd, Mead, New York. 275 p.

Thompson CJS. 1934. *The Mystic Mandrake*. Rider, London. 253 p.

Thorndike L. 1946. *The Herbal of Rufinus*. University of Chicago Press, Chicago. 476 p.

Thornton RJ. 1814. *A Family Herbal*, ed 2. B & R Crosby, London. 901 p.

Thorwald J. 1962. *Science and Secrets of Early Medicine: Egypt, Mesopotamia, India, China, Mexico, Peru*. (Translated by R & C Winston). Thames & Hudson, London. 331 p.

Tobe JH. 1969. *Proven Herbal Remedies*. Provoker Press, St Catherines, Ontario. 304 p.

Turner NJ. 1974. Plant taxonomic systems and ethnobotany of three contemporary Indian groups of the Pacific Northwest (Haida, Bella Coola, and Lillooet). *Syesis* **7** (suppl 1): 1–104.

Turner W. 1568. *The First and Seconde Partes of the Herbal. . . .* A Birckman, Collen, England.

Uphof JCT. 1968. *Dictionary of Economic Plants*, ed 2. Verlag von J Cramer. Stechert-Hafner, New York.

Wade C. 1970. *Natural and Folk Remedies*. Parker, West Nyack, NY. 210 p.

Webb WH (ed). 1916. *Standard Guide to Non-poisonous Herbal Medicine*. "Visiter" Printing Works, Southport. 371 p.

Weiner MA. 1972. *Earth Medicine-Earth Foods*. Collier Books, New York, and Collier-Macmillan, London. 214 p.

Wesley J. 1768. *Primitive Physick*, ed 13. W Pine, Bristol. 140 p.

Wheelwright EG. 1935. *The Physick Garden*. Houghton Mifflin, Boston and New York. 288 p.

Williams TI. 1947. *Drugs from Plants*. Sigma, London. 119 p.

Woodville W. 1790–1793. *Medical Botany*. 3 vols. J Phillips, London.

Wren RC. 1950. *Potter's Encyclopaedia of Botanical Drugs and Preparations*. Potter & Clarke, London. 415 p.

GEOGRAPHICALLY LIMITED

NORTH AMERICA (NORTH OF MEXICO)

Barbeau M. 1958. *Medicine-men on the North Pacific Coast*. National Museum of Canada, Bull 152, Anthropological Series No 42. Department of Northern Affairs and National Resources, Information Canada, Ottawa. 95 p.

Barton BS. 1810. *Collections for an Essay Towards a Materia Medica*, ed 3 (2 parts). Earle, Philadelphia. 53 + 53 p.

Barton WPC. 1817–1818. *Vegetable Materia Medica of the United States; or Medical Botany*. W Carey, Philadelphia. Vol 1. 273 p; Vol 2, 239 p.

Beach W. 1833. *The American Practice of Medicine*. Vols 1–3. Betts & Austice, New York. Vol 1, 679 p; Vol 2 630 + 84 p; Vol 3, 279 p.

Bigelow J. 1817–1820. *American Medical Botany*. Vols 1–3. Cummings & Hilliard, Boston. Vol 1, 1817; Vol 2, 1818; Vol 3, 1820.

Brendle TR, Unger CW. 1935. *Folk Medicine of the Pennsylvania Germans. The Non-occult Cures*. Proceedings and Addresses of the Pennsylvania German Society (Reading) 45: part 2. 303 p.

Brown OP. 1867. *The Complete Herbalist*. OP Brown, Jersey City, NJ. 407 p.

Burlage HM. 1968. *Index of Plants with Reputed Medicinal and Poisonous Properties*. Austin, Tex. 272 p.

Charter JMG. 1888. *A Synopsis of the Medical Botany of the United States*. George H Field, St Louis. 176 p.

Clapp A. 1852. A synopsis; or systematic catalogue of the indigenous and naturalized, flowering and filicoid medicinal plants of the United States. *Trans Am Med Ass* 5: 689–906.

Chesnut VK. 1902. Plants used by the Indians of Mendocino County, California. *Contr US Nat Herb* 7: 295–408.

Corlett WT. 1935. *The Medicine-man of the American Indian and His Cultural Background*. Charles C Thomas, Springfield, Ill. 369 p.

Curtin LSM. 1947. *Healing Herbs of the Upper Rio Grande*. Laboratory of Anthropology, Sante Fe, NM 281 p.

Cramp AJ. 1936. *Nostrums and Quackery and Pseudo-medicine*, Vol 3. American Medical Association Press, Chicago. 232 p.

Creighton H. 1950. *Folklore from Lunenburg County, Nova Scotia*. National Museum of Canada, Bull 117, Anthropological Series 29, Ottawa. 163 p.

Darlington W. 1859. *American Weeds and Useful Plants: Being a Second and Illustrated Edition of Agricultural Botany*. O Judd, New York. 460 p.

Dunglison R. 1839. *New Remedies*. A Waldie, Philadelphia. 429 p.

Fogel EM. 1915. *Beliefs and Superstitions of the Pennsylvania Germans*. American Germanica Press, Philadelphia. 387 p.

Gibbons WP. 1889. Report on indigenous medical botany. *Trans Med Soc Calif* 1889: 143–158.

Gilmore MR. 1933. Some Chippewa uses of plants. *Papers Mich Acad Sci Arts Lett* 17: 119–143.

Good PP. 1845. *The Family Flora and Material Medica Botanica*. Vols 1–2. PP Good, Elizabethtown, NJ.

Griffith RE. 1847. *Medical Botany: Descriptions of the More Important Plants used in Medicine, with their History, Properties, and Mode of Administration*. Lea & Blanchard, Philadelphia. 704 p.

Gunther E. 1973. *Ethnobotany of Western Washington*, rev ed. University of Washington Press, Seattle and London. 71 p.

Henry S. 1814. *American Medical Family Herbal*. S Henry, New York. 392 p.

Hocking GM. 1956. Some plant materials used medicinally and otherwise by the Navaho Indians in the Chaco Canyon, New Mexico. *El Palacio* 63: 146–165.

Howard H. 1852. *An Improved System of Botanic Medicine*, ed 3. J Kost, Cincinnati.

Hudson IB. 1950. *Medicinal and Food Plants of British Columbia*. The author, Victoria, BC. 70 p.

Hunton A. 1855. On some of the medical virtues of indigenous vegetables grown in the United States. *NJ Med Rep* 8: 69–73.

Hutchens AR. 1969. *Indian Herbalogy of North America*. Homeo House Press, Kumbakonam, S India. 492 p.

Hyatt HM. 1935. *Folk-lore from Adams County Illinois*. AE Hyatt Foundation, New York. 723 p.

Ives E. 1850. Experience on the virtues of certain plants. *Trans Am Med Ass* 3: 311–316.

Jacobs ML, Burlage HM. 1958. *Index of Plants of North Carolina with Reputed Medicinal Uses*.

Chapel Hill, NC, Austin, Tex. [no publisher given.] 322 p.

Johnson L. 1884. *A Manual of the Medical Botany of North America.* William Wood, New York. 292 p.

King J. 1854. *The American Eclectic Dispensatory.* Moore, Wilstach, Keys, Cincinnati. 1391 p.

Kost J. 1858. *The Elements of Materia Medica and Therapeutics,* ed 2. Moore, Wilstach, Keys, Cincinnati. 829 p.

Krochmal A, Krochmal C. 1973. *A Guide to the Medicinal Plants of the United States.* Quadrangle/The New York Times Book Co, New York. 259 p.

Lee CA. 1848. *A Catalogue of the Medicinal Plants, Indigenous and Exotic Growing in the State of New York.* Langley, New York. 64 p.

Lick DE, Brendle TR. 1922. *Plant Names and Plant Lore Among the Pennsylvania Germans.* Proceedings and Addresses of the Pennsylvania German Society (Reading) 33: part 3. 300 p.

Lloyd, JU, Lloyd CG. 1884–1885. *Drugs and Medicines of North America.* Vol 1, *Ranunculaceae.* Clarke, Cincinnati. 304 p.

Mattson M. 1845. *American Vegetable Practice,* ed 2. Vols 1–2. Johnson, Boston. 708 p.

McKechnie II RE. 1972. *Strong Medicine.* JJ Douglas, Vancouver, BC. 193 p.

Meyer C. 1973. *American Folk Medicine.* Thomas Y Crowell, New York. 206 p.

Meyer JE. 1918. *The Herbalist and Herb Doctor.* Indiana Herb Gardens, Hammond. 400 p.

Miller ME. 1958. A folklore survey of Dickson County, Tennessee. *Bull Tenn Folklore Soc* **24**: 57–71.

Millspaugh CF. 1887. *American Medicinal Plants.* Vols 1–2. Boericke & Tafel, New York and Philadelphia.

Millspaugh CF. 1892. *Medical Plants, an Illustrated and Descriptive Guide to Plants Indigenous to and Naturalized in the United States which are Used in Medicine.* Vols 1–2. John C Yorston, Philadelphia.

Morton JF. 1974. *Folk Remedies of the Low Country.* EA Seemann, Miami, Fla. 176 p.

Pereira J. 1843. *The Elements of Materia Medica and Therapeutics,* Vols 1–2. Lea & Blanchard, Philadelphia.

Porcher FP. 1849. Medicinal plants of South Carolina. Indigenous and introduced. *Trans Am Med Ass* **2**: 683–862.

Porcher FP. 1854. On the medicinal and toxicological properties of the cryptogamic plants of the United States. *Trans Am Med Ass* **7**: 167–284.

Porcher FP. 1869. *Resources of the Southern Fields and Forests.* Walker, Evans & Cogswell, Charleston, SC. 733 p.

Puckett NN. 1926. *Folk Beliefs of the Southern Negro.* University of North Carolina Press, Chapel Hill. 644 p.

Rafinesque CS. 1828–30. *Medical Flora; or Manual of the Medical Botany of the United States of North America.* Vols 1–2. Atkinson & Alexander, Philadelphia.

Randolph V. 1947. *Ozark Superstitions.* Columbia University Press, New York. 367 p.

Robinson S. 1832. *A Course of Fifteen Lectures, on Medical Botany, Denominated Thomson's New Theory of Medical Practice.* Pike, Platt, Columbus, Ohio. 206 p.

Rogers EG. 1941. *Early Folk Medical Practices in Tennessee.* Mid-South Publ Co, Murfreesboro, Tenn. 68 p.

Schoepf D. 1787. *Materia Medica Americana.* JJ Palm, Erlangen, Germany. 170 p.

Scully V. 1970. *A Treasury of American Indian Herbs.* Crown, New York. 306 p.

Smith E. 1830. *The Botanic Physician.* Murphy & Bingham, New York. 624 p.

Smith EL. 1968. *Early American Home Remedies.* Applied Arts Publ, Witmer, Pa. 42 p.

Smith P. 1901. *The Indian Doctor's Dispensary.* Lloyd Library Bulletin 2, Cincinnati. 108 p.

Speck FG, Hassrick B, Carpenter ES. 1942. Rappahannock Herbals, folklore and science of cures. *Proc Delaware Co Inst Sci* (Media, Pa) **10**: 7–47.

Stearns S. 1801. *The American Herbal or Materia Medica.* Carlisle, Walpole, Mass.

Strong AB. 1846–1849. *The American Flora.* 3 vols. Strong & Bidwell (Vol 1) or Green & Spencer (Vols 2–3), New York. Vol 1, 1846, 137 p; Vol 2, 1848, 192 p; Vol 3, 1849, 184 p.

Stuhr ET. 1927. *Medicinal Plants of Florida.* Thesis, University of Florida.

Stuhr ET. 1933. *Manual of Pacific Coast Drug Plants.* Science Press, Lancaster, Pa. 189 p.

Tantaquidageon G. 1942. *A Study of Delaware Indian Medicine Practice and Folk Beliefs.* Department of Public Instruction, Pennsylvania Historical Commission, Harrisburg. 91 p.

[Tennent J]. 1734. *Every Man His Own Doctor: or, The Poor Planter's Physician,* ed 2. William Parks, Williamsburg & Annapolis. 56 p. Reprinted by St Louis Medical Museum, St Louis.

Thomas DL, Thomas LB. 1920. *Kentucky Superstitions.* Princeton University Press, Princeton, NJ. 334 p.

Thomson S. 1841. *The Thomsonian Materia Medica,* ed 12. Munsell, Albany, NY. 834 p.

Train P, Heinrichs JR, Archer WA. 1957. *Medicinal Uses of Plants by Indian Tribes of Nevada,* rev ed. US Department of Agriculture, Beltsville, Md. 139 p.

Vogel VJ. 1970. *American Indian Medicine.* University of Oklahoma Press, Norman. 583 p.

Welsh JM. 1882-1883. The medical flora of Kansas. *Trans Nat Eclect Med Ass* **10:** 458-472.

Wieand PR. 1961. *Folk Medicine Plants.* Wieand's Pennsylvania Dutch, Allentown, Pa. 48 p.

Williams SW. 1849. Report on the indigenous medical botany of Massachusetts. *Trans Am Med Ass* **2:** 863-927.

Williams TI. 1947. *Drugs from Plants.* Sigma, London. 119 p.

Wyman JC, Harris SK. 1941. Navajo Indian medical ethnobotany. *Univ NM Bull* **3**(5): June 1.

Youngken HW. 1924-25. The drugs of the North American Indian. *Am J Pharm* **96:** 483-502, 1924; **97:** 158-185, 257-571, 1925.

EUROPE

Agnus Castus. 1950. *A Middle English Herbal.* ed G Brodin, Uppsala. 328 p.

Culpeper N. 1652. *The English Physician.* London.

Culpeper N. 1820. *The British Herbal and Family Physician to which is Added a Dispensatory for the Use of Private Families.* M Garlick, Halifax. 410 + 317 p.

Hool RL. 1924. *Health from British Wild Herbs,* ed 3. The "Visiter" Printing Works, Southport. 43 p + 31 plates.

Jones IB. 1937. Popular medical knowledge of fourteenth century English literature. *Bull Hist Med (Johns Hopkins)* **5:** 405-451, 538-588.

Kourennoff PM. 1971. *Russian Folk Medicine.* Pyramid, New York. (Translated by G St George) 287 p.

Larsen, H. 1931. *An Old Icelandic Medical Miscellany.* J Dybwad, Oslo. 328 p.

Lawrendiadis G. 1961. Contribution to the knowledge of the medicinal plants of Greece. *Planta Med* **9:** 164-169.

Logan P. 1972. *Making the Cure.* Talbot Press, Dublin. 178 p.

Ossadcha-Janata N. 1952. *Herbs Used in Ukrainian Folk Medicine.* (Translated by N Rubinstein), Research Program on the USSR (East European Fund), New York. 114 p.

Short T. 1749. *Medicina Britannica.* London. Reprinted B Franklin & D Hall, Philadelphia. 339 p + appendix + Bartram's appendix (7 p).

LATIN AMERICA (INCLUDING CENTRAL AND SOUTH AMERICA, WEST INDIES)

Aces RP. 1939. *Plantas Utiles de las Antillas.* G Martinez Amengual, Havana. 200 p.

Altamirano F. 1904. *Materia Médica Mexicana.* Mexican National Commission, St Louis. 78 p.

Amadeo AJ. 1888. The botany and vegetable materia medica of the island of Porto-Rico. *Pharm J* **18:** 771-772, 881-882, 906-907.

Arias H, Costas F. 1941. *Plantas Medicinales.* Biblioteca Practica, Buenos Aires. 153 p.

Asprey GF, Thornton P. 1953-1955. Medicinal plants of Jamaica. Parts 1-4. *W Indian Med J* **2:** 233-252, 1953; **3:** 17-41, 1954; **4:** 69-82, 145-168, 1955.

The Badianus Manuscript (Codex Barberini, Latin 241). An Aztec Herbal of 1552. 1940. (Translated by EW Emmart.) Johns Hopkins University Press, Baltimore. 341 p.

Cabrera LG. 1950. *Plantas Curativas de Mexico,* ed 4. Cicerón, Mexico, DF. 384 p.

Cainas F. 1937. *Plantas Medicinales de Cuba.* Havana. 204 p.

Catalogo de Plantas Reputadas Medicinales en la Republica de Guatemala, ed 2. 1929. Tipo Nacional, Guatemala. 55 p.

Combs R. 1897. Some Cuban medical plants. *Pharm Rev* **15:** 87-91, 109-112, 136.

Cruz M de la. 1939. *The de la Cruz-Badiano Aztec Herbal of 1552.* (Translated by W Gates). Maya Society, Baltimore. 143 p.

Ernst A. 1865. Plants used medicinally at Caracas, Venezuela, South America, and their vernacular names. *J Bot (London)* **3:** 143-150, 277-284, 306-322.

Fernandez Moro W. 1927-1928. Estudios de Etnografia y Medicina Salvaje. *Bol Soc Geog Lima* **43:** 1-29, 149-164, 1926; **44:** 75-90, 1927; **45:** 119-138, 1928.

Fonseca ET da. 1940. Plantas medicinais. *Campo (Rio de Janeiro)* **11**(129): **20;** (130); **28;** (131): **26.**

Freise, FW. 1933. Plantas medicinales Brasileiras. *Bol Agric (São Paulo)* **34:** 252-494.

Domínguez JA. 1928. *Contribuciones a la Materia Médica Argentina*. Penser, Buenos Aires. 433 p.

Gonzalez M, Lombardo A, Vallarino AJ. 1939. *Plantas de las Medicina Vulgar del Uruguay*. Talleres Graficos, Montevideo. 141 p.

Gracia Alcover B. 1950. *Medicina Herbaria Chilena*. La Vida Naturista, Mexico. 315 p.

Hernández F. 1942–1946. *Historia de las Plantas de Nueva Españã*. Imprenta Universitaria, Mexico. 1104 p.

Hoehne FC. 1939. *Plantas e Substãncias Vegetais Toxicas e Medicinais*. Graphicars, São Paulo and Rio de Janeiro. 355 p.

Instituto Medico Nacional. 1894–1908. *Datos para la Materia Médica Mexicana*. Oficio tripo de la secret de fomento, Mexico City. Part 1, 1894; part 2, 1898; part 3, 1900; part 4, . . . ; part 5, 1908.

Kelly I. 1965. *Folk Practices in North Mexico*. University of Texas Press, Austin. 166 p.

Manfred L. 1958. *Siete Mil Recetas Botanicas a Base de Mil Trescientas Plantas Medicinales*. Kier, Buenos Aires. 668 p.

Martinez M. 1939. *Plantas Medicinales de Mexico*, ed 2. Sanchez, SCL, Mexico City. 628 p.

Martius CEP de. 1843. *Systema Materiae Medicae Vegetabilis Brasiliensis*. F. Fleischer, Leipzig, and F Beck, Vienna. 155 p.

Maza MG de la. 1889. *Ensayo de Farmacofitoligiá Cubana*. Havana. 112 p.

Maxwell N. 1961. *Witch Doctor's Apprentice*. Houghton Mifflin, Boston. 353 p.

Monardes N. 1577. *Joyfull Newes Out of the Newe Founde Worlde*. (Translated by J Frampton). W Norton, London.

Murillo A. 1889. *Plantes Medicinales du Chili*. de Lagny, Paris. 234 p.

Oakes AJ, Morris MP. 1958. The West Indian weedwoman of the United States Virgin Islands. *Bull Hist Med* **32:** 163–170.

Pardal R. 1937. *Medicina Aborigen Americana*. J Anesi, Buenos Aires. 377 p.

Peckolt T, Peckolt G. 1888–91. *Historia das Plantas Medicinaes e Uteis do Brazil*, parts 1–4. Laemert, Rio de Janeiro. 227 + 635 p.

Pérez Arbeláez E. 1934. *Plantas Medicinales Mas Usadas en Bogotá*. Suplementa al Biolgia de Agricultura (Republica de Colombia) No 32 (Apr). 112 p.

Pérez Arbeláez E. 1956. *Plantas Utiles de Colombia*, ed 3. C Roldan, Bogotá. 831 p.

Pittier H. 1908. *Ensayo Sobre Las Plantas Usuales de Costa Rica*. McQueen, Washington, DC 176 p.

Pittier H. 1926. *Manual de las Plantas Usuales de Venezuela*. Litografía del Comercio, Caracas. 458 p.

Pompa G. 1875. *Coleccion de Medicamentos Indigenas*, ed 5, Rójas Hermanos, Caracas. 175 p.

Reitz PR. 1950. Plantas medicinais de Santa Catarina. *An Bot Herb "Barbosa Rodrigues"* **2:** 71–116.

Risquez FA. 1898. *Farmocopea Venezolana*. Tipo Americano al Vapor, Caracas. 489 p.

Roig y Mesa JT. 1945. *Plantas Medicinales*. Guerrero Casa Mayor, Havana. 872 p.

Rodriguez PM. 1915. *Plantas Medicinales de Paraguay*. C Estrella, Montevideo, La Mundial and Asuncion. 142 p.

Schendel G. 1968. *Medicine in Mexico*. University of Texas Press, Austin. 329 p.

Teixeira de Fonseca E. 1940. *Plantas Medicinales Brasilenãs*. Almeida Marques, Rio de Janeiro. 102 p.

Valdizán H, Maldonado A. 1922. *La Medicina Popular Peruana*. Vols 1–3. T Aguirre, Lima. 475 + 3, 529 + 92, 487 + 38 p.

Williams RO, Williams RO Jr. 1951. *The Useful and Ornamental Plants in Trinidad and Tobago*, ed 4. Guardian Commercial Printery, Port-of-Spain, Trinidad. 335 p.

Wright W. 1787. An account of the medicinal plants growing in Jamaica. *London Med J* **8:** 217–295.

Ximenez F. 1888. *Cuatro Libros de la Naturaleza y Virtudes de las Plantas y Animales, de Uso Medicinal en la Nueva España*. Oficio tipo de la secretarie de fomento, Mexico City. 342 p.

Zin J. 1930. *La Salud por Medio de las Plantas Medicinales por un Sacerdote Salesiano*, ed 5 rev. La Gratitud Nacional Esc Tipo, Santiago de Chile. 701 p.

MIDDLE EAST AND NORTH AFRICA

Budge EAW. 1913. *Syrian Anatomy, Pathology and Therapeutics, or the Book of Medicines*. 2 vols. Oxford University Press, London.

Fahmy IR, Ahmed ZF. 1963. Drug plants of Egypt. *Planta Med* **11:** 202–224.

Hooper D. 1937. Useful plants and drugs of Iran and Iraq. *Field Mus Nat Hist (Bot Ser)* **9**(3): 69–241.

Levey M. 1966. *The Medicinal Formulary or Aqrabadhin of Al-Kindi*. University of Wisconsin Press, Madison, Milwaukee, and London. 410 p.

Levey M. 1971. *Substitute Drugs in Early Arabic Medicine*. Wissenschaftliche Verlagsgesellschaft, Stuttgart. 102 p.

Moldenke HN, Moldenke AL. 1952. *Plants of the Bible.* Ronald Press, New York. 328 p.

The Papyrus Ebers, the Greatest Egyptian Medical Document. 1937. (Translated by B Ebbell). Oxford University Press, London. 135 p.

Parsa A. 1959–60. Medicinal plants and drugs of plant origin in Iran. 1–4. *Qual Plant Mat Veg* **5**(4): 375–394, 1959; **6**(1): 69–96, 1959; **6**(2): 137–156, 1959; **7**(1): 65–136, 1960.

Sobhy GPG. 1938. Remains of ancient Egyptian medicine in modern domestic treatment. *Bull Inst Egypte* **20**: 12–18.

SUB-SAHARAN AFRICA

Ainslie JR. 1937. A list of plants used in native medicine in Nigeria. Institute paper 7, Imperial Forestry Institute, Oxford University. 92 p.

Bally PRO. 1937. Native medicinal and poisonous plants of East Africa. *Kew Bull Misc Inf Fasc* **1:** 10–26.

Bryant AT. 1966. *Zulu Medicine and Medicine-men.* C Struik, Cape Town. 115 p.

Dalziel JM. 1937. *The Useful Plants of West Tropical Africa.* Appendix to J Hutchison and JM Dalziel, *Flora of West Tropical Africa.* Crown Agents for the Colonies, London. 612 p.

Gelfand M. 1956. *Medicine and Magic of the Mashona.* JC Juta, Cape Town. 256 p.

Gelfand M. 1964. *Medicine and Custom in Africa.* E & S Livingstone, Edinburgh and London. 174 p.

Gelfand M. 1964. *Witch Doctor, Traditional Medicine Man of Rhodesia.* Harrill Press, London. 191 p.

Gitchens TS. 1949. *Drug Plants of Africa.* University of Pennsylvania Press, Philadelphia. 125 p.

Haerdi F, Kerharo J, Adam JG. 1964. Afrikanische Heilpflanzen *Acta Trop,* Suppl 8, Verlag fur Recht and Gesellschaft AG, Basel. 334 p.

Harley GW. 1941. *Native African Medicine.* Harvard University Press, Cambridge, Mass. 294 p.

Hewat ML. 1908. *Bantu Folk Lore.* TM Miller, Cape Town. 112 p.

Irvine FR. 1961. *Woody Plants of Ghana.* Oxford University Press, London.

Jones GI. 1951. *Basutoland Medicine Murder.* HM Stationery Office, London. 104 p.

Kokwaro JO. 1976. *Medicinal Plants of East Africa.* East African Literature Bureau, Nairobi. 384 p.

Smith A. 1895. *A Contribution to South African Materia Medica,* ed 3. JC Juta, Cape Town. 238 p.

Watt JM, Breyer-Brandwijk MG. 1962. *Medicinal and Poisonous Plants of Southern and Eastern Africa,* ed 2. E & S Livingston, Edinburgh and London. 1457 p.

SOUTHERN ASIA

Ainslie W. 1813. *Materia Medica of Hindoostan.* Government Press, Madras. 301 + 48 p.

Ainslie W. 1826. *Materia Indica,* Vols 1–2. Longman et al, London. 654 + 604 p.

Attygalle J. 1917. *Sinhalese Materia Medica.* Gunosena, Colombo. 243 p.

Caius JF. 1936–1940. The medicinal and poisonous (plants) of India. A series of papers on specific plant groups. *J Bombay Nat Hist Soc* **39–41**.

Chakraberty C. 1923. *A Comparative Hindu Materia Medica.* RC Chakraberty, Calcutta. 198 p.

Chopra RN. 1933. *Indigenous Drugs of India.* Arts Press, Calcutta. 655 p; ed 2, Chopra RN, Chopra IC, Handakh et al., UN Dhur, Calcutta.

Chopra RN, Nayar SL, Chopra IC. 1956. *Glossary of Indian Medicinal Plants.* Council on Scientific and Industrial Research, New Delhi. 330 p.

Das SK. [no date.] *Medicinal, Economic and Useful Plants of India.* PO Bally, Howrah District, West Bengal. 128 p.

Dash B. 1971. *Concept of Agni in Ayurveda.* Chawkhamba Sanskrit Series Office, Varanasi. 265 p.

Dastur JF. 1962. *Medicinal Plants of India and Pakistan,* ed 2. DB Taraporevala Sons, Bombay. 317 p.

Datye PM. 1970. *A Glance at Ayurved, Science of Life.* By author, Bombay. 148 p.

Dey KL. 1898. *The Indigenous Drugs of India,* ed 2. Thacker, Spink, Calcutta. 387 p.

Drury A. 1963. *The Useful Plants of India.* Asylum Press, Madras. 559 p.

Dutt UC. 1877. *The Materia Medica of the Hindus.* Thacker, Spink, Calcutta. 354 p.

Dymock W. 1885–86. *The Vegetable Materia Medica of Western India,* ed 2. Bombay and London. 1012 p.

Dymock W, Warden CJH, Hooper D. 1890–1893. *Pharmacographia India.* Vols 1–3. Education Society's Press, Bombay. Vol 1, 599 p, 1890; Vol 2, 643 p, 1891; Vol 3, 642; 1893.

An Eight-Hundred Year Old Book of Indian Medicine and Formulas. 1937. (Translated by E Sharpe). Luzac, London. 135 p.

Fleming J. 1810. *A Catalogue of Indian Medicinal Plants and Drugs.* AH Hubbard, Calcutta. 72 p.

Gupta SM. 1971. *Plant Myths and Traditions in India.* Brill, Leiden. 117 p.

Jaggi OP. 1973. *Folk Medicine. History of Science and Technology in India.* Vol 3. Atma Ram & Sons, Delhi. 228 p.

Kirtikar KR, Basu ED. 1918. *Indian Medicinal Plants,* 2 parts. Indian Press, Allahabad. 1419 p.

Lewis F. 1934. *The Vegetable Products of Ceylon.* Associated Newspapers of Ceylon, Colombo. 402 p.

Medicinal Plants of Nepal. Bulletin 3, Department of Medicinal Plants. 1970. HM Government of Nepal, Ministry of Forests, Katmandu.

Mohan BS. 1930. *Medicinal Drugs of India.* Hindi Eclectic Press, Lahore. 256 p.

Mooss NS, 1953. *Ayurvedic Flora Medica,* part 1. Kottyama, Travancore, India. Vaidyasarethy. 128 p.

Murray JA. 1881. *The Plants and Drugs of Sind.* Education Society Press, Bombay. 219 p.

Nadkarni KM. 1927. *The Indian Materia Medica.* SK Bijur, Bombay. 1142 + 169 + 88 p.

Nordel A. 1963. *The Medicinal Plants and Crude Drugs of Burma. I. Collection of Research Material from Indigenous Sources during the years 1957–1961.* Hellstrøm & Nordahls Boktr As, Oslo.

O'Shaughnessy WB. 1841. *The Bengal Dispensary and Pharmacopoeia.* Bishop's College Press, Calcutta. 794 p.

Roberts E. 1931. *Vegetable Materia Medica of India and Ceylon.* Plate, Colombo. 437 p.

Said HM (ed). 1969. *Hamdard Pharmacopoeia of Eastern Medicine.* Times Press, Karachi. 500 p.

Sanyal D, Ghose R. 1934. *Vegetable Drugs of India.* S. Chatterji, Calcutta. 590 p.

Sharma PV. 1972. *Indian Medicine in the Classical Age.* Chawkhamba Sanskrit Series Office, Veranasi. 261 p.

Shin Naga Thein. 1971. *Illustrated Pharmacopoeia,* 4 vols [for Burma]. Mingala Press, Rangoon. (in Burmese).

Srivastave GP. 1954. *History of Indian Pharmacy,* Vol 1, ed 2. Pindars, Calcutta. 276 p.

Stewart JL. 1899. *Punjab Plants.* Government Press, Lahore. 269 + 106 p.

Waring EJ. 1874. *Remarks on the Uses of Some of the Bazaar Medicine and Common Medical Plants of India,* ed 2. J & A Churchill, London. 212 p.

Watt G. 1882–1896. *A Dictionary of the Economic Products of India,* 6 vols. Delhi (reprinted 1972).

EASTERN ASIA

Burkill IH. 1935. *A Dictionary of the Economic Products of the Malay Peninsula.* 2 vols. Crown Agents for the Colonies, London. (Reprinted Ministry of Agriculture, Kuala Lumpor, Malaysia.)

Croizier RC. 1968. *Traditional Medicine in Modern China.* Harvard University Press, Cambridge, Mass. 325 p.

Gimlette JD, Thomson HW. 1939. *A Dictionary of Malayan Medicine.* Oxford University Press, London. 259 p.

Guerrero LM. 1921. Medicinal uses of Philippine plants. *Bull Bur For Manila* 3(22): 149–329.

Holmes EM. 1892. *Malay Materia Medica. Bull Pharm* 6: 108–117.

Hooper D. 1929. On Chinese medicine: drugs of Chinese pharmacies in Malaya. *Gardens' Bull, Straits Settlements* 6: 1–163.

Huard P, Wong M. 1968. *Chinese Medicine.* (Translated by B Fielding.) McGraw-Hill, New York. 256 p.

Jaspan MA. 1969. *Traditional Medical Theory of South-East Asia.* University of Hull, England. 36 p.

McClure FA, Hwang T. 1934. The flora of a Canton herb shop. *Lingnan Univ Sci Bull* 6: 1–32.

Pardo de Tavera TH. 1901. *The Medicinal Plants of the Philippines.* (Translated by J B Thomas Jr.) Blakiston, Philadelphia. 269 p.

Quisumbing E. 1951. *Medicinal Plants of the Philippines.* Technical Bulletin 16, Department of Agriculture and National Resources, Philippines.

Risse GB (ed). 1973. *Modern China and Traditional Chinese Medicine.* Charles C Thomas, Springfield, Ill. 167 p.

Smith FP. 1969. *Chinese Materia Medica,* ed 2 revised by D Wei. Ku T'ing, Taipei. 558 p. Original ed by GA Stuart, American Presbyterian Mission Press, Shanghai, 1911.

Soepardi R. 1967. *Medicines from Forest Products.* Translation Series 24, Institute of Advanced Project, East-West Center, Honolulu. (Translated by S Notoatmodjo of *Obat-obatan dari hasil Hutan,* published by Government Publishing House, Djakarata, 1957.)

Steenis-Kruseman MJ van. 1942. *Select Indonesian Medicinal Plants.* Organization for Scientific Research Indonesia Bulletin 18. 90 p.

Takatori J. 1966. *Color Atlas Medicinal Plants of Japan.* Hirokawa, Tokyo.

Wallnöfer H, Rottauscher A von. 1965. *Chinese Folk Medicine.* (Translated by M Palmedo.) Bell, New York. 184 p.

AUSTRALIA AND OCEANIA

Brooker SG, Cooper RC. 1961. *New Zealand Medicinal Plants.* Unity Press Auckland. 46 p.

Gardner CA, Bennetts HW. 1956. *The Toxic Plants of Western Australia.* West Australian Newspaper, Perth. 253 p.

Kaaiakamanu DM, Akina JK. 1968. *Hawaiian Herbs of Medicinal Value,* facsimile reprint. (Translated by A Akana). Pacific Book House, Honolulu, and Charles E Tuttle, Rutland, Vt, and Tokyo.

Maiden JH. 1888. Some reputed medicinal plants of New South Wales (indigenous species only). *Pharm J* **19:** 116–119, 133–136, 150–152, 178–180.

Maiden JH. 1889. *The Useful Native Plants of Australia.* Turner & Henderson, Sydney. 696 p.

Safford WE. 1905. The useful plants of the island of Guam. *Contr US Nat Herb* **9:** 1–416.

Webb LJ. 1948. *Guide to the Medicinal and Poisonous Plants of Queensland.* Bulletin 232, Center for Scientific and Industrial Research, Melbourne.

Glossary

The wide range of subject matter in *Medical Botany* requires the inclusion of a small glossary for the convenience of the reader. It is not all-embracing, however, and the user may also find valuable a good general dictionary such as *Webster's New Collegiate Dictionary* (G & C Merriam Co., Springfield, Mass, 1974).

Following the definitions is information on the derivation of words, which may be particularly helpful in understanding the origins of the compound words widely used in medical and biological terminology. Scientific words are chiefly from Greek (Gr), the Greek letters being transliterated into the English alphabet, and Latin (L) in our listing, with fewer derivations from Arabic (Ar), Anglo-Saxon (AS), Carib, French (Fr), Italian (It), Sanskrit (Sansk), Scandinavian (Scand), and Urdu sources. Commonly known synonyms are also given as appropriate.

Å: = ångström unit, one tenth part of a millimicron (mμ).

abortus: a fetus weighing less than 500 g when eliminated from the uterus with little chance of survival [L].

achene: small, dry, indehiscent fruit with one seed [Gr a- not, *chainein* to gape].

achlorhydria: the absence of hydrochloric acid from gastric secretions, because of gastric mucosal atrophy [Gr a- not, *chloros* green, *hydrios* water].

actinomorphy: radial symmetry, that is,

466

floral parts are regular or similar from a central axis [Gr *aktis* ray, *morphe* form].

actinomycosis: infection induced by bacterial species of *Actinomyces* [Gr *aktis* ray, *mykes* fungus, *-osis* condition].

addiction: unable to resist indulgence in some habit, especially strong dependence on a drug [L *addictum* from *addicere* to devote].

adipose: fat [L *adeps* lard].

afferent: conveying toward a central direction [L *afferre* to bring].

aflatoxin: specific mycotoxin produced by *Aspergillus*; a potent liver toxin that can induce liver tumors (hepatomas) [L *a-* from, *fla* from species *flavus*; Gr *toxikon* poison].

alkaloid: basic organic nitrogenous compound of plant origin that is pharmacologically active and bitter tasting [Ar *alqaliy* potash; Gr *eidos* form].

allergen: substance capable of inducing an allergic response [Gr *allos* other, *ergon* work, *genein* to produce].

allergy: hypersensitivity of the body cells to specific substances as antigens and allergens, resulting in various types of reactions (anaphylaxis, atopic diseases, contact dermatitis) [Gr *allos* other, *ergon* work].

alterative: agent presumed to correct a disordered bodily function [L *alterare* to change].

alternation of generations: alternate production of haploid sexual and diploid asexual generations in life cycles typical of plants.

amebiasis: amebic infection especially with *Entamoeba histolytica* [Gr *amoibe* change; L *-iasis* condition].

ament: = catkin.

analeptic: agent that excites and stimulates; in high doses it causes generalized convulsions [Gr *ana-* up, *lambanein* to take].

analgesic: pain reliever that does not induce loss of consciousness [Gr *a-* not, *algos* pain]; anodyne.

anaphrodisiac: repressor of sexual desire [Gr *an-* not, *aphrodisiakos* sexual].

anaphylatoxin: substance produced during the fixation of complement in C_3 and C_5 fragments that causes inflammation; indirectly, through mast cell degranulation and histamine release, it causes increased vascular permeability [Gr *ana-* up, *phylax* protect, *toxikon* poison].

anaphylaxis: see **hypersensitivity.**

anemia: condition induced when the equilibrium between blood production and blood loss is disturbed, causing a reduction either in the number of erythrocytes, the quantity of hemoglobin, or the volume of packed red blood cells [Gr *a-* not, *haima* blood]. **hemolytic a.:** uncompensated decrease in red blood cell survival due to heredity, infections, or toxic causes [Gr *hemo-* blood, *lysis* dissolution]. **macrocytic a.:** characterized by abnormally large red blood cells and due to deficiency of vitamin B_{12} or folic acid [Gr *makros* large, *kytos* cell]. **megaloblastic a.:** characterized by the presence of megablasts in the bone marrow [Gr *megas* large, *blastos* germ]. **pernicious a.:** chronic disorder due to the atrophy of the stomach mucosa and its failure to produce a factor necessary to absorb vitamin B_{12} [L *perniciosus* destructive].

anemophilous: wind-pollinated [Gr *anemos* wind, *philein* to love].

anesthesia: induction of the loss of tactile sensibility, especially in relation to the sensation of pain [Gr *a-* not, *aisthesis* sensation].

aneuploidy: increase or decrease in chromosome number by less than a whole genome [Gr *a-* not, *eu-* well, *aploos* onefold].

aneurysm: local dilation of a segment of

a blood vessel, often the aorta [Gr *aneurysma* dilation].

angina pectoris: severe though temporary attack of cardiac pain, an indication of coronary insufficiency [L *angere* to strangle, *pectoralis* of the chest].

angiodema: temporary swelling of skin or mucous membranes associated with urticaria and erythema; of allergic, neurotic, or unknown origin [Gr *anggeion* vessel, *oidema* swelling].

angiosperms: flower-bearing plants; ovules are enclosed in an ovary that forms the fruit after fertilization [Gr *anggeion* vessel, *sperma* seed].

angstrom: = Å.

animism: the attribution of a soul or spirit to any natural object [L *anima* soul].

annual: plant living for one year (from seed to maturity and death) [L *annus* year].

anodyne: = analgesic.

anorexia: loss of appetite [Gr *a-* not, *orexis* appetite].

anthelminthic: = vermifuge.

antianginal agent: drug alleviating anginal pain (marked by spasmodic suffocative attacks) [Gr *anti-* against; L *angere* to strangle].

antiarrhythmic agent: drug preventing or alleviating cardiac arrhythmia [Gr *anti-* against, *a-* not, *rhythmos* rhythm].

antibody: immunoglobulin molecule that is found normally in the body or is elicited after contact with an antigen. The specific amino acid sequences the antibody contains are designed to interact with the eliciting antigen in some demonstrable way; the antibody is frequently classified according to this ability (e.g., neutralizing, lysing, agglutinating) [Gr *anti-* against; AS *bodig*].

anticoagulant: agent preventing or retarding blood clotting [Gr *anti-* against; L *coagulare* to curdle].

anticonvulsant: agent that prevents or stops convulsion [Gr *anti-* against; L *convulsus* shaken].

antifebrile: = antipyretic.

antigen: any substance (usually a protein or high molecular weight carbohydrate) that when introduced into the body will elicit an antibody response [Gr *anti-* against, *genein* to produce].

antihypotensive agent: drug that increases blood pressure [Gr *anti-* against, *hypo-* below, *tendere* to stretch]. See **hypertensive, vasoconstrictor, vasopressor.**

antihypertensive agent: drug that lowers blood pressure [Gr *anti-* against, *hyper-* above, *tendere* to stretch]. See **hypotensive.**

antipsychotic: = neuroleptic.

antipyretic: agent relieving or reducing fever [Gr *anti-* against, *pyretos* fever]. Antifebrile, febrifuge.

antirheumatic: agent that prevents or relieves the pain of rheumatism [Gr *anti-* against, *rheuma* flux].

antitoxin: antibody to the toxin of a microorganism, phytotoxin, or zootoxin that can neutralize its toxicity *in vitro* or *in vivo* [Gr *anti-* against, *toxikon* poison].

antitussive: agent that prevents or relieves cough [Gr *anti-* against; L *tussis* cough].

apatite: calcium phosphate complex, a mineral constituent of bone and teeth [Gr *apate* deceit—because the material is easily misidentified].

aperient: = purgative.

aphrodisiac: stimulator of sexual desire [Gr *aphrodisiakos* sexual].

aril: outgrowth or appendage of a seed [Fr *arille*].

arrhythmia: lack of regular heart rhythm [Gr *a-* not, *rhythmos* rhythm].

arteriosclerosis: see **atherosclerosis.**

arthritis: inflammation of joints [Gr

arthron joint, *-itis* inflammation]. **os-teoarthritis:** degenerative arthritis, chiefly of the aged [Gr *osteon* bone]. **rheumatoid a.:** chronic disease marked by inflammatory changes of the synovial membrane lining the joints and by atrophy of bones [Gr *rheuma* flux, *eidos* form]. See **rheumatism.**

asthma, bronchial: chronic hypersensitive respiratory ailment caused by exposure of the respiratory epithelium to allergens; accumulation of mucus with wheezing and overinflation of the lungs are significant clinical features [Gr *asthma,* panting].

astringent: agent contracting organic tissue, thereby lessening secretion [L *astringere,* to bind together].

ataxia: disorder of muscle control resulting in jerky, irregular movements [Gr *ataxia* disorder].

atheroma: deposit of hard lipoid yellowish raised plaques in the inner arterial walls [Gr *athere* meal, *-oma* tumor].

atherosclerosis: a condition characterized by thickening and loss of elasticity of arteries as a result of accumulation of lipoid substances and progressive decrease in the size of the lumen [Gr *athere* meal, *sklerosis* hardening]. **arteriosclerosis.**

atopic: genetic or constitutional ability to develop immediate hypersensitivity (allergic) states [Gr a- not, *topos* place].

atrium: cavity, specifically the upper two cavities of the heart [L *atrium* chamber].

autoimmunity: specific humoral- or cell-mediated immunity to constituents of the body's own tissues (autoantigens) [Gr *autos* self; L *immunis* exempt].

Ayurvedic medicine: indigenous Indian system of medicine based on the Hindu scriptures or Vedas; used interchangeably in text with Hindu medicine [Sansk *áyurveda* the science of life].

bacteriophage: = phage.

bariatrics: study of the overweight condition [Gr *baros* weight, *iatrikos* healing].

basophil: see **leukocyte.**

B cell: bone marrow derived cell; lymphocyte derived from bone marrow found in peripheral lymphoid tissue that, on differentiating into a plasma cell, can produce immunoglobulins.

berry: fleshy fruit with a succulent pericarp (fruit wall) [AS *berie*].

biennial: plant living for two years [L *bis* twice, *annus* year].

blade: flat, expanded portion of the leaf, usually green [AS *blaed* leaf].

blephoroconjunctivitis: inflammation of the eyelids and conjunctiva [Gr *blepharon* eyelid; L *conjunctivus*; Gr *-itis* inflammation].

bract: modified leaf found in the inflorescence [L *bractea* thin metal plate].

bradycardia: slow rate of cardiac contraction [Gr *bradys* slow, *kardia* heart].

bronchiectasis: following infection, dilation of bronchi associated with fetid breath, paroxysmal coughing, and mucopurulent (pus-filled) discharge [Gr *brogchos* windpipe, *ektasis* dilation].

bronchiole: minute subdivision of the bronchus that terminates in the lung alveoli or air sacs [Gr *brogchos* windpipe].

bronchitis: inflammation of the bronchi [Gr *brogchos* windpipe, *-itis* inflammation].

bronchoconstriction: constriction of smooth muscles of the bronchus [Gr *brogchos* windpipe; L *con-* together, *stringere* to draw]. **bronchostenosis.**

bronchodilator: agent that dilates the bronchi [Gr *brogchos* windpipe; L *dilatare* to spread wide].

bronchus: one of two tubes that is a division of the trachea or wind pipe and conveys air to the lung [Gr *brogchos* windpipe].

bryophytes: mosslike plants; mosses and liverworts are simple green plants tied to a moist habitat by their motile sperm and their lack of a vascular system [Gr *bryon* moss, *phyton* plant].

bulb: organ of storage and asexual reproduction consisting of a small flattened stem bearing fleshy leaves with. buds in their axils [L *bulbus* globular root].

bulla: large watery blister [L].

calculus: calcified accumulation of salivary proteins, bacterial deposits, stain, and plaque on a tooth surface [L small stone].

calyx: sepals; the outer whorl of the floral envelop that is often green [Gr *kalyx*].

candiasis: infection with the yeasts of *Candida* species. **candidosis, moniliasis.**

capsule: dry, usually dehiscent fruit derived from a compound ovary [L *capsula* little box].

cardiotonic: having a tonic effect on the heart [Gr *kardia* heart, *tonikos* tonic].

caries: bacterial infection of the enamel and dentin of the tooth leading to decalcification and cavitation [L decay].

cariogenic: promoter of caries [L *caries* decay; Gr *genein* to produce].

carminative: substance that relieves excessive amount of gas in the stomach or intestine [L *carminare* to cleanse]. See **flatulence.**

catarrh: inflammation associated with free discharge of mucous membranes especially those of the upper respiratory tract [L *catarrhus* from Gr *katarrhein* to flow down].

cathartic: = purgative.

catkin: unisexual, unbranched, elongate inflorescence with sessile flowers usually wind-pollinated [AS little cat]. **ament.**

celiac: pertaining to the abdominal cavity [Gr *koilia* belly].

cellulitis: diffuse inflammation of loose subcutaneous tissue associated with bacterial infection [L *cellula* small cell; Gr -*itis* inflammation].

cerebral cortex: thin, convoluted, gray matter covering the largest, uppermost part of the brain, the cerebrum [L *cerebrum* brain, *cortex* bark].

cerebral hemorrhage: stroke resulting from the bleeding of a vessel into the brain [L *cerebrum* brain; Gr *haima* blood, *rhegnynai* to burst].

cerebral thrombosis: stroke resulting from a blood clot blocking a cerebral vessel [L *cerebrum* brain; Gr *thrombos* clot, -*osis* condition].

cerebrovascular stroke: when blood flow is compromised through intravascular blockage among vessels leading to the brain, the portion affected dies and a stroke results [L *cerebrum* brain, *vasculum* small vessel].

cheilosis: fissured condition of the lips and angles of the mouth [Gr *cheilos* lip, -*osis* condition].

chelate: to combine with a metallic ion in which the metal is part of a ring, as a chelating agent [Gr *chele* claw].

chemotacticity: ability of chemical substances to enhance the migration of cells, particularly polymorphonuclear leukocytes or macrophages, toward or away from other substances [Gr *chemeia* chemistry, *taxis* arrangement].

cholelithiasis: stones in the gallbladder or bile ducts [Gr *chile* bile, *lithos* stone; L -*iasis* condition].

cholesterol: principal animal sterol, $C_{27}H_{46}O$, found in the fat and oil of blood, bile, brain tissue, liver, kidney, egg yolk, and others, that can crystalize and concentrate in the inner walls of blood vessels and in gallstones [Gr *chole* bile, *stereos* solid].

chorea: disease characterized by spasmodic, irregular movements beyond control [Gr *choreia* dance].

cirrhosis: fibrotic degenerative changes of any organ, especially the liver [Gr *kirrhos* orange-yellow, *-osis* condition].

colostrum: viscid yellow milk, high in protein and IgA, produced by the postpartum mother [L].

coma: complete loss of consciousness [Gr *koma* deep sleep].

complement system: enzymatic system of 9 separate components (C_1–C_9) and 11 serum proteins that is activated by antigen-antibody reactions to act sequentially, and to activate and amplify the activity of successive components, referred to as a cascade, thus affecting bacteriolysis, opsonization, chemotaxis, and immune cytolysis can take place.

convulsant: agent that causes convulsion [L *convulsus* shaken]. See **analeptic.**

corm: solid bulblike organ consisting of a large stem with obscure leaf scales bearing buds in their axils [Gr *kormos* trunk].

corolla: petals; the inner whorl of the floral envelope that is often showy and colored [L *corolla* small crown].

coronary thrombosis: = heart attack.

corticosteroid: sterol produced by the adrenal cortex [L *cortex* bark; Gr *stereos* solid].

corymb: flat or convex indeterminate inflorescence [Gr *korymbos* cluster of flowers].

cotyledon: seed or embryonic leaf [Gr *kotyledon* cup-shaped cavity].

counterirritant: agent for the induction of superficial irritation to relieve another irritation [L *contra-* against, *irritare* to irritate].

curare: crude dried extract obtained from the bark and stems of *Chondodendron tomentosum* and several species of *Strychnos*, the most important constituent being tubocurarine used to secure muscle relaxation [Carib].

cyme: flat determinate inflorescence with pedicels of equal length [L *cyma* young sprout].

cystitis: inflammation of the bladder [Gr *kystis* bladder, *-itis* inflammation].

dentifrice: tooth cleaners and polishers containing abrasive, binding, detergent, and flavoring compounds [L *dentrifricium*].

dentin: chief tissue of the tooth; it surrounds the pulp and is covered by enamel or cementum [L *dens* tooth].

depressant: agent that reduces functional activity [L *deprimere* to keep down].

dermatitis: inflammation of the skin. **contact d.** or **contact hypersensitivity:** local allergic reaction provoked by skin contact with chemical substances that act as antigens or haptens [Gr *derma* skin, *-itis* inflammation].

diabetes (mellitus): metabolic disorder affecting insulin production and resulting in faulty carbohydrate metabolism, giving rise to sugar in the urine and imperfect fat metabolism with acidosis, lipemia, ketonuria, and other symptoms leading to coma and death if treatment is not obtained [Gr *diabainein* to cross through].

diaphoretic: that which promotes perspiration, especially when it is profuse [Gr *dia-* through, *phorein* to carry].

diarrhea: abnormal frequency and fluidity of stool discharges [Gr *diarrhoia* a flowing through].

diastole: dilation or relaxation phase of the cardiac cycle [Gr *diastole* difference].

dicotyledons: angiosperms having two cotyledons (seed leaves), usually the leaves are net-veined and floral parts in fours or fives [Gr *di-* two, *kotyledon* cup-shaped cavity].

diplopia: double vision [Gr *diploos* double, *opsis* vision].

diuretic: agent that increases urine flow [Gr *diouretikos*].

DNA: deoxyribonucleic acid, a giant molecule representing the repository in the cell nucleus for genetic information that is replicated and transmitted to daughter nuclei, consisting structurally of two spirals.

dopa: an amino acid, 3,4-dihydroxyphenylalanine, produced by the oxidation of tyrosine by tyrosinase; it is the precursor of dopamine and an intermediate in the biosynthesis of norepinephrine, epinephrine, and melanin.

dropsy: = edema.

drupe: fleshy fruit with a stony endocarp (inner fruit wall) [Gr *dryppa* olive].

dysgammaglobulinemia: abnormality of gamma globulins in the blood [Gr *dys-* difficult, *haima* blood].

dyspareunia: difficult or painful coitus [Gr *dys-* difficult, *pareunos* lying beside].

dyspepsia: indigestion [Gr *dys-* difficult, *peptein* to cook].

dyspnea: difficulty in breathing [Gr *dys-* difficult, *pnoia* breath].

dysuria: urination that is painful [Gr *dys-* difficult, *urino* urine].

eczema: noncontagious, itching, inflammatory skin eruption characterized by papules, vesicles, and pustules that may also be associated with edema, scaling, or exudation [Gr *ek* out, *zeo* boil].

edema: abnormal accumulation of fluid between cells [Gr *oidema* swelling]. **dropsy.**

efferent: conveying outward from a center [L *efferre* to carry away].

embolism: obstruction of a blood vessel by a clot [Gr *embolos* plug].

emetic: agent that induces vomiting [Gr *emetikos* provoking sickness].

emphysema: distension by gas of the tissues [Gr *en-* in, *physema* a blowing].

pulmonary e.: distension in the alveoli that may be adjacent to areas in which there is partial obstruction of a bronchus or bronchiole [L *pulmonarius* lung].

encephalitis: inflammation of the brain [Gr *enkephalos* brain, *-itis* inflammation].

encephalomyelitis: inflammation of the brain and spinal cord [Gr *enkephalos* brain, *myelos* marrow, *-itis* inflammation].

endocarditis: inflammation of the endocardium (inner lining of the heart) [Gr *endo-* within, *kardia* heart, *-itis* inflammation].

endodontics: the study of the tooth pulp and adjacent tissues [Gr *endo-* within, *odous* tooth].

endothelium: epithelial cell layer lining the blood and lymph vessels, heart, and serous cavities [Gr *endo-* within, *thele* nipple].

enteritis: inflammation of the intestines [Gr *enteron* intestine, *-itis* inflammation].

enterotoxin: heat-stable proteinaceous exotoxin produced by toxigenic strains of *Staphylococcus aureus*; on ingestion, causes violent vomiting and diarrhea [Gr *enteron* intestine, *toxikon* poison].

entomophilous: insect-pollinated [Gr *entomon* insect, *philein* to love].

eosinophil: see **leukocyte.**

epilepsy: disorder characterized by severe muscular spasms, loss of consciousness, and abnormally large discharges of electricity [Gr *epilepsis* seizure].

ergotism: chronic poisoning marked by spasms, cramps, dry gangrene, and various cerebrospinal symptoms due to excessive use of medicinal ergot or of eating ergot-contaminated grain, the contamination due to the fungus *Claviceps purpurea* [Fr *ergot* spur].

erysipeloid: dermatitis or cellulitis due to infection with *Erysipelothrix rhusiopathiae*, usually beginning in a wound and remaining localized [Gr *erythros* rod, *eidos* form].

euphoria: well-being [Gr *eu-* well, *pheresthai* to turn out].

exanthem: skin eruption or rash [Gr eruption].

expectorant: agent that ejects sputum from the air passages [L *expectorare* to drive from the breast].

extrasensory perception (ESP): knowledge of or response to an external thought or event not obtained from a stimulation of the sense organs [L *extra-* beyond, *sensorius* sensory, *perceptio* a gathering together].

Fab: fragment of immunoglobulin G (IgG), resulting from papain digestion, that possesses the antigen-combining sites.

favism: induction of an acute hemolytic anemia in individuals who have inherited biochemically defective erythrocytes and ingest fava beans (*Vicia faba*) or inhale their pollen [It *fava* bean].

Fc: fragment of immunoglobulin G (IgG), resulting from papain digestion, that possesses sites for complement fixation and placental transmission.

febrifuge: = antipyretic.

flatulence: see **carminative.**

follicle: dry, dehiscent fruit derived from a simple ovary and splitting along one suture [L *folliculus* small sac].

fruit: matured ovary-containing seeds, the wall (pericarp) being either dehiscent (regularly opening) or indehiscent (not opening) [L *fructus*].

furunculosis: condition of having boils [L *furunculus* boil; Gr *-osis* condition].

GABA: gamma-aminobutyric acid.

gametophyte: haploid, gamete-forming phase in the alternation of plant generations [Gr *gamete* wife, *gametes* husband; *phyton* plant].

ganglion: a mass of nerve tissue [Gr *ganglion* a swelling].

gangrene: tissue death resulting from inadequate blood supply, direct injury, or infection [Gr *gangraina*].

gastroenteritis: inflammation of the stomach and intestines induced by bacteria, viruses, or toxins [Gr *gaster* stomach, *enteron* intestine, *-itis* inflammation].

gingivitis: inflammation of the gums [L *gingiva* gum; Gr *-itis* inflammation].

glaucoma: group of diseases characterized by increased intraocular pressures causing defects in vision [Gr *glaukos* blue-green].

glomerulonephritis: nonsuppurating, bilateral inflammation of the glomeruli of the kidney [L *glomus* ball; Gr *nephros* kidney, *-itis* inflammation].

glossitis: inflammation of the tongue [Gr *glossa* tongue, *-itis* inflammation].

glycoside: naturally occurring substance consisting of sugars combined with nonsugars (aglycones). **anthraquinone g.:** yellow substance derived from the oxidation of anthracene. **cardiac g.:** substance having a stimulating effect on the heart. **cyanogenic g.:** substance yielding hydrocyanic acid (HCN) on hydrolysis. **lactone g.:** substance yielding the aglycone coumarin. **saponin g:** substance yielding the aglycone sapogenin [Gr *glykys* sweet].

glycosuria: abnormal amount of sugar in the urine [Gr *glykys* sweet, *ouron* urine].

gout: painful disease involving joint inflammation and chalky deposits as a result of the disturbance of purine metabolism (high blood levels of uric acid) [L *gutta* drop].

gymnosperms: cone-bearing vascular plants; the seeds are exposed and the endosperm is formed before fertilization [Gr *gymnos* naked, *sperma* seed].

hallucinogen: agent inducing false perceptions that occur without true sensory stimuli [L *hallucinari* to wander in the mind].

hapten: immunologically active substance that can promote antibody production only if bound to a carrier protein (e.g., pneumococcal polysaccharide) [Gr *haptein* to touch].

hay fever: pollen- and spore-induced allergic reaction resulting in nasal congestion and conjunctivitis [AS *heg* hay; L *febris*].

heart attack: following an intravascular blockage in the circulation of the heart muscle, the portion affected dies; the patient's survival depends on the severity of the attack [AS *heorte*]. See **coronary thrombosis, myocardial infarction.**

heart failure, congestive: inadequate functioning of the heart resulting in blood congestion in the lungs or build up of blood pressure in the veins.

hematopoiesis: formation of blood [Gr *haima* blood, *poiesis* production].

heme: pigment-carrying portion of hemaglobin, an iron protoporphyrin [Gr *haima* blood].

hemochromatosis: hereditary defect in iron metabolism resulting in brown pigmentation of the skin due to deposition of iron in the tissues, especially the liver, where cirrhosis may occur [Gr *haima* blood, *chroma* color, *-osis* condition].

hemoglobin: oxygen-carrying pigment in the red blood cells [Gr *haima* blood; L *globus* ball].

hemoglobinuria: hemoglobin in the urine [Gr *haima*; L *globus* ball, *urina* urine].

hemolysis: disintegration of elements in the blood [Gr *haima* blood, *lysis* loosening].

hemorrhoid: dilation of veins around the anus [Gr *haima, rheein* to flow]. **piles.**

hemostatic: agent that arrests bleeding [Gr *haima* blood, *-stasis* standing].

herbology: study of herbs; traditional medical use of herbs that are not well known scientifically [L *herba*; Gr *logos* word].

herpetic gingivostomatitis: cold sores of the gums (gingiva), lips (stoma), and oral mucosa produced by herpes simplex virus [Gr *herpein* to creep; L *gingiva* gum; Gr *stoma* mouth, *-itis* inflammation].

high blood pressure: = hypertension.

Hindu medicine: = Ayurvedic medicine.

histamine: naturally occurring vasoactive amine released through anaphylatoxin or combination of allergen with tissue-bound IgE from tissues, and especially from mast cells that cause vasodilation and smooth muscle contraction [Gr *histos* web, *ammoniakon* resinous gum].

HLA: histocompatibility locus A; group of transplantation isoantigens belonging to a genetic system important in tissue rejection phenomena.

homeostasis: tendency to stabilize the internal environment of an organism [Gr *homoios* like, *-stasis* standing].

hyperactivity: abnormally high level of activity accompanied by inability to concentrate and learn, usually abating during adolescence [Gr *hyper-* above; L *activus* active].

hyperglycemia: high level of sugar in the blood [Gr *hyper-* above, *glykys* sweet, *haima* blood].

hyperlipidemia: excessive lipids in the blood [Gr *hyper-* above, *lipos* fat, *haima* blood]. **hyperlipoproteinemia:** excessive lipoproteins in the blood.

hypercholesterolemia: inherited tendency toward high cholesterol levels [Gr *hyper-* above, *chole* bile, *stereos* solid, *haima* blood].

hypersensitivity: increased reactivity to antigen, mediated through humoral or cellular immunity, that incites an allergic response. Five categories have been designated: **Type I, the anaphylactic or immediate type** reaction mediated by allergen that reacts with antibody (IgE, IgG) bound by its Fc portion to mast cells and basophils, and results in the release of vasoactive amines (e.g., histamine) that causes an immediate clinical response that may be generalized (anaphylaxis) or limited to target sites like the nasopharynx (hayfever), lungs (asthma) or skin (hives); **Type II, the cytotoxic or cytolytic reaction** mediated by specific antibody (IgG, IgM) that attaches to cell surface antigens, or antigens and haptens intimately associated with the cell (usually formed elements of the blood) and serves to attract either phagocytic or 'killer' lymphoreticular cells that with, or without complement, produce cell death in hours to days, and elicit symptoms of either hemolytic anemia or exanthemous skin reactions that are characteristic of certain drug reactions or hemolytic diseases of the newborn; **Type III, the immune complex or Arthus reactions** that are due to immune complexes of usually precipitating antibody (IgG, IgM, IgE) with antigen and leads to activation of the complement system and platelet aggregation with release of vasoactive substances and lysosomal enzymes to produce in minutes or days the tissue inflammation and vasculitis characteristic of streptococcal glomerlonephritis and hypersensitivity pneumonitis; **Type IV the delayed hypersensitivity reaction** due to sensitized T-lymphocytes with specific surface receptors that are stimulated by antigen to release lymphokines that mediate antigen-associated cell destruction and produce symptoms within 24–48 hours, of pruritis, stinging, erythematous macules, papules, vesicles, exudation and crusting of contact dermatitis or by foreign tissue transplantation or tumor antigens that cause sensitized T-cells to transform into blast-like cells capable of killing graft or tumor cells; and **Type V, the stimulatory hypersensitivity reaction** that results from the activity of antibodies directed against cell membrane components that cause the cells to divide rather than die as in thyrotoxicosis [Gr *hyper-* above; L *sentere* to feel].

hypertension: abnormally high constrictive tension in blood vessels, usually revealed as high blood pressure [Gr *hyper-* above; L *tendere* to stretch].

hypertensive agent: = antihypotensive.

hyperuricemia: excessive uric acid in the blood, a characteristic of gout [Gr *hyper-* above; L *urina* urine; Gr *haima* blood].

hypnotic: sleep-inducing drug [Gr *hypnos* sleep].

hypochondriasis: excessive anxiety concerning one's health, often associated with symptoms unattributed to organic disease (so-called because the hypochondrium was thought to be the seat of this disorder) [Gr *hypo-* under, *chondros* cartilage, *-iasis* condition].

hypoglycemia: deficiency of normal glucose levels in the blood, low blood sugar [Gr *hypo-* under, *glykys* sweet, *haima* blood].

hypoparathyroidism: underactive parathyroid glands resulting in a decrease of serum calcium, leading to muscle spasms and a rise of serum phosphate, which produces increased density of bone due to lack of bone resorption [Gr *hypo-* under, *para* near, *thureoeides* shield-shaped].

hypotension: abnormally low tension in blood vessels characterized by capillary permeability and fragility; revealed as low blood pressure [Gr *hypo-* under; L *tendere* to stretch].

hypotensive agent: = antihypertensive.

hypothalamus: portion of the midbrain nearest the pituitary gland [Gr *hypo-* under, *thalamos* chamber].

Ig: = immunoglobulin.

immune: resistance to a disease due to the formation of humoral (fluid) antibodies, the development of cellular immunity, or other mechanisms such as interferon activity in viral infections [L *immunis* exempt].

immunoglobulin (Ig): family of proteins composed of light and heavy chains linked by disulfide bonds that usually act as antibodies; five distinct classes (IgA, IgD, IgE, IgG, and IgM) are based on the differences within the heavy chains [L *immunis* exempt, *globulus* little ball].

impotence: lack of copulative power or virility in the male [L *impotentia* inability].

infarction: death of tissue due to loss of blood supply [L *infarcire* to stuff into].

inflorescence: manner of flower bearing, the flowering shoot. **determinate i.:** central flower maturing first with no further elongation of the central axis. **indeterminate i.:** lateral or lower flowers maturing first with continued elongation of the central axis [L *inflorescere* to begin to blossom].

interferon: class of low molecular weight proteins, induced in an animal cell by viral infection, that interferes subsequently with viral replication; it is animal species specific, not virus specific.

intraocular: within the eye [L *intra-* within, *oculus* eye].

jaundice: condition characterized by a raised level of bilirubin (breakdown product of hemaglobin) producing a yellowness of mucous membranes, including the eyes, because of deposition of the pigment [Fr *jaune* yellow].

karyotype: chromosomal constitution of a nucleus [Gr *karyon* nucleus, *typos* model].

keratolysis: softening and dissolution or peeling of the horny layer of the epidermis [Gr *keras* horn, *lysis* dissolution].

ketosis: a condition characterized by an abnormally high concentration of ketone bodies (acetone, acetoacetic acid, β-hydroxybutyric acid) in the body tissues and fluids, a complication of diabetes and starvation [keto, denoting the carbonyl group :C:O; Gr *-osis* condition].

lathyrism: development of spastic paraplegia, pain, hyperesthesia, and paresthesia leading to death, after ingestion of seeds of *Lathyrus* species (Fabaceae) [Gr *la* addition, *thouros* irritant, *-ism* condition].

leaflet: distinct and separate segment of a leaf [AS *leaf*; Fr *-let* little].

lectin: protein that affects agglutination, precipitation, or other phenomena resembling the action of a specific antibody [L *legere* to choose].

legume: dry, dehiscent fruit derived from a simple ovary and splitting along two sutures [L *legumen* pulse].

leukocyte: white blood cell and precursors [Gr *leukos* white, *kytos* cell]. Leukocyte types—**eosinophil:** polymorphonuclear (pmn) leukocyte containing eosinophilic granules whose numbers increase in allergic conditions (6% is normal) [Gr *eos* dawn, *philein* to love]. **basophil:** pmn of myeloid series containing basophilic granules that contain heparin, histamine, and vasoactive amines [Gr *basis* base, *philein* to love]. **monocyte:** large, motile phagocytic cell of RES, 2–10% total white blood cells in peripheral blood; related to macrophages [Gr *monos* single, *kytos* cell].

leukorrhea: whitish vaginal discharge [Gr *leukos* white, *rheein* to flow].

L-form: filterable forms of bacteria containing L (Lister) bodies characterized by amorphous cytoplasm and great size variation.

lipoproteinemic: lowering the lipoprotein level in the blood [Gr *lipos* fat, *protos* first, *emia* blood].

low blood pressure: = hypotension.

lumbago: lower back and buttock pain associated with poor blood circulation, such as in terminal aortic occlusion [L *lumbus* loin].

lycanthropy: delusion that one is a wolf [Gr *lykos* wolf, *anthropos* man].

lymph: fluid of lymphatic vessels [L *lympha* water].

μ: micron, one thousandth (10^{-3}) part of a millimeter.

macropsia: vision disturbance in which objects are perceived as larger than they actually are [Gr *makros* large, *opsis* vision].

macule: nonelevated discolored spot of skin [L *macula* spot].

manic-depression: mental disorder in which the patient alternates between phases of excitement and depression [Gr *mania* madness].

meatus: opening or channel [L].

medulla oblongata: portion of the hindbrain lying between the pons (above) and the spinal cord (below) [L *medulla* marrow, *oblongus* rather long].

meningitis: inflammation of the meninges (the three membranes covering the brain and spinal cord) [Gr *meninx* membrane, *-itis* inflammation].

meningococcemia: acute fulminating (developing rapidly) or insidious infectious disease resulting from the presence of *Neisseria meningitidis* in the blood [Gr *meninx* membrane, *kokkos* berry, *haima* blood].

metastasis: transfer of disease from one part of the body to another not directly connected with the first, usually by blood or lymph [Gr *meta-* change, *stasis* stand].

micron: = μ.

migraine: periodic severe headache, commonly involving only one side of the head [Fr].

milk sickness: poisoning resulting from ingesting dairy products from livestock having eaten white snakeroot, *Eupatorium rugosum*.

millimeter: = mm.

millimicron: = mμ.

miosis: contraction of the pupil of the eye [Gr *meiosis* diminution].

mitogen: substance that stimulates mitosis and cell transformation [Gr *mitos* thread, *genein* to produce].

mm: = millimeter, one thousandth (10^{-3}) part of a meter (m).

monocotyledons: angiosperms having one cotyledon (seed leaf), usually the leaves are parallel-veined and floral parts in threes [Gr *monos* single, *kotyledon* cup-shaped cavity].

monocyte: see **leukocyte**.

Moslim medicine: = Unani medicine.

mucolytic: that which dissolves mucus [L *mucus*; Gr *lysis* loosening].

muscular dystrophy: syndrome associated with the progressive degeneration of the musculature, eventually causing death [L *musculus* muscle; Gr *dys-* faulty, *trophe* nourishment].

mutagen: agent that elicits a mutation [L *mutare* to change; Gr *genein* to produce].

myalgia: muscle pain [Gr *mys* muscle, *algos* pain].

myasthenia gravis: disorder marked by fatigue and exhaustion of the muscular system resulting in progressive paralysis of muscles [Gr *mys* muscle, *astheneia* weakness; L *gravis* heavy].

mycotoxin: toxin produced by a fungus [Gr *mykes* fungus, *toxikon* poison].

mydriasis: extreme pupil dilation [Gr].

myocardial infarction: = heart attack.

myocardium: thick, middle muscle of the heart wall [Gr *mys* muscle, *kardia* heart].

myxedema: hypothyroid-induced disorder characterized by dry waxy skin due to mucin deposits [Gr *myxa* mucus, *oidema* swelling].

necrosis: death of tissue, usually in localized areas of individual cells or small cell groups [Gr *nekros* dead, *-osis* condition].

nephron: anatomical and functional unit of the kidney, which includes the renal corpuscle, the proximal convoluted tubule, the descending and ascending limbs of Henle's loop, the distal convoluted tubule, and the collecting tubule [Gr *nephros* kidney].

nephrosis: degenerative disease of the kidney affecting the renal tubules [Gr *nephros* kidney, *-osis* condition].

neuralgia: nerve pain [Gr *neuron* nerve, *algos* pain].

neuritis: nerve inflammation [Gr *neuron* nerve, *-itis* inflammation].

neurohumoral: pertaining to a chemical substance formed in a neuron that is able to activate or modify the function of an adjacent gland, muscle, or neuron [Gr *neuron* nerve; L *humor* moisture].

neuroleptic: major tranquilizing agent, generally without hypnotic affect, the antipsychotic action affecting chiefly psychomotor activity [Gr *neuron* nerve, *lepsis* seizing]. **antipsychotic.**

nut: dry, indehiscent fruit with one seed and a hard fruit wall [AS *hnutu*].

ophthalmia: inflammation of the eye [Gr *ophthalmos* eye]. **o. neonatorum:** purulent infection of the eyes of newborn babies, acquired from the mother at birth [Gr *neos* new; L *natus* birth].

opsonization: phagocytosis of bacteria, facilitated by antibodies and other substances [Gr *opsonein* to buy victuals].

osteomyelitis: inflammation beginning in the bone marrow [Gr *osteon* bone, *myelos* marrow, *-itis* inflammation].

ovary: ovule-bearing part of the pistil (bot.); small oval bodies on either side of the uterus in which ova are developed (zoo.) [L *ovarium*].

ovule: egg-containing unit of the ovary that becomes the seed after fertilization (bot.); ovum within the Graafian follicle (zoo.) [L *ovulum*].

oxytocic: hastening childbirth [Gr *oxys* quick, *tokos* childbirth].

panacea: universal remedy or cureall [Gr *panakeia*].

pancreatitis: inflammation of the pancreas [Gr *pankreas* pancreas, *-itis* inflammation].

panicle: branched inflorescence with stalked flowers [L *panicula* tuft].

papule: small circumscribed elevation of the skin that is solid and superficial [L *pupula* pimple].

parenchyma: essential or functional cells of an organ [Gr *para-* beside, *enchyma* infusion].

Parkinsonism: group of neurological disorders causing muscular rigidity and impairing movement and equilibrium, often following *slow virus* infections [named for James Parkinson, English physician, 1755–1824].

paroxysm: spasm or seizure; symptoms that suddenly intensify or recur [Gr *paroxysmos* irritation].

parturition: labor, the function of childbearing [L *parturire* to bring forth].

pedicel: individual flower stalk [L *pedicellus*].

peduncle: main stalk of inflorescence [L *pedunculus* small foot].

perennial: plant living for three or more years [L *per-* through, *annus* year].

perianth: collective term for the two floral envelopes, the calyx (sepals) and the corolla (petals) [Gr *peri-* around, *anthos* flower].

pericardium: fibroserous sac enclosing the heart [Gr *peri-* around, *kardia* heart].

periodontium: tissue that supports the teeth [Gr *peri-* around, *odous* tooth].

peristalsis: rhythmatic contraction and relaxation along the intestine promoting movement of contents [Gr *peri-* around, *stellein* to draw in].

peritonitis: inflammation of the peritoneum [Gr *peri-* around, *teinein* to stretch, *-itis* inflammation].

petiole: leaf stalk [L *petiolus* small foot].

PHA: = **phytohemagglutinin.**

phage (bacteriophage): bacterial virus that may cause lysis of bacteria. **phage types:** strains of bacteria susceptible to lysis by specific bacteriophage [Gr *phagein* to eat].

phagocytosis: engulfment of foreign particles and bacteria by phagocytic cells [Gr *phagein* to eat, *kytes* cell, *-osis* condition].

pharmacognosy: study of natural drugs and their constituents [Gr *pharmakon* drug, *gnosis* knowledge].

pharyngitis: inflammation of the pharynx [Gr *pharygx, -itis* inflammation].

phocomelia: shortening or absence of limbs [Gr *phoke* seal, *melos* limb].

photodermatitis: inflammation of the skin resulting from activation by light of chemicals on the skin [Gr *phos* light, *derma* skin, *-itis* inflammation].

phytohemagglutinin (PHA): mitogenic lectin from plants that agglutinates erythrocytes and stimulates thymus-derived lymphocytes [Gr *phyton* plant, *haima* blood; L *agglutinare* to glue].

phytotoxin: proteinaceous toxin derived from a plant [Gr *phyton* plant, *toxikon* poison].

piles: = hemorrhoid.

piscicide: substance poisonous to fish [L *piscis* fish, *caedere* to kill].

pistil: floral organ that bears ovules in seed plants; the female sporophyll [L *pistillum* pestle].

plaque: mixed or pure colonies of bacteria and their products on the surface of teeth that adhere tenaciously to tooth surfaces [Fr].

platelet: disk-shaped structure that acts in coagulating blood; also **blood p.** [Gr *plate;* Fr *-let* little].

pneumonia: lung inflammation associated with alveolar exudate and sometimes cavitation [Gr *pneumon* lung].
bronchopneumonia: inflammation of small areas of the lung. **lobar p.:** inflammation of one or more lobes of the lung. **eosinophilic p.:** allergic inflammation of the lung associated with eosinophils in the sputa.

pneumonitis: lung tissue inflammation [Gr *pneumon* lung, *-itis* inflammation].

pollen: microspore of gymnosperms and angiosperms; the male gametophyte that develops sperm [L fine flour].

polyploidy: cell nucleus containing three or more multiples of the haploid number of chromosomes; a triploid contains three sets of chromosomes, a tetraploid four sets, and so on [Gr *polyplous* many times].

porphyria: hereditary disorder in porphyrin metabolism [Gr *porphyra* purple].

prostaglandins: group of naturally occurring related fatty acids in animals; these substances lower blood pressure, affect the action of certain hormones, and stimulate the contractability of smooth muscles including the uterus [Gr *prostates* something standing before, *aden* gland].

proteolytic: splitting or absorbing protein [Gr *protos* first, *lysis* dissolution].

prothrombin: plasma glycoprotein involved in the clotting mechanism of blood [Gr *pro-* before, *thrombos* clot].

pruritis: itching [L].

psychoactive: mind-altering drug; three broad groups are recognized in the text, depressants, hallucinogens, and stimulants [Gr *psyche* mind; L *activus*].

pteridophytes: fernlike plants; primitive vascular plants with independent gametophyte and sporophyte generations (see **alternation of generations**) [Gr *pteris* fern, *phyton* plant].

purgative: cathartic (laxative, aperient) that stimulates peristaltic action and bowel evacuation [L *purgativus*].

pyelonephritis: a type of kidney infection that spreads from the pelvis to the cortex of the kidney [Gr *pyelos* trough, *nephros* kidney, *-itis* inflammation].

pyogenic: pus forming [Gr *pyon* pus, *genesis* production].

pyorrhea: inflammation of the dental periosteum associated with pus, progressive necrosis of the alveolar bone, and looseness of teeth [Gr *pyon* pus, *rheein* to flow].

pyretic: referring to fever [Gr *pyretos* fever].

raceme: unbranched indeterminate inflorescence with stalked flowers [L *racemus* bunch].

reticuloendothelial system: system of phagocytic cells found among reticular connective tissue fibers of parenchymatous organs (e.g., Kupffer liver cells, alveolar and peritoneal macrophages, blood monocytes) [L *reticulum* little net; Gr *endon* within, *thele* nipple].

retroperitoneum: area behind the membrane lining the abdominal and pelvic cavities [Gr *retro-* behind, *peri-* around, *teinein* to stretch].

rheumatic fever: inflammation of heart fibrous tissue leading to scarring of heart valves and the joints; occurs as an immunological sequel to *Streptococcus pyogenes* infection elsewhere [Gr *rheuma* flux; L *febris*].

rhinitis: inflammation of nasal mucosa usually accompanied by increased flow of mucus [Gr *rhis* nose, *-itis* inflammation].

rhizome: horizontal underground stem distinguished from a root by scalelike leaves and axillary buds [Gr *rhizoma* root].

sciatica: pain along the course of the sciatic nerve radiating from the back to the buttock, back of thigh, calf, and foot [L *sciaticus*].

schizophrenia: group of mental illnesses involving the disorganization of personality and characterized by delusions, hallucinations, abnormal behavior, and retreat from reality [Gr *schizein* to cleave, *phren* mind].

sebum: greasy, lubricating substance secreted by the sebaceous glands, chiefly of the skin [L *sebum* suet].

sedative: agent used to relieve tension and anxiety [L *sedare* to soothe].

seed: mature ovule, the essential part being the embryo [AS *saed*].

sepsis: condition associated with pathogenic microorganisms and their products [Gr putrefaction].

septicemia: presence and multiplication of microorganisms in the bloodstream [Gr *sepsis* putrefaction, *haima* blood].

serum sickness: generalized immediate hypersensitivity reaction due to localization in tissues of immune complexes formed several days after administration of hyperimmune serum; symptoms include enlarged lymph nodes, fever, urticaria, joint swelling, and renal lesions [L *serum* whey].

shock: depression of body function involving reduction in blood pressure and circulating blood.

sickle cell anemia: inherited hemolytic anemia predominant in Negroid and Mediterranean groups; erythrocytes are crescent- or sickle-shaped.

soporific: inducing sleep [L *soporificus*].

spermatophytes: seed-bearing plants, the gymnosperms and angiosperms [Gr *sperma* seed, *phyton* plant].

spike: unbranched indeterminate inflorescence with sessile flowers [L *spica* ear of corn].

spore: simple reproductive body, usually a single cell, capable of developing into a new individual; of ferns and lower plants [Gr *sporos* seed].

sporophyte: diploid, spore-forming phase in the alternation of plant generations [Gr *sporos* seed, *phyton* plant].

stamen: floral organ that bears pollen in seed plants, the male sporophyll [L *stamen* filament].

steatorrhea: excessively fatty stool [Gr *stear* fat, *rheein* to flow].

stigma: pollen-receptive portion of the pistil [Gr *stigma* point].

stimulant: agent that exites or irritates [L *stimulare* to incite].

stomachic: substance that stimulates appetite; it promotes the functional activity of the stomach [Gr *stomachikos*].

stipule: paired structure at the base of the petiole [L *stipula* small stalk].

sublingual: beneath the tongue [L *sub-* under, *lingua* tongue].

symbiosis: living together in close association of two dissimilar organisms; each organism is called a symbiont [Gr *symbionai* to live with].

synapse: junction between two neurons between which nervous impulses are transmitted [Gr *synapsis* contact].

synesthesia: condition in which a stimulus of one sense is perceived as sensation of a different sense, as one seems to be seeing music [Gr *syn-* with, *aisthesis* sensation].

systole: contraction phase of the cardiac cycle, especially of the ventricles [Gr *systole* drawing together].

tachycardia: abnormally rapid heart beat [Gr *tachys* swift, *kardia* heart].

taxon: category into which related organisms are classified (in ascending order: species, genus, family, order, class, phylum, and kingdom) [Gr *taxis* arrangement].

T cell: thymus-derived cell; lymphoid cell found in peripheral lymphoid organs and derived from the thymus; active in cell-mediated immunological responses.

tenosynovitis: inflammation of a tendon sheath [Gr *teno* tendon; L *synovia*; Gr -*itis* inflammation].

teratogen: drug or other agent causing abnormal embryonic development [Gr *teras* monster, *genein* to produce].

thrombocytopenia: decrease in the number of platelets in the blood [Gr *thrombos* clot, *kytos* cell, *penia* poverty].

thrombophlebitis: inflammation of a vein wall in association with clot formation [Gr, *thrombos* clot, *phleps* vein, -*itis* inflammation].

thrombosis: intravascular formation of a blood clot [Gr *thrombos* clot, -*osis* condition].

thrush: infection by *Candida* species of the oral mucous membranes, usually in childhood [Scand *trøske*].

tolerance: ability to endure increasingly large doses of a drug, and to exhibit decreasing effect with continued use [L *tolerantio*].

toxicomania: periodic or chronic state of intoxication as a result of repeated use of a drug harmful to the individual or society [Gr *toxikon* poison, *mania* madness].

tuberculosis: primary pulmonary infection caused by *Mycobacterium tuberculosis*; may also be found within the skin, lymphatics, and kidney [L *tuberculum* small swelling; Gr -*osis* condition].

ulcer: an open sore [L *ulcus*]. **peptic u.:** ulceration of the stomach, esophagus, or duodenum by the action of the acid gastric juices.

umbel: flat or convex determinate or indeterminate inflorescence with pedicels arising from a common point [L *umbella* sunshade].

Unani medicine: traditional or indigenous medical system found in the Moslim world [Urdu]. **Moslim medicine.**

uremia: toxic condition due to inadequate nephron function of the kidney causing accumulation and retention in the blood of excessive by-products of protein metabolism [Gr *ouron* urine, *haima* blood].

urticaria: skin rash caused by local release of histamine and other vasoactive substances; characterized by itchy erythematous weals [L *urtica* stinging nettle, *-ia* condition].

vasoactive amines: substances, such as histamine and serotonin, that cause peripheral vasodilation and increase of small blood vessel permeability [L *vas* vessel].

vasoconstrictor agent: = antihypotensive.

vasodilator: agent causing a widening of the lumen of blood vessels [L *vas* vessel, *dilatare* to spread wide].

vasopressor agent: = antihypotensive.

ventricle: small cavity (e.g., one of the two lower muscular heart chambers) [L *ventriculum*].

vermifuge: agent that expels worms from the intestine [L *vermis* worm, *fugere* to flee].

vertigo: illusion of movement, often synonymous with dizziness and giddiness [L *vertigo*].

virus, slow: virus causing a disease typified by a very long preclinical incubation period and a very gradual progression once the symptoms appear [L *virus* poison]. See **Parkinsonism.**

vulvovaginitis: inflammation of the region of the vulva and vaginal genital region [L *vulva* covering, *vagina* sheath; Gr *-itis* inflammation].

wheal and flare: immediate response to histamine release or other minor, nonpenetrating injury to the skin, resulting in erythema followed by wheal or edema radiating from the line of injury; considered a characteristic skin lesion of immediate hypersensitivity.

withdrawal: unpleasant physiological symptoms triggered by abstention from addicting drugs, in some cases including retreat from objective reality.

wort: plant, usually herbaceous [AS *wyrt*].

xerophthalmia: abnormal dryness of the eye associated with a vitamin A deficiency [Gr *xeros* dry, *ophthalmos* eye].

zygomorphy: bilateral symmetry (i.e. floral parts are divisible into equal halves) [Gr *zygon* yoke, *morphe* form].

Index

Figures are indicated by pages in italics. Many vernacular names used in the text are given with their scientific equivalents (sometimes a vernacular name has more than one scientific name and sometimes scientific names have more than one vernacular name, so be wary of their use). In addition, all genera are listed alphabetically under their major group (e.g., *Laminaria* under Algae) so that the user may know in general the kind of organism being sought. As a cross check, the major group is also associated with each genus. For the Angiosperms only, where the majority of different genera having species of medical importance are known and where phylogenetic implications have been made throughout the text, genera are associated invariably with their family (ending -aceae). The "basic unit" for names in this text is the genus. The few species (specific epithets) listed are those of particular importance having repeated references. Others may be found by referring to the pages under their respective genera. In using the Index remember that a vernacular name must be equated to a genus name before it can be located.

Bugleweed: *Lycopus virginicus*
Bulb fingers, 78
Bulbine (Liliaceae), 342, 351
Bullera (Fungus), 69
Bull horn: *Acacia*
Bulrush: *Scirpus*
Bumelia (Sapotaceae), 267
Bunchflower: *Melanthium virginicum*
Bungwingwi: *Alsodeiopsis rowlandii*
Burdock: *Arctium lappa*
Burkea (Fabaceae), 235
Burkitt's lymphoma, 5, 114, 115,
126, 131, 265
Burning bush: *Euonymus atropur-
pureus*
Burns, 7, 336, 343-345
Burow's solution, 86
Burrow weed: *Allenrolfia*
Bursera (Burseraceae), 83, 135, 255
Burseraceae: *Boswellia, Bursera,
Canarium, Commiphora*
Burweed: *Xanthium*
Bushclover: *Lespedeza capitata* var.
velutina
Bush morning glory: *Ipomoea lepto-
phylla*
Butea (Fabaceae), 285, 291, 329
Buttercup: *Ranunculus*
Butterfly, monarch: *Danaus*
Butternut: *Juglans cinerea*
Buttonbush: *Cephalanthus occidenta-
lis*
Buxaceae: *Buxus*
Buxine, 4, 39
Buxus (Buxaceae), 4, 39, 86, 93, 135
Byrsonima (Malpighiaceae), 47

Caapi, *see* Ayahuasca
Cabbage: *Brassica oleracea*
Cacoa (tree): *Theobroma cacao*
Cactaceae: *Anhalonium, Ariocarpus,
Epithelantha, Lophophora, Opun-
tia, Pachycereus, Selenicereus,
Trichocereus*
Cactus family: Cactaceae
Cadinene, 83
Cadmium, 117, 118
Caesalpinia (Fabaceae), 42, 133, 169,
245, 254, 316, 323, 375
Caffeine, 17, 34, 93, 162, 165, 181,
191, 193, 213, 277, 312,
327, 380, 384-387
Caffeoylquinic acid, 216
Cajuput: *Melaleuca cajuputi*
Caladium (Araceae), 4, 58
Calabar: *Physostigma venosum*
Calabash (tree): *Crescentia cujete*
Calathea (Marantaceae), 413
Calcium oxalate, *see* Oxalate

Calculus, 227, 260
Calea (Asteraceae), 408
Calendula (Asteraceae), 370
Caley pea: *Lathyrus hirsutus*
California bay laurel: *Umbellularia
californica*
California bay laurel oil, 121
California incense cedar: *Libocedrus
decurrens*
Calla (Araceae), 58
Callistephus (Asteraceae), 69
Callitris (Gymnosperm), 312
Calluna (Ericaceae) *vulgaris*, 316,
316, 374
Calocarpum (Sapotaceae), 80
Caloncoba (Flacourtiaceae), 353
Calophyllum (Clusiaceae), 348, 350, 353
Calotropin, 52, 134
Calotropis (Asclepiadaceae), 18, 86
procera, 52, 350
Caltha (Ranunculaceae), 30
Caltrop: *Kallstroemia*
Calvacin, 133
Calvatia (Fungus), 133
Calycanthaceae: *Calycanthus*
Calycanthine, 28
Calycanthus (Calycanthaceae), 28
Calycogonium (Melastomataceae),
135
Calycosia (Rubiaceae), 256
Calystegia (Convolvulaceae), 313
Camellia (Theaceae) *sinensis*, 17, 93,
119, 181, 191, 243, 298, 385, 387
Camel's foot tree: *Bauhinia*
Campanulaceae: *Codonopsis, Iso-
toma, Lobelia, Platycodon*
Camphor: *Cinnamomum camphora*
Camphor (oil), 83, 94, 121, 163, 443
Campsis (Bignoniaceae), 86
Camptotheca (Nyssaceae), 133
Camptothecin, 133
Canada balsam oil, 83
Canada thistle: *Cirsium arvense*
Canarium (Burseraceae), 82, 339, 348
Canavalia (Fabaceae) *ensiformis*, 42,
96, 97, 137, 362, 387
Cancer, 105-149
bladder, 117
breast, 112
cervical, 113
colon, 112-113, 117
current therapy, 126-142
description of, 105-114
development of therapy, 122-126
digestive tract, 116, 117
epidemiology, 108-111
incidence, 106
kidney, 117
liver, 117, 121

lung, 112, 116, 118
nerve, 117
oral cavity, 112, 117
ovarian, 117
prostatic, 114
rectal, 112-113
skin, 107, 112
stomach, 116, 117
transmission of, 112
urinary, 114, 117
uterine/cervical, 113
Cancer theories, 115
Candelabra tree: *Euphorbia*
Candiasis, 262-263
Candida (Fungus), 69, 195, 263, 324,
350, 363
albicans, 262, 262, 288, 303, 313, 314
Candlewood: *Fagara xanthoxyloides*
Canizo: *Leucophyllum*
Canker sore: =Aphthous stomatitis
Cannabaceae: *Cannabis, Humulus*
Cannabis (Cannabaceae), 69
sativa, 329, 400, 427-428, *428*
Canscora (Gentianaceae), 375
Cantharides, 326
Cantharidin, 326
Cantharis (Insect), 326
Canthium (Rubiaceae), 169
Caper: *Capparis spinosa*
Caperonia (Rubiaceae), 279
Capparidaceae: *Capparis, Courbonia,
Crateava, Maerua, Polanisia*
Capparis (Capparidaceae), 36, 169,
348, 351, 353
Capraria (Scrophulariaceae), 364
Caprifoliaceae: *Sambucus, Viburnum*
Capsaicin, 85
Capsicum (Solanaceae), 250
frutescens, 85, 121, 219, 348
Caraipa (Clusiaceae), 342
Carapa (Meliaceae), 238, 344, 345,
352
Caraway: *Carum carvi*
Caraway oil, 83, 273
Carbamate, 370
Carbenicillin, 167
Carbenoxolone, 275
Carbohydrate, 93, 201, 203
Carbolic acid, 152
β-Carboline, 405, 406
Carbuncle, 349
Carcinogen, 27, 38, 39, 41, 110, 112,
115, 116-118, 118-122
Carcinogenesis, 94, 114-122
Carcinoma, 107, 112, 115, 124, 130,
265
Cardamon seed, 83
Cardiac and cardiovascular disease,
176-178